Neurosurgery in the Tropics

A practical approach to common
problems for the isolated practitioner

- Second Edition -

Jeffrey V. Rosenfeld
and
David A.K. Watters

Library of Congress Control Number:		2019913165
ISBN:	Hardcover	978-1-7960-0618-6
	Softcover	978-1-7960-0617-9
	eBook	978-1-7960-0616-2

The *First Edition* was published in 2000 by MACMILLAN EDUCATION LTD, London and Oxford.

Front Cover illustrations left to right:

CT scan with contrast showing a right-sided frontal lobe tuberculoma with surrounding oedema.

Tuberculous gibbus deformity of the thoracic spine.

A child with gross hydrocephalus positioned for insertion of a ventriculoperitoneal shunt. Scalp markings outline the lateral ventricle and the position of the shunt.

'Question mark' craniotomy incision marked on the shaved scalp for craniotomy and evacuation of an acute left sided extradural haematoma.

CT scan showing an acute left sided temporal extradural haematoma.

Print information available on the last page.

Rev. date: 10/11/2019

To order additional copies of this book, contact:
Xlibris
1-800-455-039
www.Xlibris.com.au
Orders@Xlibris.com.au
793570

Jeffrey V. Rosenfeld AC, OBE

MBBS, MD, MS, FRACS, FRCS (Edin.), FACS, IFAANS, FACTM

Senior Neurosurgeon, The Alfred Hospital, Melbourne, Australia.

Professor of Surgery, Monash University, Clayton, Australia.

Adjunct Professor in Surgery, F. Edward Hébert School of Medicine. Uniformed Services University of the Health Sciences, Bethesda, MD, USA.

Adjunct Professor, Department of Surgery, Chinese University of Hong Kong.

Honorary Professor, Faculty of Medicine, University of Papua New Guinea.

Major General, Royal Australian Army Medical Corps.

Recipient of the Royal Australasian College of Surgeons (RACS) Sir Hugh Devine Medal.

David A.K. Watters AM, OBE

ChM, FRACS, FRCS (Edin.)

Alfred Deakin Professor of Surgery, Deakin University, Australia.

Professor of Surgery, Barwon Health, University Hospital Geelong, Australia.

Formerly Professor and Head of Surgery, University of Papua New Guinea.

Past President and former Councillor of the Royal Australasian College of Surgeons (RACS).

Paul Harris Fellow, Rotary International.

To Debbie, Hannah, Alexander, and Gabriella.

To Olga, Douglas, Jeni, Anna, Jakob, Florian and Laurenz.

Thank you for your support to our careers and to our work in low- and middle-income countries.

Contents

12. Neuro-rehabilitation and medicolegal issues 628

L.R. Atkinson & J.V. Rosenfeld

APPENDICES 651

INDEX 664

Contributing Authors

L.R. Atkinson AO, MBBS, FRACS, FRCS(Ed), FACS, FAFRM, Clinical Associate Professor, University of Queensland. Director, Department of Neurosurgery, Princess Alexandra Hospital, Brisbane, Australia.

J.K.A. Clezy AM, OBE, FRCS, FRACS. General surgeon. North West Medical Centre, Box 682, Burnie 7320, Tasmania, Australia.

J.E. Jellis OBE, FRCSE. Professor and Consultant orthopaedic surgeon. Zambian-Italian Orthopaedic Hospital, PO Box 30221 Lusaka, Zambia.

L.F. Levy FRCS. (1921-2007) Professor of Surgery, Consultant Neurosurgeon, PO Box Al 78, Avondale, Harare, Zimbabwe.

S. Nade DSc, MD, BS, BSc(Med), FRCS, FRACS, MRCP(UK), FAOrthA (1939-2013). Formerly Clinical Professor of Orthopaedic Surgery, Department of Surgery, Westmead Hospital, University of Sydney, Australia. Visiting orthopaedic surgeon to Papua New Guinea.

J.D. Vince MD, FRCP. Professor, Department of Paediatrics, and Deputy Dean, School of Medicine and Health Sciences, University of Papua New Guinea.

Foreword

First Edition

This book by Jeffrey Rosenfeld and David Watters is nothing short of noble in its design, intent and execution. It offers physicians working in developing areas of the world the wherewithal to deal with a wide variety of neurological and neurosurgical problems that should not be ignored. One often encounters scepticism with regard to the concept of neurosurgery playing a role in the health care of developing nations; nations that need sanitation, infectious disease control and infrastructure far more than a neurosurgeon, who is frequently viewed as a technology-dependent luxury. There are, however, inescapable public health aspects of neurosurgery in every country of the world, including those in tropical and developing areas. Head and spine trauma occur everywhere, and increases steadily as development occurs.

Stroke and cerebrovascular disease are ubiquitous problems, amenable to both preventative and therapeutic strategies. Epilepsy occurs in every country of the world, and is responsible for considerable disability and loss of productivity. Infectious diseases, commonly affect the nervous system. This is true for HIV, for malaria, for tuberculosis, and for cysticercosis along with numerous other parasitic infestations that can affect the brain and spinal cord. One of the characteristics of developing countries is that the population is skewed to the younger age groups as the birth rate rises with development. This necessarily produces an increased burden of developmental defects such as hydrocephalus and meningomyelocele. Brain tumours occur in every land; it is important to realise that some 40 percent of intracranial tumours are benign, and with a reasonable effort in diagnosis and therapy can be successfully treated. Finally, spinal and peripheral nerve surgery can often alleviate suffering and restore disabled individuals to useful work. It is interesting to speculate on what might be necessary to support neurosurgical specialisation in a developing country. Evidently there needs to be a population base of individuals who have some access to medical or nursing care. There must be a reasonable infrastructure to provide transport to centres where neurological diagnosis and neurosurgical treatment can be done. Sophisticated neurosurgery may be beyond the resources of many developing countries, as it requires computed tomography, an operating microscope, and intensive care unit, neuro-anaesthesia, specialised nursing and rehabilitation facilities, which may be low down on the list of important medical priorities. Despite the apparent mismatch of high technology neurosurgery with the needs of developing nations, there are a number of alternatives.

Jeffrey Rosenfeld exemplifies the visiting neurosurgeon to countries like Papua New Guinea, where periodic visits are made so that a neurosurgeon can manage neurological and neurosurgical problems with whatever resources are available locally. Another strategy and one which prompted the writing of this book is to train indigenous general surgeons to work with existing equipment and to deal with basic neurosurgical problems, emphasising head and spine and trauma, and the management of infectious disease. Such training of general surgeons in the basic neurosurgical procedures is the work that Jeffrey Rosenfeld and David Watters do in the South Pacific. There are a number of organisations that attempt to provide neurosurgical education and material support to developing nations.

Regional educational courses have been designed and have been quite effective for taking an entire educational programme to a developing area so that doctors with limited financial resources can keep abreast of current concepts in neurology and neurosurgery. Adjuncts to the educational efforts include the development of a basic set of instruments that can be used for the more common neurosurgical procedures. This, along with an outline of basic training in neurological diagnosis (both available in this volume) will hopefully make a major impact on the neurosurgical and neurological health of individuals in developing nations.

Edward R. Laws Jr, MD, FACS
Charlottesville, Virginia

Foreword

Second Edition

Since the first edition of *Neurosurgery in the Tropics* in 2000, the concept of global surgery and even global neurosurgery has expanded dramatically, virtually exponentially. The greatest impetus for this tsunami of momentum was in 2015 with 4 distinct events: 1) the United Nations transitioning from the Millennium Development Goals (with little reference to surgical care) to the Sustainable Development Goals, where 9 of the 13 health goals (SDG3) are directly or indirectly related to surgical care; 2) the Lancet Commission on Global Surgery with the paradigm-shifting conclusions pertaining to surgical needs; 3) Disease Control Priorities 3rd Edition, Volume 1 *Essential Surgery*, which laid out the global needs and economic case for surgical care in the developing world; and 4) World Health Assembly resolution WHA68.15 on strengthening emergency and essential surgical care and anaesthesia as a component of universal health coverage. These events, all released within a very short interval, catapulted surgical care onto the global stage with the agenda of improving population health, especially within the context of universal health coverage (UHC).

At present, the need for surgical services is dire and growing:
- ~30% of the Global Burden of Disease is surgically related—and rising
- 5 Billion individuals lack access to safe, timely, affordable surgical and anaesthesia care (1.7 Billion are children under the age of 15 years)
- 17 million deaths/year would be averted with timely access to surgical care
- Between 1-2 million additional surgical providers are currently needed worldwide
- Provision of surgical care is greatly hindered by lack of funding
- Surgical care is an "indivisible, indispensable" part of UHC

The need for global neurosurgery is equally severe. First, traumatic brain injury is one, if not the most lethal and devastating injury in all countries, regardless of income. In low- and middle-income countries, many of these injuries are low velocity injuries that could easily be treated with adequately trained surgical care providers, assuming the patients arrived at the hospital and received treatment in a timely manner.

Second, stroke is one of the most devastating, preventable diseases causing premature death and extreme disability worldwide. Third, the consequences of spine injury and degenerative conditions are profound and require not only surgical care, but also appropriate implant hardware and significant rehabilitation. These three conditions are, without question, optimally treated through prevention; but sadly, effective programmes toward this goal are predominantly lacking. Infants, children and adolescents are a vulnerable population worldwide is. In Sub-Saharan Africa, the average is 43% of the population under the age of 15; some countries are as high as 50%. With few surgeons specifically trained in paediatric conditions, these children have even less access to critically important neurosurgical care than their adult counterparts. Each of the neurosurgical conditions outlined in this second edition will dramatically improve the health and well-being of individuals of every age group within Member State populations. This requires a systems-based approach from point of injury or diagnosis, efficient transportation systems, early triage and resuscitation in emergency receiving areas, timely and appropriate surgical care, competent peri-operative care, and at least, rudimentary, perhaps family-centred rehabilitation.

The systems-based approach with adequate infrastructure, supplies and equipment, and an appropriate health workforce, will ultimately deliver intended results, but must remain community oriented with strong and efficient referral patterns to higher levels of care. This excellent volume by Rosenfeld and Watters will well equip front line surgical providers in the essential elements of those issues that require specific expertise in neurological surgery. It should be on the reference shelf and downloaded onto the laptops in every district and regional hospital, as well as become essential reading for any students or registrars learning the art and science of neurosurgical care.

Dr Walter Johnson[1]
Lead, Emergency & Essential Surgical Care Programme, WHO

[1]The author is a staff member of the World Health Organization. The author alone is responsible for the views expressed in this article and they do not necessarily represent the decisions, policy or views of the World Health Organization.

Preface

We have frequently been asked where copies of "Neurosurgery in the tropics" can be obtained. Unfortunately, since it was first published in 2000 it went out of print within a decade. There is currently no other comprehensive textbook specifically written for surgeons in low- and middle-income countries (LMICs) which covers neurosurgical diagnosis, investigation and treatment including descriptions of the common operations in adult and paediatric neurosurgery encountered in LMICs.

We therefore felt that there was a need for a revised, second edition of "Neurosurgery in the tropics". The tropics and subtropics include most developing countries and over two-thirds of the world's population, most of whom live in LMICs. The Lancet Commission on Global Surgery (LCoGS) reported that five billion of the world's seven billion people do not have access to safe, affordable and timely surgery and anaesthesia care.[2] This is particularly true for patients suffering neuro surgically remediable pathology.

The global neurosurgery movement have estimated (in 2018) that 22.6 million patients across the world suffer from neurosurgical disorders or injuries that warrant the expertise of a neurosurgeon, of whom 13.8 million require surgery (Dewan et al, 2018). The global burden of unmet, but treatable neurosurgical need is estimated to be around 5 million persons per year. There is a world deficit of neurosurgeons which had only about 50,000 trained neurosurgeons (Mukhopadhyay, 2019) in 2018. We would need to train an additional 23,300 neurosurgeons to meet this unmet burden. Although the Bogota Declaration calls on neurosurgeons to increase their capacity to train, in the years to 2030, much clinical assessment and urgent surgery will need to be done by general surgeons. Persons with traumatic brain injury may require urgent surgery or procedural intervention. In sub-Saharan Africa only a quarter of the population has access to a neurosurgeon within 2 hours; this figure is around

---

[2]Meara JG, Leather AJM, Hagander L, et al. Global surgery 2030: evidence and solutions for achieving health, welfare, and economic development. Lancet. 2015;386(9993):569-624. http://dx.doi.org/10.1016/S1040-6736(15)60160-X

30% in East Asia and the Pacific, whereas in South Asia it is about 50% (Punchak M, 2018). In the South Pacific Island nations there are only two neurosurgeons for over 10m people. The two neurosurgeons are based in Port Moresby, Papua New Guinea and Suva, Fiji. Less than a million people have access to these two neurosurgeons within 2 hours, a coverage rate of less than 10%. Head and spinal injuries are the commonest cause of death from trauma in the world, particularly in LMICs where violence and road accidents are common. There are an estimated 69 million traumatic brain injury (TBI) cases annually. One neurosurgeon per 200,000 population who deals only with neurotrauma is recommended.

The patterns of disease and infections peculiar to the tropics combined with the problems of poverty, malnutrition, lack of medical and surgical resources create a unique set of problems. The surgeon working in the LMICs cannot be fully prepared by training only in high-income countries (HICs), nor by reading textbooks written for first world surgical practice. He or she must know how to clinically assess a patient, and what can or should not be done if imaging or equipment is not available. Neurosurgery is often considered an unaffordable luxury for the developing world. However, many disorders of the nervous system are readily amenable to surgery which, when successful, has the potential to save lives and prevent disability. Some neurosurgical operations can and must be performed by general surgeons with little or no background in neurosurgery.

In some LMICs countries over 50 percent of people living are under the age of 20 and the birth rate is high. The population growth rate is often over 2-3 per cent with population doubling times of 20-30 years. Most of the patients needing neurosurgery are children or young adults with family responsibilities, vital to the future and prosperity of their nation. Modelling suggests that the economic impact of failure to treat avertable neurosurgical disease in LMICs represents approximately a $4.4 trillion loss of GDP, 0.5-0.6% of the GDP of Low and Low Middle Income countries (Rudolfson, 2018). In addition to managing head and spinal injuries, common and less complex neurosurgery operations such as insertion of ventriculo-peritoneal shunt, drainage of a brain abscess, could also be performed by general surgeons with some basic training in these procedures. Governments of LMICs will need to provide a health system with hospitals that are adequately equipped and functional to meet these needs along with all the other emergency and essential surgical procedures. Surgical decision making will be much improved where there is CT scanning available. Cost-effective neurosurgical technology also is needed. The low-cost Chhabra Shunt [3] is a good example. The principal aim of this book is to equip the general surgeon with the necessary information to manage the common pathologies encountered. It is written for the isolated practitioner with limited resources, who needs advice on the neuroanatomy, neuropathology and operative surgery of the disordered nervous system. We hope that with this information much death and misery will be prevented.

It is not our intention to encourage general surgeons to operate when they can and should refer to a neurosurgeon with better resources for treatment. The HIC reader should remember that perhaps half of the world's inhabitants have no access to a neurosurgeon and so their choice is either no treatment at all or to be managed by a general surgeon. As a surgical service expands and develops in a tropical country there will come a time when it is appropriate for subspecialty practice in neurosurgery to begin. This is a difficult transition phase, as it is never easy to establish a new service almost from scratch. There will be a struggle for adequate resources and for recognition of the emerging subspecialty. Professor Laurence Levy (1921-2007) from Zimbabwe has written an invitation chapter discussing the likely problems encountered for the would-be neurosurgeon. Although this chapter is now largely historical as it relates to sub-Saharan Africa in the 1960's to 1980's, it still contains many important lessons in regards to setting up a neurosurgical service.

We have supplemented Levy's chapter with an account from William Kaptigau (1963-2014) who more recently (2003-2012) established a neurosurgical unit in Port Moresby, Papua New Guinea.[4] It is important that a critical mass of general surgeons are trained before attempting to develop the specialty of neurosurgery. Once this critical number is obtained, it may then be appropriate for about one surgeon in 30 to be trained in neurosurgery, assuming that general surgeons are still able to provide at least a basic neurosurgical service, particularly for emergencies. Even when the first neurosurgeon in a region is trained, general surgeons, who will provide the bulk of the surgical service, must still manage neurosurgical emergencies, select cases for referral and keep appropriate cases for the occasional neurosurgical visit by a local or international neurosurgeon or neurosurgical team. In some LMICs, a neurosurgeon could merely travel from the capital city to other hospitals in the provinces, providing the facilities are reasonable.

---

[3] G. Surgiwear Ltd., India.
[4] Kaptigau WM, Rosenfeld JV, Kevau I, Watters DAK. The establishment and development of neurosurgery services in Papua New Guinea. World Journal of Surgery. 2016;40:251-257.

This may be a better solution for the local patient and their family, rather than being transferred to the capital. The Bogota Declaration called on neurosurgeons, their professional societies and related stakeholders to take urgent coordinated action to lead and address the unmet global neurosurgical need.[5] Although there is an urgent need to train more neurosurgeons in LMIC and prevent their eventual loss and recruitment to HICs, there is still much that can and must be done by general surgeons. This book has been written and updated with that in mind. It is difficult for a book that is intended to be practical to continually update references, particularly where its champions established procedures that are applicable in low- and middle-income country (LMIC) and resource-limited settings. However, we have included some general references that relate to the practice of neurosurgery in LMICs. A few are of the more recently published ones are listed below. Others are listed in footnotes throughout the text. The references from the first edition have largely been removed as they were becoming increasingly dated despite the majority still being relevant to LMIC practice today.

Jeffrey V. Rosenfeld
David A.K. Watters

---

[5]*https://globalneurosurgery.org/bogota-declaration/*

Changes to First Edition

Much of the world's population remains too poor or living too remotely to receive neurosurgery from neurosurgeons or even sometimes general surgeons. The principal purpose of "Neurosurgery in the tropics" is to serve as a resource for the general surgeon in LMICs to diagnose and treat the common neurosurgical conditions without having the resources of the developed countries and without having to train in neurosurgery. Neurosurgeons in training from LMICs and those neurosurgeons who live and work in LMICs will also find this book to be helpful and informative. Surgical and Medical House staff and nursing staff in the hospitals of the LMICs will also find the book of relevance to performing neurosurgical assessments and making decisions as they go about their daily work. Neurosurgery is not an unaffordable luxury service in LMIC. Much can be achieved as we and others have demonstrated with limited resources and some basic training and support. Many traumatic, infectious, congenital and neoplastic conditions of the nervous system can be treated successfully in the developing world with acceptable morbidity and mortality.

Getting people back to their families from life-threatening or more chronic illness is the goal and better still getting them back to work if they are a breadwinner for the family. All of this should happen in an environment where governments are supportive and where the affected families are not crippled by unaffordable debt. The gulf between neurosurgery in the LMIC and advanced wealthy countries grows progressively wider. The power drill (craniotome) used to open a skull and which is taken for granted in the advanced countries, is usually unavailable in low income countries. Here, the surgeon relies on the Hudson brace, perforator, burrs and Gigli saw. Most neurosurgeons in HICs, and trained since the beginning of the 21st century, have never used these manual instruments. Many aspects of cranial and spinal neurosurgery have advanced significantly since the first edition of "Neurosurgery in the tropics". More advanced magnetic resonance imaging, intracranial microsurgery, innovative skull base operative approaches, neuro-endoscopic and neuro-interventional techniques with coils and stents in intracranial vessels, focussed radiotherapy (radiosurgery) using the Gamma Knife or linear accelerator-based systems and minimally invasive spinal internal fixation techniques have all transformed neurosurgery and the way it is practised in the advanced countries. Inevitably, there is great expense in setting up and providing these services which renders them unattainable in LMIC. 'Super-specialisation' in neurosurgery has become the predominant HIC model with neurosurgeons separating into spinal, neuro-oncology, cerebrovascular, neurotrauma and intensive care, paediatric, functional and spinal as the main divisions.

Unfortunately, none of this specialisation is available to the poor countries of the developing world. The neurosurgeon in these countries, if available at all, will remain a generalist and even more so for the general surgeon who covers the main neurosurgical problems in the absence of a neurosurgeon. This is how things will remain into the foreseeable future. Cost-effective innovations may bring some new capabilities to neurosurgery in the LMIC but the unmet need in manpower, training deficit, and maintenance of equipment and resupply will remain critical issues. There continues to be a severe shortage of surgeons who can provide surgery and neurosurgery in many parts of the world, whether the surgery be timely or whether it happens at all. The maintenance of a sense of purpose and morale is difficult to maintain under these conditions and with wider disparities emerging with the advanced nations.

The principles and practice of neurosurgical diagnosis, treatment and operative surgery as they are practised in LMIC have not changed much since the first edition. We have added sections on global neurosurgery, an update on HIV, needlestick and scalpel injury to the surgeon, medical and nursing staff, an expansion of the section on endoscopic management of hydrocephalus in infants including third ventriculostomy and choroid plexectomy and a section on decompressive craniectomy. This latter operation has particular relevance to blast and penetrating injury to the head. Terrorist attacks using improvised explosive devices (IEDs) have become commonplace throughout the world resulting often in mass casualties with horrendous injuries and a high death rate at the scene. Non-military general and neurosurgeons should therefore become familiar with this type of surgery (Rosenfeld et al).[6]

---

[6]*Rosenfeld JV, Bell RS, Armonda R. Current concepts in penetrating and blast injury to the central nervous system World Journal of Surgery. doi: 10.1007/200268-014-2874-7.*

The key neurosurgery questions for the surgeon of the developing world have not changed. Is this a treatable neurosurgical condition? What can I accomplish with the limited resources that I have? Should I operate on this particular patient? What are the main risks? What is the prognosis and what family and societal (if any) supports will be required if I do proceed? "Neurosurgery in the tropics" should assist in answering these questions.

Jeffrey V. Rosenfeld
David A.K. Watters
May 2019

References

Scaling up neurosurgery in LMICs

Dewan MC, Rattani A, Fieggen G, Arraez MA, Servadei F, Boop FA, Johnson WD, Warf BC, Park KB. Global neurosurgery: the current capacity and deficit in the provision of essential neurosurgical care. Executive summary of the global neurosurgery in initiative at the program in global surgery and social change. Journal of Neurosurgery. 2018;1:1-10.

Kaptigau WM, Rosenfeld JV, Kevau I, Watters DAK. The establishment and development of neurosurgery services in Papua New Guinea. World Journal of Surgery. 2016;40:251-257.

Mansouri A, Ibrahim GM. Moving forward together: The Lancet Commission on Global Surgery report and its implications for neurosurgical procedures. British Journal of Neurosurgery. 2015;29(6):751-752.

Muir RT, Wang S, Warf BC. Global surgery for pediatric hydrocephalus in the developing world: a review of the history, challenges, and future directions. Neurosurgical Focus. 2016;41(5):E11.

Mukhopadhyay S, Punchak M, Rattani A, Hung YC, Dahm J, Faruque S, Dewan MC, Peeters S, Sachdev S, Park KB. The global neurosurgical workforce: a mixed-methods assessment of density and growth. Journal of Neurosurgery. 2019;4:1-7.

Park KB, Johnson WD, et al. Global Neurosurgery: The Unmet Need. World Neurosurgery. 2016;88:32-35.

Prabhu VC. Neurosurgery Initiatives in Global Health. World Neurosurgery. 2015;84(6):1544-1546.

Punchak M, Mukhopadhyay S, Sachdev S, Hung YC, Peeters S, Rattani A, Dewan M, Johnson WD, Park KB. Neurosurgical care: availability and access in low-income and middle-income countries. World Neurosurgery. 2018;112:e240-254.

Ravindra VM, Kraus KL, et al. The Need for Cost-Effective Neurosurgical Innovation--A Global Surgery Initiative. World Neurosurgery. 2015;84(5):1458-1461. https://globalneurosurgery.org/

Rudolfson N, Dewan MC, Park KB, Shrime MG, Meara JG, Alkire BC. The economic consequences of neurosurgical disease in low and middle-income countries. Journal of Neurosurgery. 2018;1:1-8.

Warf BC. Who Is My Neighbor? Global Neurosurgery in a Non-Zero-Sum World. World Neurosurgery. 2015;84(6):1547-1549.

Acknowledgments

First Edition

We thank our secretaries Ms Felicity Braun and Ms Vaporo Rei for their considerable help with typing and preparation of the manuscript.

JVR wishes to acknowledge the generous support of the Papua New Guinea Medical Officer Nursing and Allied Health Science Training Project (MONAHP), an AusAid programme of the Department of Foreign Affairs, Commonwealth of Australia; which has enabled the multiple visits to Papua New Guinea.

Our thanks also go to the Neurosurgical Society of Australasia for their Asian-Australasian Travelling Fellowship, which enabled JVR to visit, teach and work in Vietnam; and to Professor Wu Cheng Yuan, Director of the Department of Neurosurgery, Shandong Medical University, for supporting JVR's visit and work in China. We would also like to thank Helalo Guba and Mr Vincent Tomaur, the medical illustrators at the University of Papua New Guinea for their help with photographic illustrations.

We thank the medical illustrator at the Royal Children's Hospital Mr Bill Reid for the line diagrams, and Ms Janna Stickland and Mr Pierre Smith at The Royal Melbourne Hospital for their assistance with the preparation of the figures.

Dr Caroline Thew, Consultant Endocrinologist, The Royal Melbourne Hospital, has assisted with the preparation of Table 6.4.

We wish to thank the Foundation for International Education in Neurological Surgery Inc. for their generous grant towards the publication of this book.

Acknowledgments

Second Edition

We thank Dr Eileen Mary Moore PhD, Department of Surgery, Deakin University based at the University Hospital, Geelong. EM provided a Google docs version of the text, rescanned images or inserted new ones and managed the process and final submission.

Our thanks also to Mrs Anne Vandewater, University Hospital Geelong, for her assistance.

We would also like to thank Dr Su Mei Hoh FRACS, University Hospital Geelong, for her input to the cover design of the second edition and Dr Lynn Koyama, Neurosurgery Registrar at Melbourne's Alfred Hospital, for preparing the normal CT and MR images in Chapter Two.

Developing a neurosurgical service

Laurence F. Levy (1921-2007)

In the late 1950's there was no neurosurgical service on the east side of Africa between Johannesburg in the south and Cairo in the north a distance of over 6000 km. The same situation has held for large areas of Asia and the Far East as well as parts of South and Central America. Now there are centres to be found in all the capital cities and university towns of Eastern Africa. In these countries' neurosurgery has a hold (albeit tenuous in some places) but is steadily expanding to answer the people's needs. Every neurosurgeon who has embarked on his/her specialty in an underdeveloped region where there has not been anyone before, faces the same problems. For success, the criteria are, availability at all times, the willingness to take on any case that is offered, reasonable diagnostic and surgical skills, and the ability to apply simple (or old fashioned) diagnostic manoeuvres to provide the answers - all with a smiling face. The surgeon who is unable to do this will not make a success of his mission and will end up with dis-illusionment for himself, criticism from his colleagues, and disrepute for his specialty.

The young neurosurgeon who has trained only in the First World with its exotic equipment and adequate staff is in for a bad culture shock when he or she arrives in a low- or middle-income country. Much more so than in the 1960's or 70's when the difference between the types of equipment available, par-ticularly on the diagnostic side, was so much less. In the so called, developed world, reliance upon magnetic resonance imaging (MRI), computed tomo-graphy (CT), somatosensory studies, and nuclear medicine has almost replaced the clinical skills - many of these items of equipment are not avail-able in the Third World, or only in a very restricted fashion. However, there will be many acute situations demanding immediate action with which the neurosurgeon will be called upon to cope and the ability to function indepen-dently and to be self-reliant is paramount. In the first decades of the 20th century 'Air studies', Ventriculography (1917) and Pneumo-encephalography (1925), which were introduced by Dr Walter Dandy, were the standard diagnostic manoeuvres of neurosurgery. In these tests, air was used as the contrast medium. It was injected into the ventricles, either through a burr hole with a needle passed into the ventricle, or through the lumbar route with the patient in the sitting position. Sometimes air, combined with radio-opaque oils (Lipiodil, Myodil), and served to outline, in a relatively crude sort of way, the shape of the ventricular system on an X-ray of the skull. The neurosurgeon could then evaluate:

1. were the ventricles normal in size and shape, and
2. were they in their correct position,
3. and, if not, from what direction came the pressure.

No one can pretend that the pictures obtained were comparable in any way to those obtained by CT or MRI, but much excellent neurosurgery was done on the basis of them. Every developing world neurosurgeon should know how to do these tests and to interpret them. Cerebral angiography was introduced in the mid-1930s but did not get a hold as a diagnostic manoeuvre until after the Second World War. It is a very satisfactory test for the diagnosis of head injuries (is there or is there not a surgical surface or intracerebral clot?) and rapidly replaced air studies in the diagnosis of cerebral neoplasia. It has several advantages - the most import-ant being that it does not affect the intracranial pressure relationships. It was well known in patients with raised intracranial pressure that after an air study had been performed, the study would have to be followed by a definitive decompressive procedure or the patient's general condition would deteriorate for the worse. In this way diagnostic ventriculography and a surgical operation were inevitably locked together in a long-drawn-out surgical procedure.

Angiography does not disturb the intracranial pressure so that it can be per-formed preoperatively without placing a time pressure on patient and surgeon. It has this and other advantages over air studies, which it soon replaced to a very large extent. Nowadays neuroradiologists perform this test by long catheter inserted via the femoral artery, but for many years it was done, and still can be done very successfully, by direct puncture of the carotid artery in the neck. Despite much criticism of direct puncture, it is not a dangerous procedure- occasionally swelling of the neck region will occur temporarily from haematoma formation but it is very rare indeed for the airway to be compromised. Using 10 ml of modern intra-arterial contrast media (Omnipaque, Hypaque, Conray 280) the incidence of intracranial complication is very low. This is a test that every successful developing world neurosurgeon without modern imaging backup must be able to perform for himself using a sharp No. 19 lumbar puncture or similar needle, a small plastic connecting tube (so that when he is doing the injection the needle does not move) and a simple X-ray plant. Any X-ray machine that can take a routine skull X-ray (A-P and 'Shooting through' lateral) can be used. Needless to say, one which can recharge rapidly enough to enable sequential pictures to be taken is preferable. A manually operated cassette holder and changer can be built by any carpenter or even, in the lateral views, the cas-settes can be substituted one for another by hand. Views of arterial, capillary, venous and sinus phases can easily be obtained through usually only a later arterial/early capillary phase is required for diagnostic purposes.

Myelography is almost as important as angiography in the developing world where there is an enormous amount of spinal work to be done. This pre-supposes an X-ray table with screening facilities which can tilt at least in one direction, though with ingenuity and-careful adjustment of the position of the patient's body on a horizontal fixed table, satisfactory pictures can sometimes be obtained. Other diagnostic equipment is desirable but the problem with all sophisticated machinery is maintenance. Before embarking upon the purchase of an electroencephalogram (EEG), electromyogram (EMG) or evoked response equip-ment for example, one must be sure of a trained person to obtain the tracings and of electronics engineer to maintain it. With modular items of equipment and with rapid servicing overseas, this problem of maintenance is not so acute, though one still has to worry about foreign currency and the process to pay for it - not to mention customs problems on exit and re-entry of the goods. There are some instruments that are essential for neurosurgery, but for the straightforward work they are relatively few.

Clearly a perforator, burr and Gigli saw set are essential to let the surgeon into the skull and, in the absence of a trained nursing team, these are preferable to air and electric drills which inevitably get mistreated. Adequate suction and cautery are a must - it is true that Harvey Cushing did not have cautery and certainly not the bipolar variety- but today only a very experienced surgeon in desperate straits should embark on neurosurgical work without these. Punches, pituitary rongeurs and self-retaining retractors are likewise essential, but for the rest, one can get by with the ordinary instruments of general surgery if one is driven to it in an emergency. In the author's opinion, a great mistake would be made by the young surgeon standing his ground and saying 'I cannot and will not do this without ... '.

Developing a neurosurgical service

It is better to struggle a while and prove what can be done before demanding better and more appropriate instruments. It is certain that any surgeon starting out will have to be their own neuro-radiologist, to some extent their own pathologist, their own electroencephalographer, and even sometimes the intern and rehabilitationist, these are responsibilities that must be shouldered until neurosurgery as a speciality becomes accepted and others who are appropriately trained and experienced come along to help. Assistance in the theatre may be by the totally unskilled and the assistants will need training also. At first the work will be slow, very slow to appear, and it may even be perceived that neurosurgical problems do not exist. Nonetheless, interesting problems will make their appearance continuously, and indeed such problems will become more in number and more exotic with the passage of time. Tumours that are very large with widespread ramifications and locations are not unusual and, having previously been diagnosed as 'strokes', will have the reputation of not existing. Abscesses and trauma will make up a large part of the work.

Epilepsy is very common but the number requiring surgery or being willing to accept it are relatively few. In most parts of the tropics tuberculosis is the dominant spinal problem. Prolapsed intervertebral discs may be rare at first, but later as the society develops, they will become more common. The social aspects of surgery and indeed of medical practice in the developing take a lot of acclimatisation, rarely is a decision taken in immediately - invariably the elders of the family must be consulted and in some societies wives may not have the right to consent on behalf of the husband; if the family have not made up their minds it is futile to rush things. Then there is the problem of what operation can be done on which patient.

A child who lives many kilometres from the neurosurgical centre and whose parents can afford only one visit has only a small chance of benefiting from a shunt for hydrocephalus - these shunts need constant observation, regular review, and many need adjustments for blockage. If the child cannot be brought back for this, he is little better off than if the shunt had never been inserted.

In the same way, a patient needing a heart valve which requires controlled warfarinisation cannot go far from the cardiac centre and certainly not to some distant point where follow-up may be very difficult. Social factors therefore play a big part and must be seriously considered in every case. Other social factors are important, especially where there is poor sanitation and low levels of education, hygiene will inevitably be poor - parasitic disorders of the central nervous system are common, while parasitic diseases of the gastrointestinal tract or other organs may render surgery hazardous.

Many disorders are thought not to exist in the developing world or at least to be rare: multiple sclerosis, trigeminal neuralgia, schwannoma of the eighth cranial nerve. Are these really rare? and if so why? These are some research questions requiring answers. Western-type medicine that is moving into a previously un-serviced area will inevitably come up against established routines and attitudes. Traditional medicine will have been accepted as the norm in the region for centuries. Based on a mixture of herbalism and mysticism it is deeply rooted in the people's culture. No one will come to be seen by the western-style doctors until all aspects of this religious traditionalism have been covered. This, together with the dis-tances that have to be travelled to reach a neurosurgical unit and the natural fear and reluctance to accept an operation, combines to produce late presentation to hospital, a deteriorated patient and an aggravated clinical syndrome. These problems are little different from those encountered in the last 100 years in the now developed World by our forebears when surgery was establishing itself after the introduction of anaesthesia and aseptic techniques. Then, once surgery had established itself as a safe and humane specialty, it was time, in the second half of the 20th century for neurosurgery to emerge as its own specialty. The young neurosurgeons of the developing world will not, if they are persistent, need to wait another 50 years to see neurosurgery established in their own country.

SETTING UP A NEUROSURGICAL SERVICE IN PAPUA NEW GUINEA (2003-2012)

William M. Kaptigau (1963-2014)

By the end of the year 2000, Papua New Guinea's (PNG) MMed program had trained 42 general surgeons, including one Tongan, one Micronesian and two Solomon Islanders. With the support of the Royal Australasian College of Surgeons (RACS) Rowan Nicks and Surgeon's International scholarships, the first neurosurgeon, William Matui Kaptigau commenced training in neurosurgery in Townsville and Melbourne. Some training was conducted in-country, in Port Moresby with the support of visiting neurosurgeons. He was a general surgeon, gaining the MMed in 1999, and over the next three years sub-specialising in neurosurgery and he achieved the higher surgical postgraduate diploma in neurosurgery in 2002. For the next decade he produced detailed audits of his neurosurgical unit. For some years he had to work with limited neurosurgical instruments, donated neurosurgical patties, and a CT scan only available in the private sector. A CT scanner was introduced into Port Moresby General Hospital around 2007 for the public patients and those who could not afford private imaging. Kaptigau kept detailed records and took on the management of the majority of neurosurgical cases that required surgery, amassing over 1000 in ten years (see Table 1.1, page 7). He continued to be mentored and supported by annual or twice-yearly neurosurgical visitors from Australia. What is most remarkable about his achievements on surgical outcomes (Table 1.2, page 8) is the reduction in mortality from traumatic brain injuries (TBI). Port Moresby had previously reported its outcomes against both admission GCS and pathology. Table 1.2 on page 8 shows he reduced the mortality in severe (GCS $\leqslant$8) TBI from 55% to 31.3%. He achieved this whilst his unit still provided a general surgical service, he consulted on over 3600 cases, admitted 1618 cases and the neurosurgical POMR for all 1020 cases was 5.49%.

Table 1.1 Diagnoses, consultations, admissions and procedures in the neurosurgical unit, Port Moresby General Hospital, 2003–2012.

Pathology/condition	Consultations	Admissions	Procedures
Cranium			
Traumatic brain injury	1309	1067	442
Scalp suture			19
Cranioplasty for defect			7
Hydrocephalus	758	159	134
Ventricular tap			88
Mass lesions	361	174	81
Dermoid and scalp lumps	227	27	63
Dermoid and scalp lumps	227	27	63
Headache	149		
Neurological manifestations of other diseases	119		
Dysraphism/congenital	111	23	38
Vascular and other lesions	102	33	3
Infections including TB	66	57	62
Change of dressing 15			15
Epilepsy	54		
Cerebrovascular accident	22		
Craniosynostosis	13		
Spine Infection including TB	70	36	20
Myelopathy	66		
Trauma	54	4	3
Congenital	50	9	9
Back pain and degenerative	38		
Mass lesion	4	9	9
Other spinal procedures		10	10
Peripheral nerve	53	10	17
Total	3626	1618	1020

Not all cases admitted had a prior consultation, and not all patients with a procedure were admitted as some were operated as day patients

Developing a neurosurgical service

Table 1.2 Outcomes of neurosurgical admissions (1618) and procedures (1020) performed in the Port Moresby Neurosurgical Unit, 2003–2012.

Parameters measured	2003–2012	Outcome
N/S operations death rates	1020	56 (5.49 %)
Death rates for N/S admissions	1618	243 (15 %)
Death rates for cranial tumour operation	Operations 81	Mortality 7 (8.6 %)
Unplanned reoperation rates for cranial tumours	Operations 81	Re-operations 4 (4.9 %)
VP shunt operation—annual complication rate	Operations 134	Complications 22 (16.42 %)
VP shunt operation infection rate— cumulative	Operations 134	Infection 12 (8.9 %)
Overall mortality rate for VP shunt operation	Operations 134	Mortality 6 (4.5 %)
TBI mortality rates for mild, moderate, severe cases	Admissions (1067)	Mortality 171 (16 %)
Mild	541	18 (3.33 %)
Moderate	194	49 (35.26 %)
Severe	332	104 (31.33 %)
Nosocomial infection rates for all operations	Operations 1020	Infection 13 (1.27 %)

N/S neurosurgery, TBI traumatic brain injury, VP ventriculoperitoneal

Clinical assessment in neurosurgery:
a practical guide for the isolated doctor

BASIC ANATOMY

A knowledge of basic anatomy is essential for the surgeon assessing the neurosurgical patient. The following diagrams will provide a rapid focus on the anatomy of the brain, skull and spinal cord (Figures 2.1-2.7, pages 9-12). Further anatomical diagrams are presented in other parts of the text as a prelude to clinical discussion.

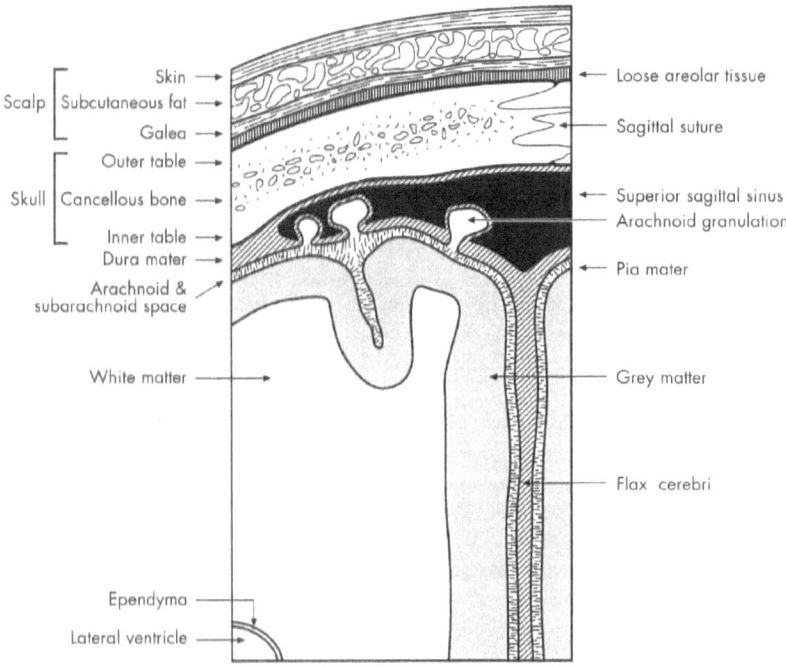

Figure 2.1 Layers of the head. Coronal section showing the layers of the head at the level of the sagittal sinus.

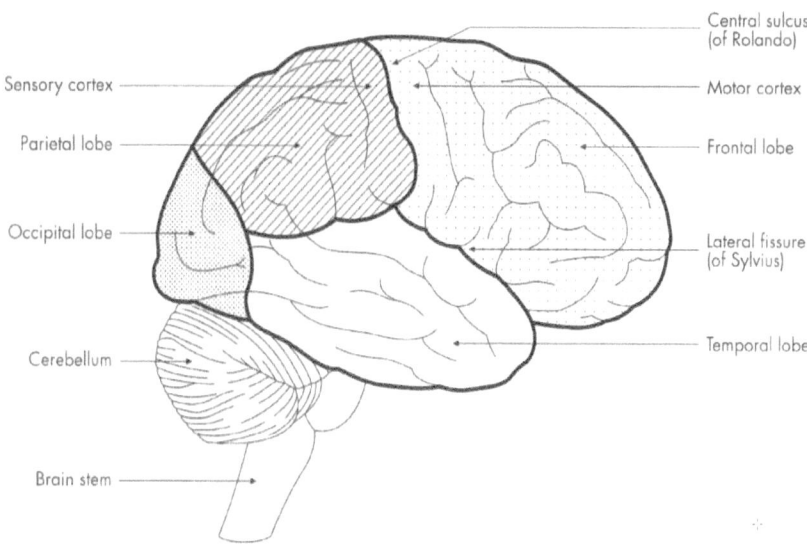

Figure 2.2 The cerebral cortex. The lobes of the brain and the two major fissures- the lateral fissure (sylvian), and the central sulcus (Rolando). The primary motor cortex lies in the pre-central gyrus and the primary sensory cortex lies in the post-central gyrus.

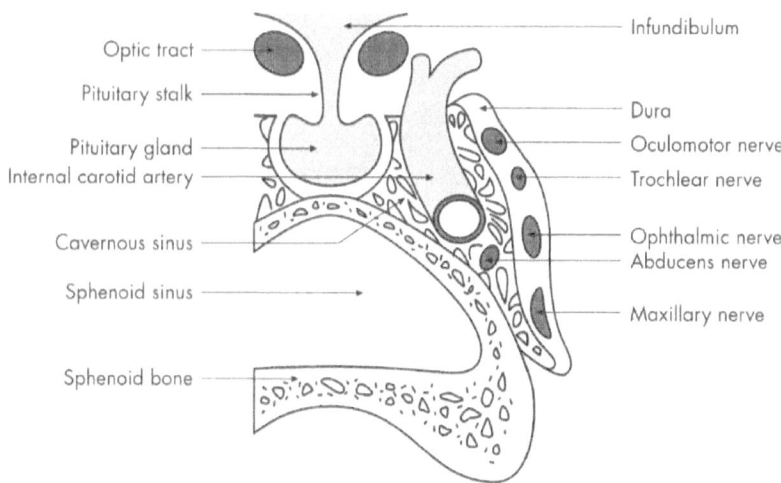

Figure 2.3 The cavernous sinus. Coronal section through the cavernous sinus showing the relation of the cranial nerves to the internal carotid artery. The relations of the pituitary gland can also be appreciated.

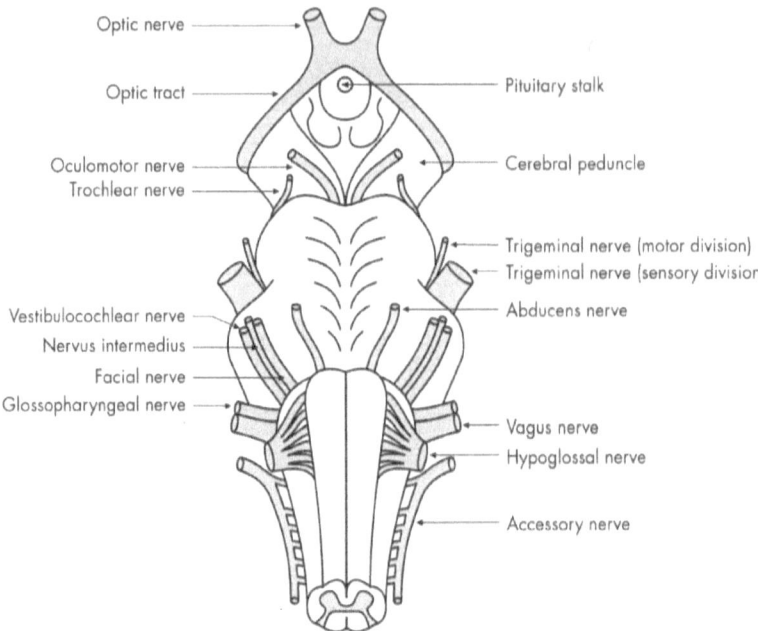

Figure 2.4 The cranial nerves and their relations to the ventral aspect of the brain stem. Note the fourth cranial nerve is the only one that arises from the dorsal aspect of the brain- stem.

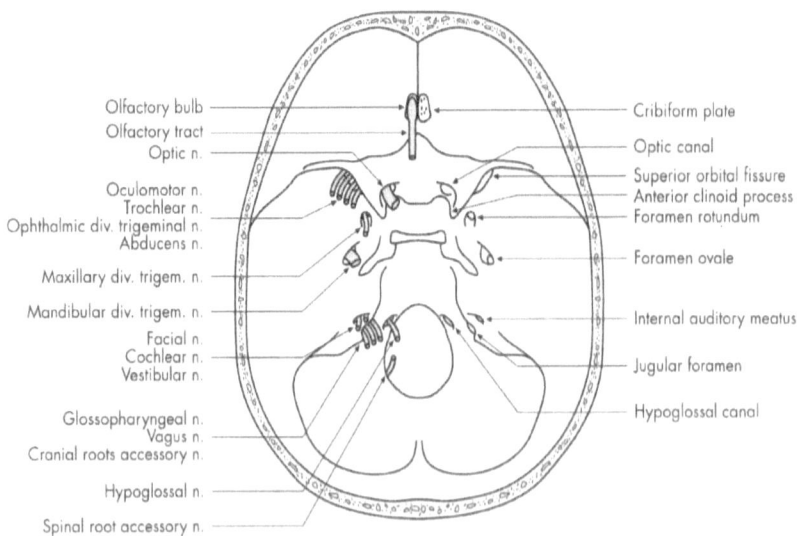

Figure 2.5 The skull base showing the locations of the cranial nerves at their respective foramina.

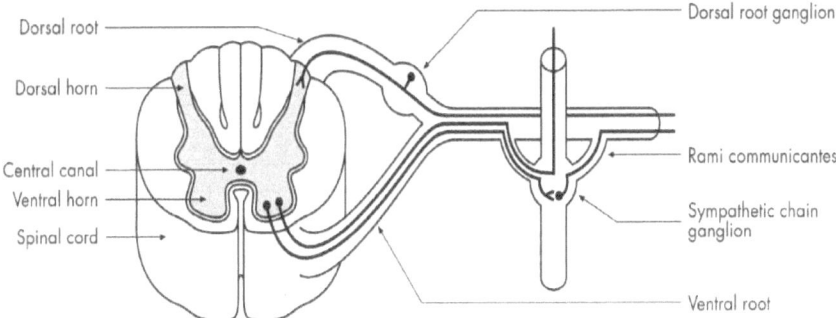

Dorsal root
Dorsal horn
Central canal
Ventral horn
Spinal cord
Dorsal root ganglion
Rami communicantes
Sympathetic chain ganglion
Ventral root

Figure 2.6 The thoracic spinal cord, ventral and dorsal roots and sympathetic chain. Note the central grey area with ventral horn containing motor neurons, and the dorsal horn containing sensory dendrites which synapse with interneurons. The main motor neurons pass from the ventral root into the peripheral nerve (bypassing the sympathetic chain) to their segmental muscle. The primary sensory neurons have cell bodies located in the dorsal root ganglion, and are pseudom-unipolar cells. There are white and grey commissures which join the two halves of the cord together with a small central canal in the centre of the cord. Sympathetic neurons pass up and down the sympathetic chain, synapse in the sympathetic chain ganglia and join the peripheral nerves via the rami communicantes.

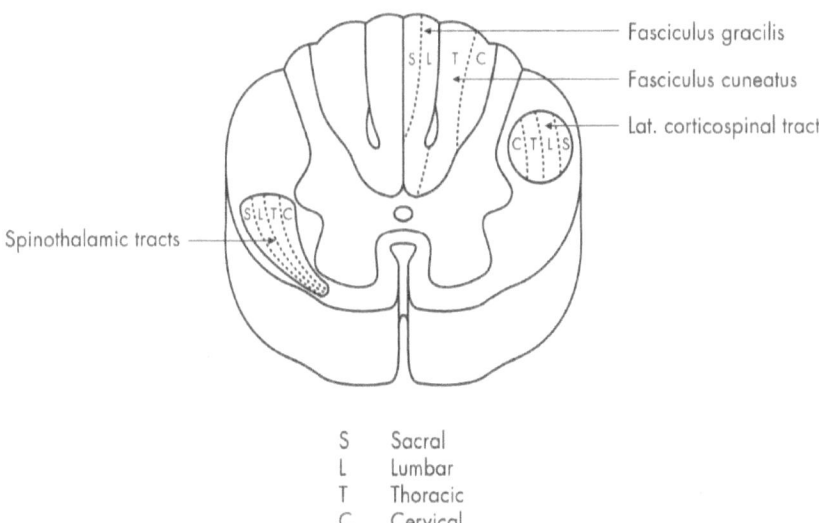

Fasciculus gracilis
Fasciculus cuneatus
Lat. corticospinal tract
Spinothalamic tracts

S   Sacral
L   Lumbar
T   Thoracic
C   Cervical

Figure 2.7 The main tracts of the spinal cord. A horizontal section of the spinal cord showing the somatotopic organisation of the main motor and sensory tracts. The fasciculus gracilis and fasciculus cuneatus form the dorsal columns.

CLINICAL ASSESSMENT

Neurological examination is a skill learned in medical school but, sadly, lack of practice means it is soon forgotten by the young graduate. Many tragic mistakes are made because basic aspects of clinical examination are not carried out. It is not difficult to perform a neurological examination but doctors avoid it because they do not feel competent or confident. The most sophisticated tool needed is an ophthalmoscope.

All too often in LMICs doctors get out of the habit of using an ophthalmoscope, it becomes the domain of the ophthalmologist. However, the clinician who wishes to diagnose and treat neurosurgical problems should make ophthal-moscopy a part of the routine examination. The other basic tools required are an auriscope, tendon hammer, stethoscope, tape measure, cotton wool, and sterile needles. All of these are readily available even in the developing world. The doctor should l keep these in a diagnostic kit and ensure that there are spare batteries and bulbs. A tuning fork is needed by the neurologist or otolaryngologist but is not essential for the general doctor.

The following clinical skills need to be revised:

Assessment of babies and young children

1. Measurement of occipitofrontal circumference (OFC) and plotting it on a growth chart (Appendices 1-2, pages 652-653).
2. Recording the developmental milestones in a baby or child (Table 2.1, page 14).
3. Examination of the skull to assess the turgor of the anterior fontanelle, which is an important means of establishing whether there is raised intracranial pressure (ICP) in a child. This should be examined with the relaxed, preferably sleeping child who is semi-erect. The suture lines can be palpated, as in raised intracranial pressure they are widened and the scalp veins may also be distended. The setting sun sign in infants with hydrocephalus is another sign that is easy to note; it is an indication of pressure directly on the upper brain stem, and leads to paralysis of upgaze, so that the eyes are pointing downwards just like a setting sun (Chapter 4).
4. Assessment of conscious level in small children (Table 2.2, page 18 and Appendix 3, page 654).

Older children and adults

The neurological history

A history should be obtained from the patient or his relatives. It is important to consider the aspects listed in the box on page 17.

The neurological examination

Level of consciousness

The level of consciousness is assessed by using the Glasgow Coma Scale (Teasdale and Jennett, 1974), is a simple objective universally accepted 15-point clinical measure in three sections - eye opening, motor responses and verbal responses (see Table 2.2, page 18 and Appendix 4, page 657). Testing the response to pain: use pressure on the mastoid process or nail- bed pressure with a pencil. When testing the response to pain using the limbs, ensure the patient is not quadriplegic due to a cervical spine injury.

Table 2.1 Main developmental milestone.

Age	Body mastery	Manipulative skills and vision	Language and hearing	Social skills and understanding
Newborn	Prone: pelvis high, knees under abdomen. Turns face to one side.	Can fixate on a visual object about 20 cm away and follows it horizontally for 90°.	Blinks or becomes quiet in response to sound.	Sleeps and feeds. Elicits affection from others.
1 month	Lifts head momentarily when held in ventral suspension. Prone: raises head momentarily.	Watches examiner intently when speaking. Regularly follows objects through 90-180°.	Soft, guttural noises when content.	May smile back at parent or examiner.

Table 2.1 *(Continued)*

Age	Body mastery	Manipulative skills and vision	Language and hearing	Social skills and understanding
2 months	In ventral suspension, keeps head in the same horizontal plane as body. Holds head erect when held upright.	Hands mostly open, grasp reflex weak. Follows moving persons with eyes.	Vocalises when talked to.	Smiles readily, starts to respond more readily to parents than to others.
3 months	Prone: lifts chest off bed, taking weight on forearms. Only slight head lag when pulled to sit.	Holds rattle placed in hand. Reaches towards objects, but unable to grasp. Starts to look at own hands.	Consistently turns to soft sound at ear level. Squeals in delight.	Pleasurable response to familiar, enjoyable situations (bottle, bath).
4 months	Rolls from front to back. Pulled to sit, only slight head lag.	Hands start to come together in the midline.	Spontaneous vocalising to self, people and toys. Laughs.	Initiates social contact with smile or vocalisation.
5 months	Rolls from front to back. No head lag when pulled to sit.	Reaches out for and grasps toys.	Babbling more tuneful.	Smiles at self in mirror.
6 months	Prone: lifts chest on extended arms. Spontaneously lifts head when supine.	Transfers objects between hands. Picks up wooden block in palmar grasp.	Turns towards soft sound at 40-50 cm on ear level.	Laughs, squeals and chuckles. May imitate sounds (cough). Fear of strangers.
9 months	Crawls. Sits unsupported for 10 min or more. Stands holding onto support.	Pincer grip developing.	Localises soft sounds at 1 m above and below ear level.	Looks for toy fallen out of sight. Plays pat-a-cake, peek-a-boo.

Table 2.1 *(Continued)*

Age	Body mastery	Manipulative skills and vision	Language and hearing	Social skills and understanding
12 months	Walks alone or with one hand held.	Repeatedly throws objects onto floor. Less likely to take all objects to mouth.	Says 2-3 words with meaning.	Drinks from cup with help. Knows and turns to own name
18 months	Jumps with both feet together. Walks backwards.	Builds tower of 3-4 blocks. Scribbles spontaneously.	Uses 5-20 words (recognises many more)	Points to 2 or more parts of the body. Indicates toilet needs.
2 years	Runs well. Kicks ball without overbalancing.	Builds tower of 6-7 blocks. Copies vertical and circular strokes.	Uses 2-3 word phrases. Starts to use pronouns.	Behaviour becoming negative. Gives first name. Begins fantasy play
3 years	Rides tricycle. Stands on one foot momentarily.	Builds tower of blocks. Copies circle.	3-5 words sentences. Uses plurals. May count to 10.	Gives full name and sex. Competent with fork and spoon.
4 years	Hops on one foot.	Copies cross. Draws person with three parts.	Asks many questions. Tells fanciful stories.	Gives age and address. Knows and names 4 primary colours. Very imaginative play.
5 years	Can skip.	Copies square. Draws person with 6 parts.	Fluent speech; good articulation.	Fluent speech; good articulation.

Reproduced from Practical Paediatrics (3rd edition) 1994 by authors Robinson M & Robertson D with permission of the publisher, Churchill Livingstone.

History of presenting complaint	*Past medical history*
Headache	Drugs
(raised ICP = worse in morning)	Alcohol
Vomiting	Diabetes
Loss of, or altered, consciousness	Hypertension
Fits, faints, blackouts	Epilepsy
Speech	Other medical illnesses
Hearing	endocrine abnormalities
Vision	pregnancy/eclampsia
Gait	Possibility of secondary
Balance	tumour from any primary TB
Peripheral nerve functions	
upper limbs	
lower limbs	*Family history*
bladder	Neurofibromatosis
bowel	Epilepsy
Vital social functions	Intracranial haemorrhage
Concentration	Brain tumours
Memory	Abnormal movements
short term	
long term	
Intellect	
Behaviour change	
Social interaction	

Table 2.2 The Glasgow Scale.

Eye opening	
Spontaneous	4
Speech	3
Pain	2
None	1

Best verbal response		*Modified for babies*	
Talking coherently	5	Fixes and follows, smiles	5
Confused conversation	4	Cries but consolable	4
Inappropriate words	3	Persistently irritable	3
Incomprehensible sounds	2	Restless, agitated	2
None		None	

Best motor response	
Obeys commands	6
Localises pain	5
Withdraws to pain	4
Flexes to pain	3
Extends to pain	2
None	

The verbal response cannot be assessed in patients with an endotracheal or tracheostomy tube. The verbal response needs to be modified for young chil·dren and babies.

Mental Status

Assessment of the mental status is important when the conscious patient has apparent cognitive problems or is mentally disturbed and is not behaving as they normally would. The change in mental status may be due to an organic problem such as a frontal or temporal lobe glioma, or dementia in an elderly patient. When organic brain pathology has been considered and excluded, consider the patient may have developed delirium or a psychiatric illness.

The mental state examination should include the following elements:

- **Cognition:** Orientation in time, place and person. Gross tests of long and short-term memory.
- **Appearance and behaviour:** Neatly dressed, well-groomed versus dishevelled, level of eye contact, motor activity -restless, slow and retarded, level of co-operation and level of aggression.
- **Speech:** Ranges from 'poverty of speech' to 'pressure of speech'.
- Assess their fluency, willingness to speak, speaking volume and expression.
- **Mood:** The patient's perception of their own mood and the examiner's perception. Judge them on a continuum of depression to elation. Any abrupt mood changes?
- **Affect:** Assess their emotional tone. Are they appropriate in their emotional reactions to your conversation?
- **Is their laughing and are they smiling appropriate?** Do they show empathy? According to the relatives, have they had a change of personality?
- **Thought form and content:** The 'form' is how their thoughts are expressed in their speech. The speech ranges from understandable to incomprehensible jumble of words. The 'content' is the actual thoughts being described. For instance, do they have delusions or obsessions?
- **Perception:** Do they have hallucinations? The most common are auditory i.e. 'hearing voices'.
- **Risk:** Is there a risk of self-harm or suicide? Are they a risk to others?
- **Insight:** Do they have insight into their own mental status?

The Mini-Mental Status Examination (MMSE) is a 30-point questionnaire that is used in clinical practice to measure cognitive impairment.[7] It was first published in 1975 and assesses orientation to time and place, repeating three named prompts, attention and calculation, recalling the three named prompts, naming objects such as a pencil and a watch, speaking back a phrase and performing complex commands. A score greater than 24 (out of 30) indicates normal cognition.[8] There are many caveats about how the test is to be administered and interpreted.

---

[7]*https://www.bgs.org.uk/sites/default/files/content/attachment/2018-07-05/mini-mental_state_exam.pdf*
[8]*Folstein MF, Folstein SE, McHugh PR. Mini-mental status: A practical method for grading the cognitive state of patients for the clinician. Journal of Psychiatric Research. 1975;12(3): 189–198. doi:10.1016/0022-3956(75)90026-6.*

Delirium

Delirium is a disturbance of consciousness, attention, cognition and perception that develops over a short period of time (usually hours or days) and tends to fluctuate during the course of a day.[9] It may be the result of the patient's condition, an infectious complication, pain or their medications. Elderly comorbid patients are at risk of developing delirium during an acute episode in hospital, particularly those already suffering from some cognitive impairment, and who are at risk of becoming disoriented to time and place. Clinical assessment of current and previous cognitive state, together with review of potential causative factors, is indicated. It is best to avoid using psychotropic medications to manage acute delirium.

Examination of the cranial nerves (Table 2.3)

Once you remember the function of a cranial nerve you can test for it. If the nerve is not working then you need to know the path of the nerve to deter-mine the possible sites of the lesion. You can look this up once you've identified that the nerve is not working. All doctors have learnt these skills as undergraduates. It is lack of practice that results in the examination being overlooked or forgotten. Table 2.3, page 20 sets out the essentials of the cranial nerve examination. The following additional points highlight aspects of the cranial nerve examination.

Table 2.3 Examination of the cranial nerves.

Origin	Nerve		Functional assessment
Forebrain	I	Olfactory	Smell (history of anosmia)
	II	Optic	Know visual pathway (Figure 2.9, page 26) Do visual fields, test vision.
Midbrain	III	Oculomotor nerve	Pupil responses (responds to light) Eye movements (look in, up, down) Palsy = ptosis, eye displaced downwards and outwards, pupil dilated and fixed.

---

[9]*https://www.safetyandquality.gov.au/wp-content/uploads/2016/07/Delirium-Clinical-Care-Standard-Web-PDF.pdf*

Table 2.3 *(Continued)*

Origin	Nerve		Functional assessment
Posterior midbrain	IV	Trochlear nerve	Eye movements (look down and in) Palsy= impaired downward movements

Pons	V	Trigeminal nerve
		  Ophthalmic division
		    Maxillary division
		    Mandibular division
			Sensory to face and cornea
			Blink or corneal reflex
			Masseter power and wasting

	VI	Abducens	Eye movements (look laterally) Palsy= inability to look outwards
	VII	Facial nerve Chorda tympani	Motor to muscles of facial expression Taste to anterior two-thirds tongue

Medulla	VIII	Auditory
		  Vestibular
		  Cochlear
			
			Balance
			Hearing

	IX	Glossopharyngeal	Gag reflex (sensory- afferent) Say 'Aah'
	X	Vagus	Gag reflex (motor - efferent) Say 'Aah'
	XI	Accessory (spinal)	Shrug shoulders
	XII	Hypoglossal	Tongue protrusion (to affected side) Tongue wasting and fasciculation

Olfaction

The sense of smell is tested with a substance of strong distinctive odour, e.g. coffee, which is placed before each nostril in turn. The patient is asked to sniff the substance with the eyes closed. Olfaction may be lost following head trauma or due to a tumour involving the floor of the anterior cranial fossa. Note that when the sense of smell is lost, there is a gross alteration in the sense of taste.

The eyes

Observe the patient. Can the patient open their eyes normally? Examine the patient for ptosis, periorbital swelling, bruising or proptosis. Subtle proptosis is often best appreciated by looking at the head from above. Ask whether the conscious patient can see. This is often forgotten in patients with trauma and results in some potentially curable eye injuries being missed. You should examine the pupils, the position of the eyelids, the eye movements the fundus and make an assessment of vision.

Practice point: ptosis

In a third nerve palsy there are impaired eye movements, the pupil is dilated and often fixed with no accommodation reflex. In Horner's syndrome there is pupil constriction (Table 2.4, below). Sympathetic nerves dilate the pupil and parasympathetic nerves constrict the pupil.

1. The pupils

Look at the size and shape of the pupils, comparing both sides. Test the response to light, including the consensual reflex (the opposite pupil constricts in response to light shone in one eye). Test the response to accommodation in a non-acute case.

Table 2.4 Homer's syndrome (lesion of cervical sympathetic).

Pupil constriction
Ptosis
Enophthalmos (eye sinking in to the orbit)
Loss of sweating on same side of face
Causes of Horner's syndrome
Brachial plexus lesion
Carcinoma of the apex of the lung (Pancoast's tumour)

Table 2.4 *(Continued)*

Cervical sympathectomy
Sympathetic chain tumour
Aortic arch aneurysm
Syringobulbia / syringomyelia

One way to confirm the diagnosis of Homer's syndrome is to put the patient in a semi-darkened room. In Homer's syndrome the pupil dilates very poorly compared with the normal side.

2. Eye movements

The eye movements are tested by asking the patient to follow the exam-iner's finger laterally, superiorly, and inferiorly on each side.

The subject should report diplopia, and the examiner should watch for the appearance of a squint in the neutral position, or at the extremes of motion. The more peripheral of the two images emanates from the affected eye. This can be discerned by covering each eye in turn, at the position of maximal diplopia. The third (oculomotor) nerve is tested by adduction, elevation and depression of the eye. The fourth (trochlear) nerve is tested by depression and adduction of the eye. The sixth (abducens) nerve is tested by the horizontal abduction of the eye (Figure 2.8, below). The diagnosis is therefore a left third nerve (oculomotor) palsy and a left seventh nerve (facial) palsy.

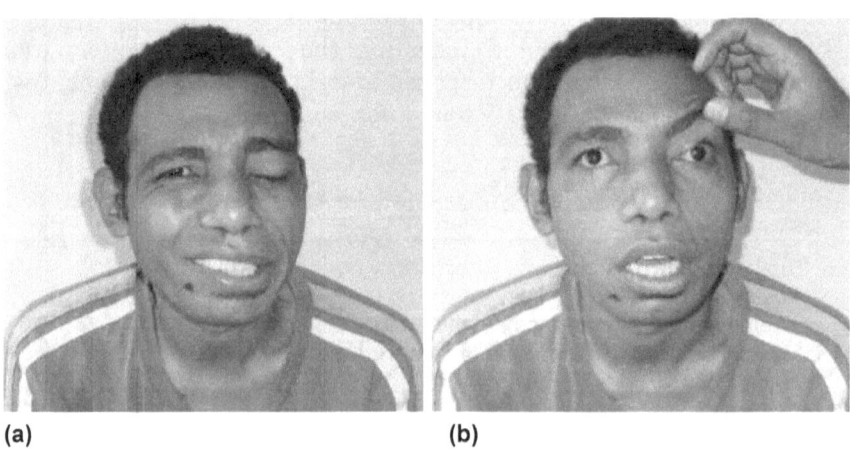

(a) (b)

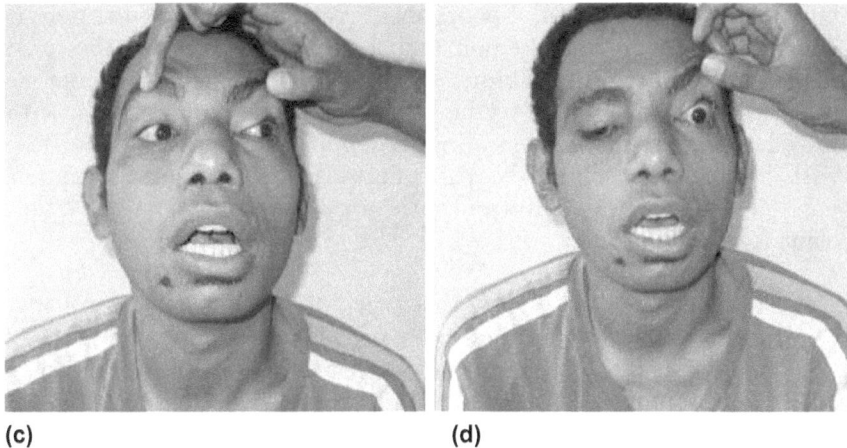

(c)   (d)

Figure 2.8 (a-d) Cranial nerve palsy for diagnosis.
Legend
(a) A young male with a complete left ptosis and drooping left side of mouth which has resulted from a head injury.
(b) He has been asked to look upwards with the left upper eyelid held open. He has a dilated nonreactive left pupil (not seen on the photograph), and the left eye cannot look upwards or inwards.
(c) He has been asked to look to the left which he is able to do due to an intact sixth cranial nerve (abducens).
(d) He has been asked to look downwards which he is unable to do on the left side.

Practice point: the cover-uncover test

The cover-uncover test may identify a latent or subtle squint, and is performed by covering each eye in turn, with the patient's eyes fixed on a target. The uncovered eye is observed for an adjusting movement which realigns the visual axis. When the cover is removed, the eye that was underneath will rotate to reacquire the target.

3. The optic fundus

The shape, colour and edge of the optic disc and appearance of the normal optic cup should be assessed. The retinal blood vessels should be assessed. It is often possible to see venous pulsation which is lost in papilloedema. Spontaneous retinal artery pulsation is abnormal. The macular region and its central fovea are the most important area of the fundus for vision. The macula is not so important for the doctor trying to assess acutely ill patients with raised intracranial pressure. Induced pupil dilation may interfere with clinical assessment of the pupils. Haemorrhages, exudates, papilloedema, optic neuritis and optic atrophy are the most important signs for the generalist.

- **Papilloedema:** swelling of the optic nerve head, most commonly due to raised intracranial pressure. There is no disturbance of visual function except in advanced cases. On examination you will see redness of the disc, blurring of its edges, starting first in the upper nasal quadrant. The optic cup flattens, the retinal veins are slighted distended and venous pulsation is lost. Haemorrhages and exudates on or around the disc may develop if the onset of raised intracranial pressure is rapid. It may be fol-lowed by optic atrophy.

- **Optic neuritis:** inflammatory, demyelinating or vascular diseases usually cause loss of vision with some hyperaemia and swelling of the optic disc. There may be pain on eye movements. It may be followed by optic atrophy.

- **Optic atrophy:** the disc is paler than normal. This may be due to optic neuritis, pressure on the nerve at any site, trauma or toxins. The margin of the disc is well defined.

Practice point

To differentiate early papilloedema from optic neuritis remember papilloedema affects vision minimally whereas optic neuritis causes visual loss.

4. Vision

The patient may complain of diplopia or blurred vision. Finger counting and reading for literate patients form a gross assessment of visual acuity which may be all that is necessary in the traumatised patient. You will have to specifically ask the patient if he has diplopia in some directions and not others if there is an abnormality of eye movements (ophthalmo-plegia).

If you are trying to localise an intracranial lesion then you will need to test the visual fields. This can be done by the patient staring at you and testing the patient using yourself as the normal standard and moving a pen or finger in from the periphery. Visual field mapping is beyond the scope of this chapter but should be plotted when there is a suspected pituitary fossa lesion or deteriorating vision. The visual pathway and the effect of lesions at various points are shown in Figure 2.9, below. Acute visual loss is discussed in Chapter 9 on page 460.

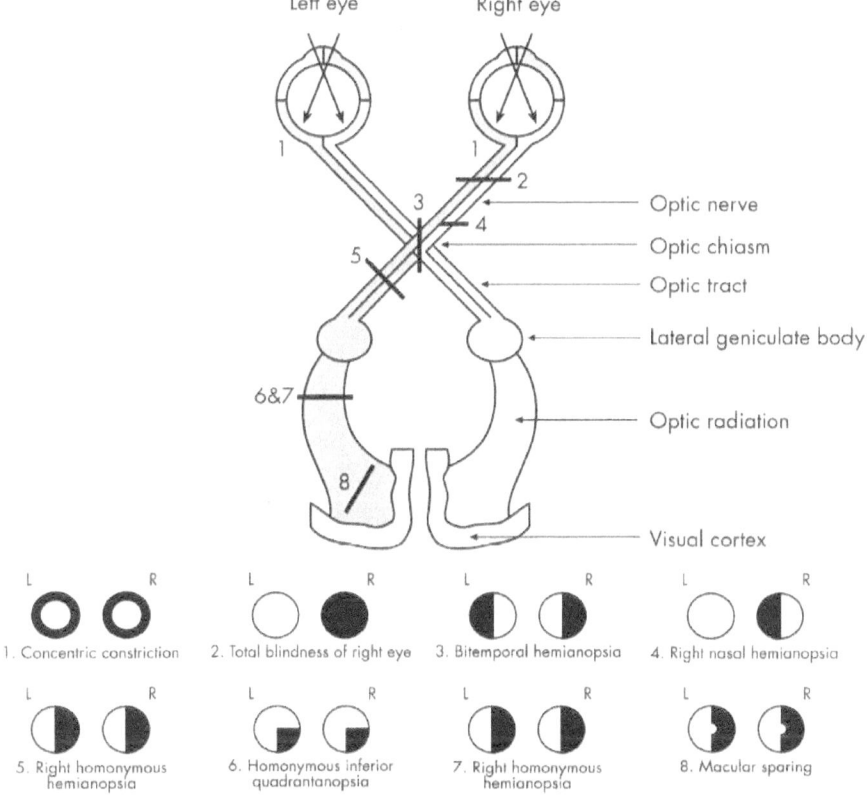

Figure 2.9 The visual pathway showing the sites of lesions and the resultant field defects.

The trigeminal nerve

The facial sensation is tested in the distribution of the three divisions: forehead for the first division, infraorbital cheek region for the second division, and mandible for the third division. The corneal reflex is tested by twisting cotton wool to a point, asking the patient to look away from the examiner and touching the lateral side of the cornea, away from the line of vision.

A blink results if the reflex arc is intact. The muscles of mastication are supplied by the motor branch of the trigeminal nerve and can be compared on each side when the mandible is opened against resistance or the teeth are clenched. The temporalis muscle and masseter are palpated to assess for wasting and strength.

Facial nerve

An upper motor neuron lesion will produce paralysis of the lower part of the face but because of bilateral innervation of the upper part of the face, occipitofrontalis muscle (action: wrinkling the forehead) will remain intact. A lower motor neuron lesion causes paralysis of the entire side of the face on the ipsilateral side. Facial palsy is described in more detail in Chapter 9, page 468.

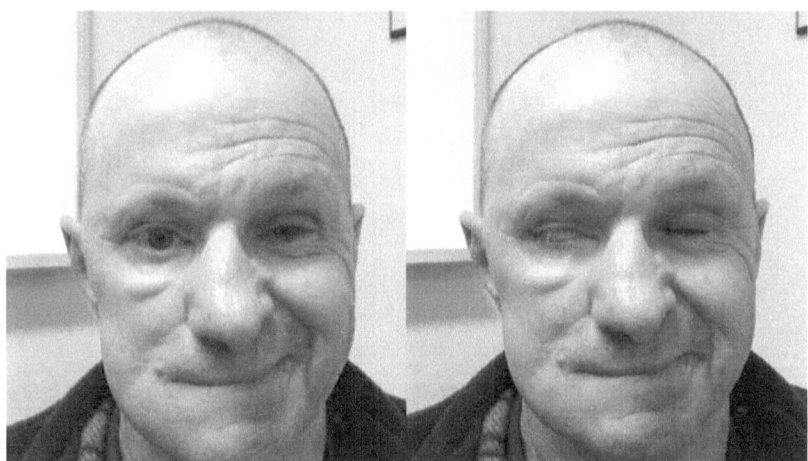

Figure 2.10 Patient has been asked to smile but has a right-sided lower motor neuron facial palsy. The right facial muscles including frontalis do not contract due to lower motor neuron facial nerve palsy (caused by an acoustic neuroma). On the right he is being asked to close his eyes and is unable to close his right eye completely due to the right lower motor neuron facial palsy. His right eye exhibits a normal Bell's phenomenon with the eye rotating upwards to reveal the sclera.

Hearing

Hearing is tested at the bedside by pushing repeatedly on the tragus of each ear in turn to block hearing, and whispering words or numbers in the other ear at varying distances, to determine if the subject can identify them.

Glossopharyngeal and vagus nerves

These are tested by asking the patient to say 'Aah' and the palate and uvula will normally move up in the midline but deviate away from the affected side when there is a lesion. The gag reflex will be depressed or absent if either nerve is affected.

Accessory nerve

The head is turned against resistance, to each side, and the power of sterno-cleidomastoid muscle noted, on the opposite side to the direction of turning. Elevation of the shoulders tests the upper trapezius muscle.

Hypoglossal nerve

A lesion of the hypoglossal nerve will cause wasting on that side of the tongue, and deviation of the tongue to the side of the lesion, when the tongue is protruded.

Examination of the peripheral nerves, cerebral and cerebellar function

This examination is best carried out in the same order each time so that important aspects are not omitted:

- inspection
- power
- sensation
- co-ordination and balance
- special tests: parietal lobe function
- tone
- reflexes
- autonomic function
- gait (see Chapter 9, page 437)

For peripheral nerves learn a key test for the ulnar, median, radial, femoral, obturator and sciatic nerves. Test the most peripheral motor and sensory functions. If they are working the nerve is likely to be intact. Look for muscle wasting in the affected muscles (see Table 2.5, below). Peripheral nerve lesions are discussed in Chapter 10, page 473.

Table 2.5 Quick test for testing the most peripheral function of peripheral nerves.

Nerve	Motor function	Sensory function
Ulnar	Hypothenar muscles	Ulnar side of palm and dorsum of the hand
	First dorsal interosseous and all interossei	
	Flexion distal interphalangeal joint 5th finger	
Median	Thenar muscles Flexion, abduction thumb	Radial side of palm
Radial	Extension of the wrist, fingers and thumb	Radial side of dorsum of hand
Femoral	Quadriceps femoris Extend the knee	Front of thigh Inner aspect of leg
Sciatic Common peroneal		
deep	Dorsiflexion of foot Palsy = foot drop	First web space
superficial	Eversion of foot	Dorsum of foot, front, lateral side of leg
Sural		Lateral side of foot
Posterior tibial	Muscles of calf and sole	Sole of foot

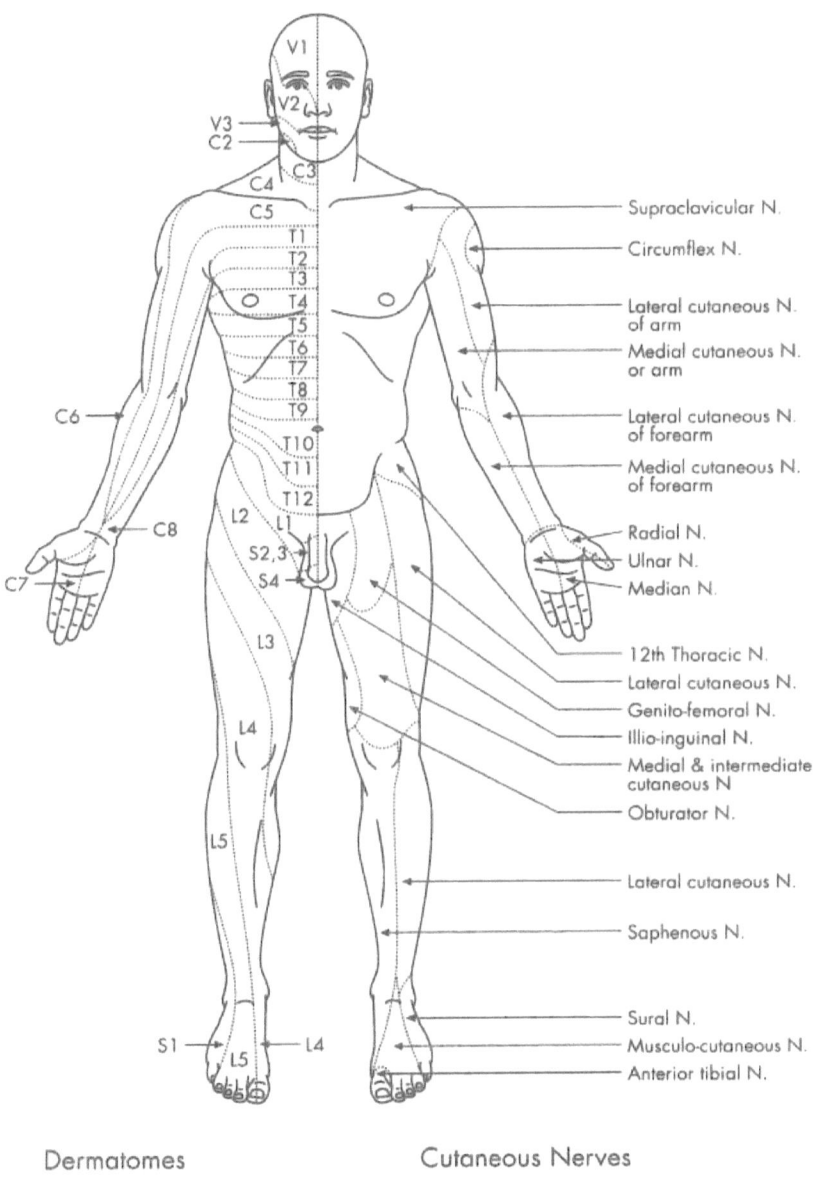

Supraclavicular N.

Circumflex N.

Lateral cutaneous N.
of arm

Medial cutaneous N.
or arm

Lateral cutaneous N.
of forearm

Medial cutaneous N.
of forearm

Radial N.

Ulnar N.

Median N.

12th Thoracic N.

Lateral cutaneous N.

Genito-femoral N.

Illio-inguinal N.

Medial & intermediate
cutaneous N

Obturator N.

Lateral cutaneous N.

Saphenous N.

Sural N.

Musculo-cutaneous N.

Anterior tibial N.

Dermatomes   Cutaneous Nerves

(a)

Figure 2.11 Dermatomes.

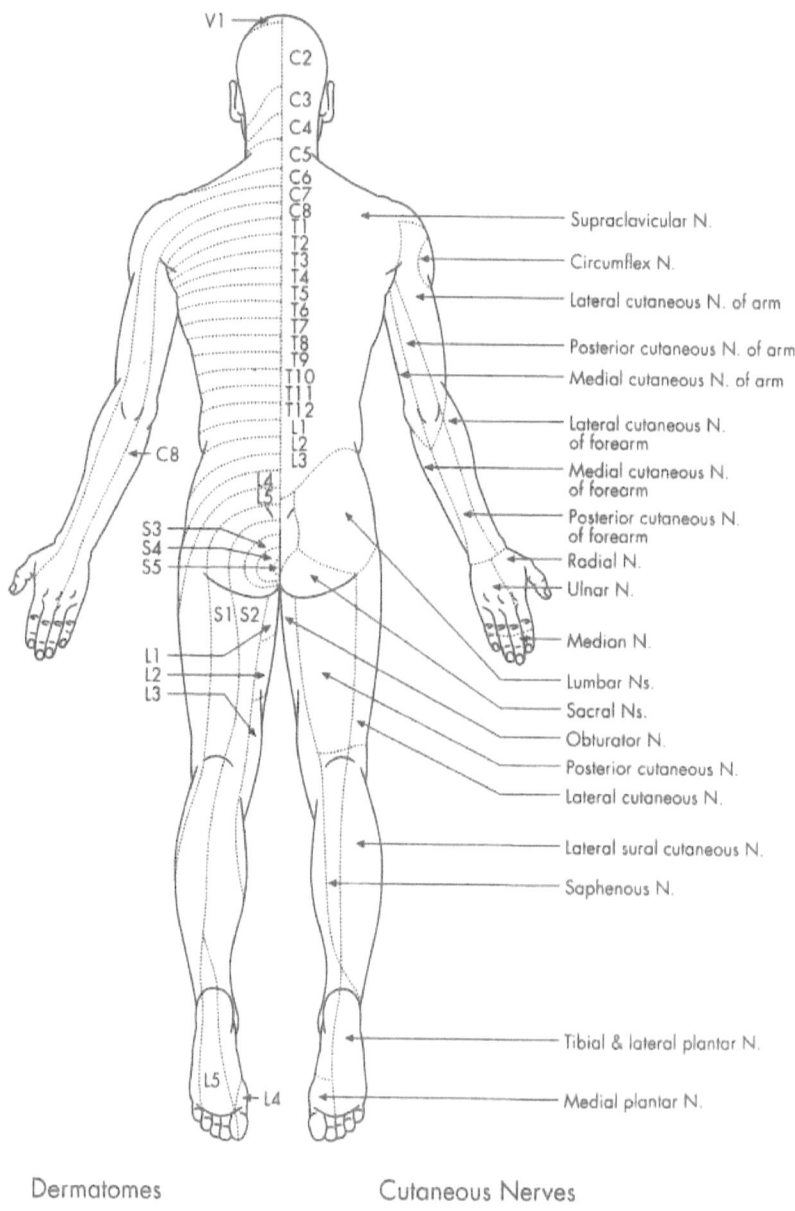

Dermatomes   Cutaneous Nerves

(b)

Figure 2.11 (a-b) The dermatome map, peripheral nerve map, and distribution of the cutaneous component of the trigeminal nerve.

To examine the peripheral nervous system, you need to know or refer to the following:
- dermatome map (Figure 2.11, page 30),
- myotome map (Table 2. 7, page 34) and reflexes (Table 2.8, page 36),
- nerve function (Table 2.5, page 29),
- nerve pathway: refer to an anatomy book.

Motor function

Grade muscle power 0-5 (see Table 2.6, below). Test the power at all major joints in the upper and lower limbs. You will need to test power in the affected limb and compare this with the other side and the other limbs. Do not forget to look for proximal lesions (weakness of the hips or the shoulders) as well as testing power in the most peripheral myotomes (movements of the fingers and toes). When a patient complains of loss of function, you must differentiate between a central and peripheral nerve lesion and an upper/lower motor neuron lesion (Table 2.9, page 36). The upper motor neuron lesion may be delayed in developing the full-blown picture. Thus, in spinal cord injury there is a period of spinal shock where there is flaccidity, paralysis and areflexia (the appearance of a lower motor neuron type lesion) and it may take several days or weeks for the spasticity to develop fully. In lower motor neuron lesions, it may take some time for muscle wasting to be obvious. The Babinski sign is negative, i.e. the great toe goes down or does not react at all.

Table 2.6 Grading of muscle power.

Grade	Finding
0	No movement at all
1	Flicker of movement
2	Movement but cannot oppose gravity
3	Can oppose gravity
4	Less than full power
5	Full power

Sensory function

Refer to anatomy of the pain pathway (see Figure 2.11, page 30 and Chapter 10, page 485).

- **Pain and temperature:** (pin-prick and a cold metal object for spinothalamic tract function)
- **Dorsal column function:** light touch (cotton wool or paper), vibration and joint position sense. Sparing of sensation to light touch can be a sign of an incomplete cord lesion because light touch sensation is carried in the spinal cord in both the lateral and posterior columns.
- **Sacral sparing:** may occur within a widespread area of sensory loss caused by an intramedullary (internal spinal cord) lesion, and is due to the laminar arrangement of the fibres in the spinothalamic tract. The sacral segments are lateral in the tract. It thus means there is an incomplete spinal cord problem and may be the only sign of this.

Coordination and balance

Examine proprioception, by finger to nose, heel to toe testing, Romberg's sign (standing upright, feet together, arms outstretched and eyes closed the patient rocks and sways because of loss of postural sensation (dorsal column function)).

Autonomic function

- Sweating,
- vasoconstriction (not very helpful),
- pupil constriction (parasympathetic),
  pupil dilatation (sympathetic),
- skin temperature, colour, sensitivity (see sympathetically maintained pain section in Chapter 10, page 474).

The spinal cord in the adult ends around Ll-2 in the adult. Then the nerve roots of the cauda equina can exit the lower end of the spinal cord at the conus medullaris, which lies at the Ll- 2 level and below this level are the roots of the cauda equina (see Figure 2.12, page 38). Lesions at the level of the conus cause a mixture of upper and lower motor neuron signs whereas lesions below the level of the conus are purely lower motor neuron. Cauda equina lesions cause lower motor neuron lesions. Bladder and bowel function may be disturbed with lesions affecting the cauda equina because of sacral nerve root involvement and also lesions affecting the spinal cord including the conus.

Anal reflex: (S4,5): contraction of the subcutaneous portion of the external sphincter in response to scratching the perianal skin.

Cremasteric reflex: (L1): a light scratch along the inner aspect of the upper thigh causes contraction of the cremaster and elevation of the testis. If this reflex is intact it indicates that the lesion is below the level of L1.

Bulbocavernosus reflex: (S2,3,4): contraction of the bulbocavernosus muscle (identified by palpation) on squeezing the glans.

1. Micturition

There are three main functions of the bladder: filling, voiding and control. The pelvic parasympathetic nerves are responsible for smooth muscle contraction. Smooth muscle fibres in the external sphincter enable continence to be maintained when asleep through parasympathetic control.

The pudendal nerves (also S2,3,4) are responsible for voluntary continence by innervating the external sphincter and the pelvic floor musculature. The bladder is a low-pressure storage organ with the smooth detrusor muscle relaxing to enable the bladder to fill. The bladder neck (internal sphincter) remains closed while the bladder is filling. The internal sphincter is better termed the bladder neck mechanism and consists of trigonal and detrusor muscle bundles.

Once a stretch reflex is stimulated by increasing bladder volume afferent impulses pass to spinal cord (S2,3,4) and parasympathetic impulses (pelvic nerves from S2,3,4) cause detrusor contraction, opening of the bladder neck mechanism and micturition. Cortical control prevents relaxation of the external sphincter and inhibits parasympathetic motor activity.

Table 2.7 Myotomes.

Joint and movement	Nerve root	Main muscles involved
Upper limb		
Shoulder		
Abduction	C5	Deltoid, supraspinatus
Adduction	C6,7	Pectoralis major

34

Table 2.7 *(Continued)*

Joint and movement	Nerve root	Main muscles involved
Elbow		
Flexion	CS,6	Biceps
Extension	C7,8	Triceps
Wrist and forearm		
Palmar flexion	C6,7	Flexors
Dorsiflexion	C6,7	Extensors
Pronation	C6	Pronator teres, quadratus
Supination	C6	Supinator
Fingers		
Flexion	C7,8	Flexor digitorum and pollicis
Extension	C7,8	Extensor digitorum and pollicis
Abduction	T1	Interossei
Adduction	T1	Interossei
Lower limb		
Hip		
Flexion	L2,3	Iliopsoas
Extension	L4,5	Gluteus maximus, hamstrings
Knee		
Extension	L3,4	Quadriceps
Flexion	LS,S1	Hamstrings
Ankle, foot and toes		
Inversion	L4	Tibialis anterior
Eversion	LS,S1	Peronei
Dorsiflexion	L4,5	Tibialis anterior and long extensors
Plantarflexion	S1,2	Calf muscles, soleus, gastrocnemius

Table 2.8 Tendon reflexes and their spinal level.

Biceps	CS-6
Supinator (brachioradialis)	C6
Triceps	C7-8
Abdominal - upper	T7-8
Abdominal - lower	T9-12
Cremasteric	L1
Knee (quadriceps)	L3-4
Ankle (soleus/gastrocnemius)	S1

Table 2.9 Differentiation of upper and lower motor neuron lesions.

Upper motor neuron	Lower motor neuron
Hyper-reflexia	Areflexia
Increased tone	Hypotonic
Clonus	Marked wasting
Spastic paralysis	Flaccid paralysis
Wasting (late sign)	
Babinski increase	Babinski down or no react ion

- **Neurogenic bladder**

The term neurogenic bladder is used to describe bladder function in a patient with a spinal cord lesion. Many confusing terms have been used to describe the problems such as automatic, autonomous, uninhibited, upper motor neuron and lower motor neuron. One classification, which is relatively simple and practical, is to divide neurogenic bladder into sacral and suprasacral problems.

- **Sacral injury**

If the sacral segments of the spinal cord are damaged then the patient will only be able to empty his bladder by abdominal and/or manual pressure. A useful sensation of bladder fullness may still be received by sympathetic pathways, which reach the cord as high as the mid-thoracic level.

- **Suprasacral injury**

After spinal injury a state of 'spinal shock' occurs in which there is either recovery or the development of bladder function through the spinal reflex at the intact S2,3,4. Manual pressure will not be able to overcome the contraction and spasticity of the pelvic floor and external sphincter. However, the spinal reflex may be initiated by scratching the perineum or anal area and the bladder may empty.

If this is done every 2-3 hours the patient may be able to have some control of bladder emptying. He will need to be able to use his hands to achieve this for himself. Bladder emptying is often incomplete and the residual volume maybe high. A residual volume of up to 50 ml is normal, 100 ml may be acceptable.

A high residual volume predisposes to urinary tract infection and stone formation. Intermittent catheterisation performed by the patient or his relatives will minimise these problems. The catheter can be reused and does not need to be sterile, only cleaned with soap and ordinary tap water.

Practice point

The renal tract should always be screened for infection and stones in patients in patients with spinal cord paralysis. Check urine cultures and perform an ultrasound.

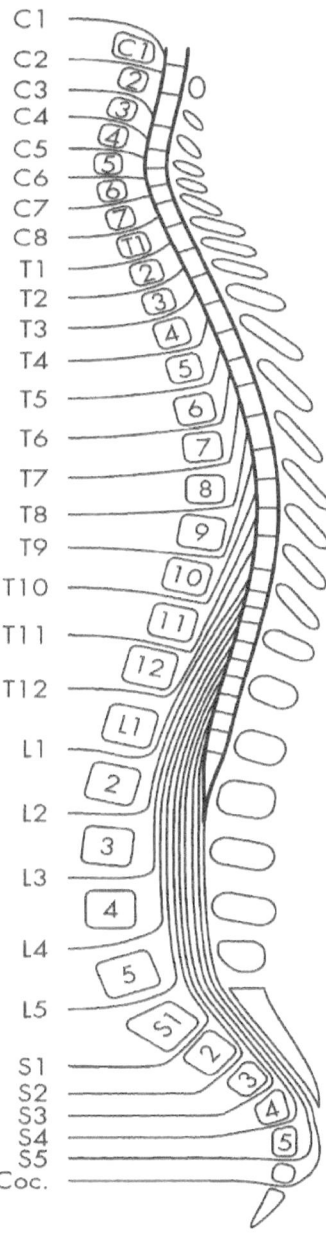

Figure 2.12 The spinal cord and spinal nerves in relation to the vertebral column. Note the termination of the spinal cord at L1-2, and the relation of the numbered cervical and lumbar nerve roots to their respective numbered vertebra immediately above.

2. Bowel function

Anal sphincter function depends largely on pelvic parasympathetics and internal pudendal Nerve (somatic). In the acute phase of spinal shock, the anal sphincter is slack and the patient cannot tighten the sphincter around the examining finger. It may also not be possible to relax the internal sphincter in response to rectal distension (rectoanal reflex). Failure to relax the internal sphincter may cause constipation and overflow diarrhoea. Failure to control the external sphincter voluntarily will result in spontaneous defecation once the rectoanal reflex is triggered. In an upper motor neuron lesion (e.g. cervical cord transection) the bladder and bowel will fail to empty. Therefore, early catheterisation is needed in spinal injury. However, the reflex for bladder and bowel emptying is a spinal reflex. If the pathway is intact all that is lost is higher cortical control. Enemas and suppositories may be needed to encourage rectal emptying initially but once the rectoanal reflex is restored the bowels should open spontaneously without voluntary control.

Practice point

RECTAL EXAMINATION must be performed in all patients with a potential lesion to the spinal cord. Anal tone and external sphincter function should be assessed. Perianal sensation can be tested at the same time.

Cerebellar function

Testing of coordination with finger-nose testing, or heel-shin movements is a good way of testing cerebellar hemisphere function. Rapid alternating hand movements and rapid pronation and supination of each forearm is also helpful. Testing of central cerebellar (vermis) function involves testing gait, with heel-toe walking. It is important to also observe gait at some point in the neurological examination (see section on gait disturbance in Chapter 9, page 437).

Parietal lobe function

Assessing the parietal lobe may help localise a cerebral lesion, but the assessment can be complicated. The simple tests are to determine:

1. **Astereognosis:** a patient can recognise an object placed in each hand while the eyes are closed.
2. **Parietal drift:** drift of the arms occurs when they are place outstretched with the palms uppermost while the eyes are closed. If one arm drifts away, usually upwards and outwards, this indicates a contralateral parietal lesion.
3. **Sensory or visual neglect:** when a sensory stimulus is placed on each side separately, it is registered by the patient, but when bilateral stimuli are placed simultaneously either in the visual field or on the skin of the arms or legs, the patient will only register one side; and this indicates a parietal lesion, contralateral to the side of extinction of the stimulus.

Higher functions and mental state

- Orientation in space and time
- Ability to carry out commands and functions
- Intellect
- Memory, short- and long-term
- Language function - naming of objects, repetition of words, content of speech and reading, writing or copying, if relevant.

Table 2.10 Karnofsky scale.

Score	Clinical status
100	Normal; no complaints, no evidence of disease
90	Able to carry on normal activity; minor symptoms
80	Normal activity with effort; some symptoms
70	Cares for self; unable to carry on normal activity
60	Requires occasional assistance; cares for most needs
50	Requires occasional assistance; cares for most needs
40	Disabled; requires special care and assistance
30	Severely disabled; hospitalised; death not imminent
20	Very sick; active supportive care needed
10	Moribund; fatal processes are progressing rapidly

Personality and mood

- Has there been a change?
- Detailed assessment is for the psychiatrist or clinical psychologist.
- Link the higher functions to a region of the cerebral hemisphere (see section: 'Localising symptoms and signs' on the next page and Figure 2.13 on page 43).

Social abilities and performance

- Ability to feed, dress, bath and go to the toilet
- Ability to be left alone, look after others, go out and about

The Karnofsky scale is a quantitative and accepted method of scoring social abilities (Table 2.10, page 40).

The localisation of intracranial and spinal lesions

General symptoms

1. Raised intracranial pressure

Headache, blurred vision, vomiting, diplopia due to false localising sixth nerve palsy. The headache is usually worse in the mornings, and continuous. The vomiting is often projectile without any preceding nausea. The blurred vision may be associated with papilloedema.

Case report

A 28-year-old male presented with a one-week history of severe headache, worse in the morning and projectile vomiting. There were no focal neurological signs. Examination of his fundi showed papilloedema. **Lesson:** *A skull X-ray showed no abnormality. CT scan showed a large tumour in his frontal lobe.*

---

2. Epilepsy

Epilepsy may be caused by a cerebral lesion. The focal lesion in the cerebral hemisphere may cause focal epilepsy to develop on the contralateral side, which may be secondarily generalised.

Case report

An 8-year-old child presented with fits and was noted to have left-side weakness. Fundoscopic examination showed papilloedema. Although the child had previously had headaches and vomiting these were thought to be due to malaria or some viral infection by the primary care doctor.

Lesson: It was only the onset of epilepsy that prompted a CT scan to be ordered. A space occupying lesion suggestive of tumour or tuberculoma found in the right frontal lobe.

Localising symptoms and signs (Figure 2.13, next page)

1. **Frontal lobe.** This is a relatively silent area of the brain and lesions usually must reach quite a large size before causing any symptoms. Large lesions in the frontal lobe, particularly if they affect both sides, may affect memory, personality, and conscious state and/or speech. Bilateral frontal lesions may produce a mute state, lack of interest in surroundings, lack of drive and initiative, a passive immobile state, or sometimes disinhibition with hypersexuality and/or aggression with lack of control over social graces; and a lack of care with appearance. Incontinence of urine and/or faeces may result from frontal lobe pathology.

2. Deterioration in higher mental function may result from frontal lobe lesions. Sub-frontal lesions may impinge on the olfactory tract and cause loss of the sense of smell either unilaterally or bilaterally. Anosmia is also not uncommon following severe head injury. These changes may be subtle and slow in developing, and therefore difficult for acquaintances of the patient to recognise them until they are quite obvious.

3. **Temporal lobe.** Lesions in the temporal lobe may be silent but if they involve the medial part of the temporal lobe, i.e. hippocampus and amygdala the lesion may result in memory disturbance and temporal lobe epilepsy (complex partial seizures), which may become secondarily generalised.

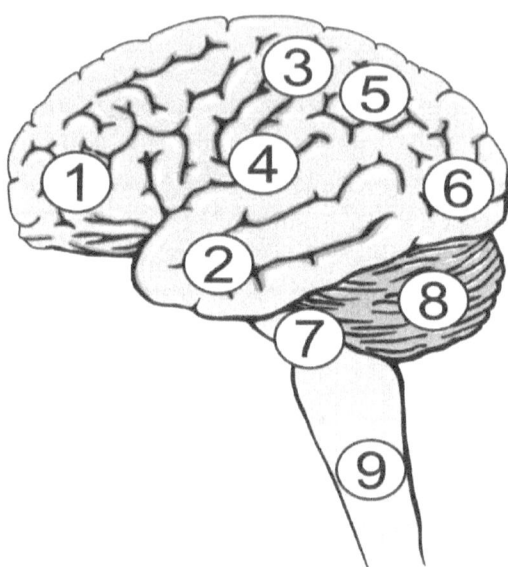

Figure 2.13 The localisation of brain function. The brain from the side with functions assigned to the different areas.

4. **Upper sensorimotor area.** A lesion in this area may cause lower limb weakness on the contralateral side, or bilateral lower limb weakness if it affects both sides of the brain, which is uncommon, but sometimes occurs with a parasagittal meningioma in this region. Sensory deficit may appear on the opposite side.

5. **Lower sensorimotor cortex.** This tends to cause contralateral weakness in the face, tongue and arm; thus, leading to slurred speech and arm weakness and clumsiness of the fingers. If the lesion extends into the adjacent speech areas, the patient may have difficulty with expressive or receptive speech if the lesion is on the dominant side of the brain, which is usually the left side. Sensory deficit may appear on the opposite side.

6. **Parietal lobe.** Lesions in the parietal lobe produce lack of coordination, lack of appreciation of where the contralateral limbs are in three dimensional space, lack of orientation in space, e.g. getting lost within a familiar environment, sensory disturbance with lack of appreciation of what is being held in the hand (astereognosis), sensory neglect on the opposite side, sometimes eye movement disorder, with difficulty following objects, receptive dysphasia with more inferior parietal lesions, and cognitive difficulties.

7. **Occipital lobe.** This is a relatively silent area, but medial occipital lesions will cause homonymous visual field defects.

8. **Brain stem.** Lesions in the brain stem may produce a multitude of cranial nerve deficits, pyramidal weakness in one or both sides, incoordination due to disruption of cerebellar pathways, and sensory deficit on one or both sides.

9. **Cerebellum.** Lesions in the vermis of the cerebellum tend to cause truncal ataxia whereas lesions in the cerebellar hemispheres tend to cause upper or lower limb ataxia. Head tilt may develop in children with cerebellar tonsillar herniation and nystagmus may develop when the eye movement pathways are disturbed.

10. **Spinal cord.** Depending on the level, if the lesion is slowly progressive upper motor neuron weakness develops below the level, sometimes lower motor neuron weakness at the level, and variable sensory loss below the level with a truncal dermatomal sensory level at the level of the lesion. Radicular pain may be associated with the lesion, if it involves the nerve roots at this level, e.g. nerve roots to the arm will produce arm pain, nerve roots to the intercostal region will produce chest wall pain, etc. Sphincter disturbance may also result from spinal cord intrinsic or compressive lesions.

11. **Suprasellar region.** Tumours of the pituitary region or adjacent structures will produce problems with the endocrine system (anterior pituitary: acromegaly, prolactinoma with galactorrhea, amenorrhoea or impotence; Cushing's disease with adreno‐corticotrophic hormone secretion; hypopituitarism; or posterior pituitary dysfunction with diabetes insipidus), optic chiasm or optic nerve compression leading to visual field loss, blurred vision and sometimes nystagmus. If the tumour is very large, it will involve the third ventricle and cause bilateral hydrocephalus.

12. **Pineal region.** Mass lesions in this region will cause obstructive hydrocephalus by blocking the aqueduct, eye movement disorder with diplopia, failure of upgaze, and sometimes endocrine disturbance or precocious puberty.

Summary

This section will have reminded you that neurosurgical examination is not complicated and that a reasonable assessment of the patient's problems can be made clinically. Most patients in tropical countries suffer because they are not properly examined not because they cannot have a CT scan. The tools needed to make a comprehensive clinical assessment are simple and inexpensive.

Practice point

You do not need to be a neurologist to work out the possible sites of a lesion clinically. Most lesions can be located by clinical examination.

INVESTIGATIONS

The investigation of central nervous system (CNS) disorders is greatly restricted in many LMICs so that careful clinical assessment becomes even more critical. Periods of observation or blind treatment trials must be more often followed because the actual pathology cannot be easily visualised owing to the unavailability of CT or MR scans. Although these imaging techniques have revolutionised the practice of neurosurgery, it is still possible to handle many clinical problems without them, even though this would be unthinkable in the HIC. High-quality myelography or angiography are also unlikely to be available. The surgeon may be able to perform these studies himself or herself because the information obtained may help decide whether an operation is necessary and gives a better idea of the nature and anatomical position of the pathology. The surgeon working in a technologically-poor environment must place his or her mindset back to the pre-CT era. Histopathology will often be unavailable and a good knowledge of gross pathology and the pattern of disease is needed to plan surgery and postoperative management.

The important investigations which will be necessary for management of CNS problems and which will usually be available are:

Microbiology

1. Lumbar puncture and CSF analysis (Table 7.2, page 366));
   - Indian ink stain for cryptococcus,
   - Gram stain, Ziehl-Neelsen stain for acid-fast organisms such as *Mycobacterium tuberculosis*,
   - culture facility,
   - cell counts,
   - protein estimation.
2. Pus/wound swab for culture - agar plates/incubator.

Serology

Serological assays on blood or CSF can be stored for later analysis if they cannot be carried out on-site. This may at least offer the possibility of a late diagnosis, particularly if a trial of treatment is unsuccessful or there is a potential public health issue.

Haematology

Full blood examination including:
- platelet count,
- clotting studies,
- slide for malaria, trypanosomes.

Biochemistry

- Serum sodium, potassium, renal function,
- blood gases - PaO2, PaCO2, pH,
- hormone studies for functioning pituitary tumours (often sent away to reference laboratories).

Radiology

Plain X-rays of skull (see Figure 2.14, next page)

- Anteroposterior (A-P),
- lateral,
- tangential for depressed fracture,
- brow-up lateral for intracranial air,
  (the patient is supine and the forehead is filmed uppermost and a shoot- through lateral is obtained),
- Towne's view - for base of skull and occipital fractures.

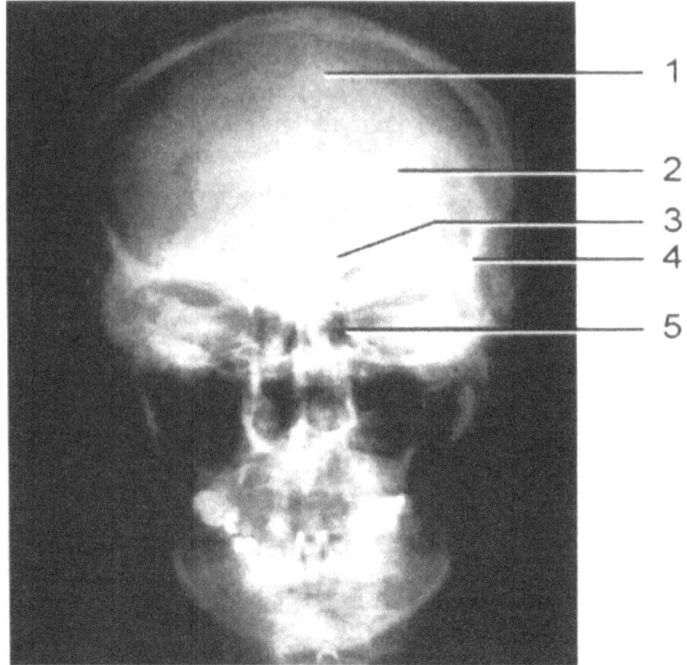

Figure 2.14 (a) A-P view.

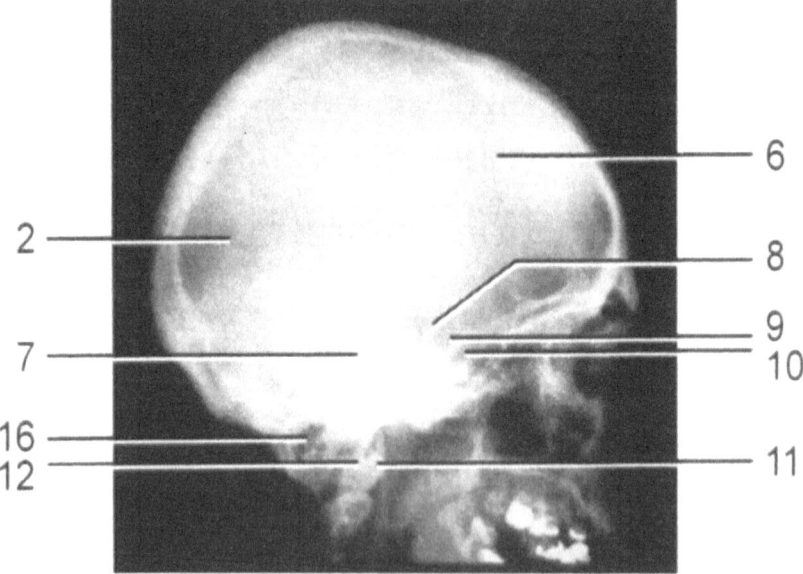

(b) Lateral view.

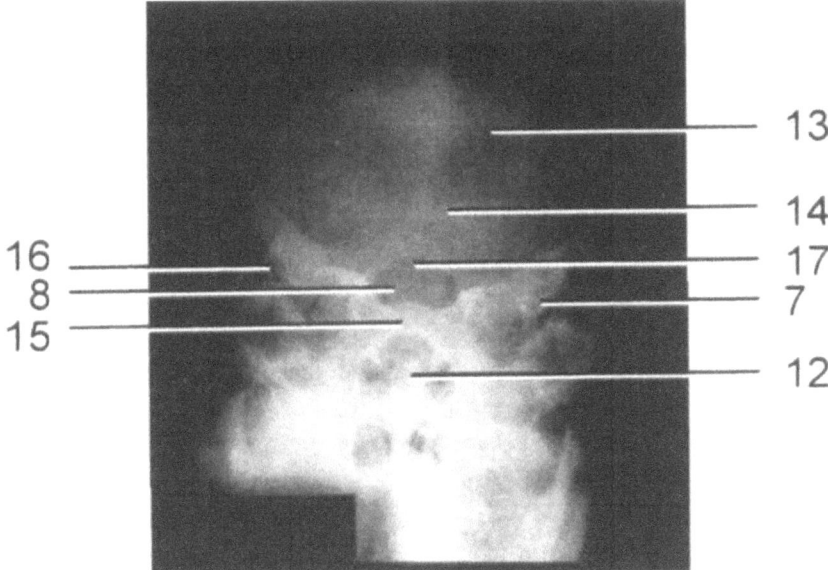

(c) Towne's view.

Figure 2.14 (a-c) The Skull X-ray.
Legend
1. Sagittal suture
2. Lambdoid suture
3. Frontal sinus
4. Lesser sphenoid wing
5. Ethmoid sinus
   (landmark of transverse sinus)
6. Coronal suture
7. Petrous temporal bone
8. Posterior clinoid process & dorsum sellae
9. Pituitary fossa
10. Sphenoid sinus
11. Anterior arch of atlas
12. Odontoid process
13. Superior nuchal line
14. Inferior nuchal line
15. Posterior arch of atlas
16. Mastoid air cells
17. Foramen magnum

Plain skull X-rays should be examined for the following features:

1. **Skull vault:**
   - Differentiate between suture lines, blood vessels and linear fractures,
   - bony erosive or lytic lesions of the skull,
   - chronic osteomyelitis, calcified tumours of the meninges such as menmgioma.

2. **Skull base:**
   - Examine the pituitary fossa for enlargement or erosion of the sell.

3. **Brain:**
   - Calcified lesions such as cysticercosis, foreign body, tumours, vascular malformations,
   - displacement of the midline calcified pineal,
   - free air bubble in the head following trauma (aerocele).

4. **Sinuses:**
   - Chronic infection, obstruction, enlargement, erosion of wall, fluid levels.

5. **Teeth and jaws:**
   - Tumours/infection/fractures.

6. **Orbits:**
   - Enlargement of superior or inferior fissure or optic foramen due to tumour,
   - tumour expansion,
   - fractures,
   - spinal X-rays,
   - these are discussed from Chapter 4, from page 163.

Ultrasound (see Figure 2.15, next page)

In many developing world hospitals ultrasound is available. It can be used providing the fontanelle is not closed. The probe can be placed on the anterior fontanelle to define ventricular size in babies, to obtain the size and position of a space-occupying lesion and to detect blood in the ventricles. The ultrasound probe can be used on the brain surface at craniotomy to help the surgeon locate a lesion below the surface inpatients of all ages.

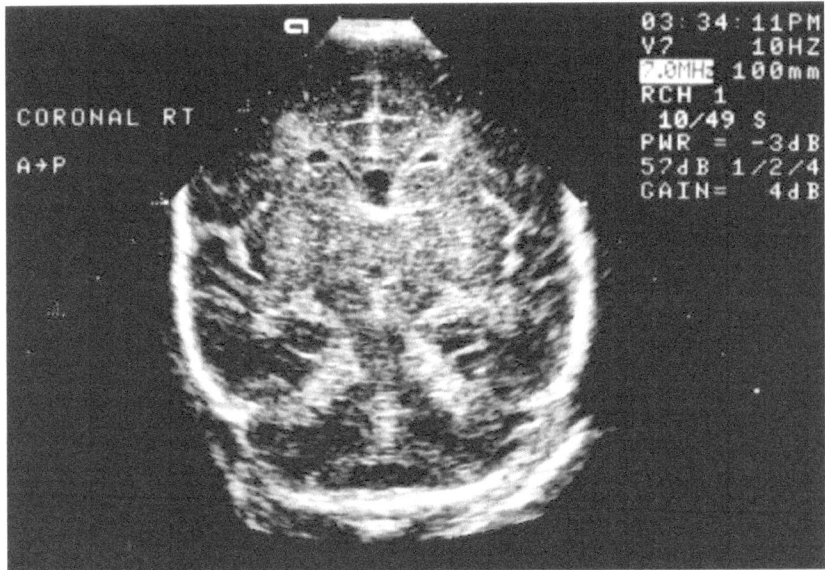

Figure 2.15 (a) Normal cranial ultrasound. Coronal projection showing small lateral and third ventricle at the top of the picture. Note the interhemispheric fissure at the centre of the top, the sylvian fissures laterally and the brainstem and cerebellum interiorly.

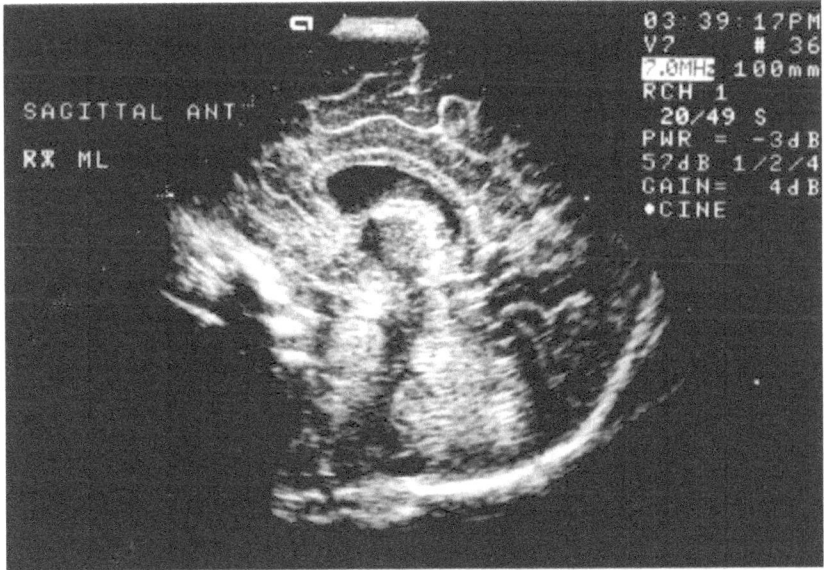

(b) Normal sagittal image. Note the lateral ventricle and the cerebral fissures above and behind the ventricle.

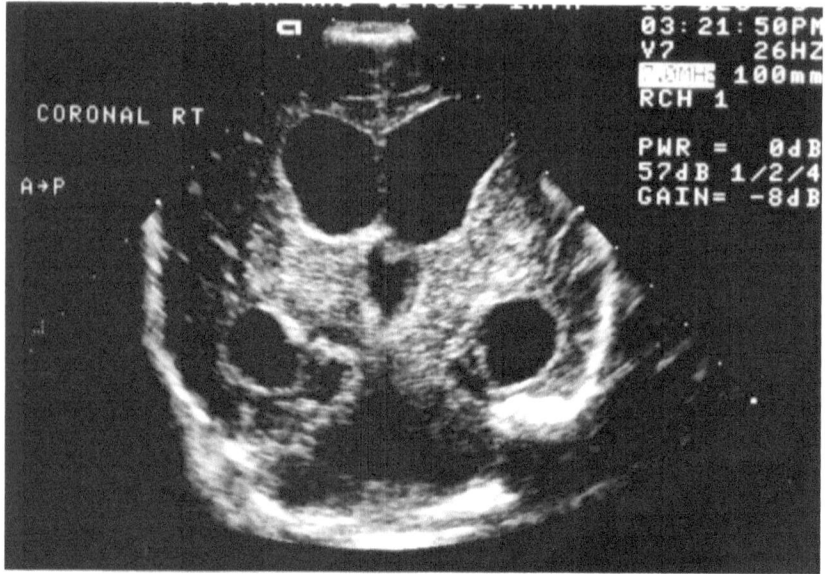

(c) i Ultrasound showing hydrocephalus: Coronal image showing dilated frontal and temporal horns and third ventricle.

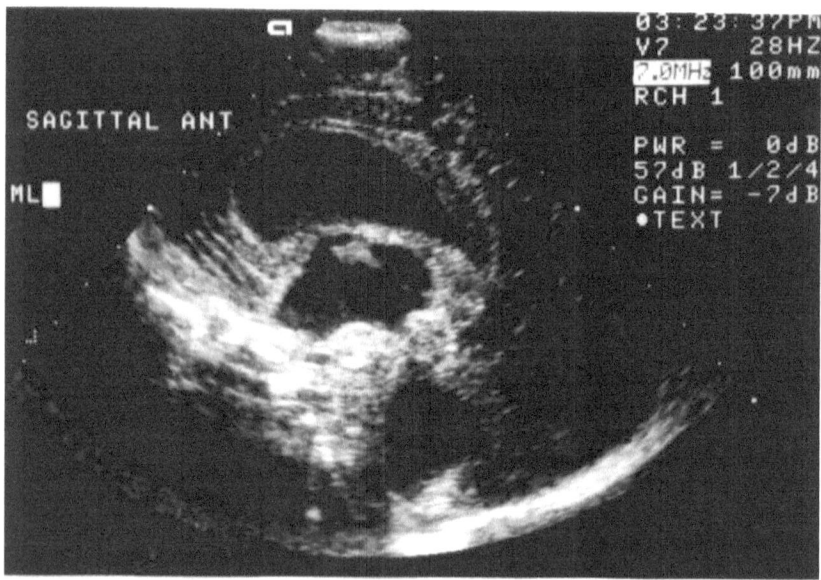

(c) ii Ultrasound showing hydrocephalus: Medial sagittal image showing dilated third and lateral ventricle above.

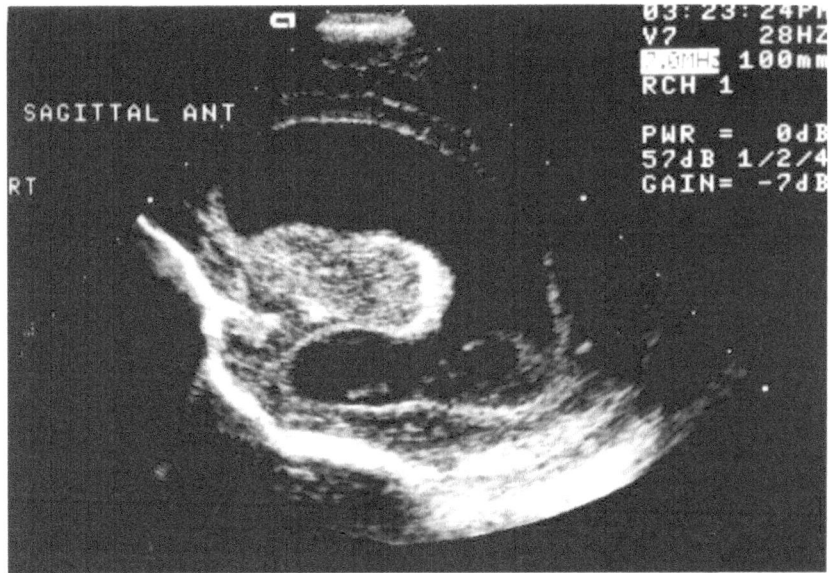

(c) iii Ultrasound showing hydrocephalus: Lateral sagittal image showing dilated lateral ventricle.

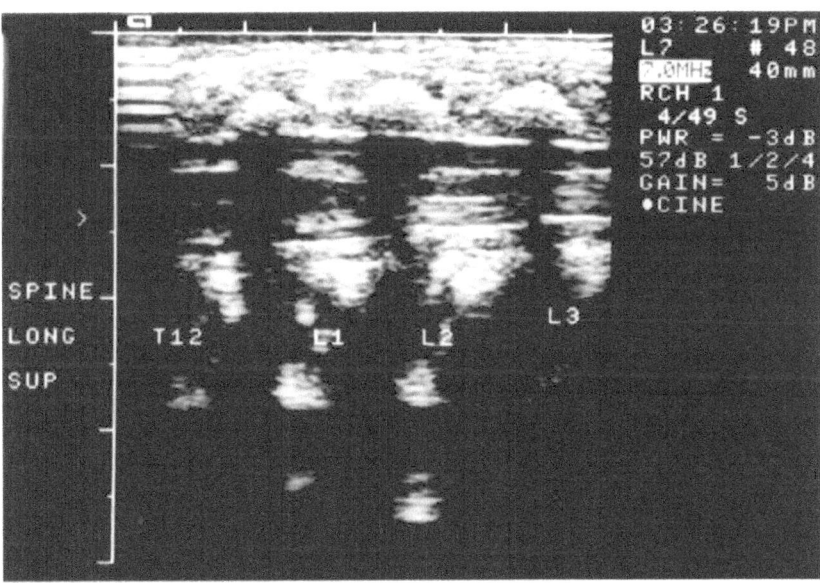

(d) Spinal ultrasound in a neonate showing the spinal cord (black signal) ending at T12-L1 with the nerve roots of the cauda equina inferior to this.

Figure 2.15 (a-d) The Cranial ultrasound.

Ventriculography & pneumoencephalography (Figure 2.16)

Air ventriculography and pneumoencephalography (PEG) were commonly performed before the advent of CT. It is however difficult to obtain useful images using these techniques and requires experience to interpret them, but they can aid the diagnosis of intracranial disorders which are difficult to diagnose clinically and where there is no CT scanner. It should be emphasized that CT or MR is much preferred. The ventricular drain can also be left in as an external drain to relieve obstructive hydrocephalus. There is also a risk of morbidity because they are invasive investigations. The use of non-ionic contrast agents, such as iopamidol for these studies will be better tolerated than air injection.

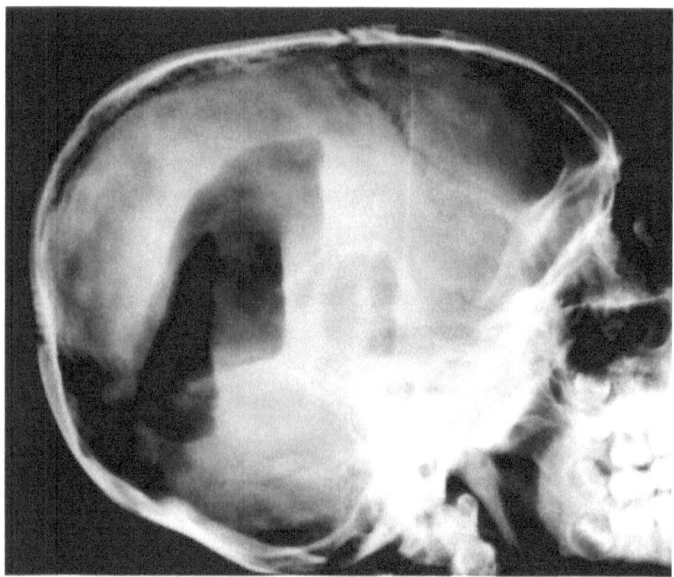

Figure 2.16 Ventriculogram. This is an air ventriculogram showing air in the posterior parts of grossly dilated lateral ventricles and a grossly dilated third ventricle. Note the splitting of the coronal suture. This was due to a malignant tumour at the level of the aqueduct which was found to be inoperable at posterior fossa exploration. No CT scanner was available.

The value of a PEG is to identify parasellar lesions, to display the basal cisterns and define subarachnoid blocks. Failure of air to enter the ventricular system may be a functional block. PEG is rarely performed as it is difficult to perform and interpret, with serious potential complications. We do not therefore advocate its general use and do not describe the technique in detail in this text. The patient is initially placed in the sitting position with the neck flexed and air enters the ventricular system from the lumbar injection. Later the neck is extended to allow filling of the subarachnoid space. The ventriculogram requires a burr hole and in the adult can be carried out under local anaesthetic., below

Occipital horn approach

Because few space-occupying lesions occur in the occipital lobes, the occipital horns are usually easy to find, and if both sides are catheterised good pictures can be almost guaranteed. Under local anaesthesia biparietal burr holes are made about 6 cm above the external occipital protuberance, 3 cm each side of the midline. This can only be done if the operating table is broken to about 60°, with the patient sitting on it with the neck flexed a further 30° and resting on a firm sandbag which is strapped to the head of the table. The patient must not be allowed to slip down the table, which occurs all too easily. After the dura is opened a brain needle is passed towards the ipsilateral eyeball, into the occipital horn. CSF will gush from the needle, which should be quickly exchanged for a 5Fr infant feeding tube. As soon as free flow occurs the tube should be closed. The wound is closed and the feeding tube sutured firmly in place. The same procedure is then performed on the other side.

A volume of 10·15 ml of air is exchanged for CSF on each side, with further CSF being allowed to escape if pressure is high. Each catheter is wrapped in a sterile pack and the table flattened, keeping the patient strictly supine for transport to the X-ray room. Films are taken in A-P, Towne's and horizontal ray lateral projections. Inspection will show whether or not adequate air is in the lateral and third ventricles to allow any distortion to be recognised. If necessary, more air can be injected into one or other catheter, or rocked from one lateral ventricle to the other. In cases where there is distortion of the anterior third ventricle better views may be obtained by extending the head over the end of the table and repeating the series. When satisfactory brow-up films have been obtained the patient is rolled over and horizontal ray lateral, P-A and reversed Towne's view are obtained. Review of the whole series should allow accurate anatomical localisation of any space-occupying lesion.

Frontal horn approach

The burr hole is placed usually on the right (non-dominant) side in the midpupillary line just behind the hairline. A brain needle is passed through the frontal cortex into the frontal horn of the right lateral ventricle, then removed and a Size 5 Fr or 8 Fr infant feeding tube passed along the track of the brain needle into the ventricle, 10-20 ml of air or 10 ml of contrast are injected slowly after removing an equal volume of CSF, and a lateral and A-P radiograph obtained. The patient should be held face down, neck flexed over the end of the trolley, further A-P and lateral views obtained, and then placed supine with head arched back over the end of the table to force the air or contrast into the far reaches of the ventricular system. Asymmetry and distortion in the ventricular shape, with obliteration of segments and shifting from the midline give an indication of the position of a space occupying lesion.

Ventriculography complications

1. Epilepsy: the risk is 1-2 per cent. Prophylactic anticonvulsants should be used.
2. Infection: prophylactic broad-spectrum antibiotics should be given.
3. Intracerebral haemorrhage: careful single passage of the brain needle into the ventricle should avoid this. Extracerebral haemorrhage (subdural, extradural) may also occur if haemostasis at the burr hole site is not meticulous.
4. Headache and vomiting after the procedure may indicate raised pressure from an air collection which will require aspiration. The alteration in pressure may cause a deterioration in the patient's conscious state so generally, definitive surgery for a space-occupying lesion should be performed within 24 hours of the procedure.

Pneumoencephalography (PEG) complications

1. Headache: post lumbar puncture headache, which is minimised by keeping the patient lying flat for 24 hours following lumbar puncture.
2. Coning: may occur if ICP elevated significantly. **Do not perform a PEG if papilloedema is present.**
3. Meningism, vomiting and headache.

Interpretation

Supratentorial masses

1. A frontal lobe lesion may compress the frontal horn, and may shift it posteriorly and medially.
2. A deep frontal lesion may distort the third ventricle and may occlude one or both foramina of Monro and cause hydrocephalus of one or both lateral ventricles.
3. A temporal lesion may compress or obliterate the temporal horn and shift it posteriorly.
4. A parietal lesion may compress the trigone (body) of the lateral ventricle.
5. An upper brain stem or pineal region lesion may compress the aqueduct and cause hydrocephalus of the third and lateral ventricles.

Posterior fossa masses

1. Pontine or medullary brainstem lesions tend not to cause hydrocephalus.
2. Midline cerebellar lesions tend to displace the fourth ventricle forwards and obliterate it.
3. Lateral cerebellar lesions tend to displace the fourth ventricle laterally to the opposite side.
4. Secondary obstructive hydrocephalus will result from obstruction to the fourth ventricle.

Cerebral angiography (see Figure 2.17, next page)

In the absence of CT, it is useful to diagnose suspected intracranial extracerebral collections such as a chronic subdural haematoma where it will show displacement of the cerebral vessels away from the inner tables of the skull. The carotid angiogram is also useful for diagnosing an intracerebral mass lesion - it will show displacement of the intracerebral vessels away from it, and in some cases a tumour 'blush' if there is an increased tumour circulation. It is the definitive investigation (with or without CT) to demonstrate aneurysms in patients with subarachnoid haemorrhage, arteriovenous mal-formations and carotid-cavernous fistulae.

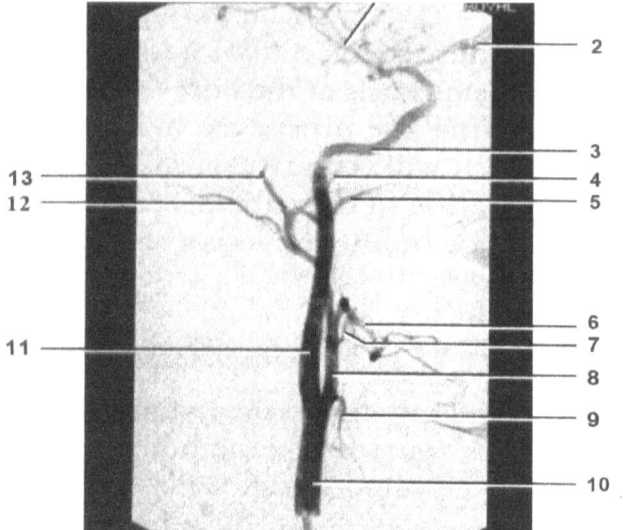

Figure 2.17 (a) Carotid angiogram including cervical carotid.
Legend
1. Middle cerebral artery
2. Anterior cerebral artery
3. Internal carotid artery petrous segment
4. Superficial temporal artery
5. Internal maxillary artery
6. Facial artery
7. Lingual artery
8. External carotid artery
9. Superior thyroid artery
10. Common carotid artery
11. Proximal internal carotid artery
12. Occipital artery
13. Posterior auricular artery

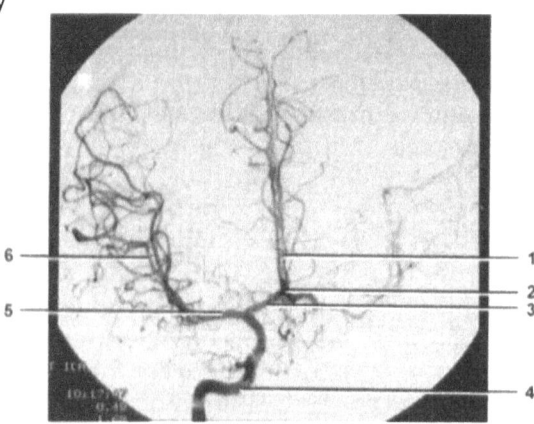

(b) Carotid angiogram A-P view.
Legend
1. Anterior cerebral artery
2. Anterior communicating artery
3. Proximal anterior cerebral artery
4. Cavernous segment of the internal
   sylvian fissure
5. Middle cerebral artery
6. Middle cerebral artery branches in
   carotid artery

Clinical assessment in neurosurgery

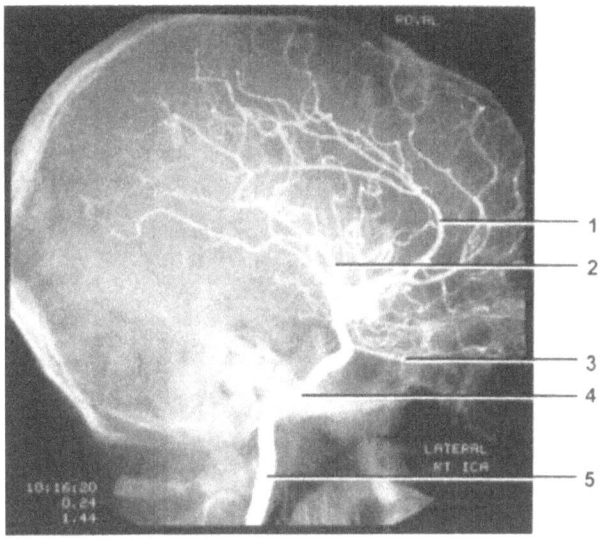

(c) Carotid angiogram lateral view.
Legend
1. Anterior cerebral artery
2. Middle cerebral artery
3. Ophthalmic artery
4. Petrous segment of internal carotid artery
5. Internal carotid artery

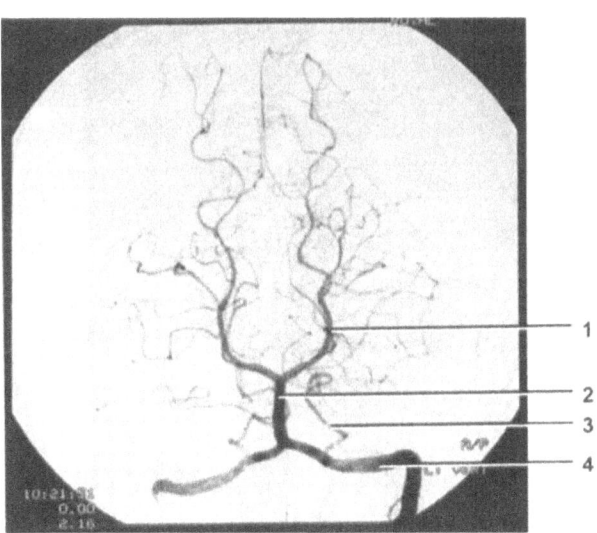

(d) Vertebral angiogram Towne's view.
Legend
1. Posterior cerebral artery
2. Basilar artery
3. Posterior inferior cerebellar artery
4. Vertebral artery

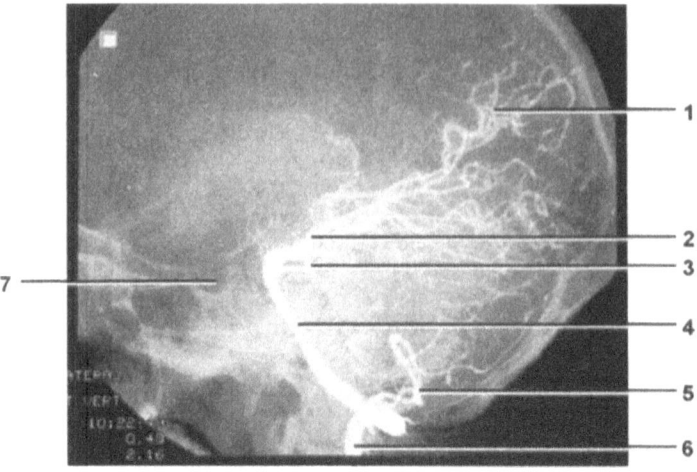

(e) Vertebral angiogram lateral view.
Legend
1. Posterior cerebral artery distal branches
2. Posterior cerebral artery main trunks
3. Superior cerebellar arteries
4. Basilar artery
5. Posterior inferior cerebellar arteries
6. Vertebral artery
7. Pituitary fossa

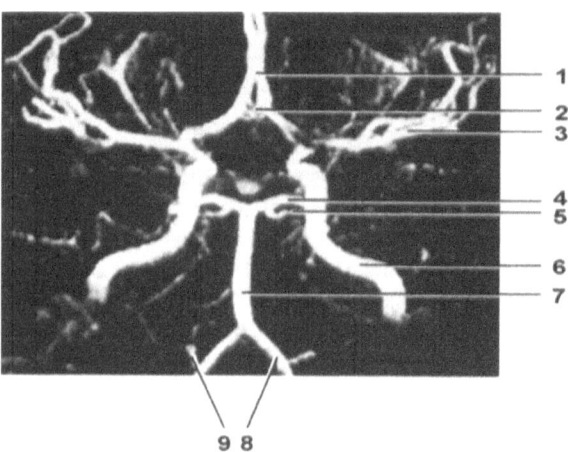

(f) Magnetic resonance angiogram showing the circle of Willis.
Legend
1. Anterior cerebral arteries
2. Anterior communicating artery
3. Middle cerebral artery branches
4. Posterior cerebral artery
5. Superior cerebellar artery
6. Internal carotid arteries
7. Basilar artery
8. Vertebral artery
9. Posterior inferior cerebellar artery

Figure 2.17 (a-f) Angiogram.

When angiography catheters and radiologists are unavailable this is best performed via a direct common carotid artery puncture (see Figure 2.18, below).

Technique of direct carotid artery puncture

1. Usually performed under local anaesthesia unless the patient is a child or is restless and unco-operative.
2. Prepare 20ml iopamidol or Conray 280 in a sterile syringe. Do not use stronger solutions as they may cause cerebral vasospasm.
3. Pass a lumbar puncture needle size 19-gauge, length 5-8 cm directly into common carotid artery. You should have a plastic connection tubing to avoid moving the tip of needle when injecting.
4. Inject 10 ml contrast.

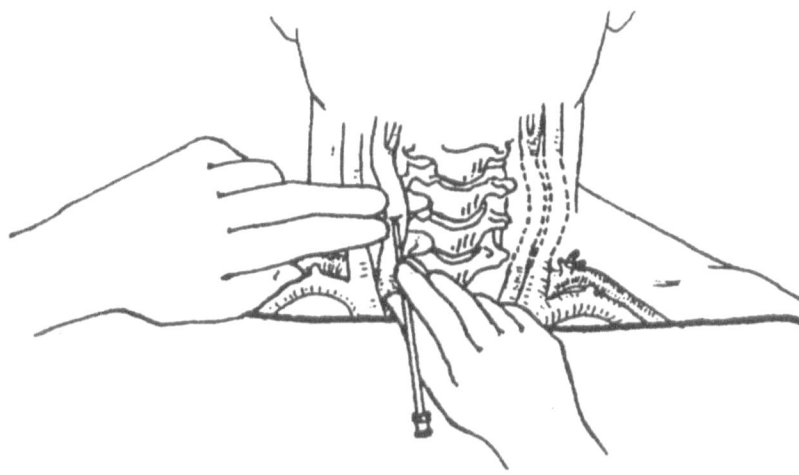

Figure 2.18 Direct puncture of the common carotid artery.

5. Rapid manual change of films:
   - while injecting and after 5 ml,
   - then every 2-2-3 seconds depending on ability of machine to change over.

   If rapid change is not possible then A-P and lateral plain films of the skull can be taken. Inject rapidly, in one to two seconds and shout as the last of the injection is going in. This will give an arterial phase. Capillary and venous phases can be obtained by repeating the injection and counting slowly to 3 or 6.
6. Repeat the procedure with 10 ml contrast and films in a lateral projection.

7. Pressure over the injection site for 10 minutes or longer if necessary, to control ooze or haematoma development.

This injection technique may fill the posterior circulation via the posterior communicating arteries. If CT scanning is available, **CT angiography** replaces standard angiography in many cases because it is non-invasive and just requires an intravenous injection of contrast. The images of CT angiography are shown in the CT images below (Figure 2.20, page 68).

Myelogram (see Chapter 5 Figures from page 249 onwards)

Indications

- Progressive neurological deficit in the limbs suggestive of an intraspinal lesion: e.g. quadriparesis, paraparesis,
- acute spinal cord compression,
- sciatica which is not settling with conservative management.

Method

- Lumbar puncture L4-5 level with the patient in a lateral position
- inject 20 ml iopamidol,
- for lumbar myelogram: take A-P and lateral soon after injection,
- for thoracic and cervical myelogram: ask the patient to kneel on the table bend the arms and place the head down - the dye should run up the spinal canal,
- take more films A-P and lateral.

Cervical puncture carries more risk than lumbar puncture and requires special training to perform. The needle is introduced just beneath the occipital bone - through the atlanto-axial membrane in the midline, or laterally at Cl-2. This could be performed when there is poor contrast filling of the cervical canal from below or when the upper level of a spinal block needs to be defined. However, it should not be necessary for the surgeon to perform this manoeuvre in the developing world setting because the clinical findings will be enough to give a guide to which is the appropriate level of the cervical spine to explore, with the added information of the myelography from lumbar injection.

Interpretation

Cord compression

Will show a complete or partial block in the spinal canal and give some indication as to whether the pathology is intradural, extramedullary or intramedullary or whether extradural. But this distinction is not crucial - the most important information is the anatomical level of pathology, particularly in the thoracic region.

Root compression

The posterolateral disc prolapse or rupture may obliterate the adjacent nerve root sheath and produce a filling defect on the myelogram. The nerve root may be compromised in a canal rendered narrow by bony osteophyte, ligament hypertrophy and disc. The bony foraminal narrowing may be seen on the oblique cervical X-rays. A nerve root tumour e.g. schwannoma may also cause compression of the nerve root and produce a filling defect on the myelogram.

Nerve conduction studies

The site and severity of a peripheral nerve lesion can be determined. The studies can generally be performed using surface rather than needle electrodes that involves little discomfort to the patient.

The three main types of nerve conduction measurement are:
1. A purely sensory branch of a nerve is stimulated (e.g. a digital nerve in the index finger) and a recording is made from the nerve.
2. A mixed motor and sensory nerve is stimulated (e.g. median nerve at the wrist) and a recording is made from the nerve.
3. A motor or mixed nerve is stimulated and a recording is made from one of the muscles it innervates.

Most entrapment syndromes can be investigated and show a slowing of conduction. However, meralgia paraesthetica and spinal root compression are not worth investigating in this way. Nerve conduction studies are not usually available in LMIC; however, the clinical assessment will suffice.

Nuclear scan

Radioisotope is injected into the bloodstream, to examine for tumour deposits in bone, cerebral lesions and cerebral blood flow. It has application particularly in patients with epilepsy and demonstrates hyperperfusion during a seizure and hypoperfusion after a seizure. It also has relevance in cases of cerebral ischaemia or stroke to examine areas of hypoperfusion. It may also be used to study CSF dynamics or identify CSF leaks, when the isotope is injected into the CSF via lumbar puncture. Nuclear scanning is not readily applicable in the developing world because of a lack of nuclear medicine facilities and isotopes. Good neurosurgical care can be practised without the need for nuclear medicine investigation.

Computed tomographic (CT) scan (Figure 2.19, next page)

The clinical application of computed tomography developed in the 1970s and revolutionised the management of patients with brain disorders and was later applied to many other regions of the body. The rotation and movement of multiple X-ray tubes around the head or other body part produces a series of small cubes of information (pixels) which contain attenuation coefficients for the particular tissues, and these are assembled by a computer into tomographic images which represent slices of tissue 2-15 mm thick. The images are usually obtained in an axial (horizontal) dimension although direct coronal images can also be obtained.

Reconstructions in the coronal or sagittal planes can be obtained but are quite blurred with poor resolution depending on the type of CT scanner. Bone and calcium appear white, the brain varying degrees of grey, the CSF dark grey to black and air and fat are black. Intravenous contrast administration enhances tumours, vascular lesions, and regions of blood-brain barrier breakdown. A series of axial images ('cuts') illustrates the normal cross-sectional anatomy of the brain (see Figure 2.19, next page).

The newer spiral CT scanner is faster than the preceding CT scanners with high resolution and enhanced capacity for subtraction studies so that angiogram images can be generated following the administration of intravenous contrast. Computed tomographic angiography (CTA) (see Figure 2.20, page 68) can be obtained by injecting an intravenous contrast agent at the time of the CT.

Although DSA with intra-arterial contrast remains the 'gold standard' for blood vessel imaging, CTA gives a clear display of the cerebral vasculature both in arterial and venous phases without the need for arterial puncture. CTA can replace DSA in many situations. CT scanners are still not widely available in the developing world, and where it is, the great majority do not have access because of the cost. The diagnosis and management of CNS disorders has been significantly improved by CT so that the development of a neurosurgery service will usually go hand in hand with the introduction of CT.

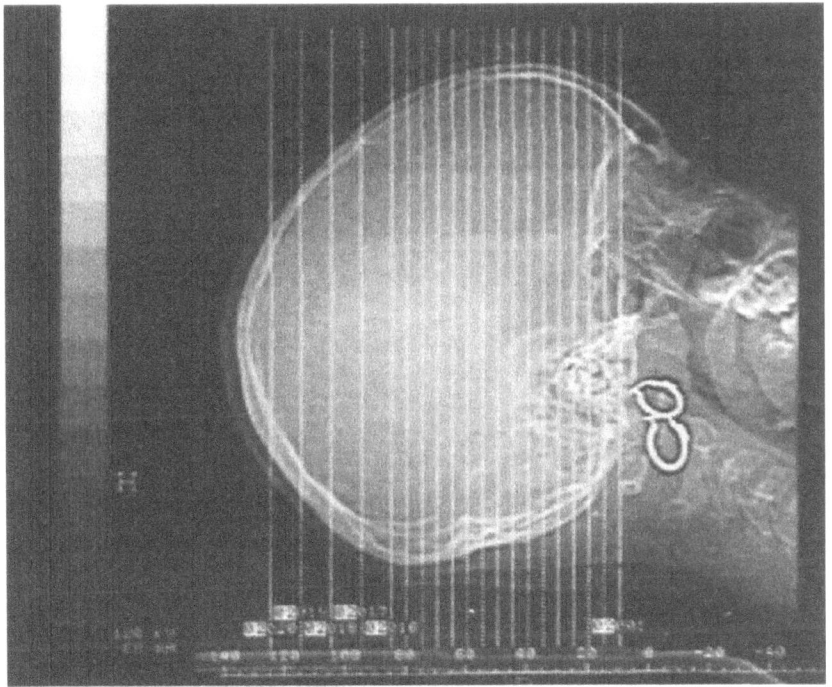

Figure 2.19 (a) Scout view with horizontal lines indicating position of tomographic cuts.

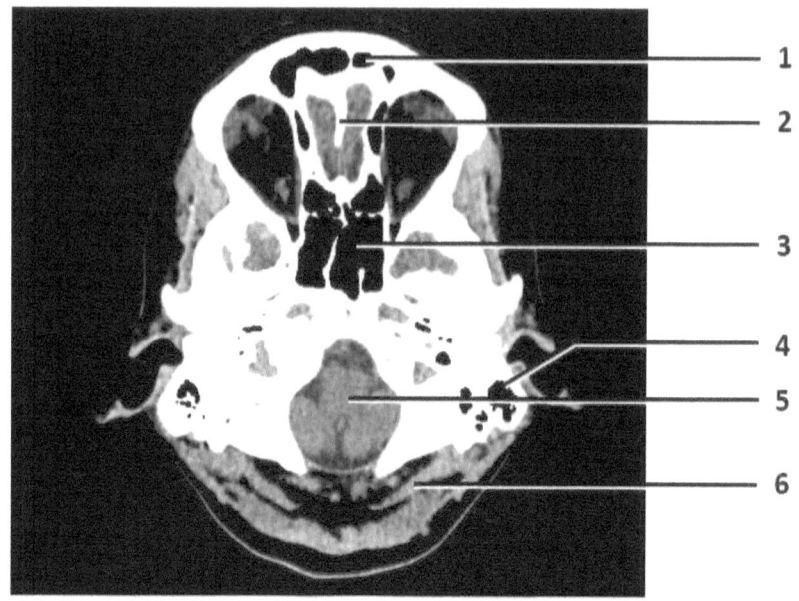

(b) i

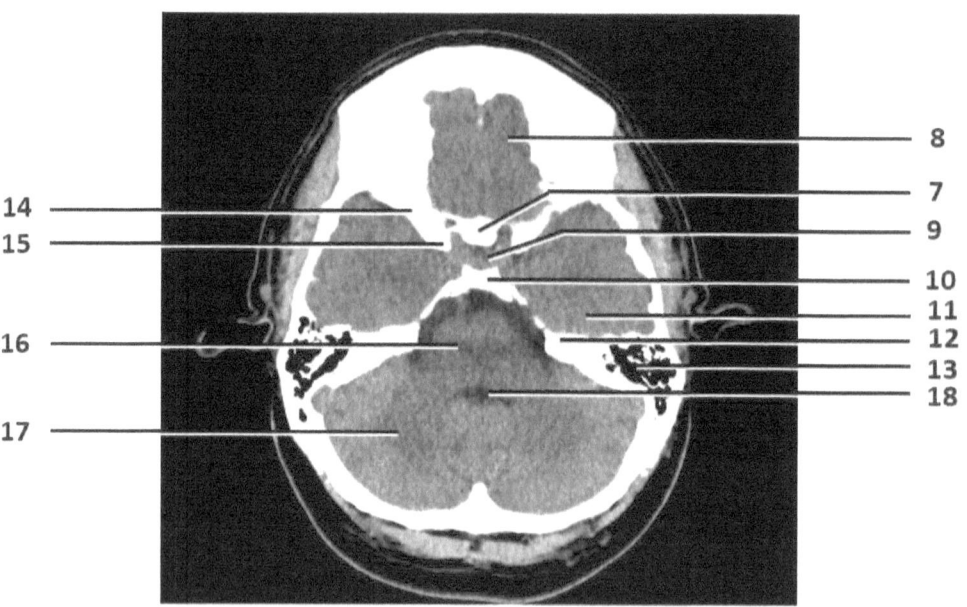

(b) ii

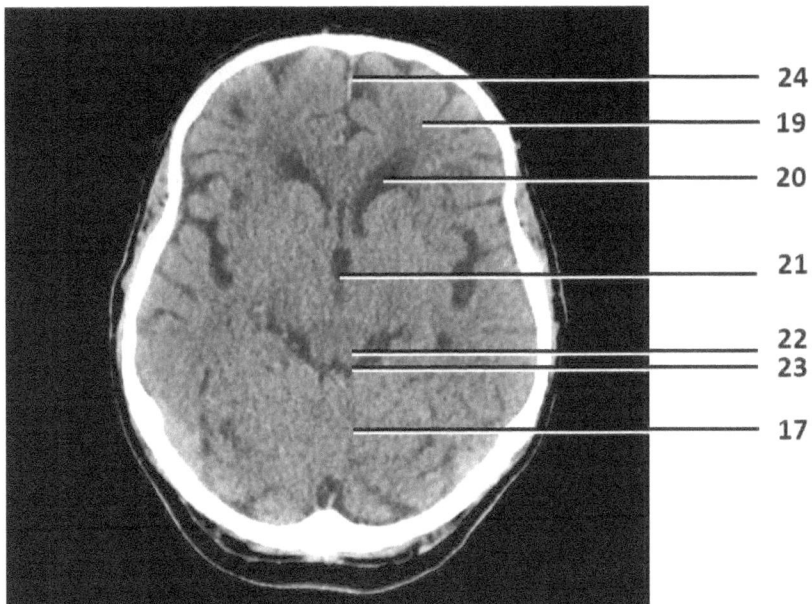

24
19
20

21

22
23

17

(b) iii

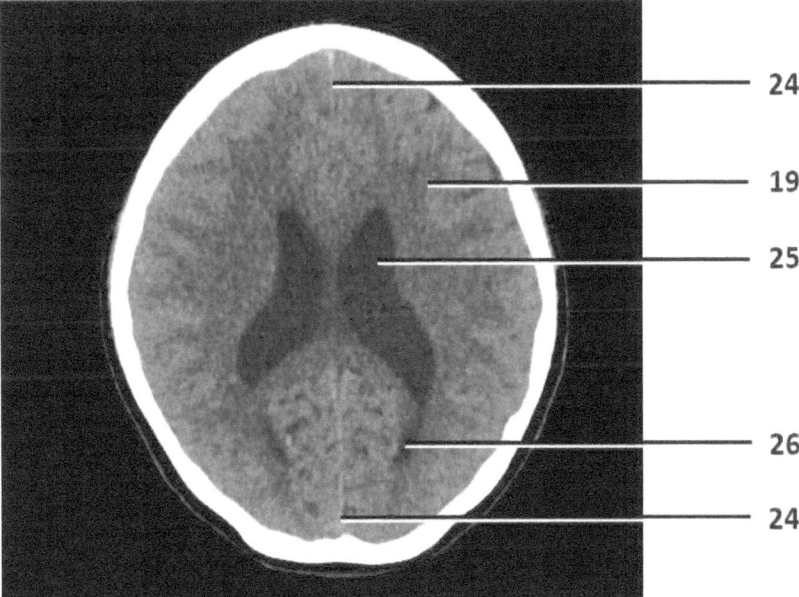

24

19

25

26

24

(b) iv

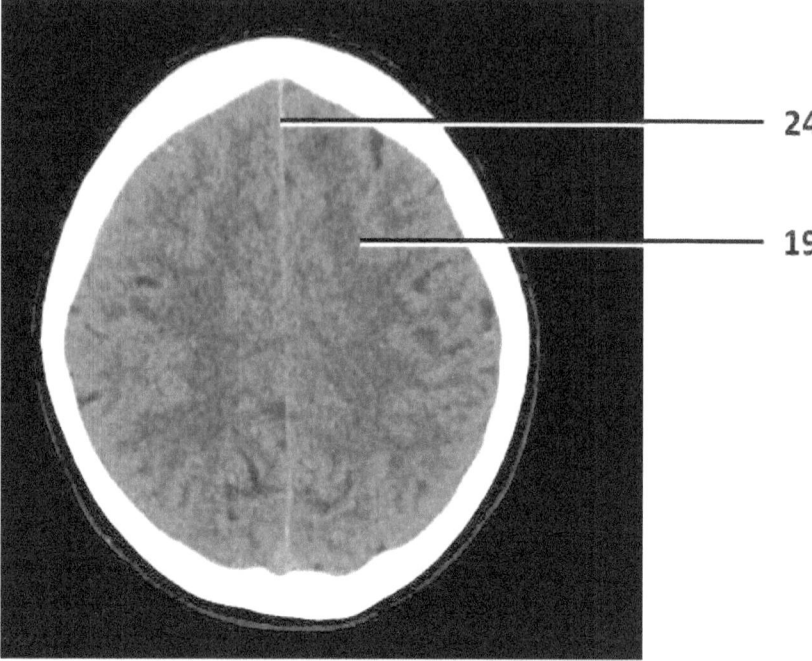

(b) v

(b) i-v Selected axial images from the base of skull to the vertex.

Figure 2.19 (a-b) Computed tomographic scans (CT).
Legend

1. Frontal sinus
2. Cribriform plate
3. Sphenoid sinus
4. Mastoid air cells between cortex
5. Lower medulla/upper cervical spinal cord
6. Nuchal muscles
7. Tuberculum sellae
8. Frontal lobe
9. Pituitary fossa
10. Dorsum sellae (upper end of clivus)
11. Temporal lobe
12. Petrous apex
13. Mastoid air cells
14. Lesser sphenoidal wing
15. Anterior clinoid process
16. Pons with horizontal bony artefact

17. Cerebellum
18. Fourth ventricle
19. Grey/white junction
    (the border between cortex
    and white matter)
20. Frontal horn of the lateral
    ventricle
21. Posterior end of the third
    ventricle
22. Posterior midbrain
    (quadrigeminal plate)
23. Quadrigeminal cistern
24. Falx cerebri
25. Body of the lateral ventricle
26. Occipital horn of the lateral
    ventricle

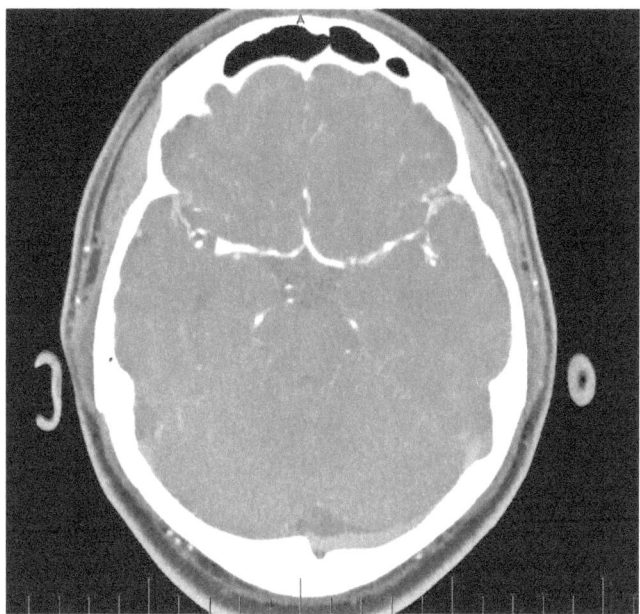

Figure 2.20 (a) Axial CTA showing the horizontal segments of the middle cerebral arteries (M1s) and the proximal anterior cerebral arteries (A1s). There is some filling of the posterior cerebral arteries at the sides of the midbrain.

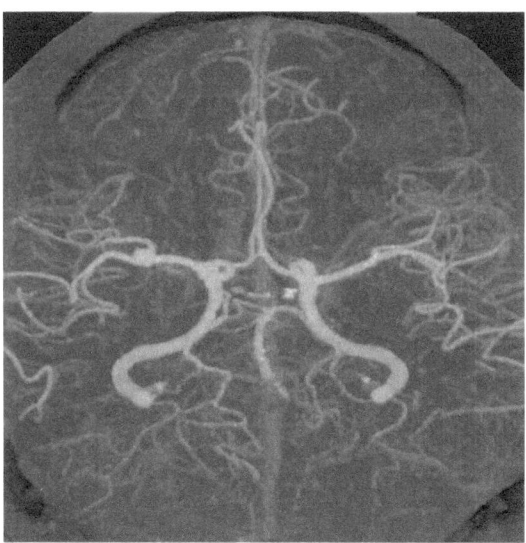

(b) CTA with the brain signals subtracted showing the cerebral arteries. Note the right the right sided middle cerebral artery (MCA) aneurysm.

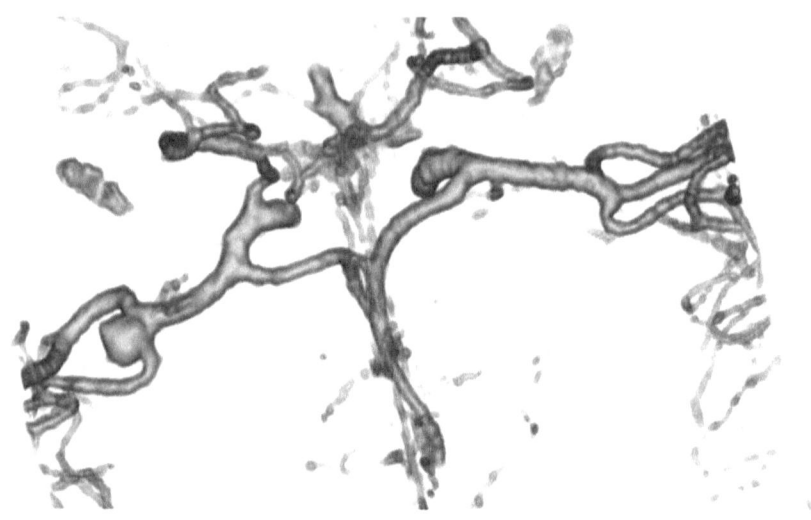

(c) CTA reconstruction of the Circle of Willis (COW) and its branches. This can be rotated on the computer screen and the vessels examined from different angles. Note the right sided MCA aneurysm.

Figure 2.20 (a-c) Computed tomographic angiogram (CTA).

Magnetic resonance (MR) imaging (Figure 2.21)

Even though magnetic resonance (MR) imaging is not often available in the developing world, we feel it is important to describe this technique because it is now such an integral part of managing the neurosurgery patient, and there are increasing numbers of patients in the tropics who travel abroad to obtain MR scans and bring them back home with the expectation that their own doctors will be able to interpret them. It is also for this reason that we present the normal brain on MR imaging and illustrate some of our descriptions in the other chapters with MR scans. Magnetic resonance imaging was developed in the 1970s and became clinically available in the 1980s. Improved resolution and speed of imaging has occurred in the 1990s. MR imaging relies on a strong magnetic field which aligns the axes of spin of atomic nuclei within the magnetic field. These axes are distorted with radiofrequency transmission which is then turned off, and the relaxation of the axes back into alignment will release radiofrequency signals which induce a voltage in the receiver coil and eventually produce the images. This is clearly very different from the standard X-ray or CT machine. Magnetic resonance imaging has provided clinicians with unprecedented accuracy in imaging internal bodily structures, without the need for ionising radiation. Another advantage of MR is its brilliant capability of producing image slices in various axes without the need for reconstruction, which is not the case with CT. It is also possible to study the real-time movement of fluid and blood with cine-MR, perform MR angiography by special subtraction techniques without the need for contrast agents, and to study the metabolism of tissue including CNS tumours, with MR spectroscopy (MRS) which shows the chemical makeup of tissues in graphical form. It is now also possible to study the function of the nervous system, with functional MRI (fMRI) which identifies parts of the nervous system that are specifically activated at the time of the study, e.g. the motor or speech cortex can be identified using this technique although there are many technical aspects that need to be considered to produce accurate images.

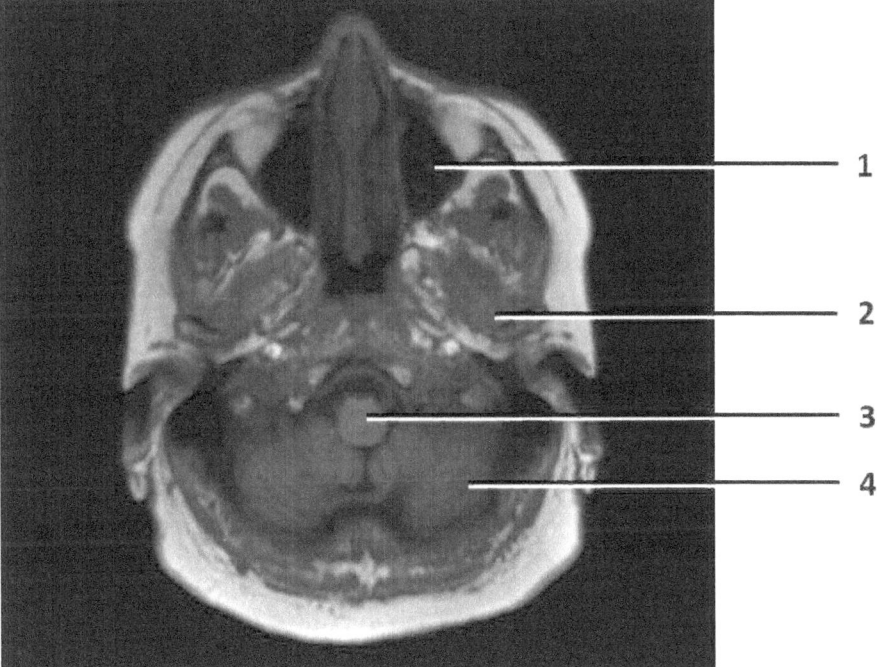

Figure 2.21 (a)

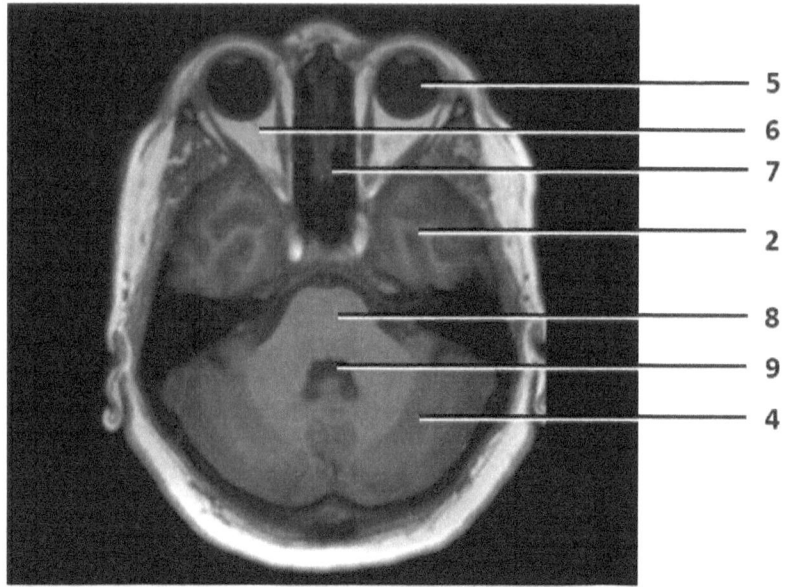

5
6
7
2
8
9
4

(b)

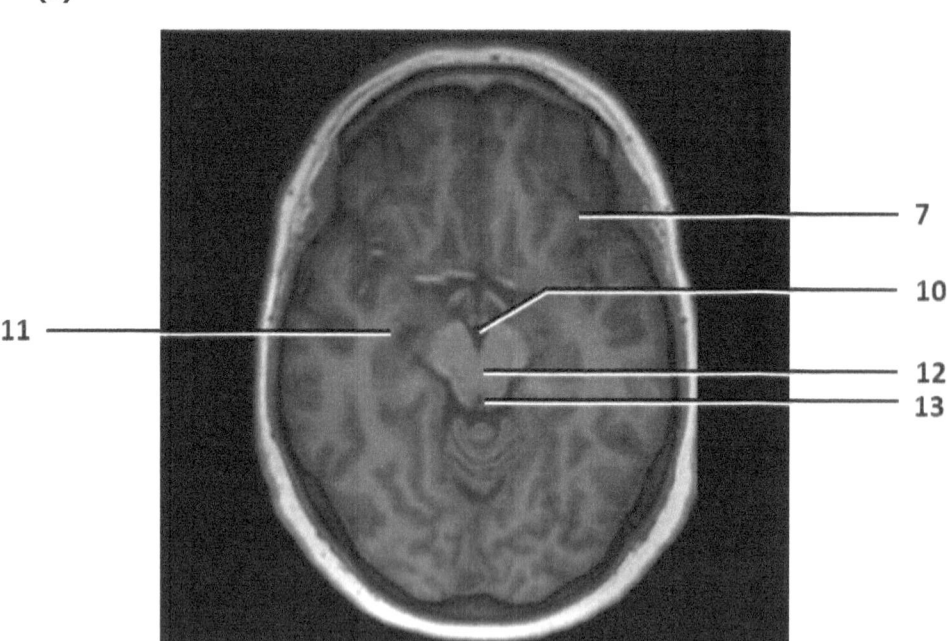

7
10
11
12
13

(c)

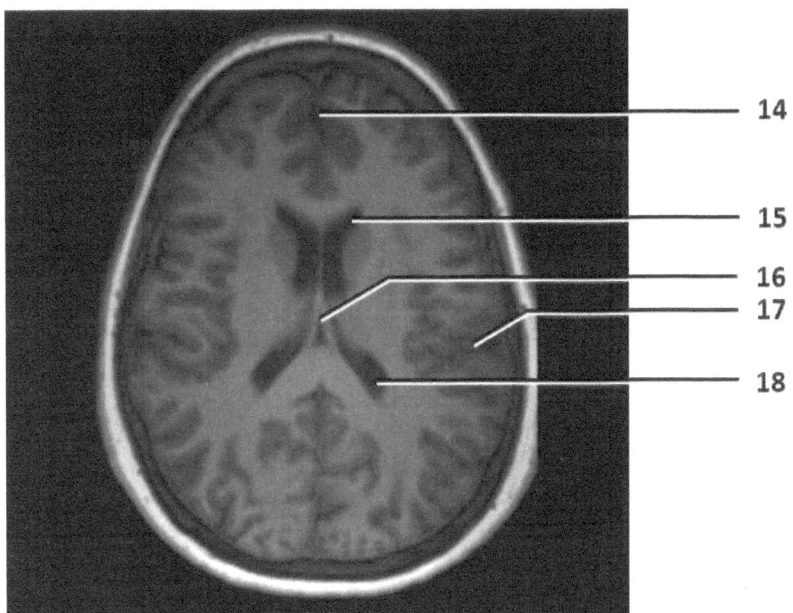

— 14

— 15

— 16
— 17

— 18

(d)

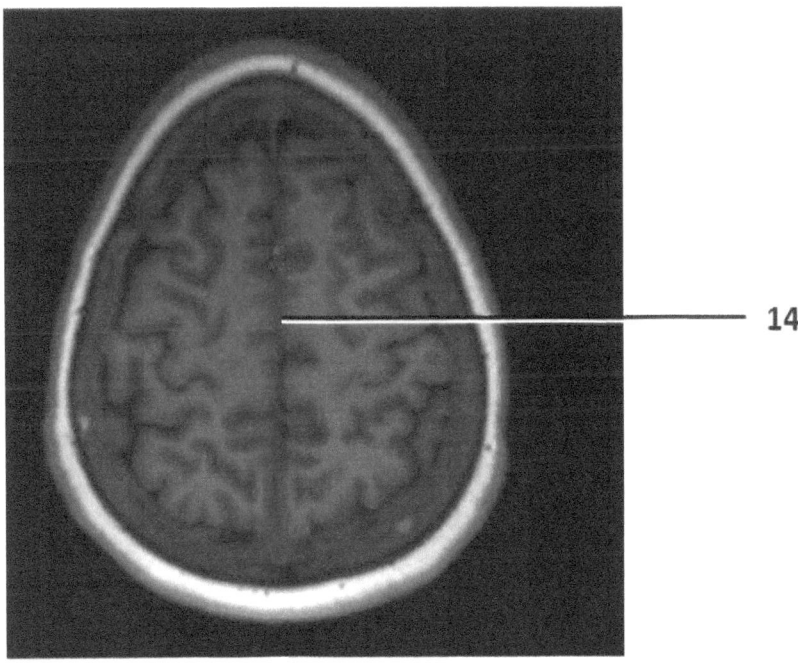

— 14

(e)

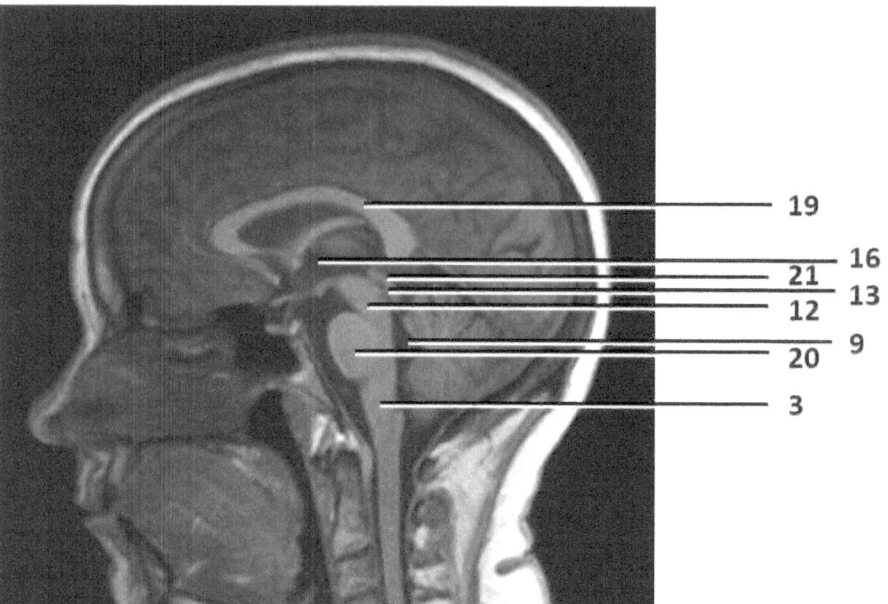

(f)

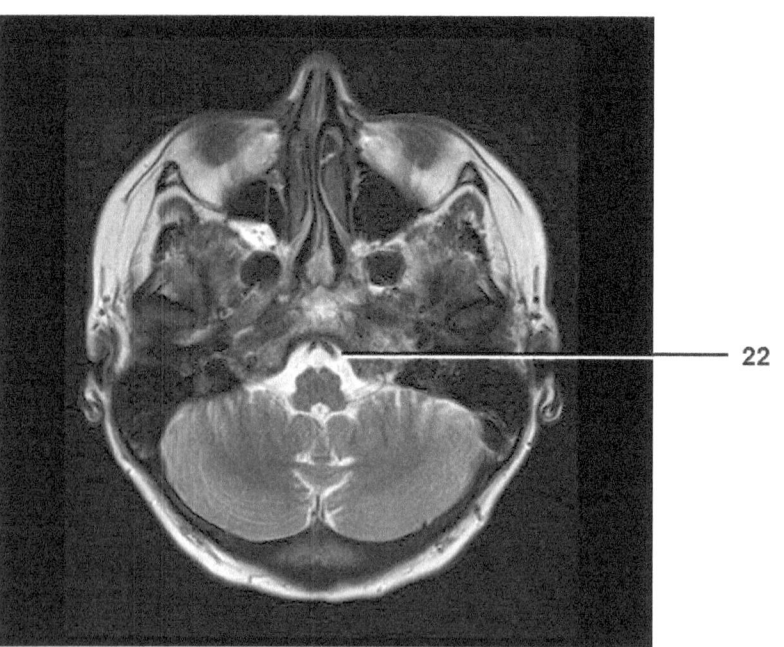

(g)

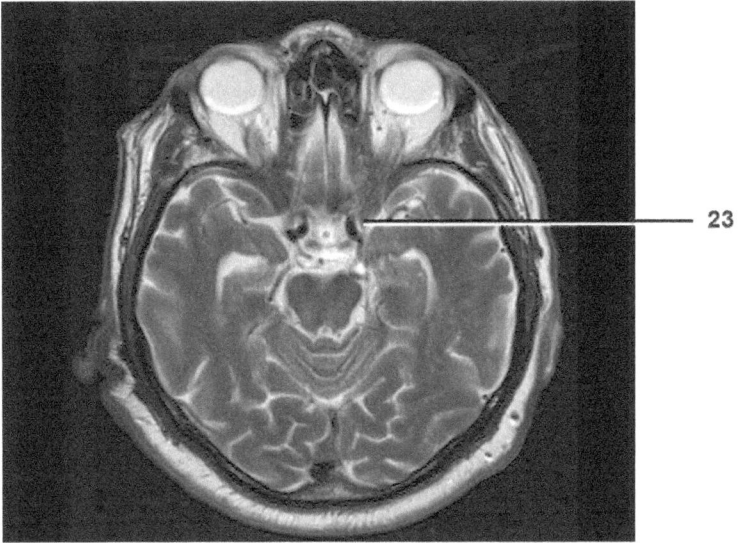

23

(h)

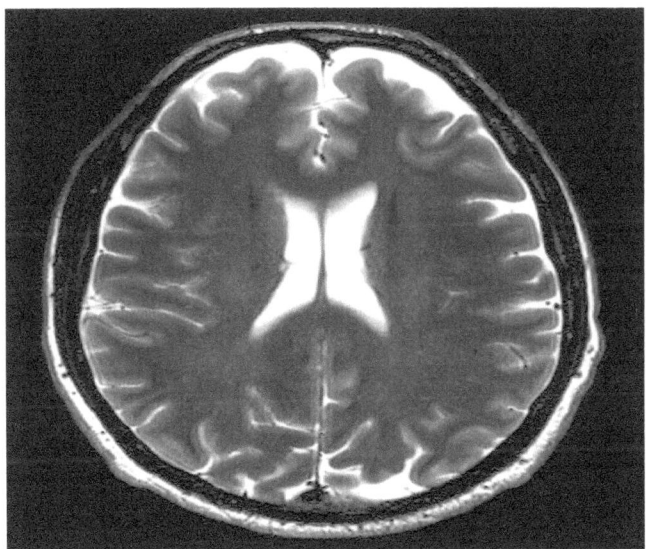

(i)

Figure 2.21 (a-i) Magnetic resonance (MR) imaging.
Legend
1. Maxillary sinus
2. Temporal lobe
3. Medulla
4. Cerebellum
5. Globe of eye

13. Cerebral aqueduct
14. Interhemispheric fissure
15. Frontal horn lateral ventricle
16. Third ventricle
17. Sylvian fissure

Figure 2.21 *(Continued)*
Legend
6. Optic nerve and retro-orbital fat
7. Frontal lobe
8. Pons
9. Fourth ventricle
10. Interpeduncular fossa (CSF cistern)
11. Temporal horn of lateral ventricle
12. Midbrain at red nucleus level

18. Posterior horn of the lateral ventricle
19. Corpus callosum
20. Pons
21. Pineal gland
22. Left vertebral artery
23. Left internal carotid artery

T1 weighted images (a-f) show air in the sinus and CSF as black. The brain is light grey and the fat in the scalp, subcutaneous tissues and orbits are white. The bone is black. The T1 weighted images are best used for the identification of normal anatomical structures. T2 weighted images show the CSF to be white and the brain architecture shows clearly as varying shades of grey and the blood vessels and bone are black. The T2 weighting is preferred for examining pathology in the brain. The lowest T2 image (g) clearly shows the vertebral arteries rising in front of the medulla to form the basilar artery. Note the lenses of the eyes are also clearly seen. The middle T2 cut (h) shows the two black internal carotid arteries in the suprasellar cistern of CSF. The cisterna magna, a large CSF cistern, may be seen posterior to the cerebellum in the midline in some the lowest MR axial cuts (Black on T1, White on T2 sequences). The uppermost T2 weighted image (i) shows the two lateral ventricles and very clear grey/white differentiation. The MR scans pass from inferior to superior with a single sagittal image through the midline (f).

Electroencephalogram (EEG)

Electroencephalography records electrical brain wave activity. It involves sticking multiple electrodes on the scalp, either during a seizure (ictal recording) or between seizures (interictal recording). The electrodes are placed in set positions (montage) so that the recordings can be compared with the normal patterns. Epileptic activity will be identified as abnormal waveforms such as spike/wave complexes and will help localise a focal area of epilepsy, demonstrate generalised epilepsy, or show abnormal waveforms associated with brain damage. It is a simple test to carry out, but requires the necessary electrical apparatus, which is expensive, and also requires the expertise and training of a neurologist who can interpret the study. It is of value in the diagnosis of epilepsy and various types of brain damage, but the vast majority of neurosurgical and neurological problems do not essentially require an EEG. Imaging with CT will answer many questions, hitherto reliant on EEG for diagnosis. Electro-encephalography is not often available in the developing world setting.

Head injury

EPIDEMIOLOGY

About 50 to 60 million new traumatic brain injury (TBI) cases are estimated to occur globally every year. 90% of trauma related deaths occur in LMIC. Head injuries are the most important cause of death from trauma in LMIC. 90% of trauma related deaths occur in LMIC. In Papua New Guinea TBI accounts for 60 percent of trauma deaths, many of which occur before the patient reaches hospital. Unfortunately, the majority of deaths are due to the severity of the primary brain injury and are therefore not preventable (once the injury has occurred). However, a proportion of patients die or are disabled from secondary brain injury and it is the prevention and treatment of secondary problems that is the focus of head injury management. The commonest causes of head injuries are assault, motor vehicle accidents and falls. In urban areas motor vehicle accidents are an important cause of severe head injury and in the tropics many people travel unprotected by seat belts or helmets or unrestrained and crowded in the back of open pick-up trucks. The introduction and enforcement of safety regulations such as seat belts or bicycle helmets is also much less prevalent in developing countries (see Figure 3.1, next page). In rural areas falls from trees or falling coconuts cause a number of head injuries.

PATHOPHYSIOLOGY

Primary brain injury

Primary brain injury occurs at the moment of impact and consists of tearing of neurons, particularly at the grey-white matter junctions, at the level of the corpus callosum and the posterior midbrain region. Although strategies are being developed to try and lessen the primary brain injury by using neuronal protective agents, these are still experimental; and primary brain injury in the remote or low resource setting should often be regarded as an irreversible component of the injury.

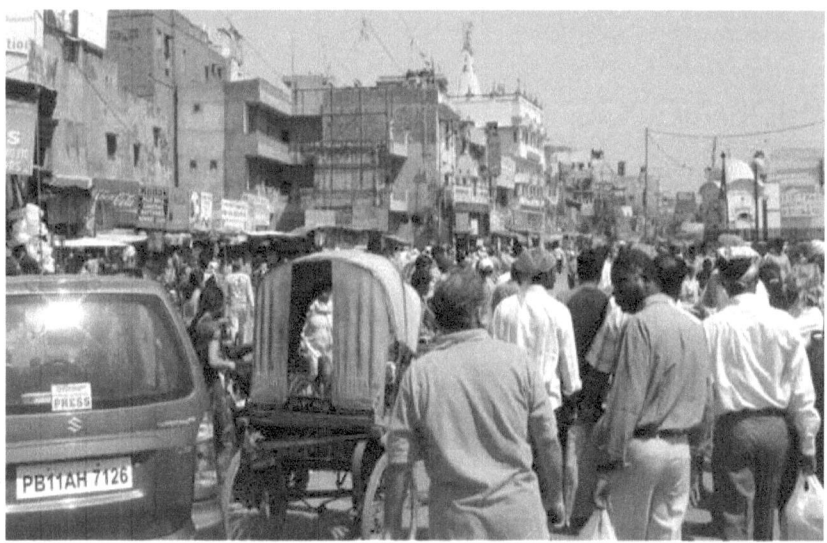

Figure 3.1 (a)

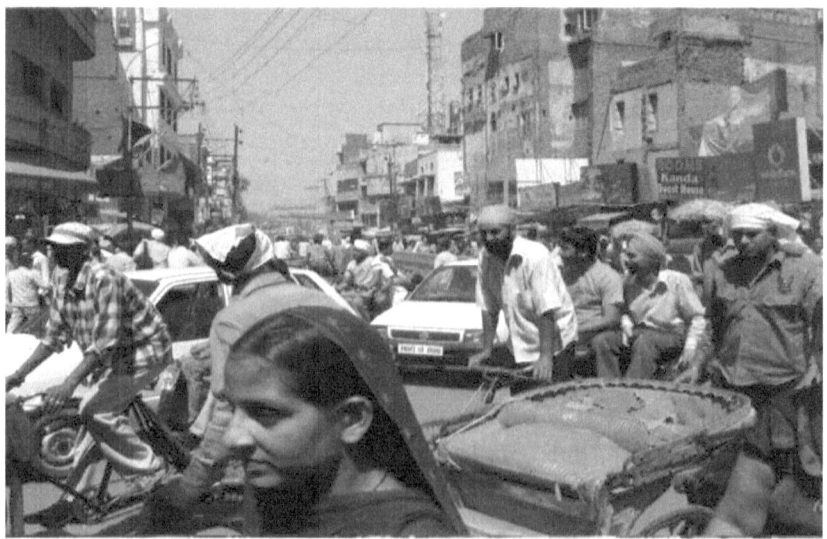

(b)

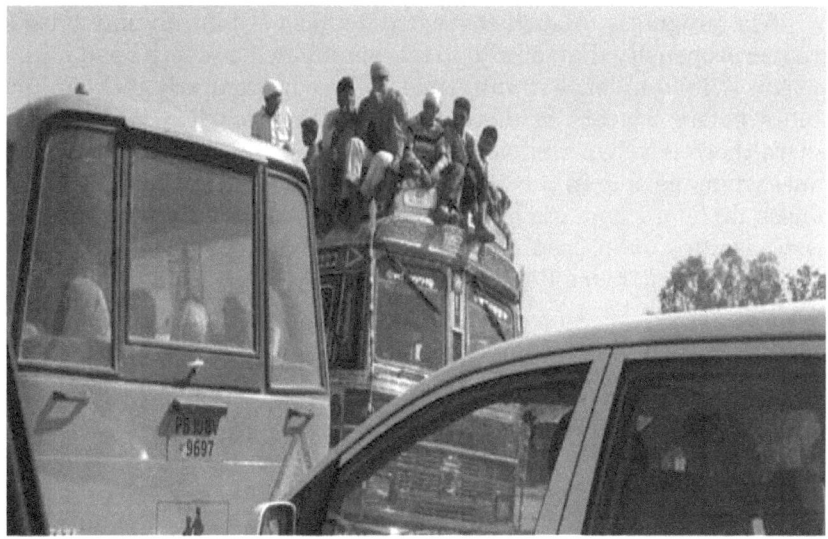

(c)

Figure 3.1 (a-c) With crowded streets, overloaded vehicles and a lack of road safety enforcement, road traffic accidents are common in low- and middle-income countries where head injuries are usually the commonest cause of death in young, economically active adults (Photo: Lhudiana, Punjab, India. Source: JV Rosenfeld).

When someone is struck on the head, they may suffer brain injury at the site of impact (coup). The injured brain may bleed or swell. Vessels on the surface of the brain may be torn. If the brain bounces off the opposite side of the cranium it may also be injured or bleed (contrecoup). In a road traffic accident at high speed, the force of the impact stops the skull but the brain may continue to travel momentarily because it is not fixed completely to the cranium. It may spin causing shearing of blood vessels and neurons or suffer multiple points of impact against the tentorium or the inner table of the skull. Such high velocity crashes may result in diffuse brain damage both to the cerebral hemispheres and to the brain stem with axonal damage (diffuse axonal injury, DAI) (Figure 3.2, next page).

DAI can be recognised on a CT scan by multiple petechial haemorrhages and general brain swelling, with effacement of the basal cisterns, reduction in the subarachnoid space, narrow 'slit' ventricles, and loss of grey-white differentiation. The haemorrhages are particularly located at the grey-white interface, subcortically near the corpus callosum and near the posterior aspect of the midbrain (Figure 3.2, next page).

The prognosis in such cases is often poor. Children may have a greater propensity than adults to recover following severe head injury but are still often left with multiple deficits particularly if the injury occurs before 2 years of age. Missile (bullet) injuries are common where there is urban strife or war. A low velocity penetrating injury causes damage only in the track of penetration. A high velocity bullet causes far more damage because it tilts and yaws its way through tissue sending out pressure waves which result in damage outside the track of the bullet (see Figure 3.3, page 81).

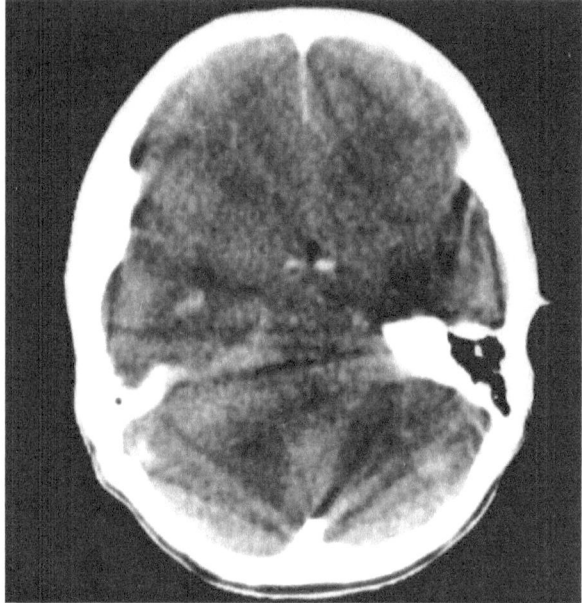

Figure 3.2 (a) CT scan showing diffusely swollen brain. Obliteration of basal cisterns. Deep right temporal lobe contusion.

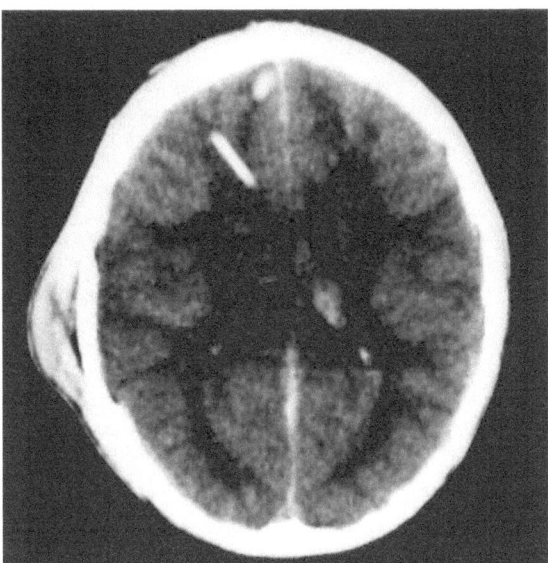

(b) CT scan of a patient with severe head injury showing evidence of diffuse axonal injury with small haemorrhages in the white matter, including the left side of the corpus callosum just above the ventricle. A ventricular catheter is placed in the right frontal horn. Right scalp haematoma and blood along the falx is seen.

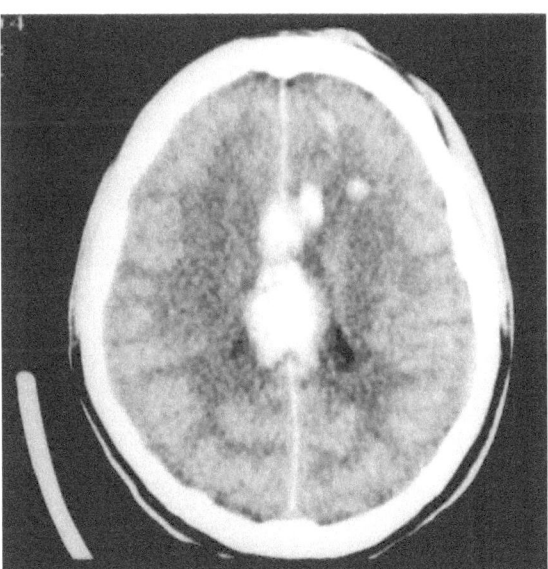

(c) CT scan showing diffuse axonal injury with extensive haemorrhage in the corpus callosum region.

Figure 3.2 (a-c) Diffuse axonal injury.

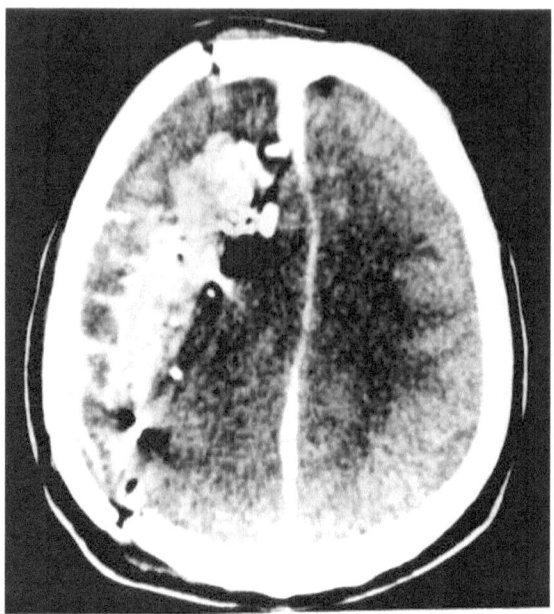

Figure 3.3 Missile injury. CT showing the haemorrhagic track of the bullet with multiple fragments. Secondary brain injury.

The three principal causes are cerebral ischaemia/hypoxia, raised intracranial pressure or mechanical brain shift, including coning (see Figure 3.4, next page).

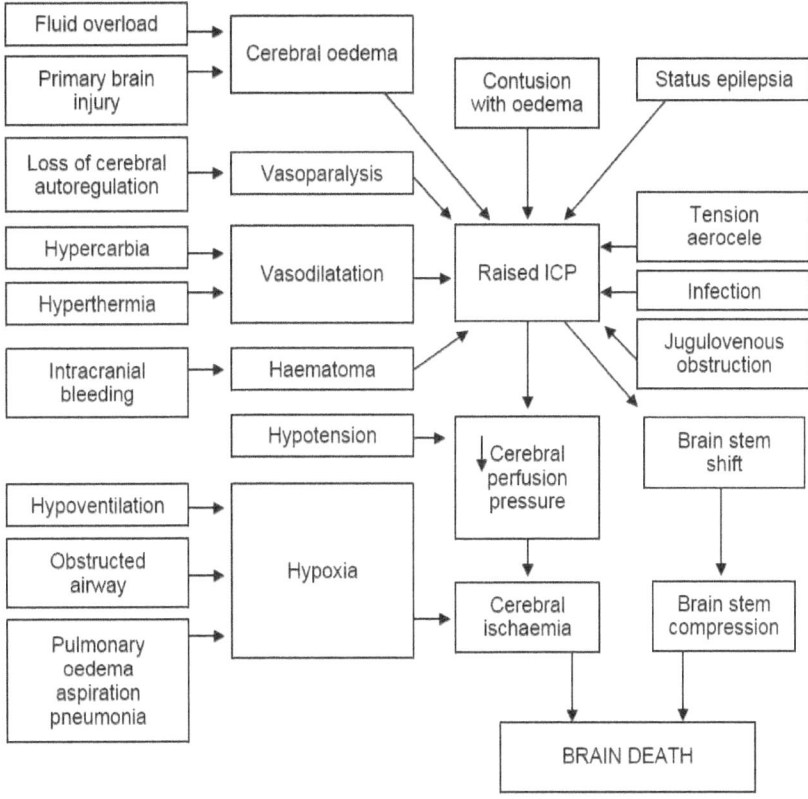

Figure 3.4 The causes of secondary brain injury.

Cerebral ischaemia/hypoxia

This may be due to:
- hypoxia due to inadequate gas exchange with hypoventilation and/or obstructed airway,
- hypoperfusion due to inadequate cerebral perfusion pressure,
- increasing cerebral oedema reducing oxygen levels to the neurons,
- vasospasm of main feeding vessels following traumatic subarachnoid haemorrhage.

The injured brain loses normal cerebral autoregulation. The cerebral circulation is normally tightly regulated, such that the cerebral blood flow remains constant over a wide range of blood pressures (Figure 3.5, next page). This is called autoregulation.

Autoregulation is disturbed following severe TBI with the normal curve becoming more linear so that the brain is more ischaemic than the normal brain at the same blood pressure up to the crossover point of the curves. Therefore, hypotension is even more damaging in the injured brain than it would be in a normal brain.

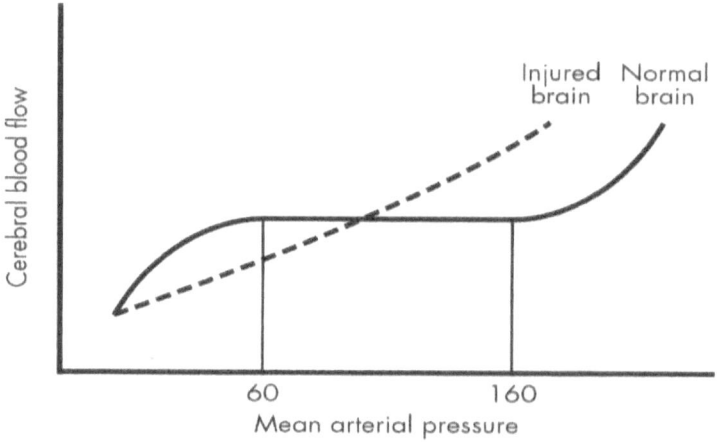

Figure 3.5 Autoregulation curve. The cerebral blood flow is maintained at a steady level, over a wide range of blood pressure, but when autoregulation is lost following brain injury, the curve assumes a more linear relationship and hypotension causes more profound reductions in blood flow, compared with the normal brain. Raised intracranial pressure (Figure 3.6, next page).

The cranium acts like a closed box. There is little room for expansion after the fontanelle and sutures close. Fluid is incompressible so if there is any extra fluid collection in the cranial cavity, be it haematoma, increasing cerebral oedema or vascular engorgement due to vasoparalysis and loss of autoregulation, it causes a disproportionate rise in intracranial pressure (ICP). Thus, when the compensatory mechanisms are exhausted, any increase in intracranial volume causes an exponential rise in ICP. A rise in ICP has two effects. First it reduces cerebral perfusion pressure (CPP) and may cause hypoxia of the brain secondary to impaired cerebral perfusion. The minimum CPP for brain survival is around 50-55 mmHg and 60-70 mmHg is preferable.

$$CPP = MAP - ICP \qquad [MAP = \text{Mean arterial pressure}]$$
$$MAP = \frac{\text{Systolic pressure} + (\text{Diastolic pressure} \times 2)}{3}$$

The normal ICP is around 5-10 mmHg and the MAP is normally about 90 mmHg. If the MAP drops to around 60 mmHg (BP of 80/50) and the ICP rises >20mmHg, the cerebral perfusion is severely compromised. The causes of raised intracranial pressure after head injury may include haematoma, increased cerebral blood flow due to cerebral vasodilatation (when the temperature is >38°C, hypercarbia, 'vasoparalysis'), epileptic activity, brain swelling secondary to injury, or the late complications of abscess formation and hydrocephalus. The commonest cause of hypercarbia is underventilation due to airway obstruction or inadequate breathing, which in turn results from an impaired central respiratory drive due to sedation, opiates, brain stem compression or injury.

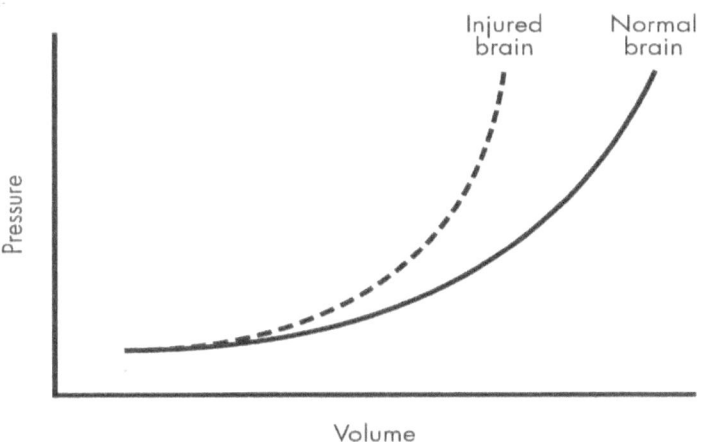

Figure 3.6 Pressure-volume curve. The injured brain loses compliance and becomes stiffer with the pressure volume curve shifting to the left. Thus, intracranial pressure rise is more severe for the same levels of intracranial volume. Mechanical brain shift and coning (see Figure 3. 7, next page).

Displacement of the brain stem downwards or laterally will impair conscious state and may lead to permanent brain stem injury with infarction or death. When the intracranial pressure rises and the intracranial contents can no longer accommodate the rise in pressure (usually due to an expanding haematoma) then coning may occur, usually with fatal results if left untreated. If the expanding lesion is in the supratentorial compartment the medial portion of the temporal lobes herniates through the tentorial hiatus.

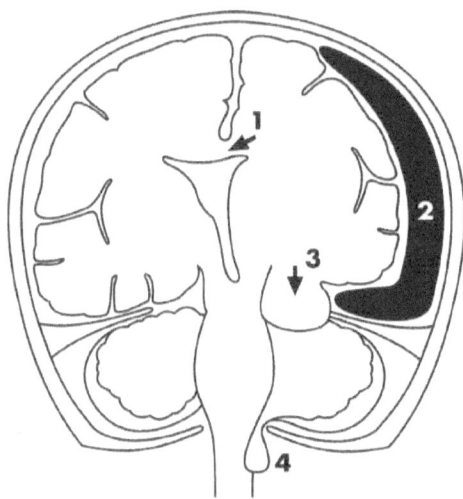

1.   Parafalcine herniation
2.   Subdural haematoma
3.   Uncal herniation
4.   Tonsillar herniation

Figure 3.7 Diagram showing sites of pressure coning due to an acute mass lesion and raised intracranial pressure.

Practice point

The earliest signs of coning are deteriorating conscious state or increasing restlessness.

A later sign is dilatation of the pupil due to pressure on the third nerve on the side of the haematoma. An expanding lesion in the posterior cranial fossa causes herniation of the cerebellar tonsils through the foramen magnum with pressure on the brain stem. Later signs of coning are irregular breathing, bradycardia and hypertension, deepening coma, and dilatation of the other pupil. A contralateral hemiparesis usually occurs with these other features but it may be ipsilateral if the cerebral peduncle on opposite side to the collection is compressed against the tentorial edge.

INTRACRANIAL HAEMATOMA

Intracranial haematoma from injured brain or meninges is an important cause of secondary brain injury because it is potentially treatable, particularly in the case of extradural haematoma. The techniques for surgical drainage of these conditions are described in the operative surgery chapter (Chapter 11, page 513). An **extradural (or epidural) haematoma** arises usually from branches of the middle meningeal artery (a branch of the external carotid artery that enters the skull through the foramen spinosum). A blow on the head with an underlying skull fracture is the most common cause. Deterioration in conscious level is usually rapid but the patient may be walking and talking shortly after injury and then develop unconsciousness within minutes or hours. The patient may initially lose consciousness, then awaken (lucid interval) and then deteriorate as the haematoma enlarges. As the bleeding develops the blood compresses the underlying meninges and brain (causing a shift of the midline structures). Downward pressure leads to herniation of the medial portion of the temporal lobe across the tentorium and coning. It is treatable by urgent evacuation of the clot by craniotomy or craniectomy and the prognosis is good. In LMICs about 80 per cent of patients have a good outcome. The sooner the collection is relieved, the better the prognosis because the underlying brain is usually in good condition (Figure 3.8, below).

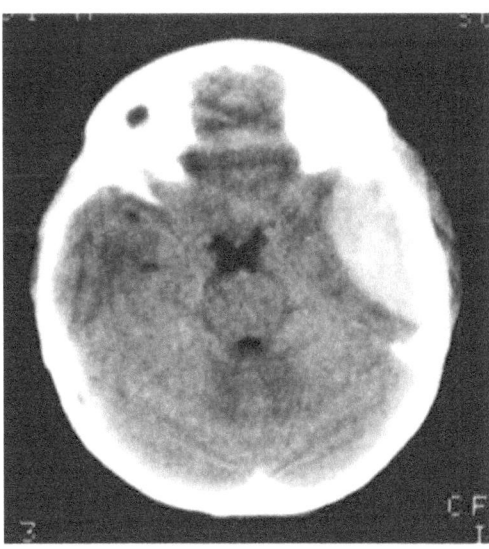

Figure 3.8 (a) Middle fossa extradural haematoma.

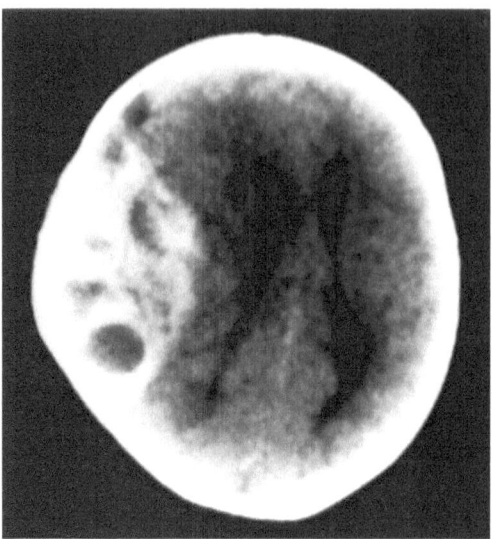

(b) A large frontoparietal extradural haematoma in an infant who fell off a change table onto a concrete floor. The child rapidly became comatose with fixed dilated pupils. Urgent evacuation of the collection produced a full recovery. Note the variegated appearance of the collection, which occurs when there is acute bleeding proceeding while the scan is being performed.

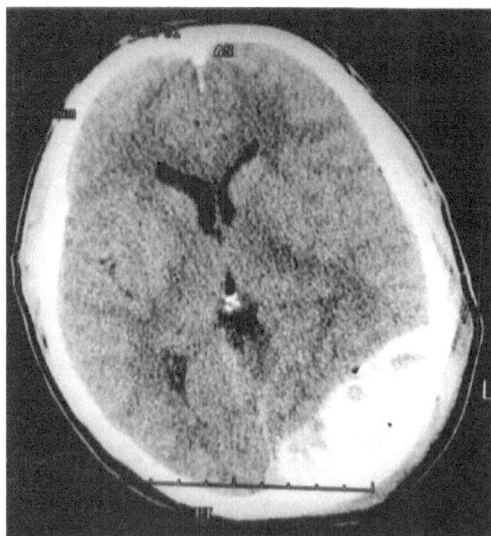

(c) Occipital extradural haematoma which is an unusual site, but underlay a parieto-occipital fracture in this case. Note the biconcave lens shape of the collection.

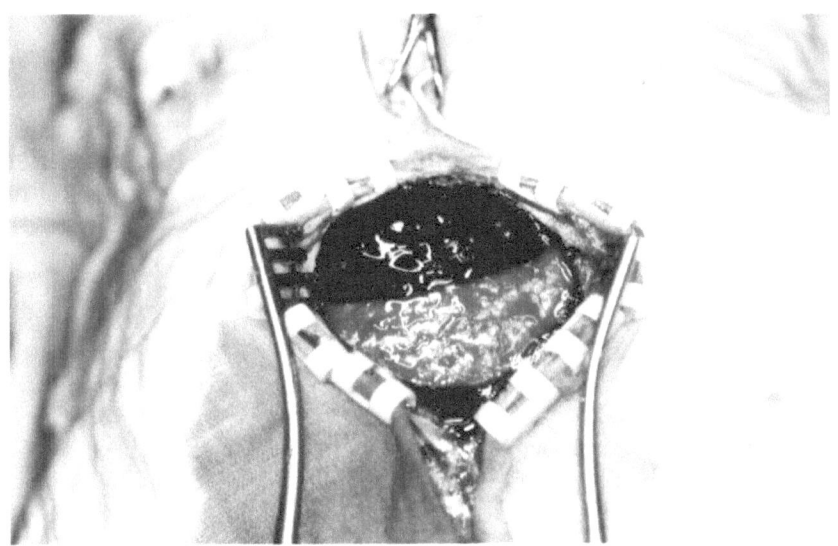

(d) Operative photograph of temporal craniotomy showing a solid dark epidural haematoma which was bulging out of the craniotomy and the adjacent oozing dural surface. Note the clear demarcation of the blood clot.

Figure 3.8 (a-d) Extradural haematoma.

Case report

*A 20-year-old man was struck on the head. He was seen in the emergency department an hour later where he was found to be drowsy but still able to talk and say what happened. He was able to walk. Fifteen minutes later the patient was comatose with a GCS of 6, his right pupil dilated and he had a left hemiplegia. The left pupil was also starting to dilate. He was rushed to the operating room but by the time he reached there, his GCS was 3 and both pupils were dilated. Right sided burr boles were immediately performed without anaesthetic, starting with a temporal burr hole. A large extradural haematoma was evacuated. At this point the patient woke up, tried to get off the operating table and was anaesthetised. The bleeding branch of the middle meningeal was ligated after raising a flap and the patient ultimately made a full recovery. **Lesson:** An extradural haematoma often causes rapid deterioration.*

An **acute subdural haematoma** develops as a result of bleeding from the vessels on the surface of the brain, bridging vessels between brain and dura or venous sinuses or the venous sinuses themselves. The temporal lobe bursting against the sharp edge of the lesser sphenoid wing in a deceleration injury, is also a common cause. There is a frequently a significant underlying primary brain injury (DAI) with the acute subdural haematoma.

The mechanism of injury is frequently a high velocity impact such as a high-speed motor vehicle accident. Acute subdural haematoma has a high mortality (36-79%) even in HICs with plenty of resources and neurosurgeons. They frequently result in considerable morbidity in survivors, who may suffer neurological disability and impairment and require considerable rehabilitation and subsequent support for daily living. Mortality is reduced considerably if surgery is performed within four hours of the injury. Only 15-30% of patients will have a good outcome (Figure 3.9, next page).

Subacute subdural haematoma by definition develops 2-10 days after head injury. There will be delayed deterioration in conscious level often with focal neurological signs.

A **chronic subdural haematoma** develops 10 days to 3-6 months after a head injury which has often appeared trivial.

It particularly affects the very young and the very old because the subarachnoid space is relatively large and therefore the bridging veins more susceptible to rupture when the brain suddenly moves following trauma. By the time it develops the patient may have forgotten the original injury and present with neurological signs, unexplained coma or a change in behaviour. Always consider the diagnosis in a patient with unexplained drowsiness or coma. A chronic subdural haematoma is a mimicker of other neurological conditions and may present with headaches, hemiparesis, cognitive decline, balance disturbance, seizures, and in an infant, enlarging head size (Figure 3.10, next page).

An **intracerebral haematoma** is difficult to recognise without a CT scanner because the haematoma develops within the brain substance. It needs to be suspected and, if present, an attempt made to evacuate it if the patient is deteriorating with focal signs. The likely scenario would be that the craniotomy has been performed, an extracerebral collection evacuated (or no collection is identified) and the brain remains very tense and bulging out of the craniotomy, a brain needle is passed into the brain and aspirated in different directions to detect the haematoma. The prognosis is poor if the haematoma is large and untreated (Figure 3.11, page 91).

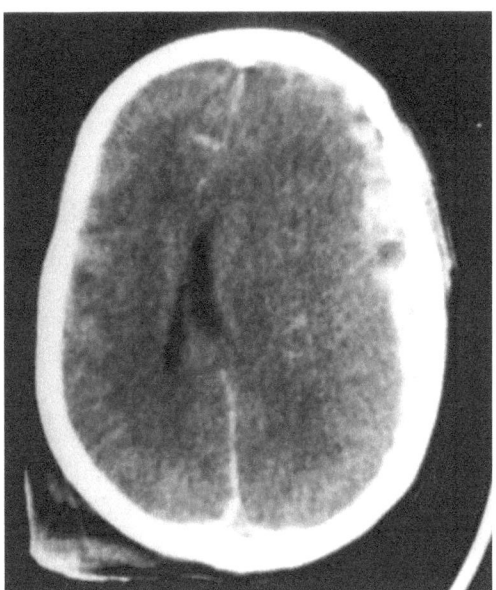

Figure 3.9 Acute left subdural haematoma. Axial CT scan. Note the convex shape following the curve of the skull. Note also the swollen hemisphere beneath the haematoma with shift and compression of the ventricles and midline structures to the opposite side.

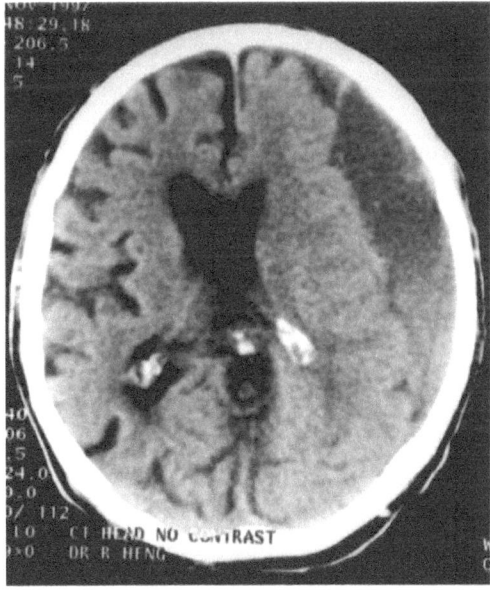

Figure 3.10 Chronic left subdural haematoma, showing hypodense extracerebral convex collection following the line of the skull. CT scan.

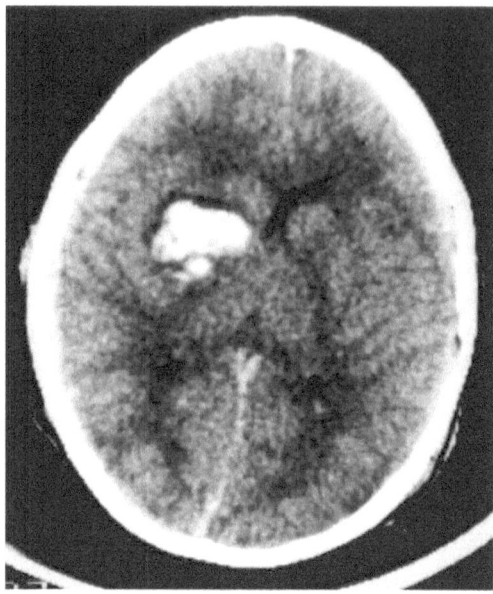

Figure 3.11 Traumatic intracerebral haematoma. CT scan. This 7-year-old boy suffered a closed head injury and progressively deteriorated 24-48 hours following the injury and was found to have an enlarging frontal haematoma. This was evacuated via craniotomy and he recovered, but was left with a contralateral spastic hemiparesis and some cognitive difficulties.

Concussion

'Concussion' represents a disturbance in conscious state and a period of post-traumatic amnesia (PTA) following a head injury. There is no observable pathological finding in mild concussion and any imaging performed in this situation does not show any abnormality. The severity of PTA can be assessed objectively with the Westmead Post Traumatic Amnesia Scale. See Appendix 5, page 658.

MANAGEMENT

Early management

The doctor who first sees the patient with a head injury must attend to the ABCs. The airway must be safeguarded whilst ensuring the cervical spine is controlled. A senior person should maintain in-line stabilisation of the cervical spine (i.e. in a neutral position) while intubation, if necessary, is being carried out. A surgical airway is sometimes required, by cricothyrotomy, if the patient cannot be intubated. Patients with a fracture to the middle third of the face may be difficult to intubate. The breathing must also be adequate, so tension pneumothorax and massive haemothorax must be drained urgently.

Patients who breathe poorly will need to be ventilated and ventilation can be achieved temporarily with an oral or nasal airway and 'bag and mask'. Hypotension and shock must be aggressively treated so that the cerebral perfusion pressure is adequate. Hypotension is a bad prognostic factor whether it occurs in the prehospital phase, in the emergency room during resuscitation or intraoperatively. The mean arterial blood pressure (MAP) should be kept above 70 mmHg (90/60) and preferably around 90 mmHg (110/80).

Practice point

Hypotension must be aggressively managed to avoid secondary brain damage from cerebral ischaemia.

The patient should then be assessed with a secondary survey from head to toe to exclude or treat other life-threatening injuries. Examination of the head injured patient involves recording the conscious level using the Glasgow Coma Scale (GCS) (Table 2.2, page 18), pupil size (Figure 3.12, next page) and reaction to light, and noting any neurological signs. Ask every conscious patient if they can see and test their eye movements. A common cause of missed eye injury is failure to ask the patient if they can see. Counting fingers is usually adequate. The entire scalp should be examined for lacerations or depressions (Figure 3.13, page 94). Look at the ear and nose for blood or CSF which may indicate a base of skull fracture. Look behind the ear for bruising around the mastoid (Battle's sign) and look for a retro-orbital haematoma (subconjunctival haemorrhage with no posterior limit). Both these signs suggest a fractured base of skull. Raccoon eyes (bruising around both orbits) indicate a fractured anterior cranial fossa. Where there is the possibility of a fractured base of skull a nasogastric tube is contraindicated as it may enter the cranial cavity via the fracture line in the anterior cranial fossa through the roof of the nose. An orogastric tube can be inserted as an alternative. Head injury patients are prone to develop paralytic ileus so gastric decompression may be a wise precaution even if other injuries do not demand it. The same tube may later be used for enteral feeding if the patient does not soon regain consciousness.

Practice point

Severe head injuries require gastric decompression. Pass an orogastric rather than a nasogastric tube if there is a fractured base of skull or fracture of the maxilla.

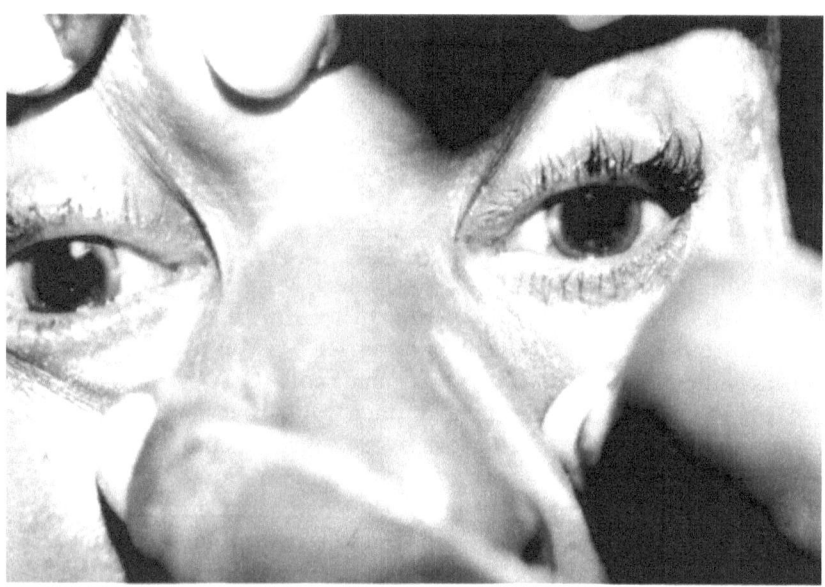

Figure 3.12 Patient with severe head injury, Glasgow Coma Score 3, and widely fixed dilated pupils. Note the eyes are slightly divergent, which occurs in deep coma with the eyes in their neutral relaxed position.

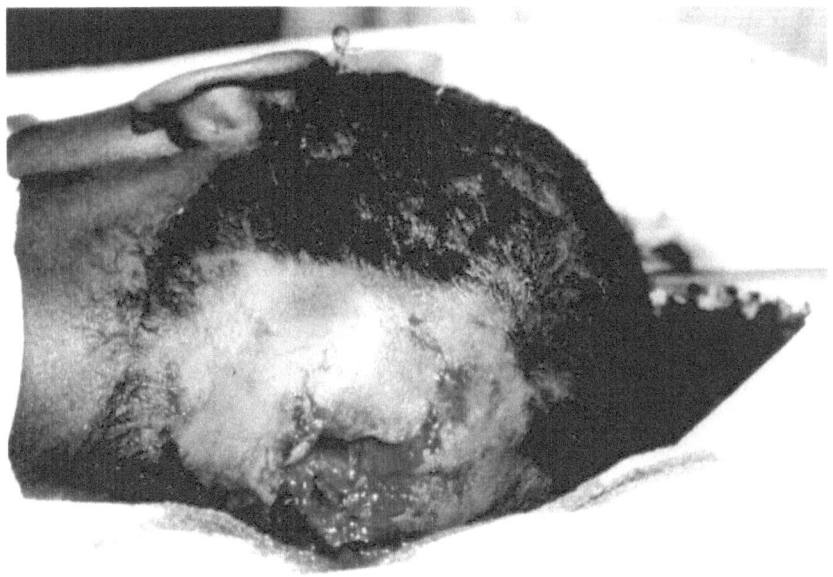

Figure 3.13 Compound depressed fracture of the occiput, which is easily missed if the patient is not log-rolled, and the posterior aspect of the head examined.

Practice point

Eye injuries: Ask every conscious patient if they can see and test their eye movements. A common cause of missed eye injury is failure to ask the patient if they can see. Shine a light in their eyes to look not only at pupillary reaction but also for hyphaema (blood in the anterior chamber) or unsuspected penetrating injuries.

When the patient is stable a lateral view of the cervical spine, an A-P and lateral of the skull are ordered if indicated. All unconscious patients should have an X-ray of their cervical spine. All seven cervical vertebrae and the top of T1 should be seen. A normal cervical spine X-ray does not exclude a cervical spine injury but has at least a 90-95 percent accuracy. A repeat X-ray with the shoulders pulled down or a swimmer's view (through the axilla with one arm above the head) can be made if all seven cervical vertebrae are not seen (Figure

5.5, page 223). The interpretation of cervical spine X-rays is discussed from page 221 onwards.

Table 3.1 Absolute indications for cervical spine X-ray in patients with head injuries.

1.	Unconsciousness
2.	Neck pain
3.	Restriction of neck movements or torticollis
4.	Paraesthesia or neurological signs

Practice point

The most important X-ray in an unconscious patient with a head injury is a lateral view of the cervical spine which shows all 7 cervical vertebrae and the top of T1.

A decision has to be made whether to admit the patient for observation, who to further investigate, who to transfer and who needs operative intervention.

Who should be admitted?

The indications for admission to hospital are shown in Table 3.2, next page. In countries where communication is good and there is an efficient ambulance service it may be possible to send some now alert patients with a history of unconsciousness home. However, in LMICs or where social support or transport is unreliable, it is usually safer to admit such patients for observation overnight.

Table 3.2 Indications for admission of patients with head injuries.

Unconsciousness

Altered consciousness

Restlessness and confusion

Aggressiveness

Drowsiness

Focal neurological signs

Drunk or drugged patients whom it is difficult to assess

Ongoing headache or severe headache

Ongoing post-traumatic amnesia

Dizziness

Diplopia or blurred vision

Blood or CSF draining from the ear or nose

Skull fractures

Associated injuries

Epilepsy

Young or elderly

Other medical conditions such as diabetes

Case report

A 25-year-old man was struck on the right temporal region with an iron bar. He lost consciousness and had a small laceration. He woke up on the way to hospital and was talking normally when he arrived in the emergency department. The emergency room doctor examined him, found him to be neurologically normal, sutured his laceration, prescribed tetanus toxoid and sent him home. The next morning, he was readmitted with a GCS of 5, fixed and dilated pupils and was not moving his left side. Despite evacuation of a right extradural haematoma the patient did not improve and he died 4 days later on a ventilator in the intensive care unit.

Case report *(Continued)*

Lesson: This patient should have been admitted because he had been knocked unconscious. Extradural haematoma is well known to present with a lucid interval. Had the patient been admitted, deterioration would have been noted and he could have been operated on promptly with at least an 80 percent chance of full recovery.

Further investigations

These are limited in many LMIC hospitals. CT scanning is the best method of visualising the damage but most patients with severe head injuries in low resource settings do not have access to such a service. The general surgeon is then often forced to make diagnostic burr holes. A carotid angiogram can be performed even with simple equipment (page 52) in cases where the decision to operate is difficult, but most general surgeons will still find it easier to do diagnostic burr holes. The technique of direct carotid puncture and timing of films is not always easy if it is performed rarely but when made routinely for uncertain cases it gives valuable information. The angiogram should not delay emergency surgery.

Indications for diagnostic burr holes

Deteriorating level of consciousness not due to other correctable factors such as hypoxia, hypotension. Usually a deterioration of 2 GCS points is an indication for exploration. The speed of deterioration also influences the decision.

The faster the deterioration the more strongly you should consider burr holes.

- Unconscious patient with focal neurological signs.
- Unconscious patient with a dilating pupil (in the absence of a direct injury to the eye).
- Severe head injury (GCS < 9) who develops fits or fails to improve.
- A hemiplegia that is becoming more extensive.

Siting of burr holes

Burr holes should be made in the temporal, frontal and parietal region. The most likely side to have a haematoma is selected on the basis of the site of injury and the neurological signs. If an extradural is not found the dura should be opened to look for a subdural and if this is negative then three burr holes should be made on the opposite side. A posterior fossa extradural haematoma is uncommon. If a haematoma is found it will be necessary to do a craniectomy or cut out a bone flap to completely evacuate the clot and control the bleeding (from page 500).

Who to transfer?

Where facilities for CT scanning are limited the indications for transfer to a centre with CT or a neurosurgeon are:
1. Unconscious patient who is not rapidly deteriorating.
2. Unexplained seizures.
3. Abnormal neurological signs in a stable patient.
4. Depressed fracture which might involve a venous sinus.
5. Persistent CSF leak (>7-10 days).

Local policies may dictate other criteria for transfer or for CT scanning. This will depend on the facilities and skills available. Severe head injuries (GCS < 9) do not all need to be transferred if they can be adequately nursed whilst awaiting recovery. The guiding principle is that the patient should not be made worse by transfer for a CT scan or performing any other investigation. Rapid deterioration is an indication for burr holes. Urgent surgery should not be delayed by investigations if the surgery is clearly indicated. The CT scan will need to be used selectively unless the scanner is situated in the hospital in which the patient is admitted. A doctor or senior nurse will need to accompany the patient being transferred. If you are not willing to go with the patient perhaps they do not need to be sent.

The same principles apply when considering which patient should be transferred to the care of a neurosurgeon. The decision to transfer should be discussed with the relevant specialist. Some complications of head injury discussed below such as persistent CSF leak, depressed fractures involving a venous sinus or a large aerocele may be better treated by a neurosurgeon. If no neurosurgery service or CT scan is available, the general surgeon will need to treat the patient as described in this book.

Operative intervention

The presence of an intracranial haematoma is the major indication for surgery. Often it is the possibility of a haematoma in a deteriorating patient in which hypoxia and hypotension have been corrected that is the major indication for surgery in the form of diagnostic burr holes. The indications for surgery are discussed above and the different procedures are discussed on page 463.

Oxygen, airway and ventilation management

All unconscious patients should have supplemental oxygen in the early period after head injury. A rate of 12 litres per minute is advised in the initial stages but later this can be reduced to 3·4 litres per minute depending on the condition of the patient. This aims to avoid secondary brain damage from hypoxia. Intubation or tracheostomy is indicated to safeguard the airway if the GCS is 8 or less.

Facial fractures or associated chest injuries may also make intubation advisable. Where there are adequate facilities for ventilation, patients with a GCS of 8 or less should be electively ventilated to avoid hypoxia and underventilation leading to hypercarbia and raised intracranial pressure. Hyperventilation should generally be avoided. Many LMIC hospitals do not have facilities to test blood gases to monitor the effectiveness of oxygenation or the carbon dioxide levels. If available, pulse oximeters and capnometers will enable oxygen saturation and end tidal CO_2. When the status of the cervical spine is unknown, airway management should be carried out with the neck protected, and maintained in as neutral a position as possible, avoiding twisting, rotation and excessive flexion or extension.

Patients who require diagnostic burr holes or who need to have a haematoma evacuated, should receive supplemental oxygen and be ventilated postoperatively whenever possible. The endotracheal tube should certainly be left in place to safeguard the airway. Premature extubation is a common cause of postoperative hypoxia, secondary brain injury and death. Tracheostomy needs to be considered for airway management in comatose patients who require intubation and/or ventilation for over a week. Tracheostomy makes airway toilet much easier and may reduce the length of time for ventilation. This is particularly so in the low resource settings where good ICU facilities may not exist. In these situations, perform a tracheostomy earlier rather than later. If only red rubber endotracheal tubes are available for intubation, then a tracheostomy should be done within 48 hours because the red rubber is so irritant to the tracheal lining that it will cause ulceration and, later this will heal with fibrosis and stricture. Tracheostomy offers an alternative means of airway suction if retention of secretions is the main problem.

Case report

*A patient was admitted with a severe head injury, unconscious with an obstructed airway and dilating pupils. The patient's teeth were clenched so no one was able to clear the airway and insert an endotracheal tube. All the other injuries were attended, including suturing a scalp laceration and splinting of a fractured femur. Oxygen by face mask was given. Later, when the consultant was called, he found the patient still had an obstructed airway and that much secondary brain damage must have occurred from hypoxia. The patient was intubated using diazepam (suxamethonium was not necessary) and then ventilated. By this time his GCS was 3, his pupils were dilated but slightly reactive. He made no improvement and died 48 hours later. **Lesson:** This patient suffered secondary brain damage due to hypoxia. He should have been intubated when first seen or, if intubation were impossible, a surgical cricothyrotomy could have been performed.*

Fluid management

The aim of fluid management is to ensure an adequate cerebral perfusion. Hypotension is bad but so is cerebral interstitial oedema secondary to fluid overload. A balance has to be struck. The blood pressure should be stabilised but then fluids should be restricted compatible with a urine output of 30-50 ml (0.5-1.0mg/kg) per hour in an adult (1 ml/kg in a child). Patients with severe head injuries should be catheterised to allow the urine output to be monitored hourly. 0.9% saline is preferred to dextrose which has a greater tendency to exacerbate cerebral oedema. In most low resource settings intracranial pressure will not be monitored so the pulse, blood pressure, state of the peripheral circulation (nail-bed blanching/ capillary refill and temperature of the tip of the nose or hands) and urine output will be the only way of judging fluid management. A central venous pressure line may also help guide fluid replacement therapy. Colloids and albumin solutions are avoided. Blood and fresh frozen plasma may be required in the resuscitation.

Convulsions

Convulsions cause hypoxia and the straining which occurs during the convulsion may cause a rise in intracranial pressure. Diazepam (0.1-0.2 mg/kg IV) or clonazepam (0.25mg IV repeated up to 1mg [not per Kg]), phenobarbitone (phenobarbital) (50-200 mg repeated after 6 hours if necessary), should be used to stop the convulsion (paraldehyde is an alternative for babies and young children) and further seizures should be prevented with phenytoin (100 mg 8 hourly by nasogastric tube or infusion) or levetiracetam 500 mg 12 hourly, or phenobarbitone (60 mg 8 hourly) prophylaxis. The development of seizures may be an indication for further investigations once the airway is secure and the seizure is over. These doses require adjustment for children. Seizures are not an indication for diagnostic burr holes unless the patient is progressively deteriorating, or is failing to improve. A hemiparesis following the seizure is most likely a temporary Todd's paresis and does not indicate a need for surgery.

Scalp lacerations

The presence of a scalp laceration should alert the clinician to the possibility of an open depressed fracture that requires debridement. Debridement cannot be carried out completely unless the fracture is elevated. A gloved finger can be placed in the wound to palpate the underlying bone for a depressed fracture. Scalp wounds should be cleaned, irrigated and foreign matter removed. They require minimal excision and can be primarily sutured up to 24 hours after the injury. Prophylactic antibiotics are not indicated unless there is an underlying fracture. Tetanus toxoid should be given. Scalp lacerations are a common cause of tetanus in many parts of the tropics or wherever vaccination coverage is poor, even though the incidence of tetanus itself has reduced with immunisation programmes. Scalp defects should be closed whenever possible especially when there is exposed cranium in the base of the wound. A rotation flap may need to be fashioned although healthy pericranium will accept a split skin graft (see Chapter 11, from page 540).

Cephalhaematoma

A cephalhaematoma is a collection of blood under the scalp occurring in young children or babies.

The two types are:
1. **Subgaleal or subaponeurotic haematoma** in which the galea is lifted up off the periosteum and may be associated with an underlying skull fracture in children <1 year of age. It presents as a soft fluctuant mass, which crosses the sutures and may become large enough to cause shock and anaemia. They do not calcify.
2. **Subperiosteal haematoma** most commonly seen in the newborn period with an incidence of 1 percent of deliveries, particularly following a difficult childbirth and are commonest in the parietal areas. They are usually unilateral and often enlarge in the first few days. There is an underlying skull fracture in 10-25 per cent of the cases. The blood elevates the periosteum and is limited by the sutures. It is firmer than the subgaleal haematoma and the scalp moves over it freely. They may occasionally calcify.

Treatment

The important aspect to management is not to explore the haematoma but rather, leave the scalp to tamponade the bleeder. These haematomas usually resolve within 2-4 weeks. Aspiration is not recommended because infection may be introduced, but tense collections may be relieved by aspiration at 4-5 days. Even if they calcify the skull will remodel to a normal contour within 3-6 months. Blood transfusion may be necessary for large lesions. A subgaleal haematoma may also occur in older children and adults.

Case report

It was State of Origin rugby league night in Australia and televised throughout the Pacific. A 20-year-old 'reds' fan watching with relatives who were opposition supporters, was celebrating a score when he was struck over the midline of his scalp, suffering a linear fracture over his sagittal suture which must have also opened the sagittal sinus. He presented confused, restless and distressed.

Case report *(Continued)*

The doctor first seeing him thought the patient's condition was due to a intracranial haematoma. However, when the patient reached theatre a senior surgeon looked at the large boggy swelling under his scalp and advised his junior to resuscitate the patient and defer operation.

After resuscitation the patient's condition improved, he was fully conscious and the haematoma was aspirated 5 days later. A potentially dangerous procedure was avoided. He was discharged home and made an uncomplicated recovery.

FRACTURES OF THE SKULL (FIGURE 3.14, NEXT PAGE)

Linear fractures alert the clinician to an increased likelihood of there being an underlying haematoma and to the most probable side of injury when performing diagnostic burr holes. They do not require specific treatment except the patient should be admitted for observation. Further decision making is based on the general condition of the patient, the conscious level and any neurological signs.

All open fractures of the vault should be explored and debrided. Most should be closed primarily, paying particular attention to dural closure which provides a barrier to CNS infection. Closed depressed fractures should be elevated non-urgently if the patient is otherwise well and stable.

Indications for elevation include the thickness of the depression being greater than the thickness of the skull, or the presence of neurological signs. The presence of an obvious depression, particularly on the forehead is also an indication for elevation. Beware of elevating closed depressed fractures over a venous sinus if facilities for blood transfusion are not good or if the surgeon is inexperienced. The management of venous sinus bleeds is discussed on page 501.

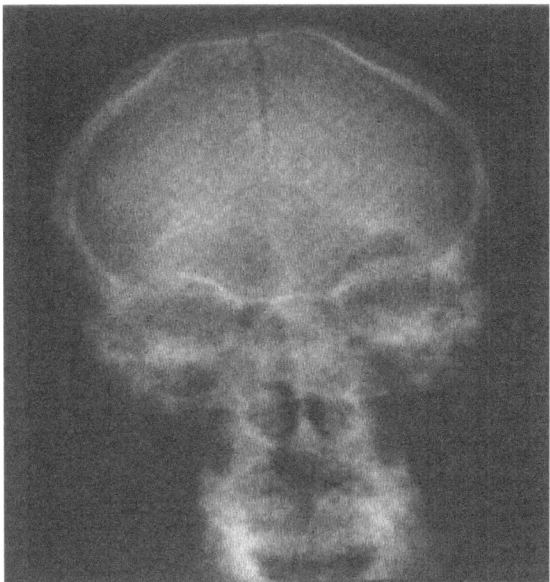

Figure 3.14 Skull fracture with diastasis of sagittal suture.

Depressed fractures, open and closed (Figure 3.15, next page and Figure 3.16, page 108)

Case report

*A young woman had been struck on the head by her husband with a bush knife. She was fully conscious but complaining of severe headache, and was bleeding from a scalp laceration. The scalp laceration was sutured by the nurse before the doctor was called. The doctor was satisfied with the patient's condition and admitted her to the ward for observation. He then attended all his other emergencies, only going to bed at 5 am. For the next two days the patient was well, but then she began to deteriorate with fever and neck stiffness. An open depressed fracture had not been elevated and the patient developed a brain abscess. **Lesson**: Always elevate an open depressed fracture. When the abscess was drained pieces of hair, scalp and wool (from a woollen hat) were found driven into the fracture and the brain substance.*

Case report

A 25-year-old male had an open depressed fracture on the midline near the vertex of his skull. He was fully conscious without neurological signs. On exploration and elevation, it was found that some of the fragments had penetrated the superior sagittal sinus. There was a shortage of the patient's blood group in the blood bank. The wound was debrided, all foreign matter was removed but some of the depressed fragments were left pressing on the sinus because of the difficulty in obtaining haemostasis. Crushed muscle and Surgicel were used to encourage clotting. **Lesson**: *It is better to stop elevating if one cannot guarantee enough blood. This patient's wound was well debrided, the underlying brain was safe and further elevation might have caused uncontrollable haemorrhage. This patient made an uneventful recovery.*

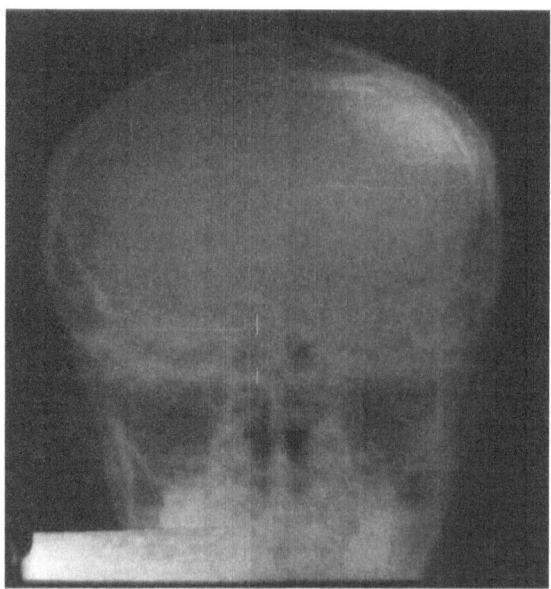

Figure 3.15 (a) Depressed fracture seen as a double image of the skull in the upper left side of the vault (poor quality radiograph).

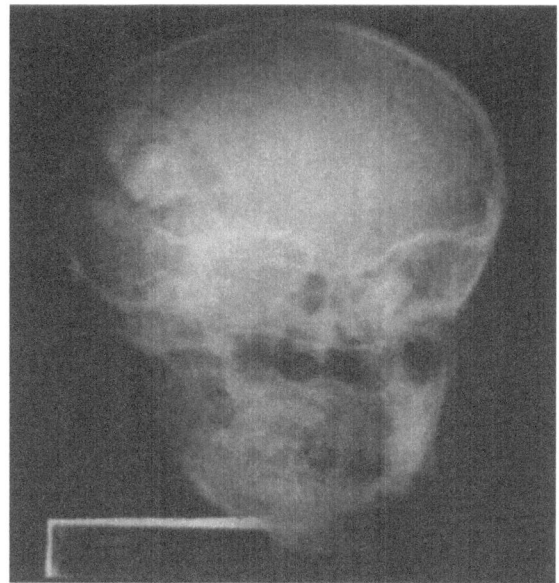

(b) Comminuted depressed right temporoparietal fracture (poor quality radiograph).

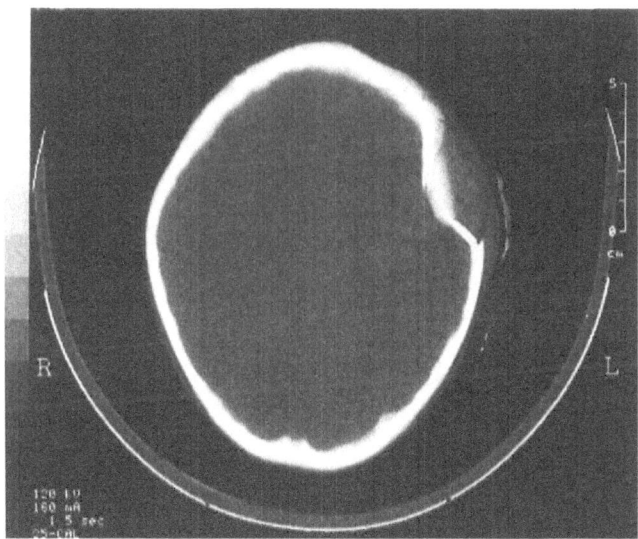

(c) Depressed fracture in the frontotemporal region causing underlying haematoma and dural tear. The child with this injury was dysphasic after being accidentally struck in the head by a cricket bat. The clot was evacuated, the dura repaired and the dysphasia largely recovered. The CT bone density images show the extent of the fracturing and the CT with brain density images.

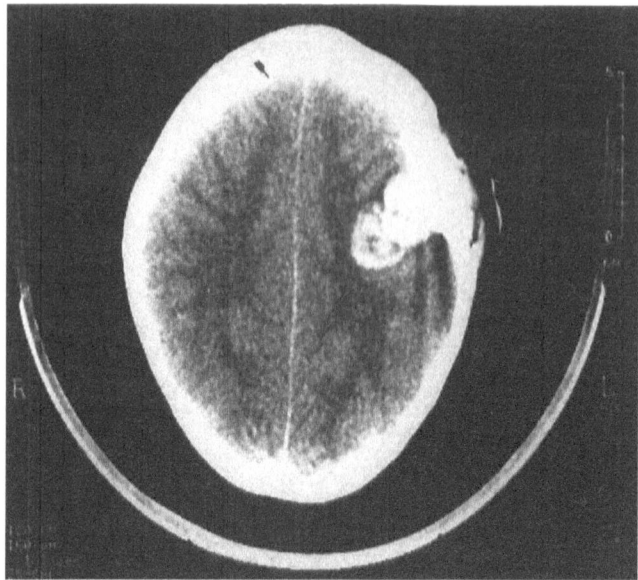

(d) Clearly shows the extent of the underlying brain injury.

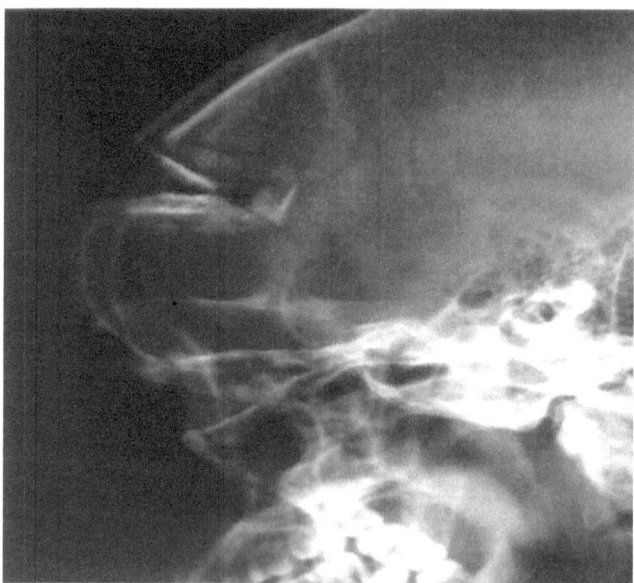

(e) Lateral skull x-ray showing a depressed fracture to the frontal bone caused by a machete blow to the head.

Figure 3.15 (a-e) Depressed fracture of the skull.

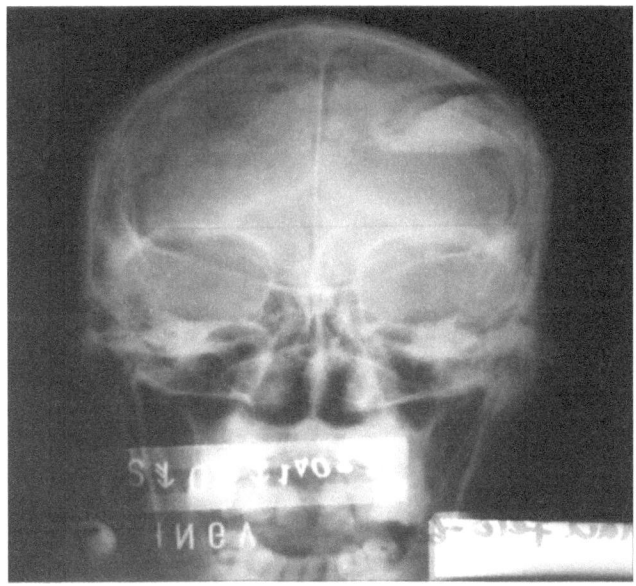

Figure 3.16 (a) AP skull radiograph showing a linear depressed fracture.

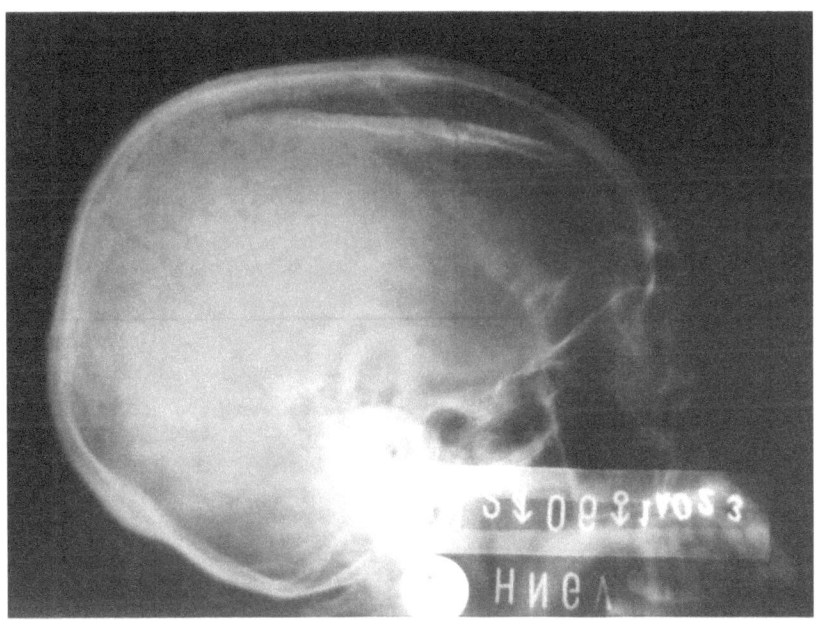

(b) Lateral skull radiographs showing a linear depressed fracture.

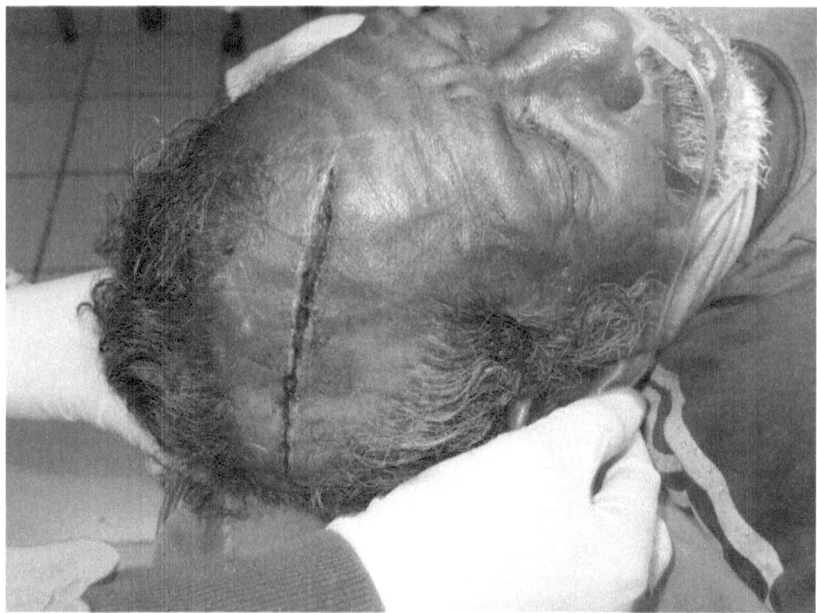

(c) Photograph showing the axe wound.

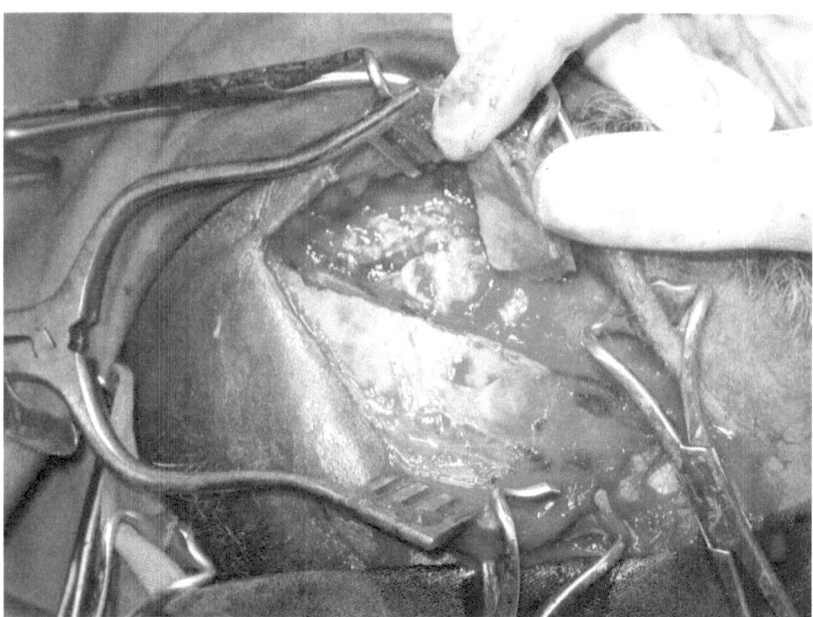

(d) Operative photograph showing the comminuted depressed fracture.

Figure 3.16 (a-d) Depressed fracture of the skull.

Base of skull fractures

These should be suspected if the patient has blood or CSF leaking from the ear or the nose. The skull X-ray often does not show the fracture. An aerocele especially on a brow-up view may indicate a fractured base of skull (air enters the cranial cavity via the sinuses or nasal passages). The air can clearly be seen on a CT scan. There is controversy over the use of prophylactic antibiotics for these fractures. Currently many neurosurgeons do not recommend their use because they may not prevent meningitis and resistant strains of bacteria may emerge. However, there are no studies from developing countries which provide hard evidence for this view and many surgeons will continue to advocate prophylactic antibiotics for all open fractures including fractures of the base of the skull. Penicillin and chloramphenicol or a sulphonamide are commonly used. Patients in deep coma (GCS 3-5) with base of skull fractures tend to do badly because they also have diffuse brain injury.

MISCELLANEOUS PROBLEMS

CSF Leak (Figure 3.17, next page)

Nasal CSF leak (rhinorrhoea) may arise from fractures through the frontal, ethmoid and sphenoid sinus, the cribriform plate, or the petrous temporal bone through the middle ear, and the Eustachian tube to the nasopharynx. CSF leak is a clinical diagnosis which is observed by the surgeon or described by the patient. Dripping of fluid from the nose may be induced by sitting the awake patient, flexing the neck and tipping the head forwards. Fractures through the cribriform plate may cause anosmia. You should examine the sense of smell.

Management

CSF rhinorrhoea - This usually ceases within a week. Prophylactic antibiotics do not need to be continued for more than 5 days. If it persists and is small it is best to wait another 1-2 weeks before proceeding to dural repair which can be performed transfrontally. The transnasal approach by an ENT surgeon may be an alternative. CSF rhinorrhoea is common after fractures of the middle third of the face (maxilla, Le Fort III) and will often close after reduction of the fracture. If a dural leak is not repaired there is a small risk of delayed meningitis. The problem with a profuse CSF leak which closes after the first week is that it may be herniated brain which finally seals the leak and the risk of delayed meningitis will be ever present. An aerocele on skull X-ray is an absolute indication for dural repair. The procedure is not beyond the capabilities of some general surgeons and is described on page 537. The procedure should preferably be performed by a neurosurgeon and transfer will need to be arranged. CSF from the ear (otorrhoea) usually closes spontaneously and does not normally require surgery.

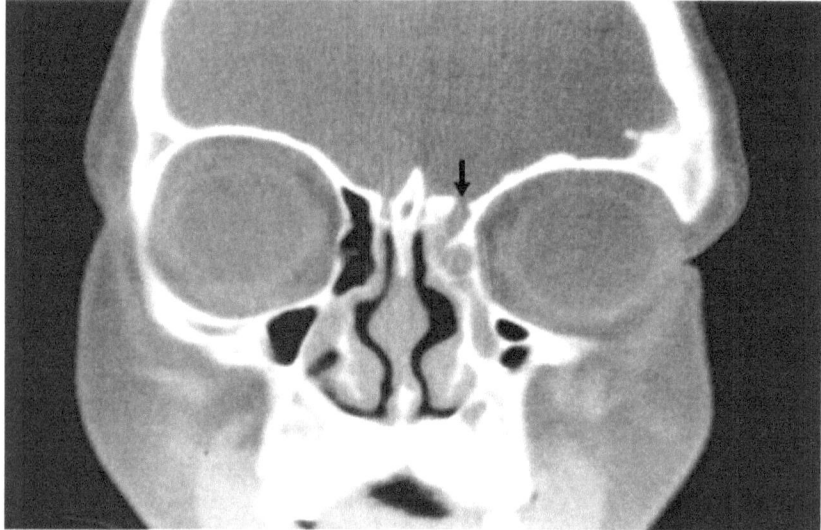

Figure 3.17 Coronal CT image (bone windows) showing bony discontinuity in the left cribriform plate region, with CSF tracking down into the ethmoid air cells. Arrow points to the defect in the skull base.

Aerocele

An aerocele is a collection of intracranial air and is an indication of an open fracture or a fracture line extending into an air sinus. The aerocele can be identified in a skull X-ray or CT scan. Prophylactic antibiotics can be given. Rarely an aerocoele may be tense, cause pressure effects and require aspiration through a burr hole.

Penetrating wounds

Penetrating wounds to the head and spine may cause immediate neurological deficit from the division of neural pathways or structures, or interruption of blood supply to the brain, or may result in enlarging haematomas, which will cause an increasing neurological deficit and require emergency evacuation. The superficial in-driven bone fragments should be extricated and a dural repair performed (Figure 3.18, below).

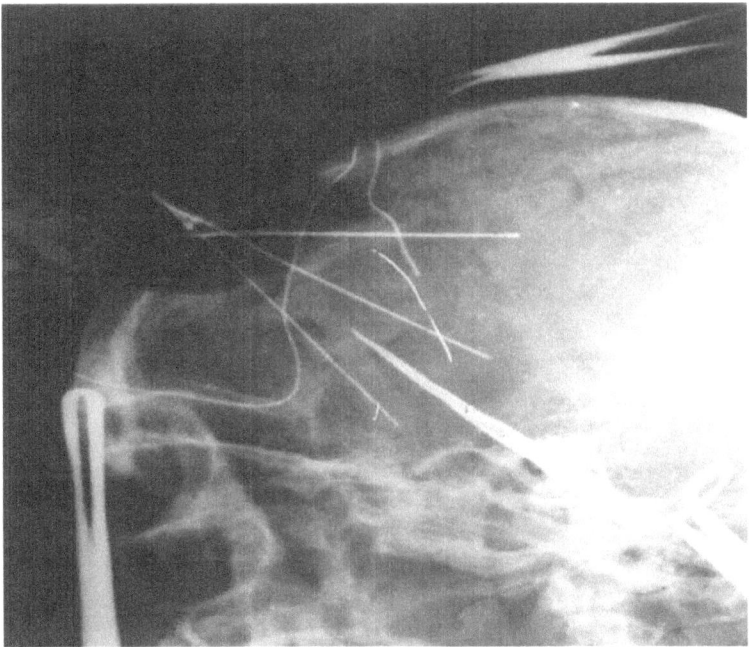

Figure 3.18 20-year-old man with an intracranial arrow head which had pierced the foramen magnum and resulted in a delayed brain abscess. The abscess was drained and the arrow removed via a frontal craniotomy.

Do not remove the spear or other implement from the head or spine until the patient is anaesthetised on the operating table and the surgeon is ready to explore the wound and obtain haemostasis. Stab wounds to the head may injure cerebral vessels causing false or pseudo-aneurysms, and arteriovenous (A-V) fistulae. False cerebral aneurysms often undergo late rupture and cause acute and life-threatening or fatal subarachnoid haemorrhage.

The A-V fistulae may progressively enlarge and eventually rupture. Early cerebral angiography, if available is helpful to diagnose these vascular injuries, and formulate a plan of management. The management of these delayed complications usually requires advanced microneurosurgery and the embolisation techniques of the interventional neuroradiologist, but accessible vascular lesions in the neck, orbit, or superficial parts of the cranium may be amenable to simple excisional surgery, even without angiography. Retained bullet fragments are often difficult to remove unless they are near the entry wound through the cranium (Figure 3.19, below). If the patient is fully conscious or stable the correct management is to debride the entry (and exit) wounds, to suck out or excise any necrotic brain but not to probe blindly for the bullet. It may migrate later, it may cause infection but, in our experience, the general surgeon and patient are better to accept the bullet is in the head and, if the patient is well, leave it there. A bullet sitting in a major venous sinus is a particularly difficult problem to manage. Ideally it should be removed but it may be wise to leave it there, particularly if blood for transfusion is scarce and surgeon is inexperienced.

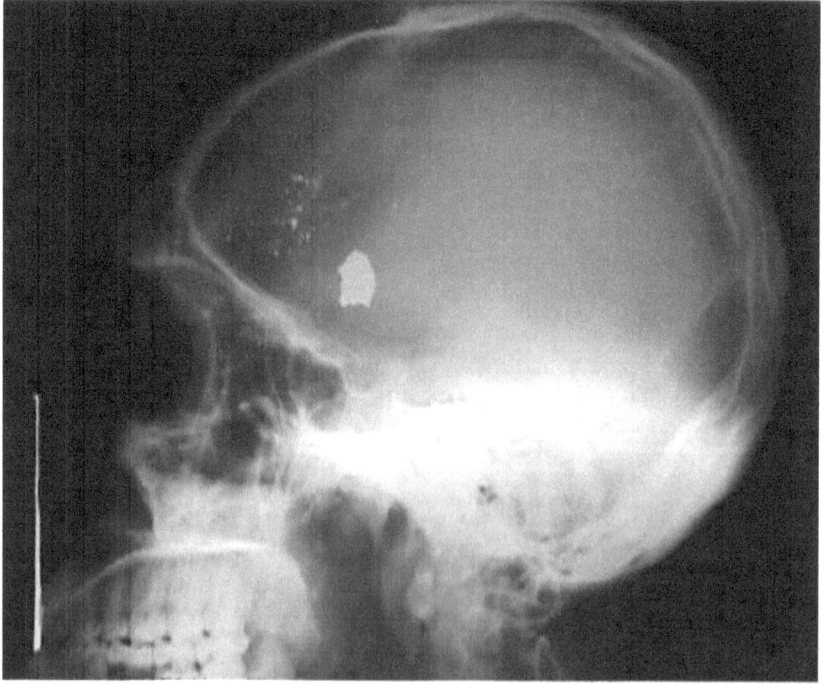

Figure 3.19 (a)

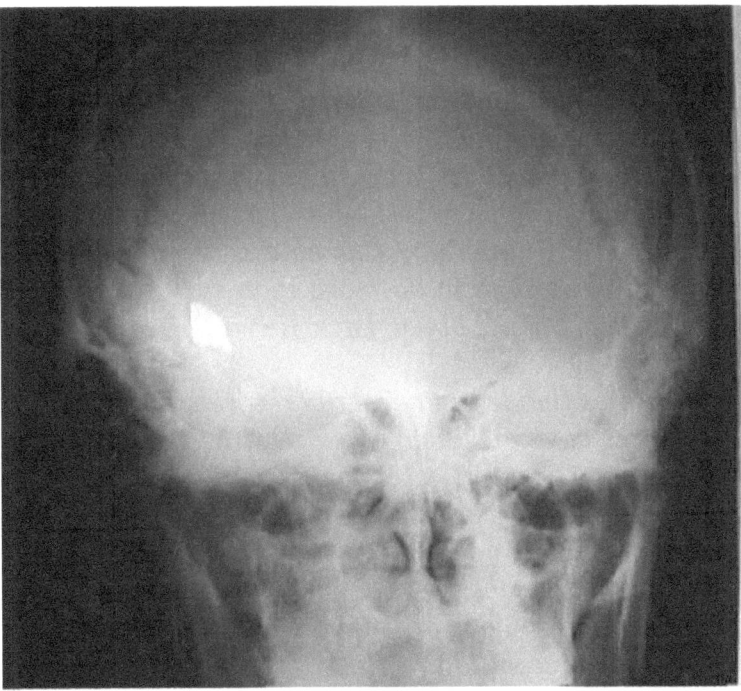

(b)

Figure 3.19 (a-b) Retained bullet fragment in left temporal region. This patient was alive and well and presented 6 years after the injury.

Case report

An 8-year-old boy was caught in cross-fire and sustained a bullet wound to the occiput in the midline. A skull X-ray showed the bullet to be lying just beneath the cranium posteriorly. The child was resuscitated (the wound had bled profusely) and was taken to theatre to remove the bullet fragment. The bullet lay half in and half out of the sagittal sinus. Removing the bullet caused massive haemorrhage.

The head of the operating table was elevated, the sinus was packed with muscle and Surgicel. Fortunately, the bleeding was controlled and the child made an uneventful recovery.

Case report

A 30-year old man was shot in the head. The bullet entered his frontal lobes and even crossed the midline. He was fully conscious. CT scanning was not available. The only investigation was a skull radiograph which showed the bullet in the middle of the contralateral frontal lobe. The entry site was debrided but the surgeon felt unable to do more than suck some liquefied, necrotic brain out of the bullet track. He was given prophylactic antibiotics for 10 days.

The patient made an uneventful recovery and 4 years after the incident is alive and well, coming to the surgical clinic for annual reviews. The bullet has not yet moved or caused infection. The general surgeon felt that removing the bullet would have done more harm than good.

Lesson: *Late sepsis is not uncommon after incomplete removal of a foreign body or weapon. Retained arrow, knife or spear-tips may present late with sepsis. Objects which traverse the nose or orbit and then enter the intracranial cavity may also result in intracranial sepsis presenting late even if they have been removed.*

BLAST INJURY (FIGURE 3.20, PAGE 118)

Bomb explosions are very common in war zones but have become more frequent occurrences in civilian settings.[10] Military neurosurgeons have treated many victims of bomb blast in the last 15 years[11] and have learnt how best to treat these complex injuries.[12] Surgeons in developing countries should also become familiar with how to manage patients with injuries due to bomb blast. Terrorist

---

[10]Bell RS, et al. Early decompressive craniectomy for severe penetrating and closed head injury during wartime. Neurosurgical Focus. 2010;28(5):E1.
[11]Bell RS, et al. Military traumatic brain and spinal column injury: a 5-year study of the impact blast and other military grade weaponry on the central nervous system. The Journal of Trauma. 2009;66(4):S104-111.
[12]Rosenfeld JV, et al. Blast-related traumatic brain injury. Lancet Neurology. 2013;12(9): 882-893.

incidents involving detonation of **improvised explosive devices (IEDs)** concealed as roadside bombs, in suicide vests or placed in vehicles have become all too common and are injuring increasing numbers of innocent civilians going about their daily lives.

The four main types of trauma caused by bomb blasts consist of combinations of primary blast injury, fragmentation injury, displacement injury from persons or objects being physically thrown by the blast and miscellaneous injury including burns[13] which may affect the face, scalp and respiratory tract.[14]

Trauma to the head and neck has been a common injury pattern following exposure to bomb blast. These bomb blast injuries are frequently associated with gross brain swelling and raised intracranial pressure. The management of these injuries frequently requires early decompressive craniectomy.[15]

These victims frequently have injuries to other body regions including penetrating neck injury, blast pulmonary injury (causing pulmonary haemorrhage and oedema), intra-abdominal solid and hollow visceral injury, peripheral vascular injury, fractures and traumatic limb amputations.

Pathophysiology of blast injury to the brain

There is a wide spectrum of injury to the brain, head and neck caused by bomb blast[16] ranging from mild concussion to severe life-threatening or non-survivable trauma.[17] This is dependent on the distance of the victim from the epicentre of the blast, whether the victim is in an enclosed or open space and the position and body disposition of the victim (standing or horizontal).

The pathophysiology of blast injury to the head has been studied extensively in rodent and pig models.[18] The over-pressure waves generated from the bomb blast epicentre results in shock waves passing through the skull and skull orifices and through the brain

---

[13]*Neuhaus SJ, Sharwood PF, Rosenfeld JV. Terrorism and blast explosions: lessons for the Australian surgical community. ANZ Journal of Surgery. 2006;76(7):637-644.*

[14]*Rosenfeld J. Neurosurgical injuries related to terror. Chapter 19 IN Essentials of Terror Medicine. Ed HJ, Shapira S, Cole LA. New York: Springer Verlag, 2009.*

[15]*Rosenfeld JV, Bell RS, Armonda R. Current concepts in penetrating and blast injury to the central nervous system. World Journal of Surgery. 2015;39(6):1352-1362.*

[16]*Bandak FA, et al. Injury biomechanics, neuropathology, and simplified physics of explosive blast and impact mild traumatic brain injury. Handbook of Clinical Neurology. 2015;127:89-104.*

[17]*Ling G, Ecklund JM, Bandak FA. Brain injury from explosive blast: description and clinical management. Handbook of Clinical Neurology. 2015;127:173-180.*

[18]*Bauman RA, et al. An introductory characterization of a combat-casualty-care relevant swine model of closed head injury resulting from exposure to explosive blast. Journal of Neurotrauma. 2009;26(6):841-860.*

and reflecting off the inside of the skull to magnify the effect. The physics of blast injury is complex and multifaceted.[19] There is diffuse brain swelling, diffuse axonal injury (DAI) and combinations of intracranial haemorrhage including epidural, subdural, intracerebral and intraventricular. The brain oedema is often severe and results in life-threatening intracranial hypertension.

This is compounded by penetrating metal fragments of bomb and skull bone fragments, often with dirt, fragments of clothing, skin and hair entering the brain in addition to the metal. These penetrating wounds are heavily contaminated. If the explosion is on the ground, the trajectory of fragments may pass from below through the facial skeleton, orbits, middle cranial fossa or posterior fossa into the brain. Complex compound depressed fractures of the cranial vault and basal skull fractures with cerebrospinal (CSF) leaks result. Pseudoaneurysms and cerebral vasospasm develop in a significant number of severe blast TBI victims[20] and may cause delayed deterioration.[21]

The eyes and ear drums, ossicles, cochlea and vestibular organs may also be injured. Victims are frequently deaf after exposure to blast. The deafness recovers to a variable degree. The structures in the neck are also vulnerable including pharynx, larynx, carotid and vertebral arteries, spine and spinal cord. High velocity missile or projectile penetrating injury involves direct pressure effects of the projectile and cavitation of surrounding brain with resultant intracerebral haemorrhage and brain swelling are both quite different from blunt injury and diffuse axonal injury (DAI) caused by deceleration.[22]

---

[19]Rosenfeld JV, et al. Blast-related traumatic brain injury. Lancet Neurology. 2013;12(9):882-893.
[20]Ling G, et al. Explosive blast neurotrauma. Journal of Neurotrauma. 2009;26(6):815-825.
[21]Bell RS, et al. The evolution of the treatment of traumatic cerebrovascular injury during wartime. Neurosurgical Focus. 2010;28(5):E5.
[22]Rosenfeld JV. Gunshot injury to the head and spine. Journal of Clinical Neuroscience: Official Journal of the Neurosurgical Society of Australasia. 2002;9(1):9-16.

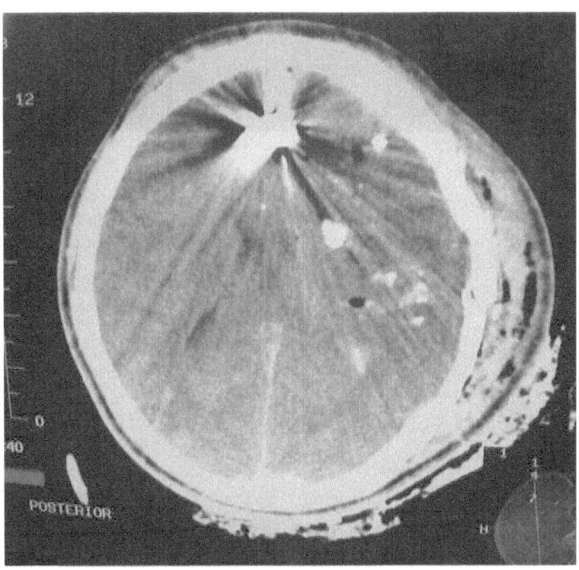

Figure 3.20 (a) Axial CT brain of a blast injury showing multiple metal fragments in the brain with scattered haemorrhages, a couple of small air bubbles (black and round) and brain swelling. The skull is fractured on the left side with gross overlying scalp swelling and subgaleal haematoma. There is scanning artefact around the metal fragments.

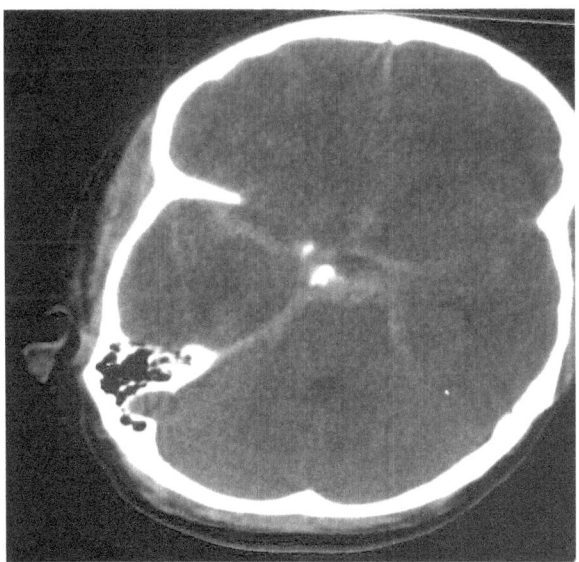

(b) Axial CT brain scan of a blast injury showing diffuse brain swelling, extensive subarachnoid haemorrhage in the basal cisterns and two metal fragments.

118

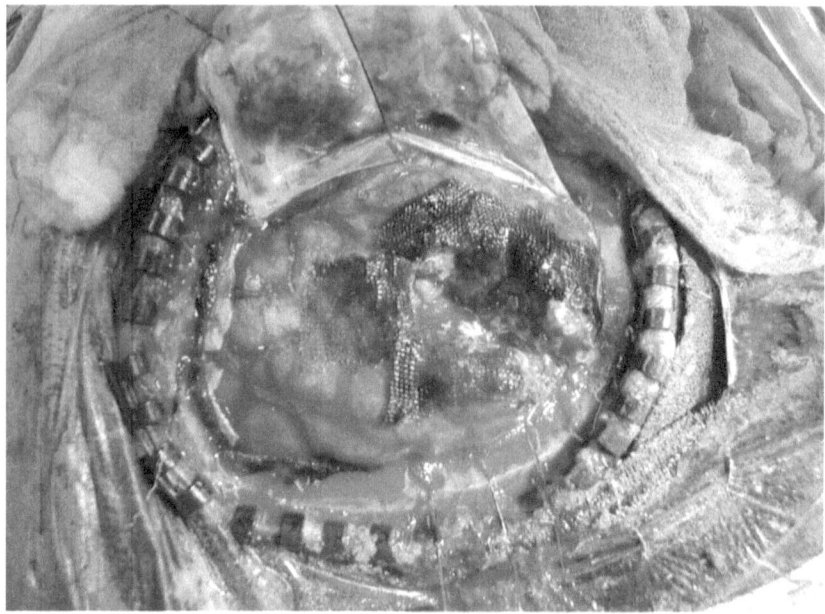

(c) The exposed brain at craniotomy following a blast injury. Note the gross swelling and congestion of the brain and the penetrating injury to the brain caused by a metal fragment. Surgicel has been placed around the edge of the brain wound.

Figure 3.20 (a-c) Blast injury to the brain.

Acute management

We have previously described the management of penetrating injury to the head including blast injury. The early surgery for severe trauma should follow the principles of 'damage control surgery' with vigorous resuscitation, rapid access to the operating room, abbreviated surgery, and continued correction of physiological derangement to prevent the lethal triad of acidosis, coagulopathy, hypothermia.

These 'damage control' principles also apply to emergency neurosurgery where emergency decompressive craniectomy has a role in the management of blast injury to the brain.[23]

---

[23]*Rosenfeld JV. Damage control neurosurgery. Injury. 2004;35(7):655-60.*

Chapter Three

Triage and initial resuscitation

The casualty should be rapidly triaged by an experienced trauma specialist. Decisions are made to provide immediate, urgent or delayed treatment. The principles of resuscitation are to stop haemorrhage, prevent hypoxia, hypercapnia and shock/hypotension are corrected. The principles of 'damage control resuscitation' follow from these goals. 'Horizontal' simultaneous procedures and treatments are carried out by a well-rehearsed trauma team rather than by following a 'vertical' step-by-step protocol. Major bleeding is controlled with torniquets to the limbs and/or direct pressure dressings and manual compression. An airway is rapidly secured.

A brief neurological assessment is made including GCS, pupil size and reactivity and weakness in the limbs (hemiparesis, quadri- or paraparesis before the patient is paralysed). If the GCS is less than 9, an endotracheal tube (ETT) should be placed using a crash induction technique to prevent laryngeal spasm, straining, coughing and jaw clamping which will cause secondary rises in intracranial pressure. If there is severe facial trauma or facial /respiratory tract burns, the casualty will require an urgent ETT before swelling and/or haemorrhage compromises the visualization of the larynx. For those with severe facial trauma or facial burns, the ETT is converted to a tracheotomy at the commencement of the operating room procedures. Adequate cerebral perfusion should be maintained when there is a severe brain injury present. Systolic blood pressure should be resuscitated to at least 100 mmHg systolic pressure.

The resuscitation of blast injury victims has been reviewed.[24] **'Permissive hypotension'** with a systolic pressure of up to 90mm has been recommended when there are multiple penetrating wounds in order to reduce blood loss but our opinion is that with rapid ongoing resuscitation available it is vital to maintain adequate cerebral perfusion, hence our recommendation for a systolic of at least 100mm Hg systolic if it can be achieved. The casualty should be kept warm with a thermal blanket to prevent hypothermia. Blood is cross-matched and blood clotting checked. Coagulopathy should be rapidly corrected with plasma, packed red cells and platelets if available

---

[24]*Dawes R, Thomas GO. Battlefield resuscitation. Current opinion in critical care. 2009;15(6):527-35.*

Medication

Prophylactic broad-spectrum antibiotics and tetanus prophylaxis are administered. We currently recommend intravenous vancomycin and meropenem prophylaxis for blast and penetrating cranial trauma in war zones because of the heavy contamination of these wounds. If these antibiotics are not available, flucloxacillin, ampicillin or gentamycin and metronidazole are alternatives.

Chloramphenicol is often available in LMIC and is another choice. Prophylactic anticonvulsants are administered with an intravenous loading dose of penytoin or levitiracetam. Intravenous mannitol or hypertonic saline may be administered as a temporizing measure if there are signs of deteriorating neurological status whilst the casualty is awaiting surgery. Steroids are not indicated.

Which first: Surgery or imaging?

If the casualty has life threatening haemorrhage, they should be taken straight to the OR for immediate damage control surgery. Otherwise a CT scan of the head and preferably neck should be obtained. If there is penetrating injury to the brain or concern about a possible vascular injury a CT angiogram should be obtained at the time of the CT. An urgent chest radiograph is obtained in the emergency room by mobile x-ray machine.

A CT scan of the chest and abdomen with or without pelvis (if CT is available), and the relevant limb radiographs are also performed. Time taken to get images should be kept to a minimum. Where a casualty has polytrauma, combined simultaneous surgery may be required to achieve the goals of rapid damage control surgery. For example, the orthopaedic surgeon is debriding and stabilizing a penetrating limb wound with compound fracture and vascular injury, the general surgeon is performing a laparotomy while the neurosurgeon is performing a decompressive craniectomy. This has been a common scenario in military settings but should also be adopted in the civilian setting.[25]

This applicability of this goal will depend on the number of surgeons available. The decompressive craniectomy should not wait until the end of a laparotomy because the brain may suffer ongoing injury from ongoing intracranial hypertension during this time.

---

[25]*Moore JM, et al. Simultaneous multisystem surgery: An important capability for the civilian trauma hospital. Clinical Neurology and Neurosurgery.2016;148:13-6.*

The acute management of accompanying injuries

The eyes are closely inspected for globe penetration or hyphema (blood in the anterior chamber of the eye) before the lids become difficult to open due to eyelid swelling. Antibiotic ointment such as chloromycetin is applied and the eye is covered with a pad dressing with the upper eyelid taped closed. A **lateral canthotomy** may be required to relieve gross orbital swelling and protect the perfusion of the globe (eyeball). This involves cutting open with a pair of sharp scissors, the lateral canthus of the eyelids along with its underlying canthal ligament. Fragments of metal in the eyes can be identified on the CT head scan. The external auditory canals are inspected for drum perforation of blood/CSF in the canals. Severe penetrating injury to the face and sinuses causes profuse haemorrhage and rapid swelling of the tissues. Local packing is placed to quell the haemorrhage until repair is undertaken.

Indications for decompressive craniectomy (DC)

1. Unilateral decompressive craniectomy (hemicraniectomy)
The blast injury is predominantly on one side of the brain with unilateral hemisphere swelling and midline shift to the opposite side. This is frequently accompanied by acute subdural or epidural hematoma. Penetrating injury may also be present on that side.

2. Bifronto-temporal decompressive craniectomy
The indications are bilateral symmetrical hemisphere swelling/ contusion, bifrontal injury, transventricular fragment trajectories. This approach also gives access to the floor of the anterior cranial fossa if there are complex anterior skull base fractures over the orbits and ethmoid and frontal sinuses. Careful attention needs to be paid to the repair of the dura over the floor of the anterior fossa as it is frequently lacerated in these injuries (see below). In more advanced settings, the floor of the anterior cranial fossa can be restored with split calvarial bone graft (in preference to titanium mesh). This prevents brain herniation and proptosis. The fronto-orbital bar of bone called the bandeau supraorbital ridge is restored with autologous bone fragments, titanium miniplates and elongated plates. This provides a cosmetic reconstruction of the facial contour.[26]

---

[26]*Ragel BT, et al. Wartime decompressive craniectomy: technique and lessons learned. Neurosurgical Focus. 2010;28(5):E2.*

3. Posterior fossa (suboccipital) decompressive craniectomy

Penetrating injury to the posterior fossa with extra-axial haemorrhage or haemorrhage / swelling in the cerebellum. If the brain stem is involved in the trajectory of a fragment or bullet, the prognosis may be very poor and decompression unlikely to improve outcome.[6] Penetrating injury across the area of brain 4cm above the dorsum sellae or 'zona fatalis' (midline skull base, thalamus, brainstem) is usually fatal and decompressive surgery is not performed.[27] The operative surgery of blast injury to the head is described from page 531.

Carotid-cavernous fistula (Figure 3.21, next page)

Carotid-cavernous (CC) fistula is an uncommon but serious complication following head injury (and sometimes occurs spontaneously in elderly people). There is a fistula between the intracavernous carotid artery or its intracavernous branches and the cavernous sinus. It usually follows a blunt injury fracturing the sphenoid bone, but may also complicate a penetrating injury. It is usually delayed in presentation to weeks or months after the injury. A unilateral pulsatile proptosis develops on the side of the fistula and may progress to visual failure.

There is chemosis (conjunctival oedema), with injection and arterialisation of the conjunctival vessels. The patient may hear the bruit in their head and it can also be heard with a stethoscope on the orbit or temple. If left untreated the other eye may be affected in the same way and the patient may gradually go blind. Small fistulae may eventually close spontaneously. The definitive management of persistent or progressive CC fistulae in advanced centres is to place a detachable balloon or metal coils in the fistula using interventional neuroradiological techniques. In neurosurgical centres with interventional imaging capability, the recommended treatment is to occlude the fistula with metal coils or muscle embolisation (Chapter 8, page 427).

---

[27] Kim KA, et al. Vector analysis correlating bullet trajectory to outcome after civilian through-and-through gunshot wound to the head: using imaging cues to predict fatal outcome. Neurosurgery. 2005;57(4):737-747; discussion 737-747.

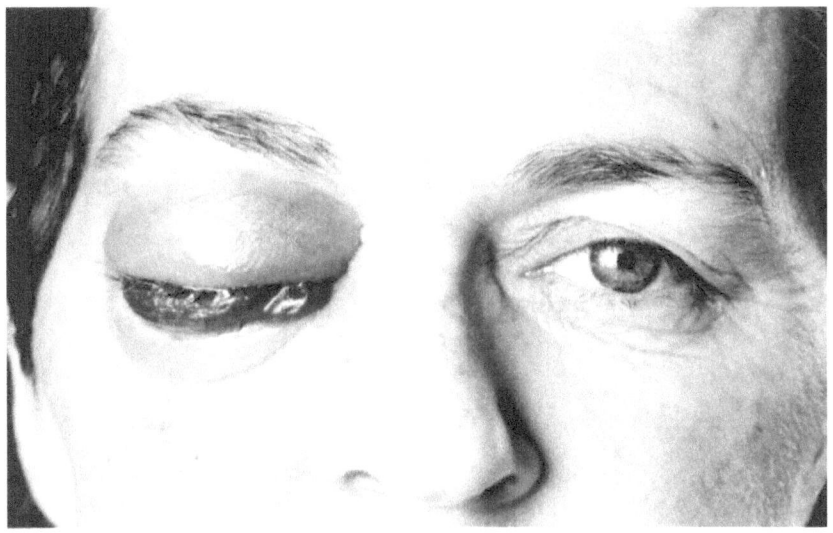

Figure 3.21 Carotid-cavernous fistula with pulsatile proptosis, chemosis and reduced visual acuity.

Child abuse and shaken baby syndrome

Child abuse commonly results in non-accidental head injury. The head may be battered or shaken. This is a well-recognised problem in many HICs, but the incidence in LMICs is unknown. A heightened awareness of this condition is important for those treating childhood injuries. The features that raise suspicions of non-accidental head injury are:

- a trivial history of trauma, the mechanism of which is inconsistent with the m1unes,
- retinal haemorrhages,
- bilateral chronic subdural haematomas in children less than 2 years of age (which can be diagnosed on ultrasound if large enough),
- skull fractures which maybe multiple, bilateral and cross suture lines,
- some child abuse cases may have evidence of malnutrition,
- previous bruising of varying ages, old (healed) long bone or rib fractures, or finger marks on the chest, neck or head.

Retinal haemorrhage may also occur after accidental head injury, in conditions where there is a sudden rise in intracranial pressure, and in haemorrhagic disease of the newborn due to vitamin K deficiency. When babies are shaken violently, the head suffers angular deceleration injury, with acute subdural haemorrhage, bilateral retinal haemorrhages, acute hemispheric or global brain swelling, and there may be few, or no external signs of trauma. The shaken baby syndrome has a significant mortality and often results in severe brain injury with a poor outcome in the survivors. Often these children are mentally retarded, epileptic, blind, sometimes deaf, and have multiple physical disabilities.

Growing skull fracture of childhood

Growing skull fractures may occur following a sizeable linear fracture in children up to 3 years of age. The fracture grows progressively in size (width) over several months. This condition is thought to arise because of the easy deformability of the young skull. The skull is suddenly forced inwards and then springs outwards and bursts, tearing the underlying dura. The pulsating brain herniates through the rent and gradually forces the bone edges further apart. The dura tends to retract well beyond the fracture margins.

The definitive treatment is wide craniotomy on either side of the fracture, exposure of the dural edges, debridement of necrotic brain, dural repair with a pericranium or fascia lata patch, and apposition of the fracture margins. The bone can be held in position with a non-absorbable thread or wire through small drill holes at the bone edge. This is a major procedure and it may be appropriate in inexperienced hands to manage it conservatively, which may leave a persistent pulsatile skull defect. If the wound is compound, the surgeon will need to at least explore, debride and close the wound, even if a definitive dural repair and cranioplasty is not carried out.

Concussion in sport

Patients with concussion should be taken off a sporting field and assessed by experienced people. "If in doubt, sit them out". The Sport Concussion Assessment Tool (SCAT) 5th Edition is now commonly used to assess the severity of concussion.[28] Patients with a significant concussion should be observed overnight in hospital and discharged in the care of a responsible relative who can report deterioration. Contact sport should be avoided until the individual is symptom free

---

[28]*Davis GA, et al. Sport Concussion Assessment Tool, 5th Edition. British Journal of Sports Medicine. Published 26 April 2017 as 10.1136/bjsports-2017-097506SCAT5. Downloaded: http://bjsm.bmj.com/*

and vigorous exercise should be avoided for 10-14 days.[29] The return to sport and to school should be graduated. 90% of individuals with concussion will make a complete recovery with rest alone. 10% of individuals have varying severity of symptoms including headaches, dizziness, fatigue and cognitive problems.

The patient has developed post-concussion syndrome if these symptoms persist. This condition is difficult to treat but requires diagnostic imaging (which is usually normal), rest, and avoidance of sport, simple analgesics, reassurance and perhaps psychotherapy if it is available. It gradually settles in most cases. Repeated concussion risks a slower recovery and may be a trigger for stopping contact sport permanently. Infrequently, there are delayed cognitive and behavioural effects or dementia many years after the sporting activities have ceased. The issue of causation is unproven in most of these cases. Boxing has also been associated with late dementia and Parkinson's disease.

General care of the comatose patient (see Chapter 9, page 431)

Psychosocial care

Assume that all unconscious patients can hear. They may derive comfort and support from relatives being at their bedside. The family will also be distressed so every effort should be made to enable a family member to be present and this person should be encouraged to talk to the patient. Later, if some recovery occurs positive stimulation through pleasant surrounds and social contact are vital. Staring at a blank wall with no pictures or colour or failure to observe the normal cycles of night and day is depressing, distressing and counter-productive. Restless or aggressive patients will require a quiet environment.

Skin care

All unconscious patients have a high risk of developing pressure sores. The patient should be turned 2-hourly to avoid their development. On each occasion the skin surface should be inspected

---

[29]*Australian Institute of Sport. Concussion in Sport Guidelines. 2019. Downloaded: https://www.concussioninsport.gov.au.*

for signs of reddening, blistering or ulceration. Any reddened areas should be protected. The findings on inspection should be recorded on a chart which lists the common pressure areas (heel, ankle, greater tuberosity, sacrum, scapula, occiput). The patient needs a sheet (in many hospitals the relatives will need to provide these), a soft mattress and should not lie on wet sheets. When turning, the patient should be lifted by three or four helpers, not dragged, which might cause a friction burn.

Bladder and bowel care

An indwelling catheter is indicated for a few days to monitor urine output. The longer this is left the more the risk of infection or irritation and ulceration of the urethra with possible stricture formation. A condom catheter or intermittent catheterisation may be indicated to avoid these problems for the patient who remains comatose for a long time.

Laxatives, suppositories and enemas should be given if there is constipation. Diarrhoea may be a sign of constipation with overflow. The abdomen should always be examined when assessing the patient.

Nutrition

A nasogastric tube allows enteral feeding to be commenced from the 72 hours. Examine the abdomen for a paralytic ileus before commencing feeds. There is some evidence that early institution of feeding in severe head injury may lessen complication risk. Feeding helps avoid hypoglycaemia, which may cause secondary brain damage. Enteral feeding neutralises gastric acid and minimises the risk of stress ulceration. There is a negative nitrogen balance after severe head injury, which causes weight loss and muscle wasting. This can be countered to some degree with enteral hyperalimentation. Enteral feeding is also important to maintain the viability of the gastrointestinal microbiome and reduce intestinal permeability and risk of sepsis. The goals are to replace 140 percent of basal metabolic requirements in patients with isolated head injury who are not paralysed, and 100 per cent of basal metabolic requirement in patients with isolated head injury who are pharmacologically relaxed. The nutritional supplementation should begin 24-48 hours post-injury in order to reach satisfactory levels by the end of the first week. The basal metabolic requirement for a 70 kg 25-year-old male is 1700 kcal/24 hour, and for a 50 kg, 50-year-old female is 1200 kcal/24 hour. Provide >15 percent of the calories as protein. The caloric requirement will increase further if multiple trauma is present.

Stress ulcer prophylaxis

A stress ulcer (Cushing's ulcer) may develop after a head injury because of reduced mucosal blood flow and increased secretion of corticosteroids, histamine and gastric acid in the metabolic response to trauma. Fasting results in less intragastric neutralisation of acid. Stress ulceration is a rare phenomenon in many tropical countries, particularly in the sub-Saharan Africa and the South Pacific. In places where stress ulceration is common (e.g. South-East Asia) antacids can be given through the nasogastric tube (30 ml magnesium trisilicate alternating with 30 ml aluminium hydroxide every 4-6 hours). Proton pump inhibitors such as pantoprazole (40 mg daily oral or IV) are given in HICs. An alternative is the H2 receptor blockers (eg cimetidine 400 mg b.d) or ranitidine (150 mg bd) by nasogastric tube. These drugs can be administered intravenously but the dose needs to be adjusted.

Avoidance of contractures

All joints should be put through their passive range of movements daily to avoid stiffness and contracture. Splintage is not normally necessary unless there are associated peripheral nerve lesions or hand injury.

Neurogenic pulmonary oedema

Damaged brain releases vasoactive products which may cause an adult respiratory distress syndrome (ARDS)-like syndrome. The management is that of pulmonary oedema and ARDS generally and will involve oxygenation, ventilation and careful control of fluids.

Disseminated intravascular coagulation (DIC)

Disseminated intravascular coagulation (DIC) may also develop due to release of thromboplastin and other products from the injured brain.

Neurogenic diabetes insipidus

Brain damage and raised intracranial pressure may affect the posterior pituitary axis resulting in a loss of antidiuretic hormone secretion. This can cause a massive diuresis. It is a poor prognostic sign in unconscious patients and is treated by avoidance of dehydration through meticulous fluid balance. Vasopressin or desmopressin can also be used if available.

Steroid administration

There is no evidence that steroids improve the outcome of head injury, and high doses of steroid depress the immune system, therefore steroids are contraindicated following head injury.

The seven deadly sins of head injury management

1. Late establishment of an adequate airway. Hypoxia causes brain injury. It must be prevented. If endotracheal intubation is not possible to make a surgical airway.
2. Hypotension and inadequate resuscitation in the shocked patient. Hypotension worsens the prognosis whether it occurs prehospital, in the emergency room or during surgery for associated injuries. A systolic blood pressure of less than 90 mmHg is associated with a worse prognosis.
3. Delay in the diagnosis and treatment of an intracranial haematoma often due to inadequate observation. The purpose of observation is to detect deterioration and act. The patient should be nursed somewhere where deterioration will be recognised and immediately reported. When a haematoma is diagnosed or suspected give the patient mannitol to temporarily reduce intracranial pressure and take the patient to theatre. In deeply unconscious patients who are deteriorating rapidly, local or no anaesthetic may be required. Do not delay evacuating a haematoma.
4. Lack of cervical spine immobilisation following severe head injury. Always consider the diagnosis of cervical spine injury. Safeguard the spine when managing the airway and always insist on seeing seven cervical vertebrae and the top of T1 on the lateral X-ray

view. Cervical spine X-rays are more important than skull X-rays in an unconscious patient.

5. Sedation of a restless head-injured patient. Restlessness or agitation following head injury may be due to raised ICP and the administration of sedatives to the patient may mask any further deterioration that is due to changing pathology in the head. Restless patients may be hypotensive or hypoxic. They might also have a distended bladder or be reacting to a blood transfusion. Never assume that aggressive or restless behaviour is due to alcohol intoxication.

6. Lack of epilepsy prophylaxis when indicated. Phenytoin is a good prophylactic agent; diazepam or phenobarbital (phenobarbitone) should be used to stop fits. Fits cause hypoxia and a rise in ICP.

7. Sending a patient home without observation when there is an indication to admit. In every series of trauma mortality there are patients who are discharged from an emergency department without an adequate period of observation. The period of deterioration is then missed and the patient is readmitted when coning has already occurred.

Practical problems

How do you manage the serious head injury who is comatose with a GCS<9?

The general approach presented here represents aggressive therapy, which is now standard practice in the developed world. It can easily be adapted for use in low resource settings, even in the absence of CT scanning. Intubate the patient in the emergency room using an anaesthetic induction technique. Preferably not with muscle relaxant or sedative alone. Then, ventilate, paralyse and sedate. Continued coughing and straining will cause severe and prolonged rises in ICP.

Do not use excessive or prolonged hyperventilation. Aim for a PaCO 2 level around 35-40 mmHg. Treat the other injuries as is appropriate. It is very important to correct shock and hypotension by replacing blood loss urgently. Aim for a systolic blood pressure >90 mmHg, and preferably >100 mmHg. Perform exploratory burr holes (see operative surgery section), to exclude an extracerebral collection if CT scanning is unavailable. Insert intracranial pressure monitor if measurement is feasible. Elevate head end of the bed 20 degrees if the blood pressure is adequate. Preferably manage the patient in the intensive care unit. Continuous intracranial pressure (ICP) monitoring following severe traumatic brain injury is standard practice in advanced neurosurgery centres and is one component of multimodality monitoring of these patients. However, ICP monitoring is not often performed in the LMICs primarily due to a lack of resources but there is also uncertainty about the efficacy. Does ICP monitoring improve the outcome following severe traumatic brain injury?

This is a controversial issue amongst neurosurgeons. There is moderate evidence that successful control of intracranial hypertension is associated with improved outcome and continuous ICP monitoring facilitates the effective and efficient treatment of intracranial hypertension.[30] However, a randomized controlled trial of ICP monitoring performed in Bolivia and Ecuador found that the ICP monitoring was not superior to care based on imaging and clinical examination.[31]

This study is not readily applicable to countries where there are advanced trauma systems with rapid prehospital transport systems and trained paramedics. It should also be noted that in many LMICs there is also no or limited CT scanning. Chesnut et al have further described a treatment algorithm for managing severe traumatic brain injury in the absence of ICP monitoring which involves imaging and clinical examination.[32]

The Latin American Neurosurgeons have now developed a consensus-based treatment protocol without ICP monitoring.[33] This protocol may have increasing application in the LMICs. **Anticonvulsants:** status epilepticus cannot be diagnosed clinically if the patient is paralysed and sedated. Administer a loading dose of phenytoin, then a maintenance dose until the sedation is tapered.

[30]Chesnut R, Videtta W, Vespa P, et al. Intracranial pressure monitoring: fundamental considerations and rationale for monitoring. Neurocrit Care. 2014;2:S64-84.

[31]Chesnut R, Temkin N, Carney N, et al. A trial of intracranial-pressure monitoring in traumatic brain injury. New England Journal of Medicine. 2012;367(26):2471-2481.

[32]Chesnut RM, Temkin N, Dikmen S, et al. A method of managing severe traumatic brain injury in the absence of intracranial pressure monitoring: the imaging and clinical examination protocol. Journal of Neurotrauma. 2018;35(1):54-63. doi: 10.1089/neu.2016.4472.

[33]Hendrickson P, Pridgeon J, Temkin NR, et al. Development of a severe traumatic brain injury consensus-based treatment protocol conference in Latin America. World Journal of Neurosurgery. 2018;110:e952-e957. doi:10.1016/j.wneu.2017.11.142.

Control of ICP

With an ICP monitor in situ

The CO2 level is maintained at 35-40 mmHg. Do not allow the PaCO2 to stay persistently below 25 mmHg. Maintain CPP 60 to 70 mmHg. Treat if ICP > 22 mmHg for >2 min, preferably with CSF venting, and mannitol or hypertonic saline bolus rather than prolonged hyperventilation.

Treating high ICP

- Make sure the patient is well sedated
- Check blood gases. Keep arterial blood oxygen saturation (SaO2) > 95% and PaO_2>60mm Hg (> 8.8 kPa).
- Check neck posture - ensure the neck is not twisted which would obstruct venous return.
- Acute hyperventilation for 30 sec for acute rises in ICP. This may be done by hand bagging the patient, i.e. connecting the ventilation circuit to a rubber bag, and manually breathing the patient. Aim for PaCO2 30-35mm Hg. When completed this short period of hyperventilation the PaCO2 should be maintained at 35 to 40 mmHg.
- Venting CSF for 5 minutes by opening the vent tap for acute rises in ICP. Venting may fail if the brain is very swollen with small slit like ventricles, which is often the case after a diffuse brain injury.
- Mannitol 0.25 to 0.5 g per kg 4-6 hourly p.r.n. Monitor serum osmolality. Keep <310 mosm/kg. Watch urine output. Beware of repeated doses aggravating cerebral swelling and ICP. Hypertonic saline is an alternative if it is available. Aim for Serum Sodium 135 to 145 mEq/L.
- Barbiturate (thiopentone) infusion or intermittent boluses if other treatments have failed. Beware of resultant systemic hypotension.
- Hypothermia using ice bags, or preferably a cooling blanket with intramuscular chlorpromazine to stop shivering, to a level of 33-35°C.
- Unilateral or bilateral temporal craniectomy has a role in allowing the brain to expand out of the cranial cavity in an attempt to lower an otherwise uncontrollable ICP. This may save a patient's life only to leave a neurologically damaged individual. If the ICP stays above 30-40 mmHg, the patient is likely to die.

Without an ICP monitor in situ

Sedation is helpful for control of ICP, but you will lose the ability to assess the patient neurologically, except for the pupil size and reaction. Try to use sedation without paralysis, so you can better assess the patient's responses when the drugs wear off. Regular mannitol - 0.25-0.5 g/kg 4-6 hourly i.v. Beware of brain swelling if this is continued for more than 4-6 doses. Maintain PaCO2 level at 35-40 mmHg. Hypertonic saline boluses are an alternative but not often available in LMIC. A difficult dilemma is presented by the very restless, agitated head injury patient who cannot be controlled without sedation in situations where CT is unavailable and intubation and ventilation with ICP monitoring are also unavailable, or where the patient is breathing satisfactorily with a patent airway. Sedation will render the patient difficult to assess clinically for deterioration. Either you will have to observe the patient closely, which will mean adequate nursing numbers and competence, and operate if there is further neurological deterioration, or preferably sedate and operate early with exploratory burr holes to detect and evacuate an extracerebral collection. There is a trend by neurosurgeons in LMIC, where CT imaging is available, to perform early decompressive craniectomy (DC) to control ICP if the CT shows brain swelling, contusions, or intracranial haematoma (see section above on management of patient with GCS<9 and Chapter 3, page 120).

THE PROGNOSIS OF HEAD INJURY

The outcome of head injury is partly related to the GCS on admission and, after stabilisation of the patient, securing the airway, breathing and circulation. The type of pathology also influences prognosis as does any associated injuries. Decision making should be linked to the prognosis as there is usually little point in performing diagnostic burr holes in a patient with a GCS of 3-5 who has not recently deteriorated or had a lucid interval. This is all the truer if the pupils are fixed and dilated or if there is a fractured base of skull. The GCS is a guide to clinical decision making and is invaluable in the absence of CT or MRI scans, which would show the actual pathology.

Glasgow Outcome Scale

1. **Favourable outcome**
   - normal
   - mild or moderate disability, patient maintains independence
2. **Unfavourable outcome**
   - severe disability resulting in loss of independent function
   - persistent vegetative state
   - death

The favourable outcome on the Glasgow Outcome Scale tends to underestimate problems with social reintegration. Moderate disability means independent but disabled. Severe disability means conscious but dependent.

Glasgow Assessment Schedule

Severe social problems due to personality or mood changes can occur after even mild head injuries. A Glasgow Assessment Schedule has been devised to try and quantify the disabilities. Aggressive behaviour, divorce or inability to concentrate may be the legacy of a head injury. Medicolegal and compensation claims may result. It is important to be aware that a head injury may have a devastating effect on a family and that the disabilities are psychosocial as well as physical (see Chapter 12).

The outcome of severe head injury

The mortality of severe head injury is on average 30-40 percent and of those who survive, 60 percent will have severe disability. There are many factors which may increase the mortality and severe disability rates further. These mortality figures may be worse in resource poor settings particularly when there are long delays getting the patient to hospital. The factors that strongly relate to outcome are: age (the elderly do significantly worse), level of coma, and duration of post-traumatic amnesia. Other important clinical factors are displayed in Table 3.3. The CRASH and IMPACT TBI are large data bases of patients with severe TBI which have been used to generate prognostic information about an individual patient based on their basic clinical parameters which are typed into the websites. These are freely available on the internet.[34]

Table 3.3 Factors affecting the outcome of severe head injury.

Pupils reacting	39%	50%
Pupils not reacting	91%	4%
Eye movement intact	33%	56%
Eye movement absent	90%	5%
Extensor response or no response	85%	8%

The prediction of outcome becomes more accurate as the time following the injury increases. Of survivors of severe head injuries at 6 months, 65 per cent have cerebral hemisphere dysfunction, 37 percent cranial nerve palsy, 9 percent ataxia, 17 per cent epilepsy, 29 percent dysphasia, and 49 percent hemiparesis. The late cranial nerve problems relate mainly to the optic nerve, deafness, extraocular muscle palsy and anosmia. Facial nerve palsies if delayed, usually recover over 6-8 weeks, and taste usually recovers before facial function. Most immediate total lesions remain permanent. Other late complications are vascular conditions, such as carotid-cavernous fistula and false aneurysm rupture, meningitis following CSF fistula, post-traumatic hydrocephalus, and epilepsy (25 per cent occurring greater than 4 years post-injury).

There is an increased risk during late epilepsy with intracranial haemorrhage evacuated within 2 weeks of injury. An early seizure (in the first week), compound depressed fracture, post-traumatic amnesia more than 24 hours, dural tear or focal neurological signs, further increase the risk. Most patients with moderately severe disability will endure it for 30-40 years, because the average age of such patients is 27 years. Neuropsychological deficit may improve over the first few years but symptom levels do not reduce after 2 years. The CT findings that correlate with poor outcome are acute subdural haematoma, a large area of contusion, absent basal cisterns, midline shift, especially if it is associated with hemisphere swelling, and new lesions appearing on subsequent scans.

---

[34]*http://www.crash.lshtm.ac.uk/Risk%calculator/index.html*
http://www.tbi-impact.org/?p=impact/calc

FURTHER READING

- Aarabi B, Simaud M. Decompressive Craniectomy. Nova Science Publishers Inc. April 2018.
- Carney N, Totten AM, O'Reilly C, et al. Brain Trauma Foundation TBI Guidelines. Guidelines for the management of severe traumatic brain injury. 4th Edition. Neurosurgery. 2017;80:6-15.
  Online: https://www.braintrauma.org/coma/guidelines
- Rosenfeld JV. Practical Management of head and neck injury. Churchill Livingstone, Elsevier. 2012.
- Rosenfeld JV, Maas AI, Bragge P, et al. Early management of severe traumatic brain injury. Lancet. 2012;380:1088-1098.
- Traumatic brain injury: integrated approaches to improve prevention, clinical care, and research. Lancet Neurology. 07 November 2017.

Hydrocephalus and congenital abnormalities

HYDROCEPHALUS

Hydrocephalus is an increased volume of CSF within the ventricles, which are enlarged. It literally means 'water in the head'.

Essential anatomy and physiology (Figure 4.1, next page)

There are two lateral ventricles in the cerebral hemispheres which communicate via the foramen of Munro with the third ventricle (located in the diencephalon between the two thalami). The aqueduct of Sylvius leads through the midbrain to the fourth ventricle in the hindbrain. The fourth ventricle is located between the cerebellum and the brain stem. CSF leaves the fourth ventricle via the two lateral foramina of Luschka or midline foramen of Magendie. CSF passes around the brain from the basal cisterns to the subarachnoid space around the brain and also into the spinal canal.

Cerebrospinal fluid cushions the brain and maintains its physiological environment. It also enables neurotransmitters to circulate. The total adult volume is about 130 ml and the normal pressure is about 130mm H_2O. It is actively secreted by the choroid plexus in the lateral, third and fourth ventricles. CSF passes passively across the ependymal lining of the ventricles from the brain parenchyma (which opens directly into the ventricles), the blood vessels and the nerve root sleeves.

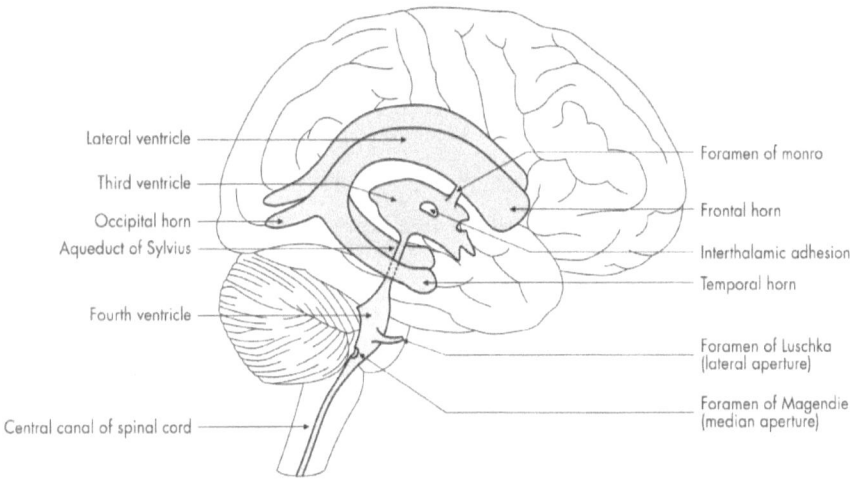

Lateral ventricle

Third ventricle

Occipital horn

Aqueduct of Sylvius

Fourth ventricle

Central canal of spinal cord

Foramen of monro

Frontal horn

Interthalamic adhesion

Temporal horn

Foramen of Luschka
(lateral aperture)

Foramen of Magendie
(median aperture)

Figure 4.1 Ventricular anatomy.

Secretion from the choroid plexus is an active process, requiring carbonic anhydrase, occurring at a rate of 20 ml per hour (about 500 ml per day). There is no feedback mechanism but normally CSF production, flow and absorption are well balanced. Absorption of CSF takes place in the arachnoid villi of the venous sinuses, is a passive process flowing across a pressure gradient (see Figure 2.1, page 9).

Surgical pathology

Obstruction to the free flow of CSF results in a raised intracranial pressure. This results in damage to the brain and loss of white matter. Hydrocephalus can be classified according to whether it is due to increased production, blockage of flow or failure of absorption. Most cases are due to blockage of flow or failure of absorption. Hydrocephalus may be classified as communicating or non-communicating.

Communication or non-communication is determined by whether CSF can flow from the ventricular system to the subarachnoid space or not. Excess formation of CSF is rare but can occur with choroid plexus tumours (papilloma and carcinoma). The causes of hydrocephalus may be congenital or acquired and are shown in (Table 4.1, next page).

Table 4.1 Common causes of hydrocephalus.

Congenital	Neonatal ventricular haemorrhage	Aqueduct stenosis or atresia
		Ependymal cyst
		Suprasellar arachnoid cyst
		Chiari malformation
		Posterior fossa cyst
Acquired	Post-infection, meningitis	Posterior fossa tumours
	Post otitic - transverse sinus	Third ventricular tumour/colloid cyst
	(following middle ear infection)	Pineal region tumour
		Chronic ventriculitis (post-infection)
	Trauma - subarachnoid haemorrhage	Acute intraventricular haemorrhage

Congenital hydrocephalus

Intraventricular haemorrhage of prematurity, and neonatal meningitis are the two commonest causes of congenital hydrocephalus to present early. Aqueduct stenosis may not present until the teenage years. These children tend to present with chronic headaches and may have papilloedema. A Dandy-Walker cyst in the posterior fossa is an uncommon cause of congenital hydrocephalus, and is accompanied by a deficient formation of the vermis of the cerebellum (Figure 4.4 (d), page 148).

Acquired hydrocephalus

The child presents with an enlarged head. This is confirmed by placing the head circumference on a standard percentile chart. The child with hydrocephalus will cross the percentile lines (Figure 4.2, next page). The anterior fontanelle will be bulging and tense.

The skull sutures will split and may become palpable. The percussion note of the head will become 'crackpot' and sound like a drum. In advanced cases the child becomes lethargic, feeds poorly, and may develop down-turned eyes (the 'setting sun' sign).

This is caused by the third ventricle bulging posteriorly and compressing the superior colliculi on the back of the midbrain which results in failure of up-gaze. The natural history of untreated hydrocephalus is to produce varying degrees of unsightly head enlargement, and mental sub-normality. In the most advanced cases, the cerebral mantle (the thickness of brain between the ventricle and the surface) becomes very thin and the child is profoundly retarded (Figure 4.3, next page).

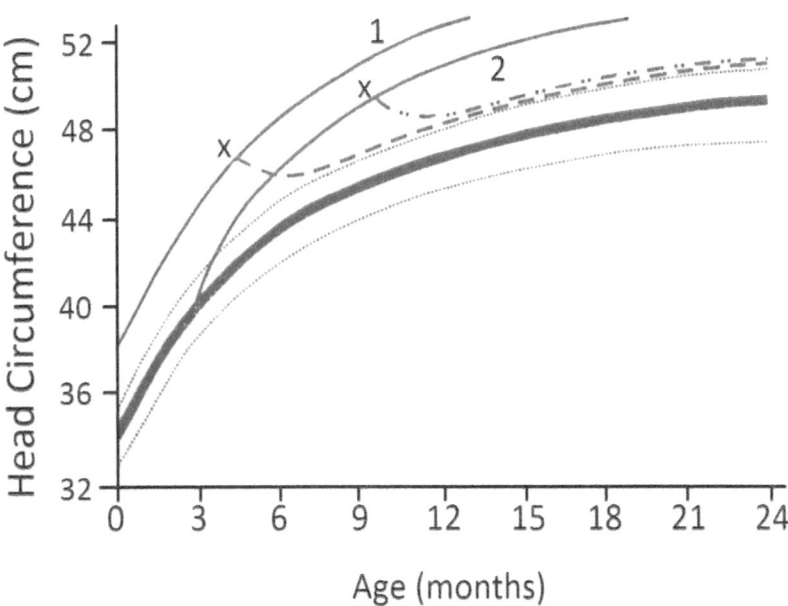

Figure 4.2 Schematic graph showing the normal occipitofrontal circumference (black line at 50th centile, fine dotted lines at the 2nd and 98th centiles). Curve 1 represents congenital hydrocephalus treated at point 'x' with the head circumference coming to rest just above the 98th centile. Curve 2 is acquired hydrocephalus treated at point 'x' with the curve of head circumference also coming to rest just above the 98th centile.

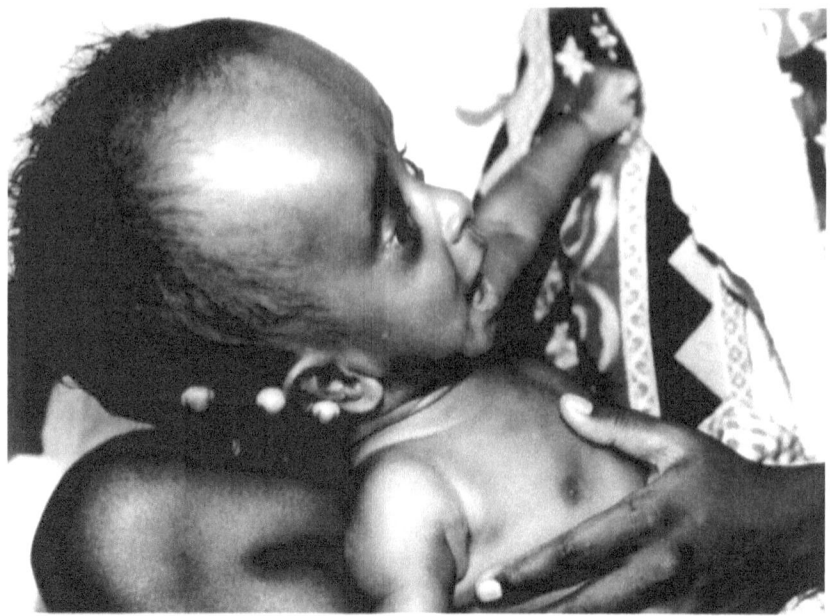

Figure 4.3 (a) Note the head enlargement is out of proportion to the body size.

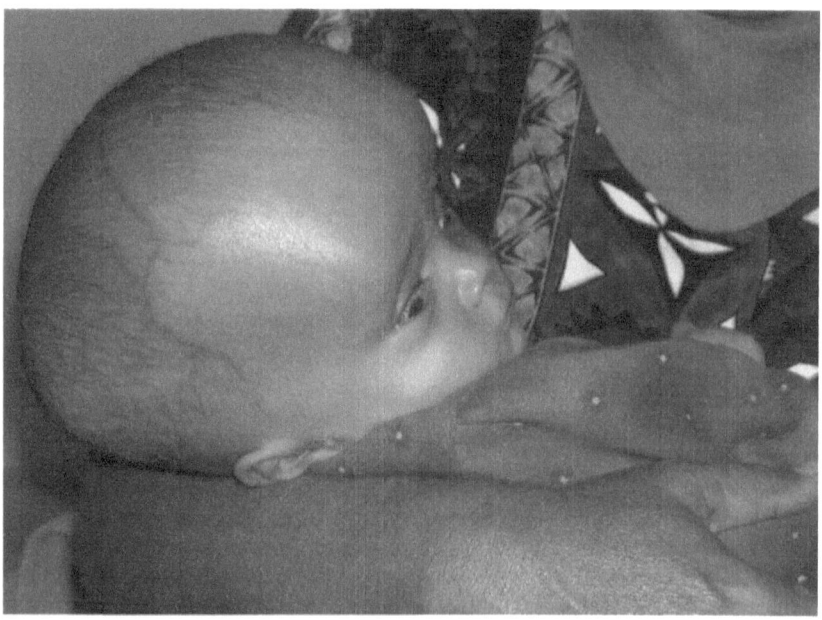

(b)

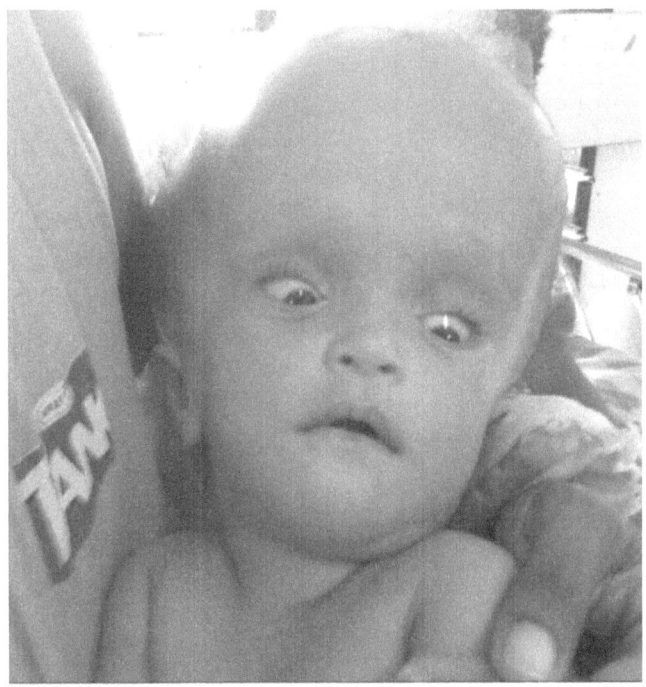

(c)

(b & c) Infants with gross hydrocephalus resulting in macrocephaly and the setting sun sign.

Figure 4.3 (a-c) Infants with gross hydrocephalus.

Arrested hydrocephalus

Arrested hydrocephalus is a non-progressive condition. A steady state of CSF production and absorption is reached. The child can have a big head but serial plotting of head circumference on a chart shows that the head now grows along a new centile line. No specific treatment is required. The ventricles may remain large, but the ICP is not raised and the brain is able to develop relatively normally.

Case report

A 4-month-old baby was seen in the central hospital. He was being observed for a large head. Weekly ultrasounds in the previous 6 weeks confirmed dilated ventricles but a normal looking brain texture. The child was able to sit, grasped objects in its hands, made normal sounds and was beginning to gain head control. At birth his occipitofrontal circumference (OFC) was on the 50th centile. At 8 weeks it was on the 80th centile and at 10 weeks it was at the 90th centile. Since then the OFC had grown along the 90th centile. **Lesson**: *This child is developing normally. His hydrocephalus may be arrested. He needs regular follow-up with recording of developmental milestones, OFC measurements and ultrasound.*

Compensatory hydrocephalus

Compensatory hydrocephalus is an increased volume of CSF secondary to loss of brain tissue. This may occur after a head injury or dementia. This has also been the cause with hydrocephalus *ex vacuo*.

Clinical recognition

The presentation of hydrocephalus depends on the age of the patient (Table 4.2, next page).

Infants

Vomiting, drowsiness, irritability, fever and seizures are the most common symptoms. Before the sutures are closed a most important part of assessment is to plot an infant's occipitofrontal head circumference (OFC) on a chart (Figure 4.2, page 140). Serial measurements will allow you to determine whether the head circumference is crossing percentile lines. Bulging fontanelles, distended scalp veins and setting sun eyes (failure of upgaze) are other important signs. Determine whether or not the child has normal developmental milestones (see Table 2.1, page 14). The cranial sutures may be widened on palpation.

Case report

A 4-month-old baby was seen in a rural clinic with a huge head and setting sun eyes. He had no head control which the mother blamed on the large head. The child fed well and his limbs were normal in tone and posture. The developmental milestones were abnormal: he only began to smile at 3 months, could not sit even with support, and failed to pay any attention to objects placed in its hand. The OFC was on the 95th centile. He was referred to the base hospital where an ultrasound confirmed dilated ventricles. Once the parents agreed to bring the child for regular review a ventriculoperitoneal shunt was inserted by the local surgeon. At one year the child was reviewed and found to have near normal milestones, and the head size was then below the upper limit of normal.

Table 4.2 Clinical features of hydrocephalus or shunt malfunction.

Infants	Toddlers	Children and adults
Head enlargement	Head enlargement	Fever
Fontanelle tense and bulging	Fever	Vomiting
Scalp veins prominent	Vomiting	Headache
Fever	Headache	Loss of coordination / balance
Vomiting	Irritability/sleepiness	Decline in academic performance
Sleepiness	Loss of previous abilities	Swelling / redness along shunt track
Setting sun eyes	Swelling and redness along shunt track	
Seizures	Fluctuant CSF collection around the valve	
Splitting sutures		
Crackpot percussion note		
Fluctuant CSF collection around the valve		

Toddlers

Fever, vomiting, headache and irritability or drowsiness are common complaints for many conditions. The child may lose certain abilities he had already developed (e.g. talking in sentences or walking). The head circumference will be increased on an occipitofrontal circumference (OFC) chart.

Children and adults

Fever and vomiting may be the only signs of mild hydrocephalus. Headache, loss of coordination or balance, and a decline in academic performance are other symptoms. Neck stiffness may occur as a result of the herniation of cerebellar tonsils through the foramen magnum onto the brain stem.

Differential diagnosis

Hydrocephalus should be distinguished from a large head for which the causes are:
1. a constitutionally large head (one or other parent may have a large head) with a normal brain;
2. benign enlargement of the subarachnoid space;
3. enlarged brain: hemi-megalencephaly or the rare Sotos' syndrome (generally large brain usually associated with a large body and mental retardation).

Case report

*A child was being reviewed in the clinic because the nurse in the outstation had recorded an OFC above the 90th centile at a 6-week check. The child was developmentally normal when seen at 8, 12 and 16 weeks. The head remained above the 90th centile. During the visits the doctor observed that the father, who only came twice to the clinic, also had a large head. Brain ultrasound showed no hydrocephalus and normal brain. **Lesson:** This is a case of a congenitally large head, which is in fact normal.*

Investigations

1. **Brain ultrasound.** This is possible when the fontanelles are still open or the sutures are sprung. Ultrasound of the anterior fontanelle will demonstrate dilated ventricles (see Figure 2.15 from page 52) and may show the cause such as a subependymal and intraventricular haemorrhage of prematurity, third ventricular cysts or a tumour of the fourth ventricle.

2. **Skull radiograph.** In babies and young children, a skull X-ray may show split sutures. Chronic pressure from the brain on the inside of the skull may cause a copper-beaten appearance. There may be bony erosion of the dorsum sellae. Calcification in a tumour or tuberculoma may cause pineal deviation.

3. **CT scan (or MR scan)** will show the degree of hydrocephalus and its cause. These are investigations of choice if the fontanelle is not available for ultrasound (Figure 4.4, below).

4. **Ventriculogram** shows the degree of hydrocephalus and may also show the site of the block.

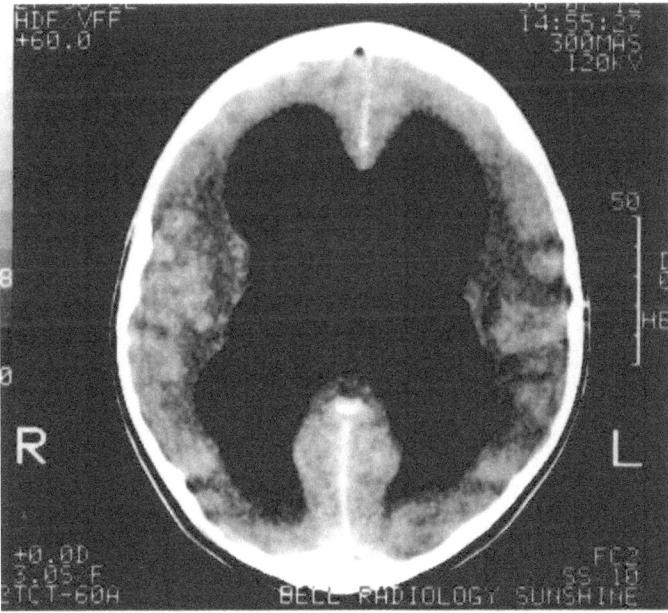

Figure 4.4 (a) CT axial scan showing dilated lateral ventricles.

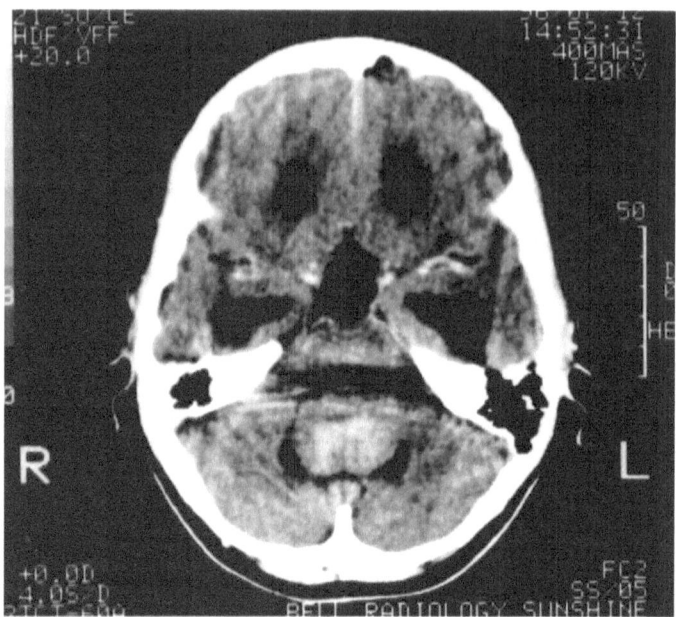

(b) CT axial scan showing dilated third ventricle, and temporal and frontal horns of the lateral ventricles. There is a tumour in the posterior fossa distorting the fourth ventricle.

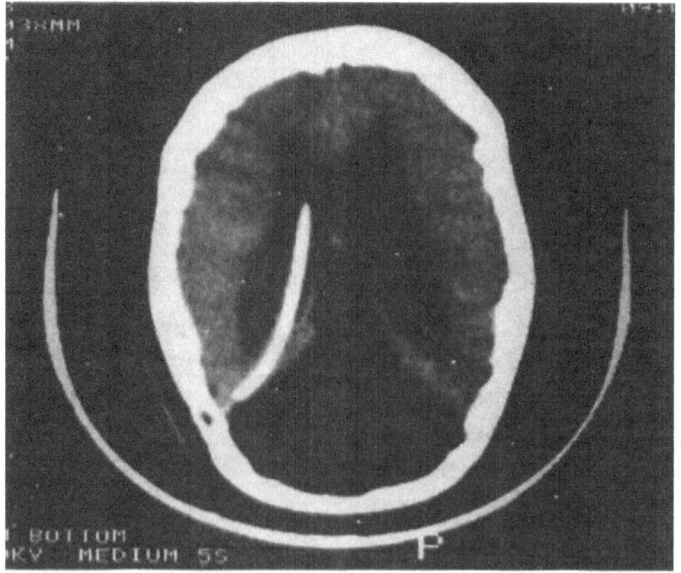

(c) CT scan showing a shunt tube in position with gross hydrocephalus and a posterior fossa Dandy-Walker cyst.

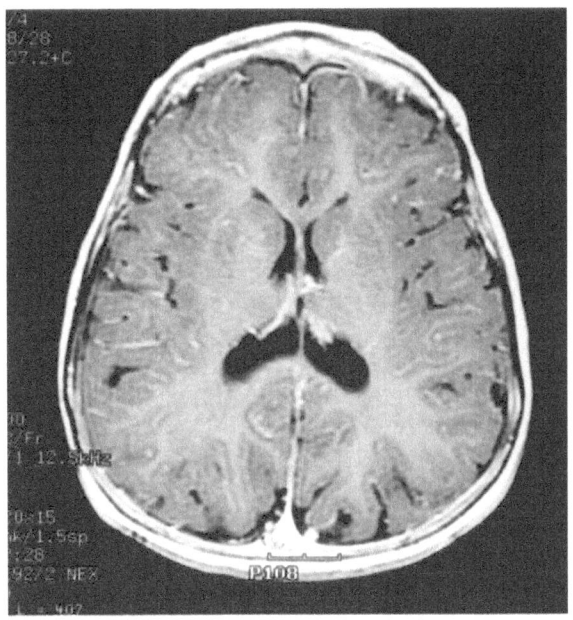

(d) Magnetic resonance scan (T1 weighted image) showing normal ventricle size.

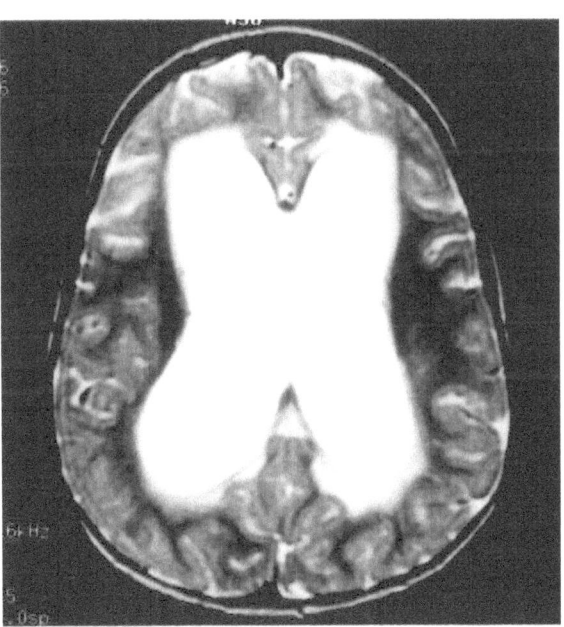

(e) Magnetic resonance scan (T2 weighted image) showing grossly enlarged lateral ventricles.

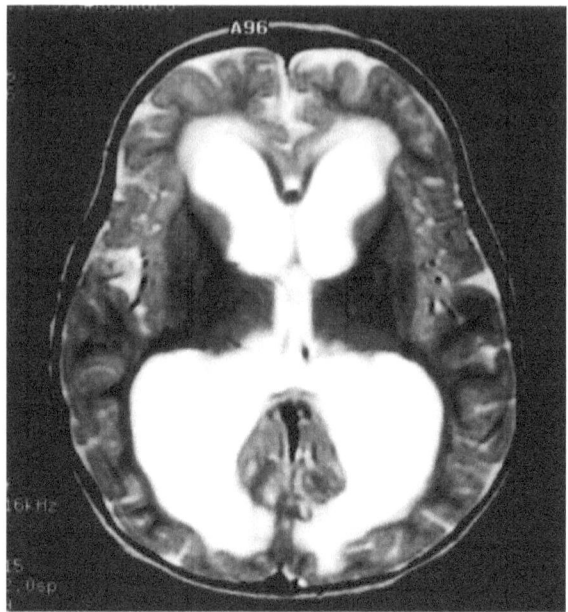

(f) Magnetic resonance scan (T2 weighted image) showing enlarged lateral ventricles and note the periventricular high signal indicating transependymal movement of CSF.

Figure 4.4 (a-f) The imaging of hydrocephalus.

Management

Diuretics

Acetazolamide is a diuretic which reduces active secretion of CSF by the choroid plexus. Furosemide (frusemide) may reduce intracranial water content. These drugs do not influence CSF production by the brain parenchyma or ependymal cells lining the ventricles. Diuretics are therefore of limited value, but they may sometimes slow or halt the progression of hydrocephalus temporarily.

Shunts

The definitive treatment for hydrocephalus is to insert a shunt. The first shunts were developed by Holter, Spitz and Pudenz in the mid to late 1950s and their valves shunted CSF from the ventricles to the right atrium (ventriculo-atrial). Nowadays, the ventriculo-peritoneal (V-P) shunt is the route of choice and the operative procedure is described in Chapter 11 on page 546. Unfortunately, many children with hydrocephalus in the developing world end up with irreversible brain damage and large heads through lack of a surgeon willing or able to attempt a shunt operation, or lack of the shunt equipment. The commercially available shunts from Europe and the United States of America (USA) are relatively expensive, but cheap shunts have been produced in India and Africa.

Even if no standard shunt is available, it is possible to use a plain length of fine plastic tubing without a valve, pass it from the ventricle to the abdominal cavity, and achieve a satisfactory reduction in the size of the ventricles. It is important for surgeons in this predicament to lobby their hospital and health authorities to provide some shunt equipment using the argument that it is much more cost beneficial to treat hydrocephalus than to have retarded children and adults who are a long-term burden on their families and society. (Addresses of shunt suppliers including charitable organisations who will sell at low cost are given in the appendix to Chapter 11, page 614). There are many potential problems of inserting a shunt in a child who must return to a remote village (page 4). Who should ·be shunted is a decision that can only be made by considering resources for treatment (the availability of shunts), the wishes of the parents and the opportunity for monitoring complications.

The complications of not shunting a child who survives are mental retardation with all its inherent costs and a large, unsightly head. A properly inserted shunt has the potential to work for many years without complication even in the tropics.

When to shunt?

Shunt the patient between 12 and 18 months if hydrocephalus progresses slowly. This gives the hydrocephalus a chance to arrest. If hydrocephalus increases rapidly in the first few months and the condition is clearly progressive with raised ICP, an earlier shunt will be required. If the cerebral mantle (the cortex and white matter overlying the ventricle) is less than 2 cm in thickness on ultrasound and the ventricles are enlarging a V-P shunt will be required. Follow-up ultrasound should be done weekly if possible, at least initially, until the decision is made to shunt. Following an intraventricular haemorrhage repeated lumbar punctures can help clear the CSF of blood, lessen the CSF build-up, and sometimes avoid a shunt. If lumbar punctures fail, a thin spinal needle can be passed from the lateral edge of the fontanelle into the lateral ventricle to aspirate CSF in the neonatal period. This may also help avoid a shunt. While the CSF is heavily blood-stained with a high protein content a shunt, if inserted, may easily block. So, it is worthwhile to delay inserting the shunt until the protein and blood content subside.

Choosing the method of shunting

Ventriculo-peritoneal (VP) shunting is the preferred method because the shunt does not need to be revised as the child grows. The tubing in the abdomen will gradually uncoil as the child's height increases. Choice of valve is discussed in Chapter 11. Ventriculo-atrial shunts need to be lengthened as a child grows and thus need multiple revisions. It is technically more difficult to insert the atrial end into the atrium and there is always the risk of septicaemia and septic emboli from endocarditis. Ventriculo-pleural shunts may also be inserted if it is difficult to establish a ventriculo-peritoneal or ventriculo-atrial shunt. They may cause a chronic pleural effusion.

Complications of shunts, their presentation and avoidance

Shunts are subject to multiple possible complications many of which can be prevented by careful surgical technique. This section describes the various complications of shunts, how they are recognised and the necessary strategies to correct the problems. Much of the corrective surgery is straightforward. Children and adults with shunts can lead normal lives but should not engage in activities that vigorously flex the neck, such as gymnastics, because this may cause a disconnection of the peritoneal catheter from the valve. They should wear a protective helmet when engaging in a contact sport. They can go swimming (but not scuba diving), and can travel in aircraft. The general symptoms of shunt malfunction are presented in Table 4.2, page 144. Fever usually only occurs if the shunt is infected, not with the other complications. Whenever a patient has a suspected shunt complication, plain X-rays of the shunt should be undertaken. Modern shunt catheters are X-ray opaque, and disconnection or migration of the tubing can be easily identified.

Testing the shunt

Compressing the shunt valve is notoriously unreliable for identifying a shunt malfunction, and repeated flushing of the valve may suck choroid plexus against the ventricular catheter perforations and precipitate a blockage. If the valve is incompressible this may indicate a distal blockage. If the valve empties and does not refill or refills very slowly, it may indicate that the ventricular catheter is blocked, although it may also indicate that the ventricles are over drained and that the CSF volume in the ventricle is very low (so called 'slit ventricles') with a functioning shunt. The valve may also appear to empty and refill perfectly well but be totally disconnected.

Prophylactic antibiotic cover

Surgical interventions including dental manipulation may cause bacteraemia particularly if there is active sepsis. This bacteraemia may seed bacteria into the shunt setting up a chronic shunt infection. Prophylactic antibiotics are therefore indicated for elective and emergency procedures. The antibiotic chosen should reflect the likely organisms, but a staphylococcal cover is most important. We suggest flucloxacillin or a penicillin, chloramphenicol combination, or cephalosporin such as cephazolin, as a single dose at the time of the procedure.

Blockage

Shunt blockage is the commonest shunt complication and most commonly affects the ventricular catheter. The choroid plexus adheres to the catheter and occludes the perforations. Placing the catheter tip in the frontal horn of the lateral ventricle may lessen this complication by keeping the choroid plexus out of contact with the catheter perforations. The peritoneal end may be blocked by greater omentum or adhesions. When there is shunt infection, a pseudocyst may form because of the surrounding adhesions. This can be diagnosed by abdominal ultrasound. It is uncommon for the valve to block. The clinical features of a shunt blockage are summarised in Table 4.2, page 144, but the presentation varies considerably in its rapidity of onset, depending on the completeness of the blockage and the degree of shunt dependency. Treating the blockage involves exploring the shunt, disconnecting it, testing the peritoneal catheter by observing the rate of fall of a column of fluid within a connected extension tubing (manometer) held vertically, and observing the flow of CSF from the ventricular catheter. If the catheter is stuck in position it can often be dislodged by passing a ventricular catheter stilette down the catheter and passing a low diathermy current down this stilette. If this fails, the catheter may have to be left in position, and a new catheter placed beside it. If the catheter is withdrawn forcefully a severe intraventricular haemorrhage may result. Once the peritoneum has been affected by peritonitis, the absorption of CSF may become ineffective and ascites may develop. The shunt will then have to be placed in the right atrium or pleural cavity.

Disconnection

Shunt disconnection is a common problem, and particularly occurs when the child is passing through a growth spurt. There is increasing tension on the valve/peritoneal catheter join, and it usually disconnects at this point with the peritoneal catheter often ending up entirely in the peritoneal cavity. Although it can be left there, it may be easy to retrieve when the new catheter is sited, or else retrieved via a laparoscope.

Case report

*A 3-year-old child had a shunt, inserted 18 months previously. He had been well and developed normally. The parents had had no cause to bring him for review until he developed a swelling over the chest wall. The local medicine man drained this and obtained water, not pus. The parents brought the child back to the hospital on the third or fourth occasion that the fluid accumulated. There the visiting missionary doctor confirmed again that it was CSF not pus and he could see the shunt tubing in the base of the wound. He phoned the referral hospital for advice. He was advised to send the child in. It was confirmed that the child was well, the shunt was not infected. On abdominal x-ray, the peritoneal end of the shunt tubing had migrated out of the peritoneal cavity in a loop, and CSF was accumulating under the skin. **Lesson**: seek and you will find the cause. Always explore when CSF is leaking, the cause could have been a disconnection (common) or a crack in the tubing (rare).*

Migration

Migration of a peritoneal catheter, or less often a ventricular catheter, will usually follow a disconnection. Uncommonly, the entire peritoneal catheter will migrate from the abdomen to wrap around the valve. It is important to anchor the valve to the pericranium to try and prevent this cart-wheel effect.

Infection

Prevention of shunt infection should be the aim. The most important time to prevent a shunt infection is when the shunt is initially inserted, as this is by far the commonest time for the bacteria to colonise the shunt (see Chapter 4, page 152). The surgeon and all the staff should try and use the highest standards of aseptic technique for shunt operations. The important steps in the method are to try and place the shunt as the first case in the day when the theatre is cleanest, with the minimal number of personnel in the room. Prophylactic antibiotics are administered. The shunt components are not taken out of their packets until the last moment, and the operators and nurses should, as far as possible, use a no-touch technique. It is probably also helpful to avoid any contact of the components with the skin edge to avoid Staphylococcus epidermidis contamination. Once the peritoneal catheter has been passed through the tunneller, it is wrapped in a pack until it is ready to be placed in the peritoneal cavity. The shunt components can also be soaked in antibiotic solution although this may not be necessary.

A shunt infection rate of greater than 10 per cent is excessive, and the techniques of insertion should be closely analysed to try and reduce the infection rate. The risk of infection is greater in neonates and young babies. Symptoms identical to those of shunt infection may occur with many types of intercurrent infections in children. Whenever a shunt infection is suspected, the child should be admitted and observed. Viral and other systemic infections will usually declare themselves over 24-48 hours (eg. pus on the tonsils) and shunt revision is then avoided. In trying to diagnose shunt infection, one should avoid placing needles directly into the reservoir (valve) to aspirate CSF, because this may introduce bacteria into a non-infected shunt. Diagnostic lumbar puncture (LP) is preferable, although a smouldering low-grade shunt infection may not show much CSF abnormality on LP. The three management options for shunt infection are: antibiotics alone, removal of the shunt, or temporary externalisation of the peritoneal catheter, then secondary replacement of the lower end (see incidental intra-abdominal sepsis section). Once bacteria colonise a shunt, they adhere firmly to the plastic and antibiotic concentrations are not sufficient to eliminate these intrashunt bacteria. Therefore, antibiotics alone are usually ineffective. For an incidental shunt infection, complete removal of the shunt will be required. While there is no shunt and intravenous antibiotics are being used to clear the CSF of infection, an external ventricular drain will be required, with the CSF draining in a closed drainage system. When the CSF cultures are negative and the cell counts satisfactory, the external drain is removed and the new shunt replaced.

Case report

A 2-year-old child had a ventriculo-peritoneal shunt in place for 6 months. He was developing normally but presented with vomiting, headache and a low-grade fever. His parents said he was very sleepy and he was walking with a limp but complained of no joint pains. He was admitted overnight, and the shunt was found to be functioning. Scars of healing impetigo were found in the scalp. Examination of the foot showed an old, neglected wound on the sole so a megaunit of i.m. benzylpenicillin was given and then i.v. cloxacillin. Irrigation and dressing cleaned up the wound but the fever continued. Three days later the child became drowsy and irritable and showed features of meningitis.

Lesson: This child presented with an infected shunt. A delay of 24 hours was appropriate to exclude and treat other causes of infection but since the wound on the foot would not cause such severe symptoms it was probably the source of contamination of the shunt (or else the previous impetigo) rather than the cause of the child's illness. Systemic antibiotics are unlikely to penetrate the shunt where the bacteria are adherent. The shunt should have been removed on the second or third day of admission and certainly as soon as deterioration occurred. External closed drainage can provide temporary relief of hydrocephalus until the child's' CSF is clear, his temperature settled and a replacement shunt can be inserted.

Overdrainage - slit ventricle syndrome

If the patient with a shunt develops chronic headache (which may be relieved to some degree by lying down), this is usually due to an overdrainage situation, with excess siphoning of CSF out of the head. A CT scan, if available, will show thin slit-like ventricles. The treatment is to change the valve to a higher-pressure valve and preferably to choose a valve which has an inbuilt anti-siphon mechanism. These valves may not be available in LMIC. The high-pressure valve without the anti-siphon mechanism may suffice. Programmable valves are now commonly used so that the pressure can be adjusted with an external magnet device but these are very expensive and not usually available in LMIC.

Case report

A 2-year-old child who had had a shunt for 1 year presented confused, irritable, drowsy and incoherent. Examination revealed no neck stiffness and there was no sign of fever. The child had been reviewed a week earlier and was fine, his developmental milestones were normal. He was referred to the base hospital where an inexperienced doctor was uncertain how to proceed. He compressed the valve vigorously a few times after he was shown how to do this by the parents and found the valve emptied but refilled very slowly.

Lesson*: The shunt was probably blocked, due to the ventricular catheter being occluded by choroid plexus. A sign of distal blockage would be inability to empty the valve. Note, vigorous compression of the valve may suck choroid plexus into the catheter but the function of the shunt must still be assessed. If the child had had symptoms of overdrainage (chronic headache, relieved by lying down) then the delay in refilling might have indicated rather empty ventricles.*

Scalp necrosis overlying the valve (Figure 4.5, next page)

A baby's scalp is thin and easily devascularised if stretched under tension. It is therefore important that when shunts are placed in infants that a scalp flap is made which is much larger than the size of the valve, otherwise the chance of scalp necrosis is high. After surgery the child should not lie directly on the side of the shunt and the dressing should not be too tight. It is preferable to use a 'low profile' valve (thin profile in vertical dimension), if it is available, which will reduce the chance of skin necrosis further. Once necrosis has occurred, the shunt will need to be inserted on the other side, the necrotic area will require excision, and probably a small rotation scalp flap to close it.

Trauma to the shunt

Trauma to the shunt causing malfunction is uncommon, but a direct blow to the shunt may damage the tubing or more likely the valve. It is also possible for the valve to be pushed partly or totally through the burrhole, and require revision.

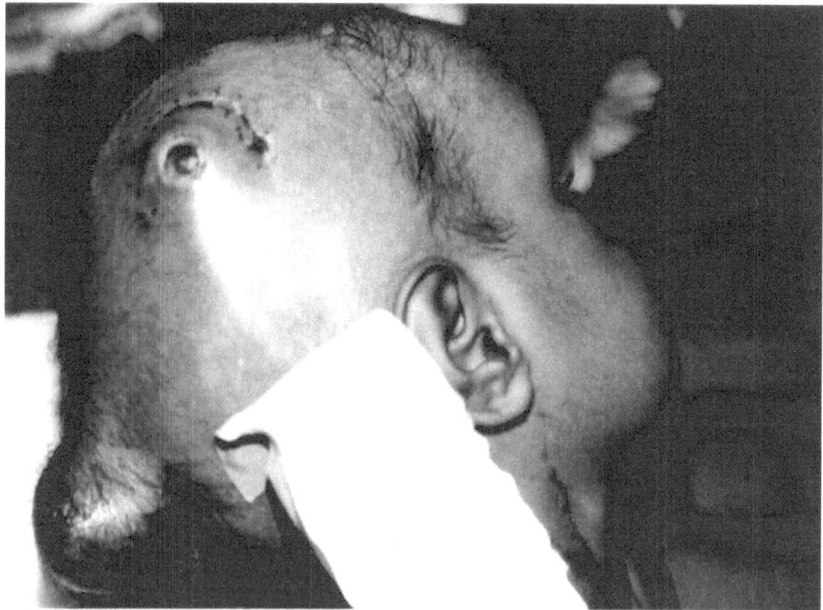

Figure 4.5 Necrotic ulcer overlying exposed shunt valve. Perhaps this was due to undue pressure over the scalp in this region. This problem necessitated removal of the shunt with replacement on the other side. Note also the presence of the occipital encephalocele which has not yet been treated.

Perforation of a viscus

This rare complication usually occurs with old style reinforced and relatively rigid peritoneal catheters. The perforation usually affects large bowel, although the small bowel may also be affected. The tip of the shunt may present per anum or the patient may develop a sudden peritonitis. Infants are especially at risk.

Management: The perforation is treated on its merits - the shunt management is described in the section on incidental intra-abdominal sepsis.

Incidental intra-abdominal sepsis: how to handle the V-P shunt

The most common situation is a patient with acute appendicitis and a shunt. The appendix or other intra-abdominal pathology is treated on its merits. The peritoneal end of the shunt can be left in situ if the sepsis was contained and away from the tip of the shunt, or there was no frank intra-abdominal suppuration or free faecal, gastric or small bowel content.

The patient should be treated with antibiotics that cover bowel flora including anaerobes. Alternatively, if the catheter has been in contact with pus or a perforated viscus, then the lower end should be externalised, i.e. brought out through a separate stab incision, and the CSF collected in a closed drainage system. Once the intra-abdominal problem has been brought under control the peritoneal catheter is replaced and at least initially, is re-sited in the peritoneal cavity (see blockage section above).

Renal disease

Glomerulonephritis is a rare autoimmune reaction to a shunt.

Hydrocele

If there is a patent processus vaginalis in an infant when a shunt is placed, the excess intraperitoneal fluid load may result in a hydrocele. The solution is a closure of the processus.

Routine surveillance of patients with shunts

There is controversy over the necessity for routine surveillance. In the developing world where access to a tertiary centre may be difficult, it is often not feasible, and the patient may only return if there is a problem. Unfortunately, this return may be delayed and parents should be strongly advised to bring their children for review.

Can the shunt ever be removed?

Shunt dependence almost invariably develops once a shunt has been in place for several years. The drainage pathways in cases of obstructive hydrocephalus tend to close up permanently, the drainage pathways in cases of communicating hydrocephalus are already deficient.

The old adage 'once a shunt, always a shunt', usually holds true, and if longstanding shunts are disconnected or removed, the patient usually develops symptoms, sometimes precipitously and may deteriorate to a comatose state within hours. Therefore, once the shunt is place, it should be regarded as a life-long companion.

Third ventriculostomy

The complications of shunts are not infrequent and may be serious. Shunt infection will be a problem in the tropics when performed by inexperienced teams. The regular follow-up of shunt patients and the prompt diagnosis and treatment of shunt complications will not be achievable in many developing countries especially with many patients living at a distance from definitive care. The cost and supply of shunts may also be a disincentive for the treatment of hydrocephalic children. For all these reasons, an alternative to the insertion of shunts would be welcome.

The third ventriculostomy may be such an alternative. An opening is made in the floor of the third ventricle using an endoscope (see description in Chapter 11, page 552). Specifically, designed neuroendoscopes are available, but the paediatric cystoscope or arthroscope are alternatives. There are reports of the correction of up to 70 per cent of selected hydrocephalus patients using this technique, but operation works best for obstructive hydrocephalus which is likely to be responsible for no more than 30 percent of cases in tropical countries. Many of the hydrocephalus cases in the tropics are communicating and follow meningitis and these cases may not respond to ventriculostomy. However, even if the response to ventriculostomy were partial, this procedure may still lead to better long-term results for these children than shunting. The operation is not simple and the surgeon attempting it needs specific training from an experienced neurosurgeon. The third ventricle must be dilated and the child should be over 6 months of age for the operation to be attempted unless the surgeon is experienced. The potential injuries to the adjacent basilar artery and its branches have a high mortality. Neuroendocrine complications may also result from injury to the hypothalamus.

Endoscopic third ventriculostomy and choroid plexus cauterization for the treatment of hydrocephalus in the developing world

There are potentially 100,000 to 200,000 new cases of infant hydrocephalus each year in sub-Saharan Africa.[35] There are 6000 infants who develop hydrocephalus each year in East Africa and a significant proportion is secondary to postnatal infection.[36] There is considerable disability associated with hydrocephalus including epilepsy, cognitive impairment and headaches but treatment to improve brain growth and restore a more normal trajectory for head growth is crucial to the child's development. It is tragic when a mother in brings their child to the clinic with massive head enlargement where the treatment provided can only be palliative. The child's brain has been irreparably damaged and stunted in growth due to the massive ventricular size.

This is all too common a scenario in the developing world. Obstructive hydrocephalus in children older than 2 years and adults are often managed with endoscopic third ventriculostomy (ETV). VP shunt remains the standard of care for children older than 2 years and adults with communicating hydrocephalus.[37] ETV alone for hydrocephalus fails is about 35% in children and most by 6 months and the risk of failure can be stratified. Infection is less common than with VP shunt occurring in less than 2% cases and basilar artery injury is rare but may have an increased risk for the inexperienced

[35] Warf BC. Congenital idiopathic hydrocephalus of infancy: the results of treatment by endoscopic third ventriculostomy with or without choroid plexus cauterization and suggestions for how it works. Child's Nervous System: Official Journal of the International Society for Pediatric Neurosurgery. 2013;29(6):935-940.
[36] Prabhu VC. Neurosurgery Initiatives in Global Health. World Neurosurgery. 2015;84(6): 1544-1546.
[37] Kahle KT, Kulkarni AV, et al. Hydrocephalus in children. Lancet. 2016;**387**(10020):788-799.

surgeon. The basilar artery apex lies below the floor of the third ventricle just posterior to where the endoscope instruments are passed to create an opening in the floor. The rate of shunt infection is 5-9% per procedure, but is higher in the first 6 months of age and is often higher in developing world settings. ETV has been combined with endoscopic choroid plexus cauterization (CPC) in the lateral ventricles to enhance the effect of ETV alone and to avoid the need for ventriculoperitoneal (VP) shunts in infants with idiopathic congenital hydrocephalus or communicating hydrocephalus.[38] The removal of the choroid plexus in the lateral ventricles using diathermy via a flexible endoscope reduces the production of CSF. Dr. Warf developed and trialled this operation in Uganda in infants with hydrocephalus. Dr. Warf has described this operation in detail.[39]

In Uganda, two thirds of infants younger than one year and more than three quarters of children older than one year have successfully avoided shunt dependence with this combined procedure. Nearly all failure occurred within 6 months.[40] Dr. Warf showed that the addition of the choroid plexus cauterization was significantly more successful in children <24 months with idiopathic congenital hydrocephalus than ETV alone. Warf et al also reported the long-term outcome for children <1 year with congenital aqueduct stenosis was significantly superior when CPC was added to ETV.[41] Warf reported ETV with CPC gave better long-term outcome than VP shunt for hydrocephalus associated with myelomeningocele and encephalocele and avoided shunt dependence in sub-Saharan Africa.[42]

The post infectious hydrocephalus is the most common cause of infant hydrocephalus in many developing countries. The outcome may be worse than in other forms of hydrocephalus because it is often accompanied by primary brain damage from the infection particularly

---

[38]Warf BC. Comparison of endoscopic third ventriculostomy alone and combined with choroid plexus cauterization in infants younger than 1 year of age: a prospective study in 550 African children. Journal of Neurosurgery. 2005;103(6):475-481.

[39]Warf BC. Hydrocephalus associated with neural tube defects: characteristics, management, and outcome in sub-Saharan Africa. Child's Nervous System: Official Journal of the International Society for Pediatric Neurosurgery. 2011;27(10):1589-1594.

[40]Warf BC. The impact of combined endoscopic third ventriculostomy and choroid plexus cauterization on the management of pediatric hydrocephalus in developing countries. World Neurosurgery. 2013;79(2):S23 e13-25. Also see: Warf BC. Who Is My Neighbor? Global Neurosurgery in a Non-Zero-Sum World. World Neurosurgery. 2015;84(6):1547-1549.

[41]Warf BC, Tracy S, et al. Long-term outcome for endoscopic third ventriculostomy alone or in combination with choroid plexus cauterization for congenital aqueductal stenosis in African infants. Journal of neurosurgery. Pediatrics. 2012;10(2):108-111.

[42]Warf BC.Hydrocephalus associated with neural tube defects: characteristics, management, and outcome in sub-Saharan Africa. Child's Nervous System: Official Journal of the International Society for Pediatric Neurosurgery. 2011;27(10):1589-1594.

if this is not treated adequately or treatment is delayed.[43] Warf et al reported on the post-infectious hydrocephalus patients in Uganda. Nearly one third of treated infants died within 5 years of surgery and at least one third of survivors were severely disabled. There was no survival benefit for the non-shunt-treated patients, but the cognitive outcome compared well with VP shunt.

Because of the large numbers of post-infectious hydrocephalus infants in the developing world, Warf raises the challenging question as to how we could increase the number of surgeons trained to perform this procedure and whether it could be done by general surgeons (who have many other responsibilities) in these countries and whether they would wish to take it on.[44] The ventricles remain enlarged following the endoscopic operation compared with a functioning VP shunt. The effect of this enlargement on long-term cognitive outcome compared with VP shunt will require further investigation. Brain volume correlates better with cognitive outcome than brain CSF volume.[45] ETV and CPC requires special equipment and specific training to perform this surgery and will need to be tested by other surgeons working in different environments to see if the excellent results of Warf can be reproduced. As for any unfamiliar procedure there is a learning curve. Based on the encouraging results of Warf, the ETV and CPC have been introduced into the USA and Canada.[46]

Courses need to be developed with simulation heads to train neurosurgeons from LMIC to perform this surgery. Specific training and supervision is required to use the flexible endoscope to perform both the ETV and the CPC. Subsidised equipment will need to be made available perhaps through the World Federation of Neurosurgical Societies.

---

[43]Warf BC, Dagi AR, et al. Five-year survival and outcome of treatment for postinfectious hydrocephalus in Ugandan infants. Journal of Neurosurgery. Pediatrics. 2011;8(5):502-508.
[44]Warf BC. Comparison of endoscopic third ventriculostomy alone and combined with choroid plexus cauterization in infants younger than 1 year of age: a prospective study in 550 African children. Journal of Neurosurgery. 2005;103(6):475-481.
[45]Mandell JG, Kulkarni AV, et al. Volumetric brain analysis in neurosurgery: Part 2. Brain and CSF volumes discriminate neurocognitive outcomes in hydrocephalus. Journal of Neurosurgery. Pediatrics. 2015;15(2):125-132.
[46]Kahle KT, Kulkarni AV, et al. Hydrocephalus in children. Lancet. 2016;387(10020): 788-799.

CONGENITAL ABNORMALITIES OF THE CRANIUM

Scalp defects

Dermoid cysts (Figure 4.6, next page)

These cysts are found along embryonic lines of fusion of the developing head and are most common at the lateral margin of the orbit (external angular dermoid), in the midline at the bridge of the nose, and anywhere from the nasion to the occipital region. Some indent the bone and extend to the dura. These lesions are best excised completely including curetting of the bone in which they sit, to prevent recurrence. They tend to enlarge progressively and contain soft keratinous white to yellow greasy material. The scalp is usually intact over their surface. Dermoid cysts occasionally occur intracranially and require craniotomy to totally excise them.

Dermoid sinus

An intracranial dermoid cyst may communicate with the surface via a sinus track, which often has fine hair protruding from it and discharges sebaceous material and/or pus. The deeper component may act as a space-occupying lesion. These are commonest in the posterior fossa and will cause cerebellar signs. Repeated meningitis is a presenting feature, which may result from secondary pyogenic meningitis or release of sterile contents which are highly irritant. A careful search is needed through the hair-bearing scalp to see the midline occipital sinus if the patient does present with recurrent meningitis.

The dermoid sinus may also present in the midline on the spine, particularly in the lumbosacral region and be associated with an intraspinal dermoid. If the skin pit is close to the anal verge, below the coccyx, it is unlikely to penetrate deeper than the subcutaneous tissue, but a sinus placed on the sacrum or above may extend deeper and should be probed.

If its lower end cannot be identified, it should be surgically explored and excised. This is often a technically difficult procedure because of adherence of the lesion to neural structures. If necessary, the track should be followed into the spinal canal following a laminectomy, and the entire dermoid excised. It is also a source of recurrent meningitis, tethering of the spinal cord and cord compression.

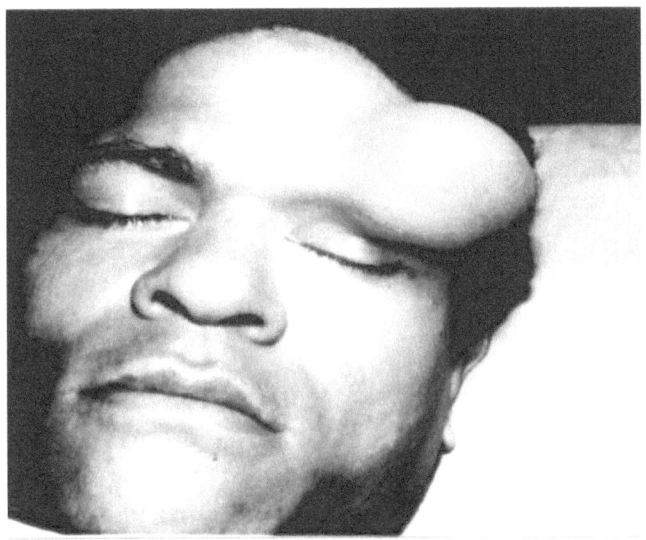

(a) Large external angular dermoid.

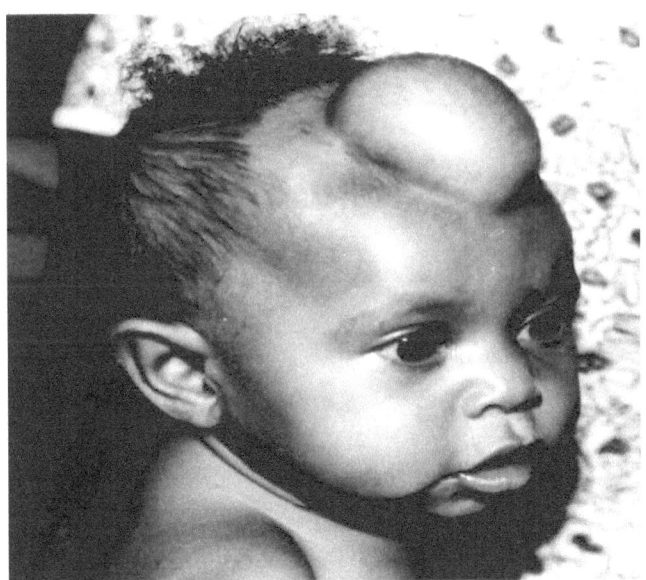

(b) Large midline dermoid of the anterior fontanelle.

Figure 4.6 (a-b) Dermoid cyst.

Haemangioma of the scalp

Small haemangiomas are common and are usually present at birth. These consist of abnormal capillaries arteries and veins raised above the skin. They are common on the face and neck (and may extend into the mediastinum). The intradermal capillary element may regress but a raised cavernous element may gradually increase in size and require excision. These should be distinguished from the port wine capillary haemangioma in the distribution of the trigeminal nerve (usually the forehead and upper face), which are a feature of the Sturge-Weber syndrome, and may indicate underlying cortical involvement with the haemangioma and cause epilepsy. Haemangioma is discussed in further detail in Chapter 6, page 340.

Cutis aplasia congenita

This is an uncommon condition. There is a congenital absence of skin and often underlying skull, over part of the vault. It often arises along suture lines and does not spontaneously close. The exposed tissue should be kept moist until closure can be performed. This could be achieved by split rib graft cranioplasty (see section on cranioplasty, page 545) and a scalp rotation flap (see section on scalp defect closure, page 540). A relatively new technique is to use tissue expanders which consist of an inflatable reservoir beneath the scalp.

The reservoir is gradually inflated, to stretch the scalp enough to cover the defect. This can create extra hair bearing tissue and prevent patches of baldness. Even though the expanded scalp looks unsightly it is usually well tolerated. Tissue expansion clearly requires a plastic surgery service. Full reconstruction requires careful planning in a craniofacial unit.

Case report

A child was born with a normal sized head but with no cranium (Figure 4.7). The parents were well educated so sought medical advice 10 days after birth. A senior paediatrician and general surgeon scratched their heads not having seen the condition before and wondered what to do. They proceeded according to first principles. First were there any other abnormalities?

Case report *(Continued)*

It seemed there were no obvious ones, at least not life-threatening ones. Was the brain normal? The plan was to observe the milestones as they developed. Clearly hydrocephalus would not be a problem. An ultrasound examination queried the integrity of the brain but confirmed normal ventricles.

A senior specialist in one of Australia's Craniofacial units was consulted by telephone. He had seen a few cases where emergency flaps were required to cover exposed brain and prevent meningitis. As in this case there was an intact scalp and, most likely, dura, no immediate action was required. The developmental milestones were observed and over the ensuing months found to be retarded. At one year of age bone grafts were cut and placed on the dura as free grafts to begin to provide a cranium to protect the brain. The child wore a protective helmet once he started crawling.

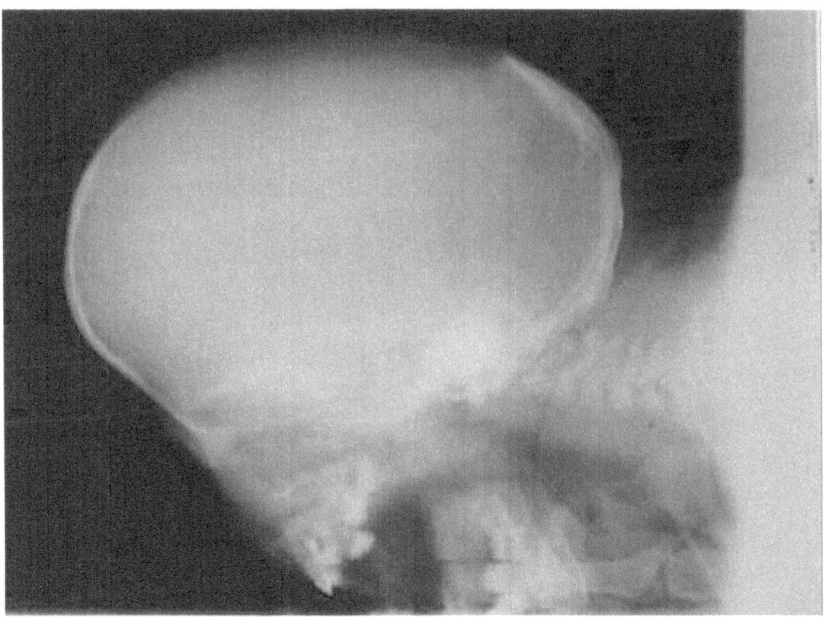

Figure 4.7 Child born with normal appearing head, but absence of bony vault (see case report).

Craniosynostosis

The sutures of the skull are lines of growth. Craniostenosis results from premature closure of a suture (craniosynostosis). This restricts the development of the region affected with compensatory growth at other suture lines, which distorts the shape of the skull. This may cause raised intracranial pressure and intellectual retardation. The more severe deformities may also result in craniocervical junction abnormalities and hydrocephalus and be associated with facial/orbital deformities. Craniosynostosis seems to be rare or under-reported in the developing world. The most common varieties are described below.

Scaphocephaly (see Figure 4.8, next page)

The sagittal suture is fused leading to a long, narrow head with prominent bulging frontal and occipital regions. There is often a palpable ridge along the fused suture line. Scaphocephaly requires early treatment at 2-3 months of age with excision of the sagittal and lambdoid sutures, a bone cut just behind the coronal suture on each side, and an out-fracturing of the parietal bone places. This leads to an immediate correction of the deformity and a good cosmetic result. Excision of the sagittal suture a lone, leads to less of an improvement, but may be appropriate for a less experienced surgeon. The bone edges can be covered with pericranium to prevent recurrence. Great care should be taken to avoid injuring the sagittal sinus and causing excessive blood loss. The operation can be done through a biparietal incision.

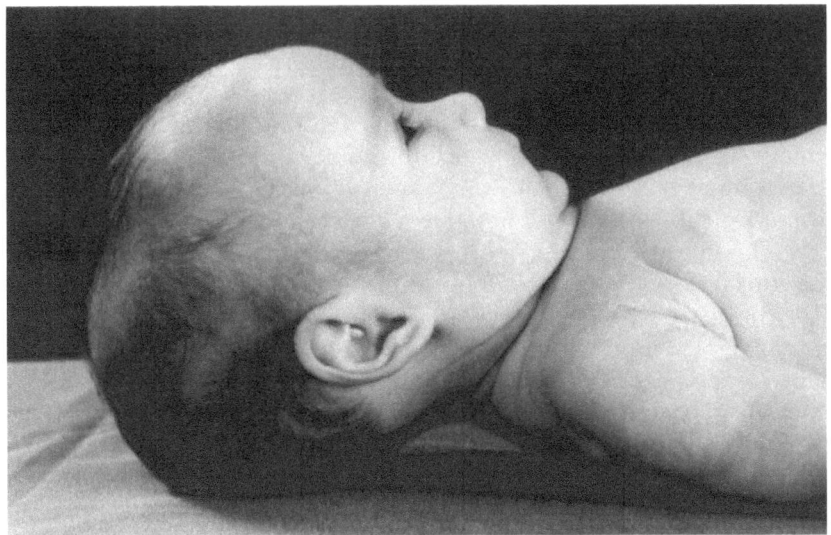

Figure 4.8 (a) Scaphocephaly. Note the elongated head in a lateral view.

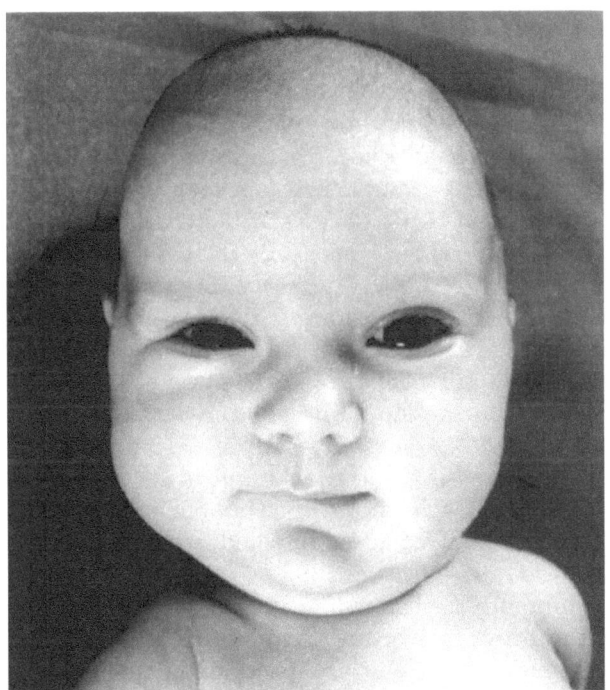

(b) Note the narrow head at the apex on A-P view.

Figure 4.8 (a-b) Scaphocephaly.

Brachycephaly

The coronal sutures are prematurely closed. The head has a short anterior-posterior, and wide biparietal, diameter. The eyes are widely separated and the orbits point upwards and laterally (harlequin eyes), which is easily seen on skull X-ray. Excising the coronal sutures alone will not give a good cosmetic result.

The operation required is a fronto-orbital advancement where the supraorbital margins and frontal bone are advanced forwards and the frontal region reconstructed. This operation is best done in a craniofacial unit and requires detailed planning, expert neuroanaesthesia and postoperative care of infants. A more extreme example of brachycephaly is turricephaly where both coronal sutures are fused and other sutures may also be involved.

Plagiocephaly (Figure 4.9, next page)

This is (a skewed head in the shape of a parallelogram) due to premature fusion of a lambdoid or coronal suture. The lambdoid synostosis results in a prominent forehead on the same side as the flattened occipital region where the lambdoid suture is abnormal. The ear on this side is placed forwards of the unaffected side and in more advanced examples, the face becomes asymmetrical with an abnormal curve to its long axis. A common problem seen in infants who sleep on the back of their head is the so-called 'sticky lambdoid suture' where there is an abnormal restriction of growth of the suture, but where it is still patent on X-ray.

There may be a sclerotic margin along the edge of the suture on the skull X-ray. This abnormal head moulding mostly results from babies lying continually in the supine position although it may result partly from intrauterine moulding and may also be associated with torticollis. It usually settles over the first 6-12 months. If the facial asymmetry is progressing and the occiput is very flattened, surgical correction involves excision of the lambdoid suture up to and including the junction of the lambdoid with the sagittal suture (lambda) (see Chapter 11, page 569).

Less commonly, the lambdoid suture is prematurely fused and this will not improve by waiting. It requires excision of the suture to correct the cosmetic deformity. Bilateral lambdoid synostosis leads to a flattened occiput. If both sutures are fused, they will require excision. To complicate matters, a flattened occiput can also be a normal variant. A unilateral coronal synostosis will also produce plagiocephaly. Unilateral closure of one coronal suture also produces under- development of the forehead and orbital roof on the affected side, with flattening of the forehead and bulging of the opposite side, and facial asymmetry. This requires freeing of the fused suture and frontal-orbital advancement

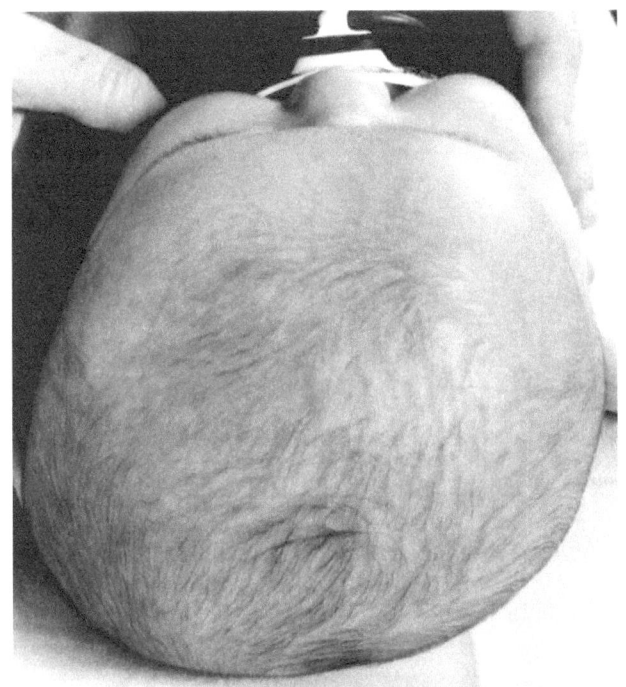

Figure 4.9 Plagiocephaly (note the flattening of the occiput).

Trigonocephaly (Figure 4.10, next page)

This occurs with a premature fusion of the metopic (frontal) suture leading to a pointed forehead. This requires re-modelling of the forehead and craniofacial surgical expertise. It is normally corrected at about 6 months of age. The eyes are closely set together. There is an association with underlying cerebral abnormalities, particularly holoprosencephaly (see below). The presence of a median cleft lip and trigonocephaly are strongly associated with holoprosencephaly.

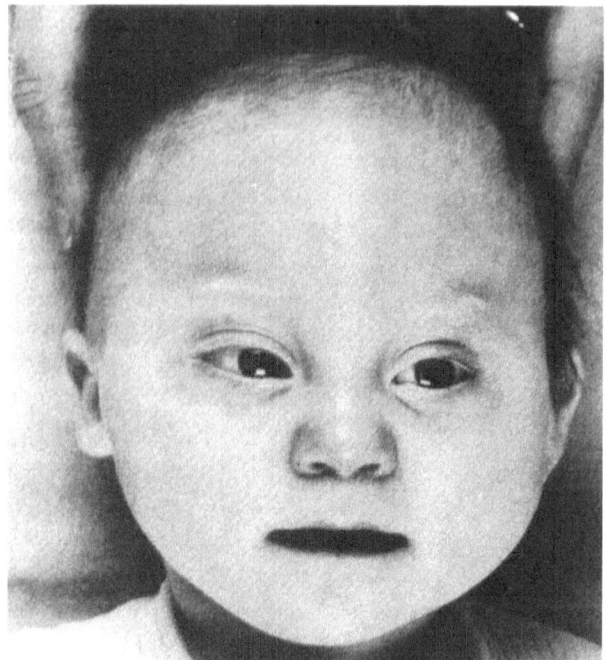

Figure 4.10 (a) Trigonocephaly.

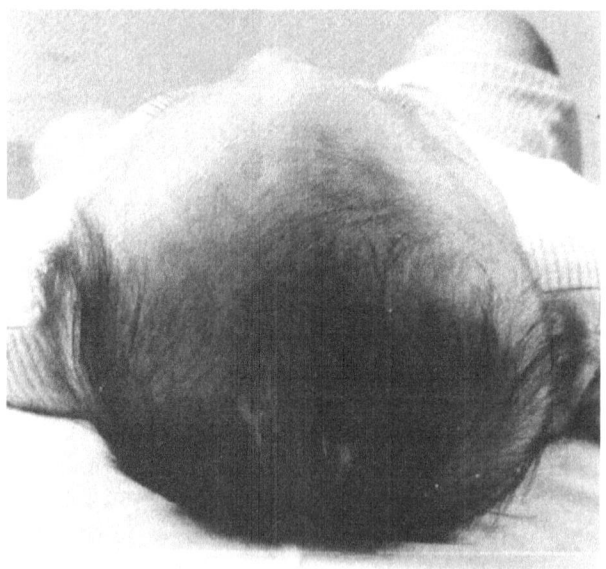

(b) Trigonocephaly.

Figure 4.10 (a-b) Note the beaking of the forehead and the close-set eyes.

Turricephaly

The coronal and sagittal sutures are obliterated. The skull enlarges vertically with a high vault (tower skull). The head is also broad and slopes backwards towards the occiput, which is less prominent than usual. The vertex of the head is further forwards near the bregma. There may be mild hypertelorism (wide separation of the orbits). The anterior fontanelle is usually small and occasionally absent. Excision of the coronal sutures and fronto-orbital advancement is required to correct this deformity.

Oxycephaly

The head is abnormally high and conical and as a result of fusion of multiple sutures. This condition requires surgical correction because the brain will not have enough room to grow and will be adversely affected. The stenosed sutures are excised, and a fronto-orbital advancement may also be required in a craniofacial unit to achieve the best result. Craniosynostosis syndromes are rare but are mentioned in Table 4.3 for reference. All these conditions require complex craniofacial and maxillofacial surgery to correct the deformities of the cranial vault and face. Multiple operations are usually required. Plastic surgery will also be required to reconstruct the syndactyly and other defects.

Brain abnormalities

Microcephaly

In microcephaly, the head circumference is small at birth in proportion to the weight and length measurements, or starts off small and gets progressively smaller. This condition is due to a small brain; as opposed to the problem of untreated craniostenosis, where the head starts off relatively normal in circumference and remains relatively static while the length and weight measurements increase at their normal rate. These two conditions should be distinguished. Evidence of sutural stenosis and increased convolutional markings on the skull X-ray, resulting in a copper-beaten appearance is typical of craniostenosis and may be associated with signs of raised intracranial pressure with papilloedema or chronic optic atrophy if left untreated. Craniostenosis is best thought of as a craniocephalic disproportion. These children will have a progressive deterioration in intellectual function. Release of the sutures is required to lower the intracranial pressure. Microcephaly on the other hand, is due to underdevelopment of the brain with secondary growth retardation of the skull. This may lead to secondary sutural synostosis, which may lead to confusion with primary synostosis, but there will be no copper-beaten appearance and no signs of raised pressure. The child will be intellectually retarded from birth and will fail to reach developmental milestones. The child may also have epilepsy and have abnormal facies and other congenital abnormalities. This condition may also result from severe intrauterine infection, or antenatal haemorrhage or placenta praevia, where there has been intrauterine anoxia. The brain imaging will be helpful to determine the cause. There is usually sign of atrophy, whereas in primary craniostenosis, there is no space around the brain. No surgery is required for microcephaly.

Table 4.3 Craniosynostosis syndromes.

Syndrome	Date	Aetiology	Common abnormalities
Saethre-Chotzen	1931-2	Autosomal dominant gene 7p21-p22	Brachycephaly Maxillary hypoplasia Prominent ear crus Syndactyly Short clavicles with distal hypoplasia
Pfeiffer	1964	Autosomal dominant fibroblast growth factor receptor mutations 8p11.22-p12 10q25-q26	Brachycephaly Craniosynostosis of coronal suture Ocular hypertelorism Small nose, narrow maxilla Broad distal phalanges of thumb & great toe Syndactyly of 2nd and 3rd fingers and toes
Apert	1906	Autosomal dominant fibroblast growth factor receptor 2 mutations 10q25-q26	Irregular craniosynostosis, especially coronal suture Midfacial hypoplasia Syndactyly Broad distal phalanx of thumb and big toe Mental retardation with mean IQ of 70 or less Short A-P diameter of skull with high forehead and flat occiput
Crouzon	1912	Autosomal dominant fibroblast growth factor receptor 2 mutations 10q25-q26	Shallow orbits, ocular proptosis Premature craniosynostosis, especially of coronal, lambdoid and sagittal sutures Conductive hearing loss Poor visual acuity, exposure keratitis Curved parrot nose with inverted V palate

Table 4.3 *(Continued)*

Syndrome	Date	Aetiology	Common abnormalities
Craniofrontal dysplasia (Cohen)	1979	X-linked dominant but occasional case in males	Craniosynostosis, brachycephaly, frontal bossing Hypertelorism Facial asymmetry, bifid nasal tip Syndactyly and broad first toe
Carpenter	1901	Autosomal recessive	Acrocephaly Variable craniosynostosis of all sutures Polydactyly, syndactyly of feet Lateral displacement of inner canthi 50% have congenital heart disease
Greig	1926	Autosomal dominant 7p13 translocation	Frontal bossing, high forehead, macrocephaly, apparent hypertelorism, broad nasal root Preaxial and postaxial polydactyly and syndactyly
Antley Bixler	1975	Autosomal recessive	Craniosynostosis (70%), brachycephaly Large anterior fontanelle, midfacial hypoplasia Depressed nasal bridge, proptosis, choanal stenosis Radiohumeral synostosis Joint contractures
Baller-Gerold	1950	Autosomal recessive	Craniosynostosis Radial hypoplasia (77%) Absent or hypoplastic thumb Anorectal anomalies (40%), renal abnormalities

Anencephaly

Anencephaly is a lethal malformation in which the forebrain, midbrain, cranial vault, overlying skin and membranes are missing. Over half the mothers have hydramnios and many have premature labour.

The anencephalic infant is usually stillborn but occasionally survives a short time. The prevalence is about 1 in 1000 births. There is a 3·5 percent chance of subsequent children having anencephaly, or other neural tube defects.

Holoprosencephaly

There is a failure of separation of the embryonic forebrain into two hemispheres. The children that survive are mentally retarded, with cerebral palsy, facial deformity and may have disturbances in temperature regulation. The olfactory nerves may be missing. The orbits are close together (hypotelorism) and rarely there is a single eye and orbit (cyclopia). The diagnosis can be made on cranial ultrasound. It is associated also with occipital encephalocele, aqueduct stenosis and systemic malformations. The frequency of the disorder is of the order of 1 in 18, 000 but is more common in the offspring of diabetic mothers (1 percent).

ENCEPHALOCELE

Encephaloceles are congenital lesions consisting of a herniation of intracranial contents from the cranial cavity, and may consist of meninges alone (meningocele), contain brain, (meningoencephalocele or encephalocele) or include the ventricle (hydroencephal-omeningocele). The embryology of the encephaloceles is complex and varies depending on the site of the defect. Only some may represent neural tube defects. An encephalocele is an ugly deformity which remains a blight on the child until repaired. If the afflicted children survive without repair in developing countries, they may be secluded in virtual isolation because of parental embarrassment or shame.

The goals of surgery include closing open skin defects to prevent infection and desiccation of viable brain tissue, preventing rupture of a thin meningoencephalocele sac, removal of non-viable extracranial cerebral tissue, watertight closure of the dura, closure of the cranial defect and reconstruction of the facial deformity.

Classification, epidemiology, pathology (Figure 4.11, page 177)

Encephaloceles are classified as occipital, basal, convexity or sincipital (anterior). The sincipital group are divided into frontoeth-moidal encephaloceles, interfrontal and craniofacial clefts. The frontoethmoidal group is further subdivided into nasofrontal, nasoethmoidal and naso-orbital types (see Table 4.4, page 180). Encephaloceles occur in 1 per 5000 births worldwide. The incidence of sincipital encephalocele compared with occipital encephalocele is significantly greater in the tropical latitudes, particularly in parts of Asia and Africa, and is also more common in parts of Russia.

For instance, in Thailand, sincipital encephalomeningocele is nine times more common than the occipital lesion. However, the occipital to sincipital encephalomeningocele ratio is reversed in North America, Australia, Europe and parts of South America, varying from 2.5:1 to 15:1. The occipital encephaloceles occur in 1-3 per 10, 000 live births.

The ratio of cranial to spinal meningocele is also reversed in Thailand (3.5:1), compared with a ratio of 1:5.2 to 1:22 in Europe, USA and Australia. The aetiology of sincipital encephalocele is unknown. There are certainly ethnic influences, but these are quite variable. An absence of familial incidence and one case of identical twins being discordant argues against a genetic influence and normal karyotypes have been noted. It is possible that diet, ambient temperature, drugs or chemicals are aetiological factors, but these are unproven. Paternal age may also be a factor resulting in a dominant inheritance pattern.

The **sincipital encephaloceles** are due to herniation of intracranial contents through a midline tunnel from the anterior cranial fossa into the facial skeleton. This defect is usually found at the foramen caecum which is normally a small pit in the frontal bone anterior to the crista galli to which the falx cerebri attaches. The sincipital encephalocele may be associated with craniofacial deformity consisting of hypertelorism, orbital dystopia, elongation of the face and dental malocclusion.

The **occipital encephalocele** may occur through the occipital bone above and/or below the transverse sinus, and therefore may involve occipital lobe and/or cerebellum. The **infratentorial or subtorcular encephaloceles** may variably contain all the posterior fossa structures and some also contain occipital lobe. This neural tissue cannot be excised. The upper cervical spine may also be involved (occipitocervical encephalocele).

The **'aborted' or atretic cephalocele** is a small midline lump usually around the vertex region, which often has a tuft of hair associated with it or a cutaneous naevus, and is exquisitely tender to touch, sending the infant into screams of discomfort. These lesions contain a small element of gliotic tissue passing through a small hole in the skull via a thin stalk, and can easily be excised down to the skull level with transfixion of the stalk and primary closure of the scalp. The parietal encephalocele is rare.

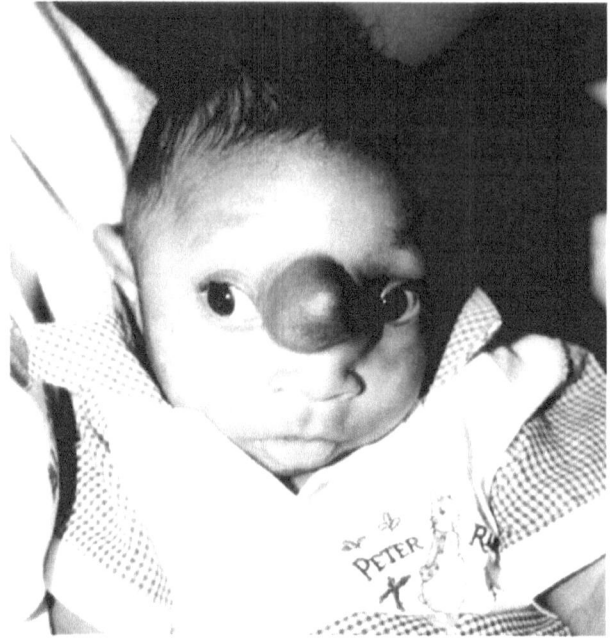

Figure 4.11 (a) Frontoethmoidal/nasofrontal.

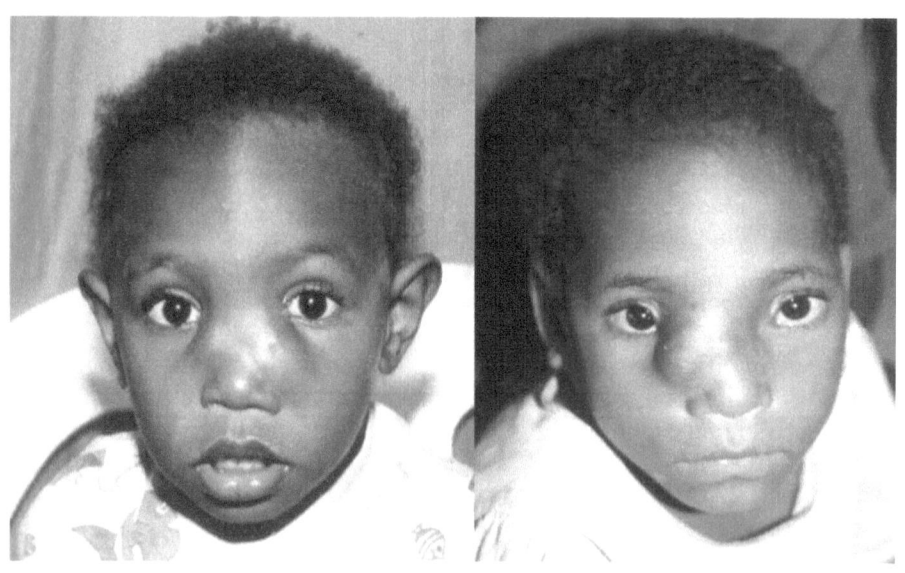

(b) Frontoethmoidal/nasoethmoidal.

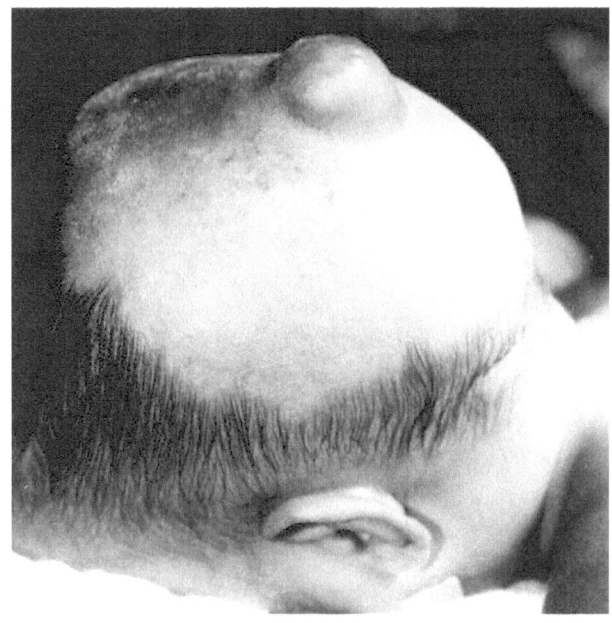

(c) High occipital. This was a small encephalocele, not quite small enough to call atretic.

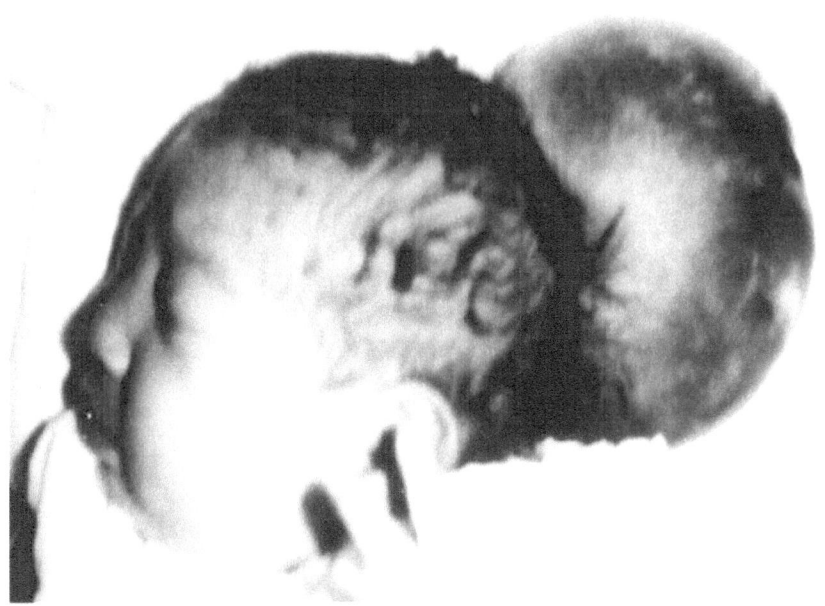

(d) Occipital/supratentorial meningoencephalocele. This lesion contained mainly CSF and the child has done very well with normal intelligence and vision.

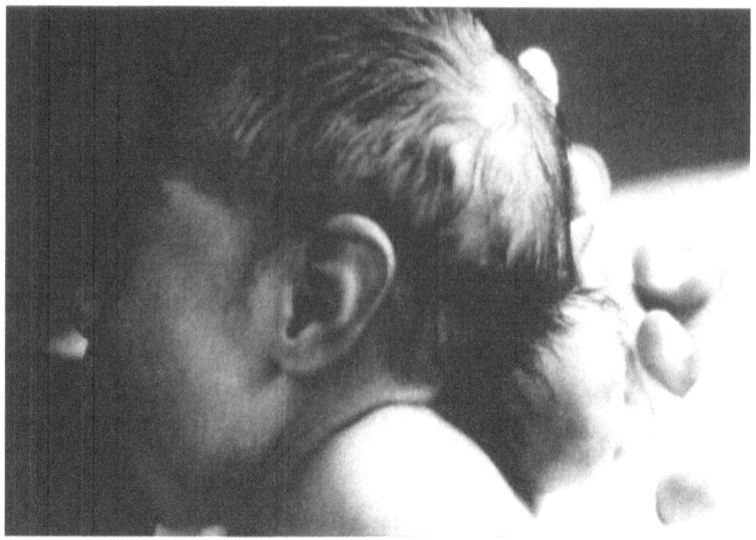

(e) i

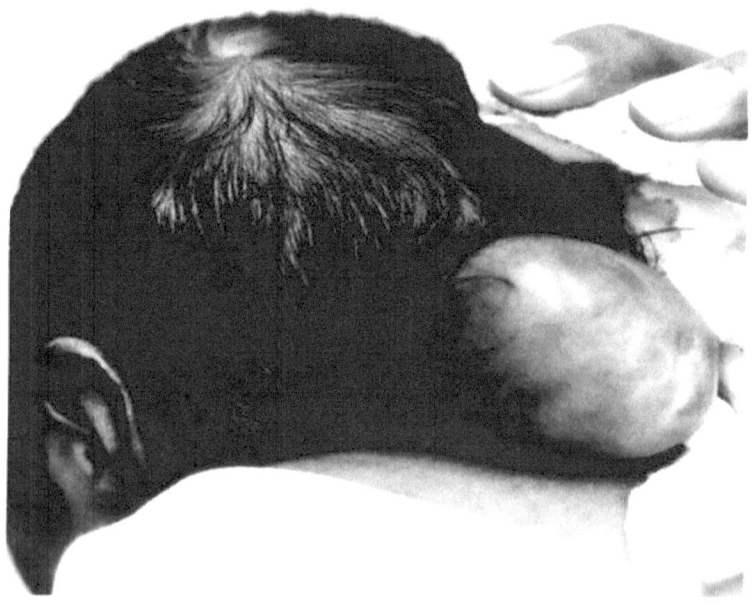

(e) ii

(e) i-ii Subtorcular occipital encephalocele.

Figure 4.11 (a-e) The types of encephalocele.

Table 4.4 Classification of encephaloceles.

Convexity
    Occipital
    Parietal
    Sagittal
    Occipitocervical

Sincipital
    Frontoethmoidal
        nasofrontal
        nasoethmoidal
        naso-orbital
    Interfrontal
    Craniofacial cleft

Basal
    Intranasal
    Spheno-orbital
    Sphenomaxillary
    Sphenopharyngeal

Atretic

Clinical assessment

The clinical examination should include a close inspection of the skin of the encephalocele for any thin or necrotic areas which would encourage the surgeon to operate sooner, any other cranial or spinal anomalies and any other congenital anomalies of organs or other tissues. The neurological problems may only become manifest as the child grows older. The head circumference is measured and the turgor of the anterior fontanelle is assessed. Hydrocephalus may develop progressively in the first few weeks.

Transillumination of the sac may help disclose how much cerebral tissue is present as opposed to CSF. Ultrasound can give an even more accurate picture of the contents particularly in a large lesion. A series of plain skull and facial X-rays including basal views for a sincipital encephalocele are helpful in delineating the size and position of the cranial defect through which the hernia passes. The ultrasound is also used to examine ventricular size. The incidence of co-existent hydrocephalus ranges from being rare to 24 percent of cases in the sincipital encephaloceles and in over 50 per cent of the occipital encephaloceles. Computed tomography (CT) including bone windows is also helpful in assessing the brain and the bony anatomy.

Surgical management

The type of operative repair depends on the anatomical pathology of the particular lesion and the surgical resources and. equipment available. Nasoethmoidal encephalocele involves a hernia through the foramen caecum to a defect between the nasal bones and the nasal cartilage. The encephalocele involves the ethmoid complex. The floor of the anterior cranial fossa tends to be steep and cone shaped, and because there is a relatively long canal from the skull to the face, trans-cranial repair is advised. Nasofrontal encephalocele involves a hernia from the foramen caecum to the junction of the nasal and frontal bones, with the nasal bones being intact at the inferior margin of the defect.

Experience of surgical repair in Papua New Guinea suggests that because of the short canal involved in this type, an extracranial transfacial repair is possible. The differentiation between these two types can be made clinically and with skull and facial X-rays. Naso-orbital encephalocele is rare and involves a defect in the medial wall of the orbit and a long tract through a bony tunnel from the anterior fossa to the orbit with nasal bones intact.

Transcranial repair is advised. In our experience, where there is a small external defect present, and the internal opening is not accessible, CSF leak and recurrence are likely if an extracranial repair is attempted. The narrow external defect usually implies a long canal between the internal and external openings of the lesion. The larger anterior defects (greater than 2- 3 cm) presenting at the bridge of the nose or in the forehead are suitable for extracranial repair. Lesions on the middle third of the nose, or medial orbit with an external defect less than 2-3 cm are best repaired intracranially.

Most authors have described a transcranial or combined transcranial/ extracranial approach for all of these lesions. Any intracranial repair or craniofacial surgery in the developing world is best performed by a visiting neurosurgeon or craniofacial teams, if unavailable locally. It is possible for visiting neurosurgeons to use basic neurosurgery instruments available in the developing world to achieve an adequate intracranial repair (Figure 4.12, next page).

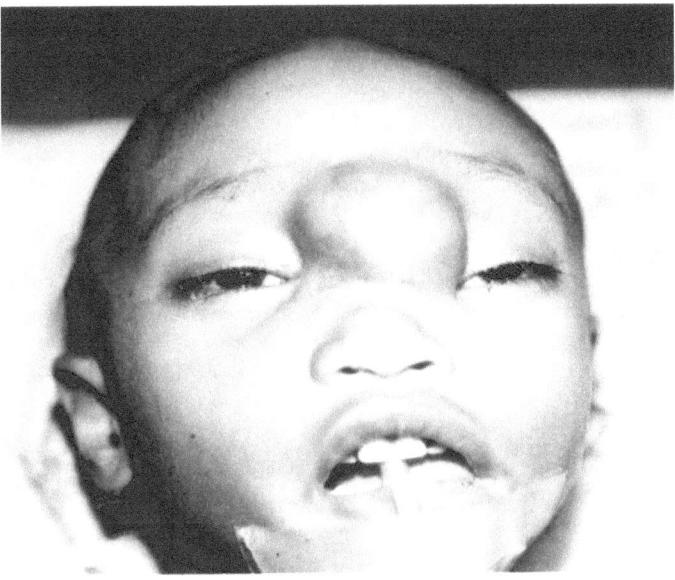

Figure 4.12 (a)

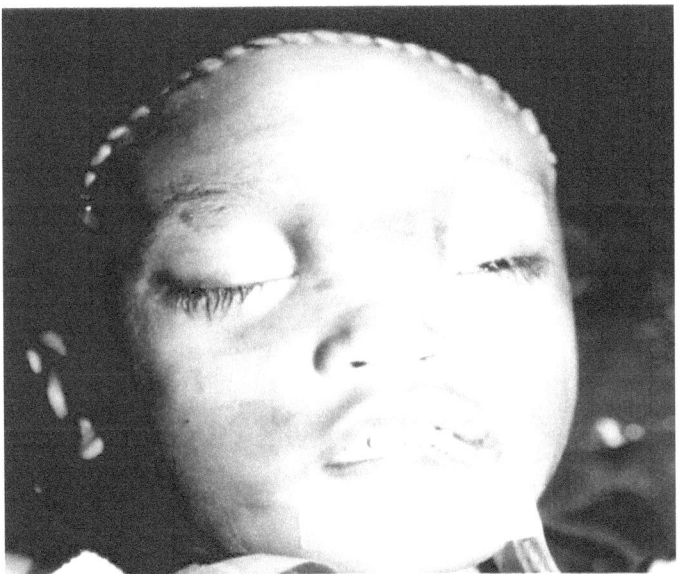

(b)

Figure 4.12 (a-b) Transcranial repair of a frontoethmoidal/nasoethmoidal encephalocele. Note the bicoronal incision and the disappearance of the lesion following repair.

The one-stage extracranial transfacial approach has been infrequently described or advocated. We have used the extracranial approach for the appropriately selected lesions, and feel that this is a relatively straightforward procedure for a general surgeon to pursue in the developing world. The sac is opened, the hernia reduced, the dura closed with a double-breasted closure, and the excess skin excised. The bony defect can also be repaired with a bone graft using split rib or a metallic implant. It is important to close the defect to avoid recurrence (Figure 4.13, next page). The frontal extracranial repair may have a significant recurrence rate. The extracranial technique is also used for the repair of occipital and parietal encephaloceles. The bony defect in newborn infants with occipital encephaloceles may close spontaneously, but if still present beyond the age of 2 years can be closed with a cranioplasty.

The extruded brain tissue in an occipital encephalocele can usually be replaced into the cranial cavity and should only be excised when necrotic or extensively gliotic or when it is impossible to reduce. Associated hydrocephalus usually requires shunting. The skin-covered sincipital encephaloceles are not repaired until at least 3 months of age, but in the developing world it is preferable to wait till the child is at least 2 years of age for an intracranial repair, to reduce the risks of surgery. A disadvantage of the extracranial anterior repair is that the associated hypertelorism and orbital dystopia are not corrected. The involvement of a multidisciplinary craniofacial team including plastic, maxillofacial surgeons and neurosurgeons is necessary to correct this deformity.

Detailed imaging with three dimensional CT scans is obtained and the lesion is approached via a forehead scalp flap which is turned down to expose the anterior skull and upper facial skeleton. These techniques are not generally available in the developing world. As an alternative, orbital osteotomies in the first year of life, which move the medial orbital walls closer together with bone grafts and canthopexies may reduce the space occupying effect of the hernia and allow early remodelling of the facial skeleton. In our cases of frontoethmoidal encephalocele repaired extracranially, the hypertelorism has not been severe, and the cosmetic result has been satisfactory. A rotation forehead flap can be used where there is a frontal skin defect at the bridge of the nose.

The intranasal encephaloceles may be accidentally discovered when nasal operations are performed, particularly for presumed nasal polyps. When the 'polyp' is grasped, a gush of CSF follows. In the developing world setting, this situation is best handled with an intranasal dural repair using fascia and /or fat from the thigh. Spinal drainage at 5-10 ml per hour, may help resolve the CSF fistula in these situations. Contraindications to reparative surgery are gross brain herniation, severe brain damage or malformation, multiple congenital anomalies with poor general prognosis for development, or an open encephalocele with meningitis.

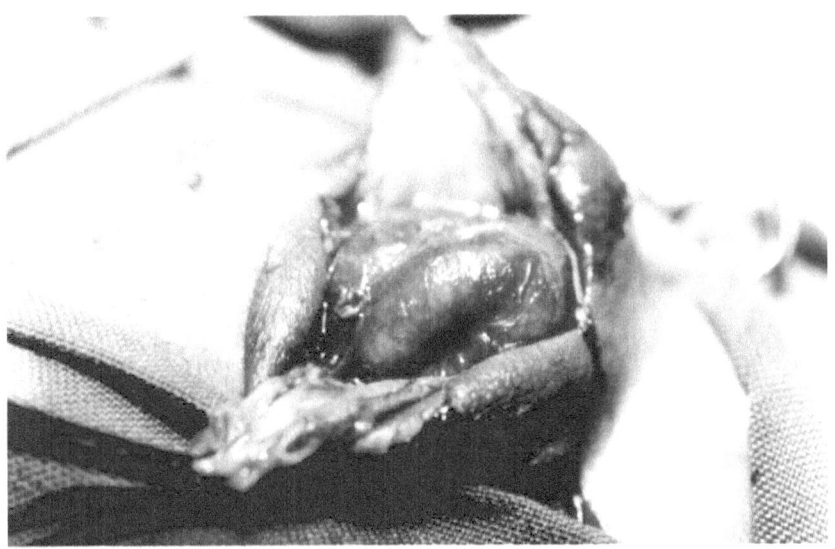

Figure 4.13 (a) The encephalocele sac is open showing the cerebral cortex.

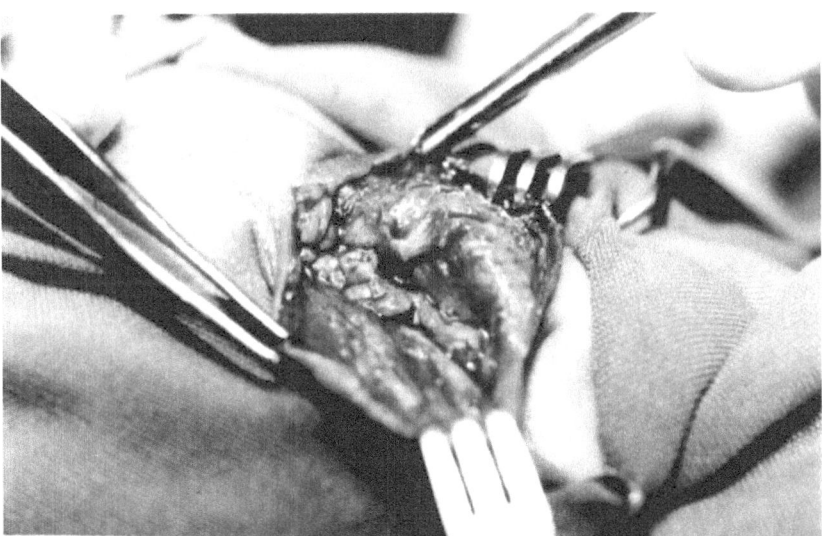

(b) Reduction of the contents into the intracranial cavity and plication of sac.

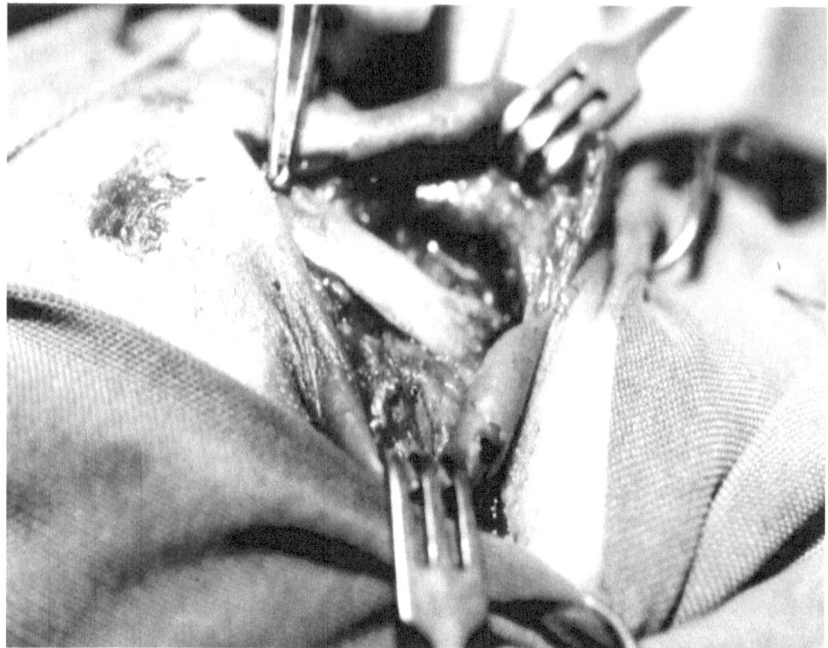

(c) The defect is repaired with a rib graft before final closure.

Figure 4.13 (a-c) Transfacial repair of a nasofrontal encephalocele. This is the same patient as shown in Figure 4.11 (a).

Prognosis

The prognosis for the sincipital or frontal encephalocele patient is generally good and is usually associated with normal intelligence and motor development. However mental retardation, epilepsy and ocular problems have been described in this group. The epilepsy may develop late. Where there is a gross brain herniation or where the extruded brain is damaged and gliotic the prognosis may be poor. The most important prognostic factors for the child with an occipital encephalocele are the presence or absence of brain tissue in the sac and the size of the infant's head. The occipital encephaloceles have a strong association with visual defects, epilepsy and mental retardation.

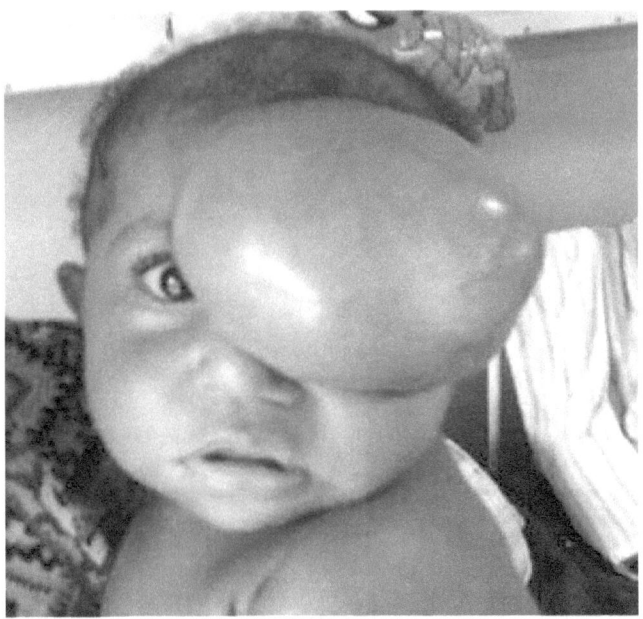

(a)

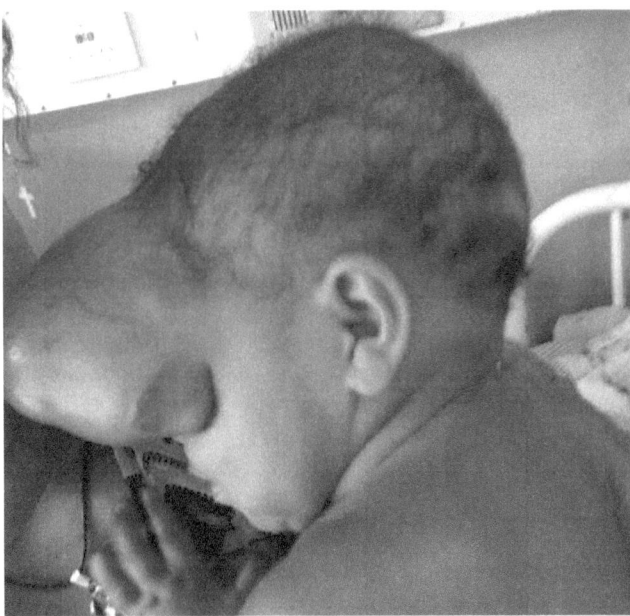

(b)

Figure 4.14 (a-b) Shows the child in front view and in profile.

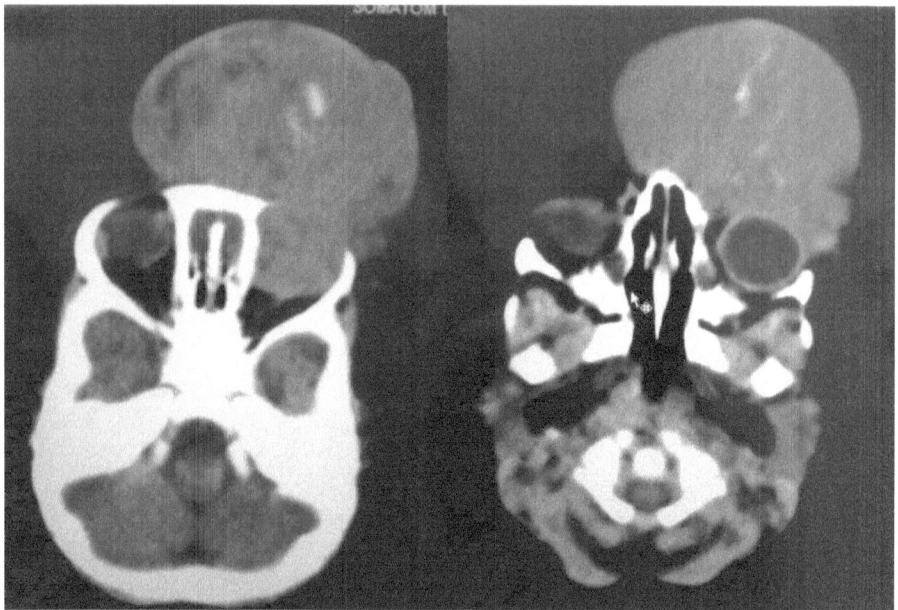

(b) Axial CT scans show the orbital tumour extending anterior to the frontal and nasal bones.

Figure 4.14 (a-b) Consider the differential diagnosis of a facial/orbital mass. A young child with a large left facial/orbital mass. It is firm and is clearly not an encephalocele. The tumour was biopsied and was most likely to be a malignant sarcoma. The child was treated expectantly as excision was not feasible in this setting. Chemotherapy or radiotherapy were not available.

Of children with occipital meningoceles (i.e. minimal or no extrusion of brain tissue), 60-80 per cent are normal, whereas only 10-25 per cent of children with occipital encephaloceles containing brain tissue are normal. To illustrate this pattern, an occipital meningoencephalocele may be larger than the child's head but have a good prognosis if the cerebral herniation is minimal and the head circumference normal, but a relatively small occipital encephalocele with a microcephalic head and a backward sloping brow carries a poor prognosis.

Overall 60-70 percent of infants with occipital encephaloceles will develop hydrocephalus that requires shunting (Humphrey, 1994). Magnetic resonance imaging, if available, helps to define the state of cerebral development, the contents of the sac, and assists with the prognostication.

NEURAL TUBE DEFECTS; SPINA BIFIDA AND MYELOMENINGOCELE

The term 'spina bifida' literally means that the spine is splayed into two parts dorsally due to a failure of bony fusion. There may be a failure of fusion of the lamina (occulta), a sac involving the meninges only (meningocele) or a sac or swelling which includes the meninges and spinal cord or cauda equina (myelomeningocele). Spina bifida is more common in Caucasians than Africans and Asians.

The opportunity to repair myelomeningoceles with shunting for hydrocephalus began in the mid to late 1950s.

Pathology and clinical presentation

Spina bifida occulta

This failure of fusion may be mild as in spina bifida occulta, a failure of bony fusion of the laminae (usually the fifth lumbar vertebra), fibrous tissue replacing bone, resulting in no spinous process evident on X-ray. The patient is neurologically normal. It occurs in up to 15 per cent of the population. It may be associated with lower back pain in adult life but the width of the spinal canal at this point also makes spinal canal stenosis unlikely. A sinus, hairy patch or pigmented naevus over the lower lumbar spine suggests occult spinal dysraphism (see below).

Occult spinal dysraphism

In occult spinal dysraphism, the bony abnormality is associated with abnormalities within the spinal canal: thick filum terminale, intradural epidermoid and dermoid cysts, intradural lipoma (lipomyelomeningocele), teratoma, diastematomyelia (midline splitting of the spinal cord by a midline bony or fibrous peg). A spinal bony defect associated with a skin abnormality, or with back pain, scoliosis, and enuresis, may be associated with a tethered spinal cord. A tethered cord usually presents in childhood (but may present at any age) with back pain, lower extremity pain and weakness, or bladder and bowel changes. There may be a subcutaneous lipoma as in lipomyelomeningocele. Surgical release and untethering the cord is associated with normal development and function.

Practice point

Never operate on a lipoma or cyst over the midline of the back unless you are prepared to release a tethered spinal cord. Always perform a full neurological assessment of patients with lesions over the spine.

Meningocele and myelomeningocele (Figure 4.15, next page)

The defect, usually posterior, involves the meninges and/or the cord. The difference between these two is determined by whether the posterior defect includes the spinal cord or cauda equina or whether it only consists of meninges. The prognosis is better for meningoceles because, providing the cord is not damaged by infection, exposure or corrective surgery, the lower limbs, bladder and bowel will be normal. They may be open or closed. **Open lesions** will become rapidly contaminated and complicated by meningitis if not closed rapidly. **Closed lesions** allow more careful assessment, providing they are not tense and about to rupture. Always beware of incising a fluctuant midline swelling over the spine. Prenatal diagnosis by ultrasound is now possible from about 12 weeks of gestation. There will also be a raised level of alphafetoprotein in the amniotic fluid of fetuses with open defects. In developed countries this has resulted in a sharp fall in the numbers of spina bifida cases, as the pregnancy can be terminated.

Management

The three crucial questions to ask are:

1. What is the spinal level affected?

2. What are the other defects?

3. Who to operate on?

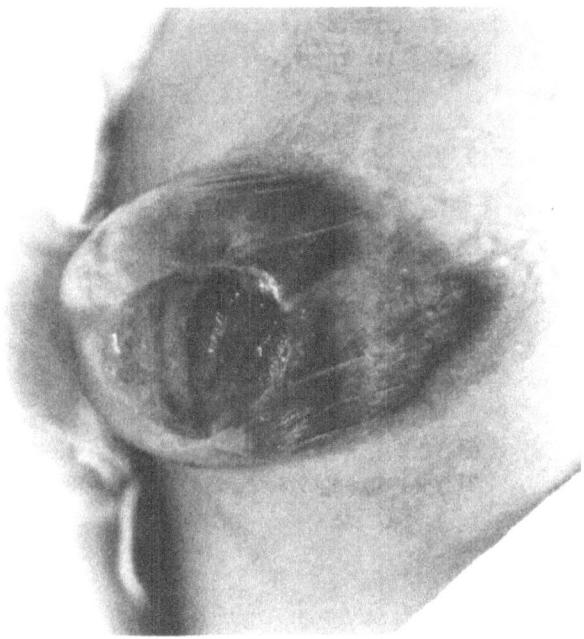

Figure 4.15 (a) Open myelomeningocele showing placode with central groove with a thin membrane surrounding the placode.

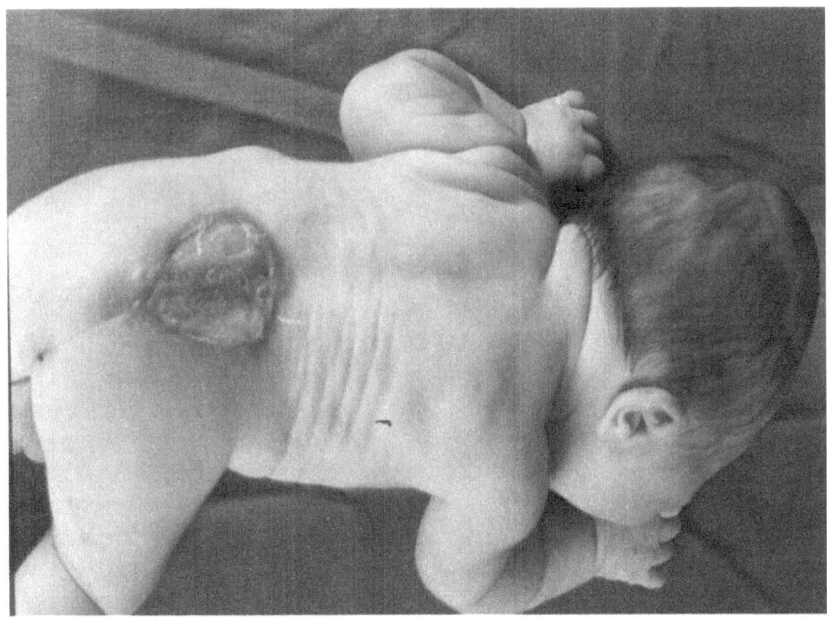

(b)

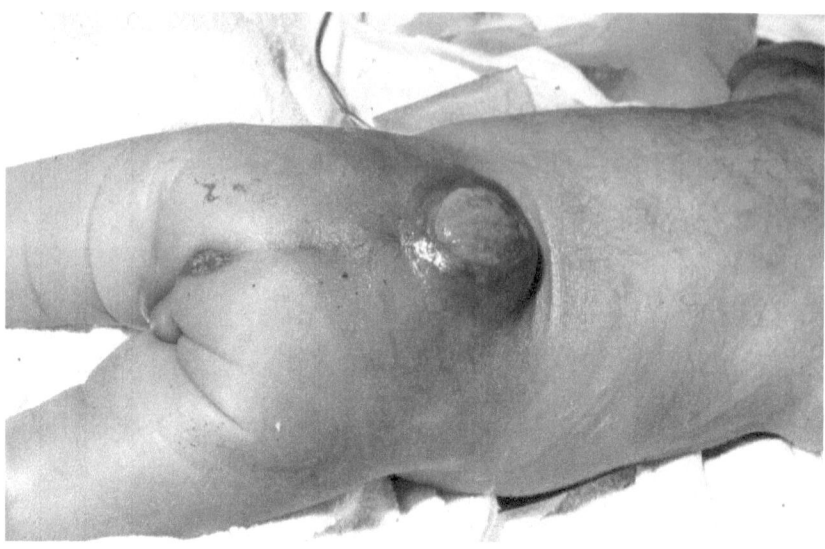

(c)

(b-c) Two infants with open myelomeningoceles. Large skin defects. Note the patulous anus in each baby.

Figure 4.15 (a-c) Open myelomeningocele.

What is the spinal level affected?

It is important to examine the child, particularly in relation to the function of the lower limbs, and determine what the motor and sensory levels are. A gentle prick of the skin with a blunted needle will allow determination of the sensory level (starting distally and moving proximally) by noting the movement of the limbs and the facial expression. Spinal reflexes involving withdrawal leg movements may be obtained with skin stimulation below the lesion level, but skin stimulation above the level of the lesion, if it is complete, will not produce any lower limb movement. A lesion with a motor level clinically above L3-4 should be considered a high lesion. The motor level can be checked by looking at which muscle groups are wasted and watching the spontaneous movements of the legs and on pain stimulation with a gentle prick. The assessment of the sphincter function is difficult in a neonate, but the continuous dribbling of urine indicates a neurogenic bladder and a patulous incontinent anus usually indicates sacral root involvement. Paraplegic babies and those with only hip flexion (Ll-2) do equally badly. The prognosis is better when there is some extension of the knees (L3-4).

What are the other defects? (Table 4.5, below)

In over 90 per cent of cases myelomeningocele is associated with some degree of hydrocephalus. The child may already have an enlarged head at presentation, and a careful search for other congenital abnormalities should be made, especially the heart and kidneys. An ultrasound will determine whether the kidneys are present. Other serious congenital anomalies will further strengthen the argument for conservative management in a neonate with a high lesion. A neonate with L5-S1 involvement may just require supportive orthotic braces to walk satisfactorily. However, once the extensors of the knees are affected (L3-4), then ambulation may become more difficult as the child gets older and heavier, and eventually the adolescent may end up requiring a wheelchair. Club feet may also need to be managed.

Table 4.5 Common congenital defects associated with myelomeningocele.

Hydrocephalus

Other brain malformations

    Chiari II malformation - cerebellar ectopia

    Absent corpus callosum

    Dysmorphic (misshapen) lateral ventricles

Renal abnormalities

Congenital heart disease

Talipes

Abnormal facies

Who should be operated on?

In the developing world where severe physical disability is very difficult to manage, if not impossible, it is reasonable to take a conservative approach to the high open myelomeningocele lesions in the thoracic or cervical region. These are all associated with total paraplegia and double incontinence. The upper lumbar spine open myelomeningocele may also have a similar effect, but the low to middle lumbar lesions are associated with a better prognosis, in terms of ambulation and other complications. This selective policy of repair was described by Lorber in Sheffield in the 1960s but is controversial in many HICs. Some authorities recommend repair of all lesions but then face the consequent management of the severely disabled child.

The conservative approach involves maintaining the child's hydration, using sedation (e.g. barbiturate) to treat any distress and letting nature take its course. Some of the less severely affected infants may survive non-operative treatment and the open spinal defect is epithelialised (Figure 4.16, below). For those lesions selected for repair, the recommendation is that the open myelomeningocele be repaired in the first 24 hours of life. A closed myelomeningocele does not need to be repaired urgently. The technique of closure is the same as for the open lesion (see page 556), but the spinal cord is usually structurally intact in these cases. The recommended management for hydrocephalus is to insert the shunt 2-3 days after myelomeningocele closure. This allows time for enough wound healing to reduce the risk of shunt infection. Insertion of the shunt at the same time as the repair, may increase the risk of infection.

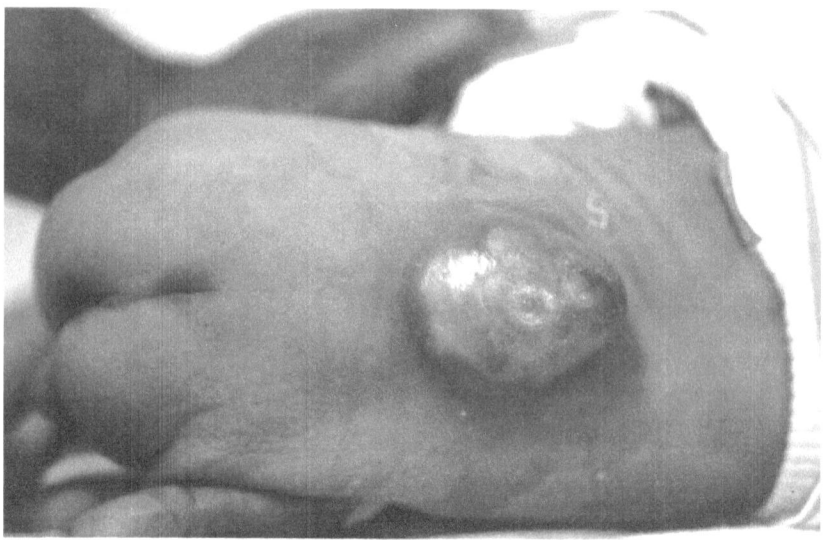

Figure 4.16 (a) An infant lying on the side. Almost completely epithelialised myelomeningocele with central eschar.

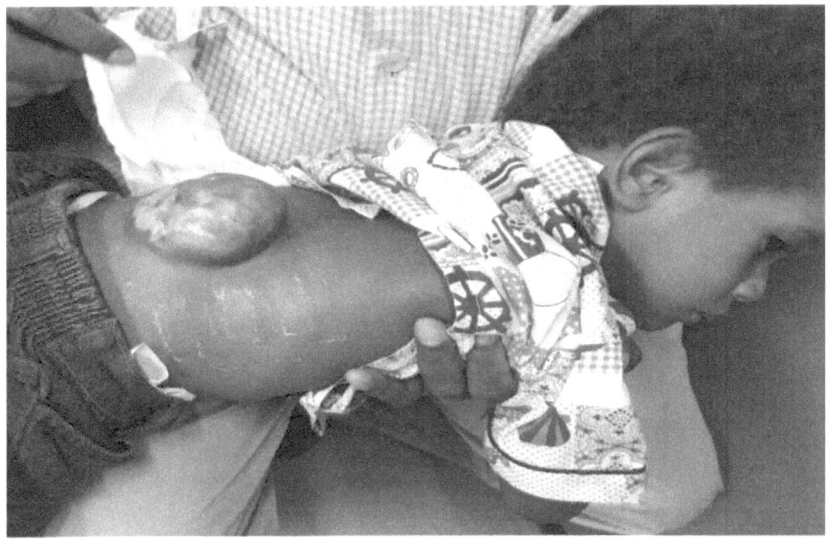

(b) A young child with a large completely epithelialised myelomeningocele. The child is paraplegic and has urinary incontinence.

Figure 4.16 (a-b) Epithelialisation of myelomeningocele as a result of conservative management.

Although most meningoceles are posteriorly located they may occasionally be anterior. An anterior sacral meningocele may present as a pelvic mass, large bowel obstruction or even form part of the differential diagnosis of a sacrococcygeal teratoma. The principles of closure of the posterior lesion are to close the neural tube (if open), then the meningeal layer, muscle and skin. The operations for closure of myelomeningocele and lipomyelo-meningocele are described in Chapter 11, page 564.

DIASTEMATOMYELIA

Diastematomyelia is an uncommon congenital malformation of the spine occurring mostly in the lower thoracic and lumbar regions, resulting in a split lower spinal cord (diplomyelia) with a cartilaginous, fibrous, or bony spur or septum passing vertically across the spinal canal between the bifid cord. A bony spur may be seen on plain X-rays. Myelography will give better definition and demonstrate a fibrocartilaginous spur and the split cord and sometimes dural sac. Widening of the interpedicular distance in the region of the spur, hemivertebra, neural arch abnormalities (spina bifida), scoliosis and kyphosis are all common accompaniments. Cutaneous abnormalities such as a hairy patch or a naevus are often present at the site of spinal abnormality. Symptoms of tethering of the cord such as back and lower limb pain, postural abnormalities, spasticity in the lower limbs and bladder disturbance are likely to develop as the child grows in length. This must be corrected if permanent deficit is to be avoided. A laminectomy is performed, the spur completely removed and a single dural tube created and the cord detethered.

TETHERED SPINAL CORD

Primary tethering of the spinal cord is due to congenital malformations such as lipomyelomeningocele, intraspinal lipoma, diastematomyelia, dermoid cyst, thickened filum terminale, or combinations of these problems. Secondary tethering may be caused by scarring as a result of previous detethering procedures for any of the above congenital disorders or years after a myelomeningocele repair. There may be a dermoid cyst at the site of tethering due to the failure to excise all skin around the placode at the time of the primary myelomeningocele repair.

The tethered cord also may be associated with the development of syringomyelia and scoliosis. Patients with tethered spinal cords develop increasing pain in the back and sciatica, paresthesia in the lower limbs, weakness and increasing spasticity in the lower limbs and finally sphincter disturbance. The features may be asymmetrical and tend to occur during growth spurts, especially in the teenage years. The patient may have had a longstanding neurogenic bladder and chronic constipation when they present. They may have developed an equinus deformity of the feet with toes curling under in flexion and trophic foot ulcers, limping, leg length discrepancy, and chronic wasting of various muscle groups in their lower limbs. Sensory loss can usually be demonstrated and the perineum and perianal area should also be tested.

There may be an old scar or cutaneous features of spinal dysraphism on their lower back. Most patients with primary tethering will present by their teens but some present with chronic problems in adulthood. The diagnosis can be confirmed with myelography and the conus is found to end at L3-4 or below. If the filum is thickened it may be difficult to determine where the spinal cord ends. MRI with sagittal images has eliminated the need for myelography in the advanced centres and gives the surgeon excellent views of the anatomy, which also aids in the planning of surgery. The treatment requires a laminectomy and removal of the cause.

The methods of laminectomy and repair of lipomyelo-meningocele are discussed in the operative surgery chapter (Chapter 11, page 564). The thickened filum which consists of fibro-fatty tissue is divided below the conus without damaging any of the roots of the cauda equina.

The nerve roots have all come off the conus and the filum below this has no attached nerve roots and so can be divided. Some surgeons recommend nursing the patient prone for a few days after surgery to try and prevent retethering of an exposed area of spinal cord following the lysis of adhesions or the removal of a lipoma, dermoid etc.

Spinal problems

CLINICAL ASSESSMENT OF THE SPINE

A patient with a spinal problem will present with a combination of sensory, motor, visceral and autonomic problems, depending on the site and extent of the lesion (Table 5.1, below). It is important to differentiate between upper and lower motor neuron lesions and recognise the difference between vertebral, radicular (nerve root) and long tract (spinal cord) symptoms. Reference to a cross-section of the spinal cord may help to understand the mix of clinical signs and symptoms. Some aspects of clinical assessment relevant to spinal problems are discussed in further detail in Chapter 2, page 9.

Table 5.1 Signs of spinal cord disease or compression.

Motor
Weakness
Upper motor neuron
Lower motor neuron
Combination
Sensory
Pain
Vertebral
Radicular
Tract
Visceral
Bladder sphincter dysfunction
Anal sphincter dysfunction
Autonomic
Sweating
Cardiovascular (hypotension/hypertension)
Sexual (impotence/priapism)
Horner's syndrome

Essential anatomy and pathophysiology

There are seven cervical vertebrae, twelve thoracic vertebrae, five lumbar vertebrae and five sacral vertebrae (Figure 5.1, page 199 and Figure 5.2, page 200). The spinal cord itself extends to the LI, L2 level where it becomes the cauda equina. In spinal injuries, the tissue damaged includes the surrounding bone, the ligaments, the intervertebral discs and the spinal cord.

Pressure on the spinal cord for more than 15 minutes is likely to disrupt the blood supply and the oxygen requirements. The spinal cord can be injured by penetrating injuries, by direct force and by associated haemorrhage. The types of injuries include flexion, flexion with rotation, compression injuries and hyperextension injuries. The most common levels of injury are around C5 and C6 causing partial or complete quadriplegia, and in the thoracic region at T12/L1 causing partial damage or a complete paraplegia. The injuries may be stable or unstable. The spinal cord injury may be complete or incomplete.

The examination of patients with spinal disorders

Watch the patient walking and undressing - this will give many clues as to what is wrong and the severity.

Spine

With the patient standing only in their underwear:

• Look for skin lesions such as a pit, sinus, hairy patch, lipoma, naevus or angioma. These may indicate underlying occult spina bifida, spinal dysraphism or tethering of the cord.

• Assess the posture, alignment, particularly for scoliosis or kyphosis. Feel for tenderness, paraspinal mass, paraspinal muscle spasm, fixed flexion deformity of the hip. Percuss for tenderness.

• Move: Assess the range of movement - forward flexion, lateral flexion, rotation and extension.

Motor function

- **Gait:** limping, rate of movement, length of stride, need for walking aid (will have already been observed). Then continue the examination with the patient lying on the couch:
- **Muscles:** muscle wasting and fasciculation (which imply denervation of muscles); tone, power, reflexes and clonus to determine whether it is an upper or lower motor neuron problem, or a mixed picture.
- Refer to **myotome map** (Table 2.7, page 34) and know which nerve roots are responsible for each reflex (Table 2.8, page 36).

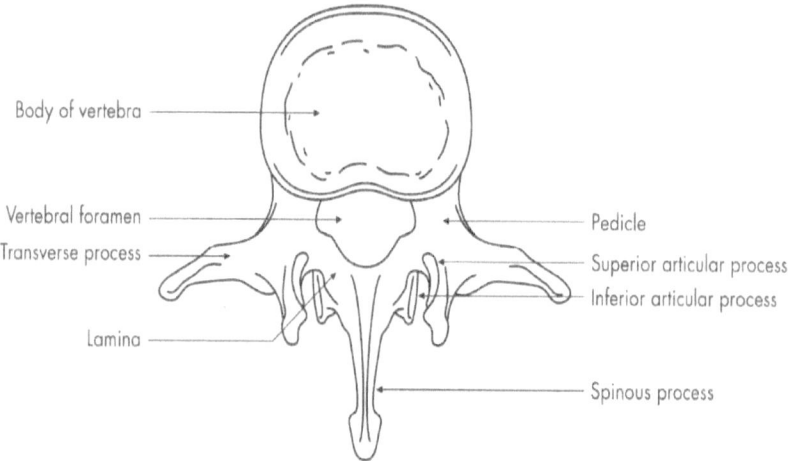

Figure 5.1 (a) The bony anatomy of a vertebra from above.

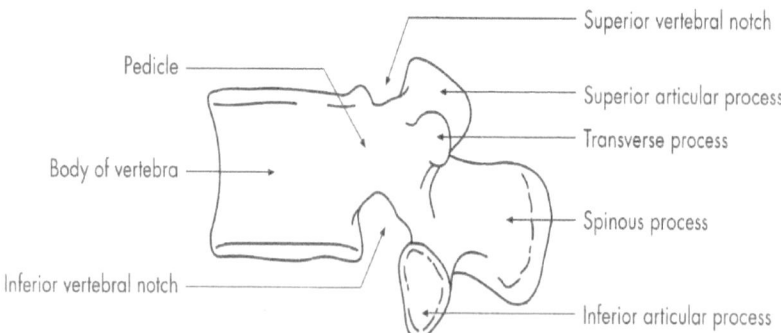

(b) The bony anatomy of a vertebra from the side.

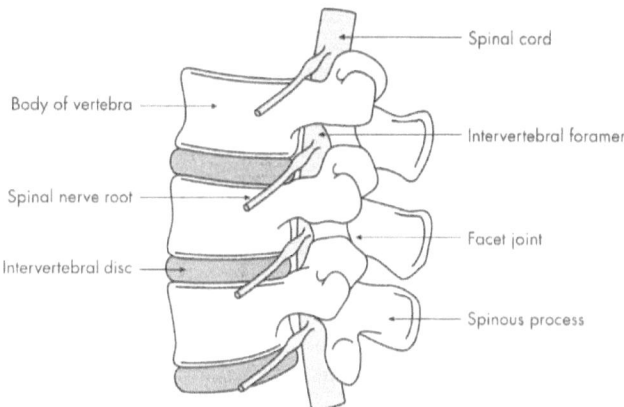

(c) The spine showing the position of the spinal cord and the nerve roots exiting their intervertebral foramina.

Figure 5.1 (a-c) Anatomy of the spine.

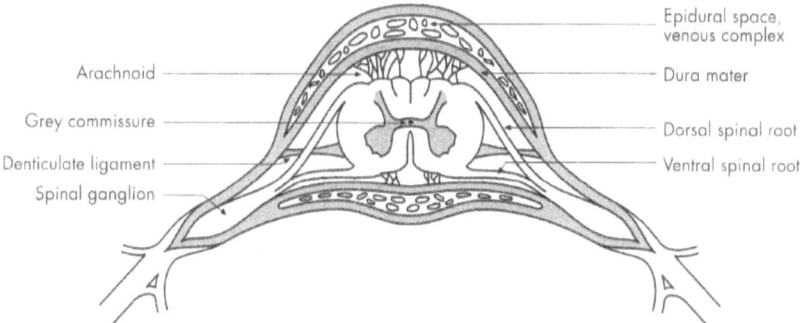

Figure 5.2 A cross section of the spinal canal showing the coverings of the spinal cord and the exiting nerve roots. The spinal ganglion is the dorsal root ganglion. The denticulate ligament anchors the spinal cord. The epidural space contains a prominent venous plexus.

Sensation

- Test pain (spinothalamic tracts), light touch and proprioception (dorsal columns)
- Do not forget to test sacral, perianal and scrotal/vulval sensation
- Establish sensory level on the trunk
- Refer to **dermatome map** (Figure 2.11, page 30).

Special tests

- **Straight leg raising** - is normally 90 degrees in the supine position. Stretches sciatic nerve roots.
- **Lasegue's stretch test** - is a test of pressure on the lower lumbar nerve roots. The ankle is dorsiflexed with the hip flexed placing extra stress on the sciatic nerve, which if it is already tethered by some pathology such as a disc prolapse will cause a sharp jab of pain.
- **Femoral stretch test** - is a test of pressure on the upper lumbar nerve roots. The patient is prone and the lower limb is extended at the hip placing tension on the upper lumbar roots.

Visceral

Rectal examination - perineal sensation, anal tone, external sphincter contraction (the patient tightens the anus with the gloved finger in the rectum), perianal sensation, prostate and pelvis. Assess the abdomen for bladder fullness and enquire about micturition.

Anal wink reflex (S4, 5) - contraction of the subcutaneous portion of the external sphincter in response to scratching the perianal skin.

Practice point

In patients with spinal problems. Do not forget to examine sacral sensation or to percuss the bladder.

Sacral sparing may occur within a widespread area of sensory loss caused by an intramedullary lesion, and is due to the laminar arrangement of the fibres in the spinothalamic tract. The sacral segments are lateral in the tract. It thus means there is an incomplete spinal cord problem and may be the only sign of this (see Figure 5.2, page 200).

Autonomic

Autonomic dysfunction will be evident from the history. Ask about impotence. Autonomic problems may manifest as abnormal hypotension, hypertension, Horner's syndrome, gastroparesis and delayed gastric emptying or impaired bowel motility and constipation. I suspected spinal cord or cauda equina pathology, examine the cremasteric and bulbocavernosus reflexes and for priapism which may follow a spinal injury (see page 218). A conus or cauda equina lesion may abolish the bulbocavernosus and anal reflexes.

Cremasteric reflex (L1): A light scratch along the inner aspect of the upper thigh causes contraction of the cremaster and elevation of the testis.

Bulbocavernosus reflex (S2,3,4): Contraction of the bulbocavernosus muscle (identified by palpation) on squeezing the glans.

General examination

Includes chest, abdomen and lymph nodes. In a patient with back or radicular pain always consider intra-abdominal and other pathologies as a cause for pain (see page 203).

X-rays

Look at:
1. Posture of the spine for scoliosis or kyphosis.
2. Soft tissue shadow indicative of a paraspinal abscess or a haematoma.
3. Vertebrae for alignment, fractures (as above),
   a. height of vertebral body, destruction, arthritic change, osteophytes,
   b. spinal canal - any narrowing,
   c. pedicles - width, integrity,
      • a malignant lesion may erode a pedicle which is absent on an A-P view overlying the vertebral body,
      • tuberculosis causes loss of vertebral body height and the intervening disc space,
      • longstanding intraspinal lesion may increase the interpedicular distance,
   d. dorsal arch - is it intact? Look at lamina and spinous processes
      • dorsal arch will be missing in spina bifida or following laminectomy surgery,
   e. transverse processes.

BACK PAIN AND SCIATICA, NECK PAIN AND BRACHIALGIA

Sydney Nade

Pain in the neck or back, with or without associated pain in the arm or leg, is a common complaint. Even in the absence of limb pain a careful examination must be made of the limbs, as the neurological signs that may be detected will often lead you to the precise site of pathology in or around the spine.

While developed countries use sophisticated radiological and electronic methods to provide anatomical images of the spine and its surrounds, an astute clinician can usually determine the cause of the pain without the help of any form of imaging, or at most a plain radiograph of the spine. On many occasions not even, that is necessary. It is important to remember that most back pain is benign in nature and cause, and usually resolves, even without treatment, in 3-4 weeks. The most important feature in the analysis of cause of back pain is the age of the patient, and careful history taking is an essential part of the diagnostic process. Careful neurological examination usually completes the diagnostic process, and declares the level of any pathology. In taking a history the sequence of questions is important, as each question leads to a rational means of not only achieving a diagnosis, but guiding treatment.

The age of the patient

Table 5.2 on the next page gives a guide to the diagnoses that are most common in each age group, and to the urgency of investigation and intervention.

Taking the history

The questions that you must ask yourself during and after you have taken a history are the following. If you can't answer them you haven't asked your patient enough questions.

Spinal problems

1. Is the pain spinal?

Remember that back pain can be caused by disorders of organs that are not part of the musculoskeletal system. Abdominal aortic aneurysm, salpingitis, renal disease, and pancreatitis are some of the visceral causes of back pain. The clues that they are the cause in your patient will come from detection of other symptoms which may relate to them. What is the relation to menstrual periods? Is there diarrhoea or constipation? Has there been weight loss? These are some of the questions that must be asked to decide whether the pain has a non-spinal cause. If that is the case your subsequent patient management will be directed at that non-spinal cause.

Table 5.2 Common causes of back pain classified by age.

Childhood	
Osteomyelitis	Always serious
Neoplasia	Investigate without delay
Leukaemia	
Adolescence	
Sports injury	Precipitating cause is usually evident
Occupational strain	Investigate if not improving or constant
Scheuermann's disorder	
Spondylolisthesis Osteomyelitis	
Active life	
Acute back strain	Cause usually evident
Postural discomfort	Investigate if not improving or constant
Disc protrusion	
Fracture	
Middle age	
Degenerative disc and joint disease	Investigate if pain is constant
Secondary neoplasia	
Old age	
Degenerative disease	Investigate
Secondary neoplasia	
Osteoporotic fracture	
Osteomyelitis	

2. Is the pain constant?

Constant musculoskeletal pain means that the cause is neoplasia or infection. 'Constant' means that the pain is there all the time, day and night, and prevents sleep. Many patients will tell you that the pain is 'there all the time' but have an uninterrupted night of sleep. Such pain is not constant and has less sinister importance. Constant back or neck pain must be investigated further, and the presence of degenerative changes on plain radiographs cannot be assumed to be the cause of the pain. Degenerative changes may be the cause of mechanical pain, which has the characteristic of varying in severity with level of activity, posture or movement, but is not present at rest in a comfortable position. Having decided that the pain is spinal the most important question you must answer is this one as all constant pain is sinister and demands investigation.

3. Is the pain acute?

This question assesses the onset of pain (not its severity). Acute pain has the characteristic of the patient being able to tell you when the pain started and what he or she was doing at the time. Acute onset of pain, at any site, implies rupture or blockage. There may be an external force that can be identified, such as lifting, bending, a fall, a vehicle accident, a sporting accident or exertion. Acute back or neck pain usually means breakage of a tissue (bone, disc, joint) rather than obstruction to a tube (thrombosis, embolism). The alternative to acute pain is chronic pain having a gradual onset which may be measured in days or weeks. Acute back or neck pain is usually caused by fracture of a vertebra, protrusion of an intervertebral disc, subluxation or dislocation of a joint, or tearing of a muscle or tendon (of which there are many in the back and neck). Pain which is not acute is chronic, and its cause should become apparent from the next questions.

4. Is the pain postural?

This means, the pain is made worse by lying, sitting or standing, or conversely the patient indicates that there are some postures which are avoided. Some patients with sciatic pain prefer to stand while you take your history as they are more comfortable that way. Most people with mechanical back pain are more comfortable when lying down, although not usually in the prone position. Posture related pain usually is associated with pain in one limb, and the comfortable posture that the patient adopts is that which causes least irritation of a nerve root in the spinal canal. The causes of pain in which there is a distinct postural relationship are facet joint degeneration (osteoarthritis), in which spinal extension is often avoided, and intervertebral disc partial rupture, or posterior protrusion in which the forward bending position is often the least comfortable.

5. Is the pain related to movement?

Pain which is related to movement, as opposed to static postural positions, usually comes from acute muscle strain, joint sprain, or fracture, or more commonly, when the pain is chronic, from degenerative disease in the facet joints. Spondylolisthesis may be free from pain, or if painful, it is usually related to movement. The pain of spondylolysis, probably due to stress fracture of the pars interarticularis of the lamina of a vertebra, if it occurs, is also related to movement, and is not postural.

6. What if the pain does not fit any of the above categories?

There are some types of back and neck pain which do not fit clearly into any of the above groups. When you have asked yourself the questions and not got a diagnosis, then think of congenital or developmental anomalies. Transitional vertebrae at the lumbosacral junction are not uncommon. They are usually free from pain, but if a traumatic incident occurs, such as a motor vehicle accident, a sporting injury, or a fall, and there is acute pain, that pain may not settle in the normal period expected for an acute back or neck strain. In such cases think of an anomaly.

Adolescent idiopathic scoliosis is not usually painful. If there is pain, the cause of the scoliosis may not be idiopathic, the spinal curvature being a postural indicator that there is underlying pathology. By the time you have taken the history in sufficient detail to answer the above questions for yourself you should have a good idea of the cause of your patient's back pain. If the patient has limb pain as well, either as a constant companion of their back or neck pain, or present some of the time the trunk pain occurs, then you must consider that a nerve root is involved with whatever pathology is causing the trunk pain. Spinal stenosis, for example, is not a cause of back pain - just the opposite, the cause of the pain has a stenotic effect on the spinal canal and its contents, and the limb pain is just an indicator of that. The site of limb pain, if anatomically in the distribution of a nerve root, will lead you to the spinal problem if you know your neurological anatomy.

Clinical examination

Do not make the mistake of only examining your patient lying on the examination couch. You will get much information watching your patient walk, undress and dress again, and move around your office. Your observations in those positions will give you a good estimate of just how severe your patient's pain is, and what is the level of disability. Then observe the way the patient stands. Is there a tilt of the trunk to one side? Are both feet placed symmetrically on the ground? Is the normal lumbar and cervical lordosis present? Is there 'spasm' of the paravertebral muscles causing a variation from the normal posture? Next, ask your patient to move: bending forwards to touch the toes, recovering to the erect posture, bending to each side asking the patient to put the fingertips on the side of the knee, rotating the trunk to each side (hold the pelvis with your hands and ask the patient to look over the shoulder at you), and leaning back towards you.

For each of these movements you should watch the rhythm and record the range (comparing it with normal is a good way, although with a tape measure you can measure to where the fingers reach). Then get the patient to lie supine. Watch the way the couch is mounted. Do a straight leg raise test, and record the angle at which pain stops the movement. Examine the movements of the hips and knees; stress the sacroiliac joints by forced abduction of the flexed hip and see if it causes pain.

Do a thorough neurological examination of the legs (or arms if the problem is neck pain) testing for muscle power, appreciation of sensation to light touch (differentiation of pin-prick, hot and cold, and pressure is only necessary if you suspect a spinal cord lesion), and test the reflexes. With the patient still supine examine the abdomen, front of chest, axillae and front of neck. It doesn't take long! Then get the patient to sit up and watch the pattern and rhythm of movement. Next ask the patient to lie prone with the arms hanging down by the sides of the couch. Locate the level of the iliac crests to approximate the space between the fourth and fifth lumbar spinous processes and then move each spinous process individually to determine the level at which movement, and/or pressure causes pain or discomfort.

By now you should have a good idea of the diagnosis, and the severity of the symptoms and disability. That will help you make the important decision of whether any further investigation is necessary, and what is the urgency of investigation and treatment. Remember, most backache or pain is musculotendinous in origin and settles promptly even without treatment, or with simple analgesics.

Case report

A 64-year-old woman presented with constant lower back pain and general weakness. She had no urinary symptoms, was not jaundiced and had no abdominal masses. Examination of the spine revealed a normal shaped spine without gibbus, kyphosis or scoliosis. She could flex and extend her spine almost normally. Straight leg raising was normal.

Examination of the lower limbs revealed no neurological signs, sensation, power, tone and reflexes were all normal. Plain X-rays demonstrated lytic lesions in the pelvis and a generally osteoporotic looking spine without fractures. The lytic lesions in the pelvis prompted a skeletal survey which showed multiple lytic lesions in the skull, a pathological fracture in a rib and an expanded lesion in the right clavicle. The total protein was raised and Bence-Jones proteins were found in the urine. A bone marrow and fine-needle aspiration of the right clavicular lesion confirmed multiple myeloma. Lesson: constant back pain suggests infection or malignancy.

__Lesson:__ In this case it was the commonest primary bone tumour in the elderly, multiple myeloma. Conditions such as myeloma and secondary carcinoma are far more common than a primary bone tumour (Figure 5.3, page 210).

Case report

A 30-year-old, previously fit, man developed severe pain in his arm radiating down the C6 root. He was unable to sleep at night because the pain was so severe. There was no pain in the neck but he had pain above his scapula. On examination there was diminished sensation in the C6 dermatome and weakness of the biceps brachii. Movements of the neck were only a little restricted. The blood supply to the limb was normal, there was no cervical rib.

Lesson: *The diagnosis, later confirmed on an MRI scan overseas, was a prolapsed cervical disc causing brachialgia and weakness. This patient was treated expectantly and his pain settled over the next 3 weeks. No surgery was required and he made a full recovery. The important management decisions were made on the basis of his history and examination and normal cervical spine radiography.*

Investigations

There are many investigations that can be done for back pain and sciatica, or neck pain and brachialgia. The aim of the investigation is to see if there is a recognisable anatomical cause for the symptoms, and whether distorted anatomy, if present, is amenable to treatment. Plain radiography which may be all that is available in the LMIC gives useful information. It is not always necessary - particularly if you think that musculotendinous strain is the cause of the symptoms, and that they are improving. Films taken in the A-P and lateral position, with special views of the lumbosacral junction are the minimum.

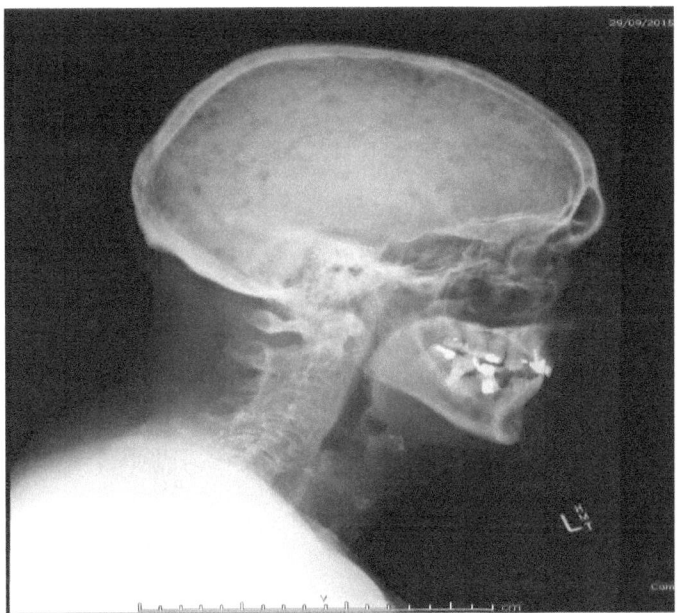

Figure 5.3 (a) Skull X-ray

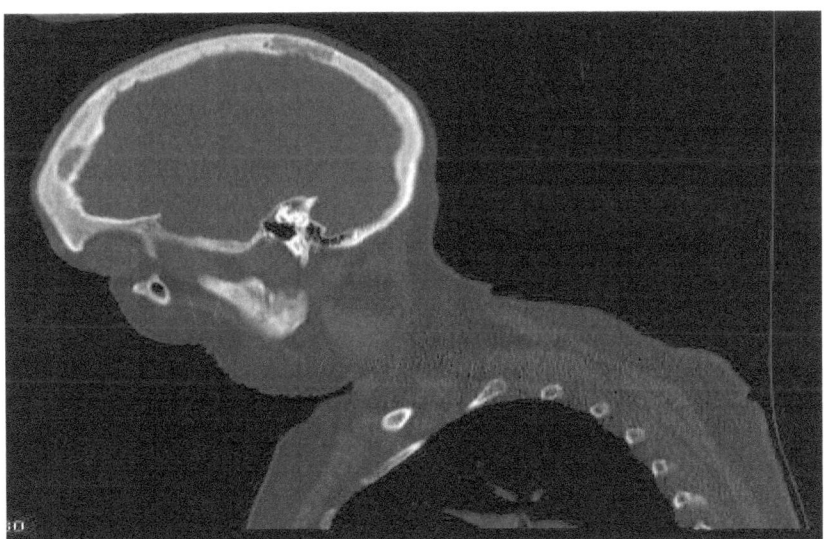

(b) CT showing multiple lytic lesions of multiple myeloma (see case report). This has been described as 'pepper pot' skull on a plain X-ray.

These are seen as black spots of varying size. The patient presented with back pain and general weakness.

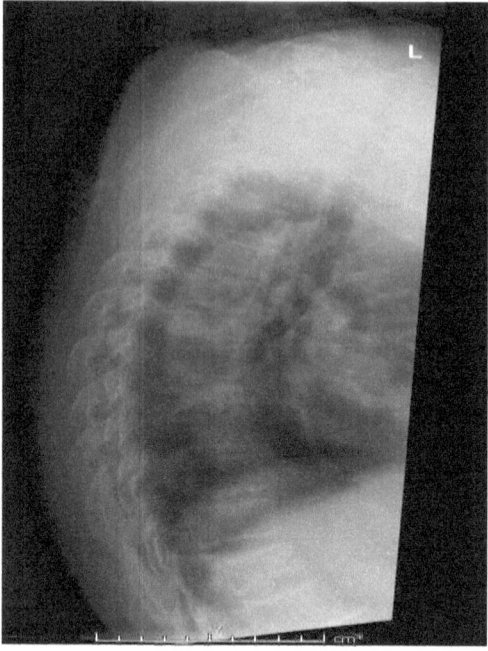

(c) Spine X-rays also showed lytic lesions with the collapse and wedging of two thoracic vertebral bodies.

Figure 5.3 (a-c) Multiple lytic lesions of multiple myeloma.

Oblique views may give added information about the synovial facet joints and intervertebral foramina. Such views can be done in static position, with the patient lying or standing, or dynamically with the erect patient flexed forwards as far as possible, then extended as far as possible. If there is an 'instability' it is more likely to show on such flexion/extension views than on static films. Loss of the normal lordosis is a good sign that the patient has quite severe pain, the muscles causing the altered posture to splint the spine. Look for tilt, or scoliosis, and the level at which it occurs. Look carefully at the intervertebral disc spaces. Narrowed discs are a feature of long-standing disc degeneration. In acute disc prolapse the intervertebral disc height remains normal. Look carefully at the height and shape of the vertebral bodies. If less than normal look at the adjacent vertebra and the disc space between them.

Infection, and remember that tuberculosis is common in the tropics, causes loss of disc as well as adjacent bone, while secondary neoplasia, which gives exactly the same symptom of constant pain, and loss of spinal movement, does not involve intervertebral discs - only the bone collapses. Anterior spondylophytes are a marker of abnormal stresses on discs, but by themselves are not a cause of pain. Synovial facet joints, which are integral parts of the axis of movement between vertebrae, are not well imaged on plain radiography, and reflect degenerative changes only if osteophytes are seen. These are much better imaged in oblique views in the cervical region than any views in the lumbar region.

Computed tomography (CT) is the best way to image the facet joints, as they are then cross-sectioned throughout their curved surfaces, and the thickness of the articular cartilage can be assessed, as well as the osteophytes. Those osteophytes may well impinge on nerve roots causing limb pain and dysfunction as part of a spinal canal stenosis syndrome. (A prolapsed intervertebral disc causing limb pain is only one cause of spinal stenosis.) Myelography is an invasive investigation, and should be reserved for those patients who are about to undergo surgery to display their spinal canal, and to provide extra information to guide the surgeon. Myelography can only tell if the shape of the dural sac is altered by extradural compression, or intradural expansion.

A good myelogram is adequate to diagnose a prolapsed intervertebral disc even if there are no CT or magnetic resonance imaging (MRI) facilities. Even when CT is possible a myelogram preceding the CT is an excellent way of displaying a compressed nerve root. A CT is performed with the contrast remaining in the intradural sac within 2 hours of the myelogram (a CT myelogram). MRI of the spine has become the investigation of choice in HIC. The axial and sagittal views give clarity on the contents of the spinal canal and whether the nerve roots are compressed. Nerve conduction studies, and/or electromyography, if available, are only useful if there is some doubt about the neurological findings on your clinical examination, and rarely have a part to play in the investigation of back or neck pain with limb symptoms. Blood investigations may help confirm your clinical suspicions but are rarely diagnostic. In multiple myeloma, the erythrocyte sedimentation rate (ESR) may be markedly raised, with an associated anaemia, and abnormal biochemical parameters. Leukocytosis is suggestive of an infective cause, but may not be present in tuberculosis. To determine the causative organism in spinal osteomyelitis a biopsy may be necessary if blood cultures do not give an answer. Biopsy by needle aspirate under radiological control may be sufficient (but requires radiography in two planes to locate the needle in the vertebra). Specimens should be assessed both by the microbiology and histopathology laboratories, as acid-fast bacilli may not grow on culture, and granulomata are useful guides to chronic infection. The spread of AIDS, and the use of recreational drugs given by vein has increased the spectrum of organisms causing spinal infection, and although they might be treated by antibiotics alone, the choice of effective antibiotic will only be from a knowledge of the causative organism.

Treatment

The choice of treatment depends on the diagnosis. However, the pragmatic way of deciding is based on answers to these questions:

1. Who needs an operation?

The only patients who need an operation are those in whom the spinal cord is at risk of permanent damage, and those in whom infection is suspected, but not proven. In the first case the operative procedure is therapeutic, while in the second it is diagnostic and may be therapeutic also. The spinal cord is at risk if it is compressed from without by an enlarging swelling. That swelling may be neoplastic, but may also be an abscess, or prolapsed intervertebral disc squeezing the central nerve roots of the cauda equina, putting the nerve supply of the bladder and bowel at risk. In general terms the cauda equina, which contains only nerve roots is far less vulnerable to compression than the spinal cord. Therefore, the critical level of lesion is at about the first lumbar vertebra. Decompression of the spinal canal depends upon your experience, and can be done from the front or back. If the impression into the canal is from the vertebral body (secondary neoplasia) it is sensible to approach from the front, thereby maintaining the integrity of the only intact supporting structures · the spinous processes, interspinous ligaments, laminae and facet joints. However, posterior decompression is a cord-saving procedure and should be the approach for prolapsed lumbar intervertebral discs, or for the inexperienced surgeon. Preserve as much of the posterior elements as is possible. Surgery for spinal cord problems and prolapsed intervertebral disc is described in more detail on page 505.

Clinical decision making for patients with prolapsed intervertebral disc is described below. In HIC, surgery for chronic low back pain frequently involves spinal fusion and, in some cases, artificial disc replacement. The outcome is uncertain and the selection of patients for surgery is crucial to success. There are some conditions such as spondylolisthesis where surgery is indicated to decompress the entrapped nerve roots and stabilise the spine, but for many patients with chronic low back pain, surgery is not the answer to their symptoms.

2. Who needs rest?

Most patients with severe back pain of musculotendinous nature need rest in a comfortable position. That need not always be in bed, but should be in a posture in which the pain is minimised. It is not necessary to put hard boards under a mattress, or to lie on the floor. In acute pain the period of rest required is seldom more than a week, and as long as the pain is decreasing its benign nature can be assumed. If the pain remains constant, or increases you may have to reconsider the diagnosis, but if the spinal cord is not at risk, if the pain is not intolerable, or if the patient is not severely ill as a result of infection in the spine, nothing needs to be done urgently.

3. Who needs physical therapy?

Physical therapy has many different modalities · thermal, movement, exercise, massage. In acute back and neck pain it is best for the patient to rest and gradually mobilise as the pain permits. There is probably no indication for physiotherapy in that acute stage. As the pain recedes, gentle massage and mobilisation of the spine and limbs from a physiotherapist can be helpful. Physiotherapists are in short supply in LMIC. Spinal manipulation by chiropractic methods has little evidence-based proof of efficacy. Thermal therapy, the application of heat or ice, may be analgesic. Exercises are not useful in acute back pain, but may have a role once it has settled to condition the many muscles, including abdominal and paraspinal muscles, protecting the spine. If the pain is constant do not ever send the patient to a physical therapist as that may cause a potentially disastrous delay in arriving at the correct diagnosis of the cause of the pain.

4. Who needs analgesia?

All of the patients who consult you about pain warrant treatment of their pain. Just what you prescribe as an analgesic medication will depend on the diagnosis, and your assessment of the severity of the pain. If the cause is an infection, the definitive treatment is that of the infection, but it is not unreasonable to treat the pain also. If the cause is a secondary neoplasm, then narcotic analgesics may have to be used. However, the vast majority of patients do not have a sinister cause for their pain, and simple analgesics should be all that are necessary, the dose dependent on the severity. The use of non-steroidal anti-inflammatory drugs (NSAIDs) is common, but as most of the causes of back and neck pain are not due to inflammation, their use, with potential side effects, is often not warranted.

Obviously, every patient responds differently to analgesics, and it is often necessary to try different drugs if the simple analgesics - paracetamol, aspirin - are not effective. Opiates may be required in the acute stage if the pain is severe which it can be with acute nerve root compression due to a disc prolapse.

5. Who needs referral?

Never hesitate to ask for advice! You can do this by telephone if necessary. The principal reason for urgent referral is if the spinal cord is at risk of permanent damage. The next most pressing indicator is if you are uncertain of the diagnosis, especially if the natural history in your patient is not the same as the natural history that you would have expected from your presumptive diagnosis. The third indicator is if you consider that the patient might benefit from a surgical procedure and you do not have the experience, or facilities, to perform that procedure.[47]

Summary and conclusions

There is a mystique about back and neck pain which is unwarranted. Part of that comes from the fact that most doctors do not see many patients with back pain during their training, part from the emotional fear of causing spinal cord dysfunction by that lack of experience, and part from the many anecdotal, and measured, bad results of spinal surgery. Such bad results probably are a residual of the days when prolapsed intervertebral disc (first reported in 1934) was the presumed cause of all back pain and sciatica, and laminectomy was the only operation done on the spine. While the indications for operation remain unclear for benign back and neck pain, the correct choice of surgery, and its performance by experts, has allowed for more successful results. There are not a lot of diagnoses to consider when assessing a patient with back or neck pain, with or without limb pain, and a systematic approach to

---

[47]Atkinson L, Zacest A. *Surgical management of low back pain. Medical Journal of Australia.* 2016;204(8):299-300. doi: 10.5694/mja16.00038

diagnosis, as outlined above, should result in the diagnosis being made much more often on clinical grounds, without the need for expensive and sophisticated imaging techniques, which often do not influence the clinical therapeutic programme advised.

They tend, in experienced practitioners, to confirm a diagnosis already made. Sometimes they can confuse, as degenerative changes are common in older people, but cannot always be assumed to be the cause of the pain which may have a pattern suggesting something more sinister. Common things occur commonly, from common causes - and acute musculotendinous strain, local trauma, sports and occupational injury, which are self-limiting and recover - will confront you more often than the other causes. Your job is not to miss the others, particularly infection and neoplasia, when confronted with them.

SPINAL TRAUMA

Early management of severe trauma

The priorities in all trauma patients are the airway, breathing and circulation. The cervical spine should always be assumed to be injured in patients who cannot give a history because they are comatose or moribund and in those complaining of neurological symptoms (numbness, paraesthesiae, spinal pain). Management of the airway should include in-line immobilisation of the cervical spine. Patients should be log-rolled when being turned to safeguard the spine, e.g. when the back is being examined during the secondary survey. Any patient with weakness of the arms or legs should be assumed to have a spinal injury.

Neurological examination should include examination of the anus and perianal sensation and percussing the bladder. The type of spinal injury will need to be determined by plain X-ray which will show the bony skeleton. The spinal cord can only be visualised if MR scanning is available. CT gives poor definition of the spinal cord in axial cuts. However, most problems can be worked out by clinical examination and plain X-rays.

Case report

A 17-year-old male was involved in a motor vehicle accident in which there was a hyperflexion injury to the spine. He developed an immediate flaccid paraplegia. Plain X-rays showed a mild wedge fracture of the lower thoracic spine. MRI scan showed acute haemorrhage in the lower thoracic cord (see Figure 5.4).

He was managed conservatively and methylprednisolone was administered. Minimal improvement ensued. This is an example of spinal cord concussion/ contusion. Probably many cases that were previously labelled concussion have had degrees of haemorrhagic contusion which can now be identified on MRI.

Lesson: *In advanced settings acute spinal cord injury such as this may have been decompressed by laminectomy and the spine stabilised using pedicle screws. This is further discussed below.*

Care of the spine

The essential elements of spinal care are:
1. The recognition of a spine injury.
2. Assuming there is a spine injury in a severely injured patient.
3. Assuming any spine injury is unstable until proven otherwise.
4. Prevention of further injury to the spinal cord by immobilisation of the neck in a collar after a serious head injury; the use of cervical traction using tongs for unstable fracture dislocation of the neck if neurosurgery is not available; and careful log rolling and log lifting.
5. Committed medical and nursing care of the paraplegic patient to prevent skin, urinary, joint and other complications, followed by early mobilisation in a wheelchair.

The clinical examination must determine the motor and sensory level of the spinal cord injury. The sensory level is identified by testing from distal areas of no sensation, in a proximal direction according to the dermatomes. If the level appears higher than the level of the injury shown on the radiograph, there may be further trauma higher up the spinal cord, which has been missed. Further imaging will be required.

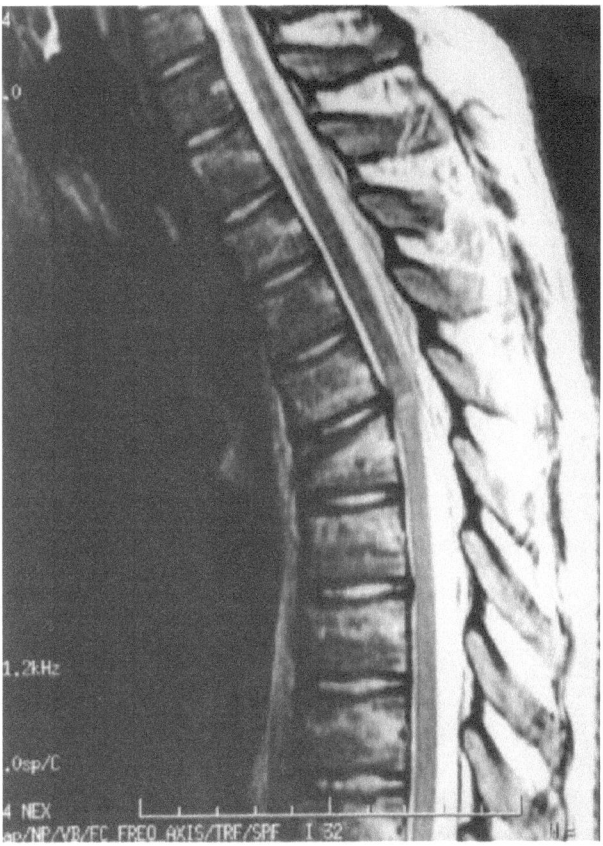

Figure 5.4 Spinal cord contusion at point of acute angulation of thoracic spine with mild wedge crush fracture and posterior thoracic disc protrusion. The patient presented with acute paraplegia, following a motor vehicle accident.

Initially, following a spinal cord injury, there will be a flaccid paresis (period of spinal shock), which is followed after several days to weeks by the development of spasticity. In the acute phase the blood pressure may fall due to vasoparalysis in the periphery, the temperature regulation below the level of injury fails, leading to hypothermia (depending on the ambient temperature), acute urinary retention develops, there is a loss of anal tone and perianal sensation, and there may be priapism. There will be obvious usage of the accessory muscles and respiratory distress if the diaphragm is paralysed.

Clinical assessment

It is helpful to recognise the clinical patterns of spinal cord injury:

1. A spinal cord injury at C5-6 results in paralysis of the hands, intercostal muscles and a partial paralysis of the diaphragm.
2. A spinal cord injury at T10-L1 (conus/cauda equina lesion) results in:
   - sacral 'saddle' anaesthesia
   - bladder: spinal cord reflex disrupted
   - there may be enough residual nerve root function to preserve walking
3. Compression below L1 results in:
   - if complete: flaccid legs (lower motor neuron lesion) - no bladder reflex
   - if partial, there may be some recovery of the motor deficit and bladder function

Paralysis with a sharp sensory level and anal and penile reflexes present indicates a complete injury. Some recovery may occur if there is some perineal, heel, and toe sensation.

History

Pain

Ask the patient where the pain is located. Suspect a cervical spine injury if there is persistent neck pain. The patient with an injury to the upper cervical spine may be sitting up, holding his neck. Pain in the neck radiating to the occipital regions may indicate an atlantoaxial fracture. Pain in other parts of the spine may also indicate an underlying spinal injury.

Mechanism of injury

First find out what caused the injury: a fall from a height, rugby scrum, motor vehicle accident at high speed etc. The mechanism of the injury, including an estimate of the force involved and the direction of deformity of the spine, can give the surgeon a good idea of the type of injury likely to be present. The mechanism of spine injury includes compression, twisting/shearing, hyperflexion or hyperextension. There may be a significant degree of spinal cord injury due to hyperextension without there being any significant bony injury, and conversely, there may be marked bony injury sparing the spinal cord. The spinal cord segment and/or nerve roots may be injured at the level of the trauma. The long tracts passing up and down the spinal cord may be interrupted at the level of the trauma.

Examination

1. An initial gross examination is helpful:
   - Can the patient move the limbs individually to command or with painful stimulus?
   - Can he feel his limbs being moved?
   - Does he feel pain?

Practice point

Do not test movement of the neck or spine.

2. A detailed neurological examination is then performed if the patient is co-operative (use a pin and light touch to test sensation).
   - C5 dislocation on C6 - biceps paralysis or weakness
   - C6 dislocation on C7 - biceps intact
   - C7 dislocation on Tl - Horner's syndrome may be present
3. Examine for other injuries if not already completed as part of the secondary trauma survey - abdomen, chest, limbs etc.
4. Examine the patient's back by log rolling them into a lateral position. (Log rolling involves 3 to 4 people to roll the patient keeping the spine stable.) Identify bruising, deformity, tenderness, or swelling and palpate all the spinous processes for a gap which indicates an underlying fracture dislocation.

The ASIA Impairment Scale

The American Spinal Injuries Association (ASIA) publishes the International Standards for Neurological Classification of Spinal Cord Injury (ISNCSCI). The ASIA Impairment Scale (AIS) is now the standard assessment tool in acute spinal cord injury. The AIS is based on a detailed clinical assessment which includes a dermatomal sensory examination, a myotomal motor examination, anal sensation and anal motor function, determination of motor and sensory levels, determination of the neurological level of injury (NLI) and whether the injury is complete or incomplete. The Scale goes from A to E: A is a complete injury; B is sensory incomplete; C is motor incomplete with sparing of voluntary anal contraction OR has some sparing of motor function and is sensory incomplete. Less than half of key muscle functions below NLI have a muscle grade ≥3; D is motor incomplete with at least half of key muscle functions below the NLI having a muscle grade ≥3. The assessment method is outlined in Appendix 6, page 659.

Assessment of cervical spine X-rays in trauma

There are seven cervical vertebrae and eight cervical cord roots. It is important to see all seven cervical vertebrae and the top of the first thoracic vertebra. A cervical spine X-ray is more important than a skull X-ray in most patients who are unconscious from a head injury.

You need to follow the following steps:

1. Is it an adequate film in that it shows all seven cervical vertebrae and the top of T1. Is the quality adequate for you to make a reasonable assessment?
2. Is there a normal lordosis? Loss of lordosis suggests pain and muscle spasm.
3. Look for prevertebral soft tissue changes such as widening between the trachea/larynx and vertebral column. Widening may be due to haematoma from a fracture of the cervical spine. The thickness of the prevertebral soft tissue shadow should be less than 5 mm between the pharynx and the vertebral body of C3. Children normally have a prevertebral thickness that is less than two-thirds of the thickness of the body of C2. Lower in the cervical spine the prevertebral thickness should be less than the width of a vertebral body. Prevertebral air may be due to oesophageal or airway injury in a patient with penetrating trauma.
4. Look for normal alignment at the front and back of the vertebral bodies, and at the back of the laminae and that the spinous processes point to a common focal point.
5. Look at the shape of the vertebral bodies and see whether there are any bone fragments in the spinal canal.

Be aware: Portable X-rays of the cervical spine may miss a fracture in 5-10 percent of cases. A normal cervical spine on X-ray does not exclude a spinal cord injury or an unstable spine that is reduced at the time of X-ray. A plain X-ray will not show what is happening to the intervertebral discs. Where available, an MRI scan shows the spinal cord and CT is very helpful in defining bony injury and both investigations help to evaluate what is happening within the spinal canal.

Radiological views of the cervical spine (Figure 5.5, next page and Figure 5.6, page 226)

1. **Lateral view** - pull down shoulders if all vertebrae not seen. Take swimmer's view if this fails.
2. **Swimmer's view** (taken through the axilla with one arm up) - This is used to show C7/T1 if it is not seen on the standard lateral projection.
3. **A-P view** - Identify the vertebral bodies, pedicles, transverse processes and spinous processes which should all be in alignment.
4. **Open mouth view for the odontoid peg (dens) (C2)** - The upper teeth are in line with the base of the skull. There is a growth plate at the base of the dens in young people which should not be mistaken for a fracture. Look at:
   • the dens
   • the lateral mass of the atlas - if spread apart - may indicate a bursting fracture of C1.
5. **Oblique views** - These will give a better view of the facet joints and the intervertebral foramina but are not essential in the early period following trauma. A more experienced radiographer will be needed to produce good quality oblique, open mouth and swimmer's views.
6. **Flexion and extension lateral views** - When indicated these should be done under medical supervision with a doctor flexing or extending the neck but stopping if there is increased pain or paraesthesia. They require an awake, alert patient who is co-operative. They are indicated to confirm stability after 6 weeks of cervical traction or in cases in which the X-ray findings are dubious or if there is persisting pain after a neck injury without X-ray abnormality (Table 5.3, page 227).

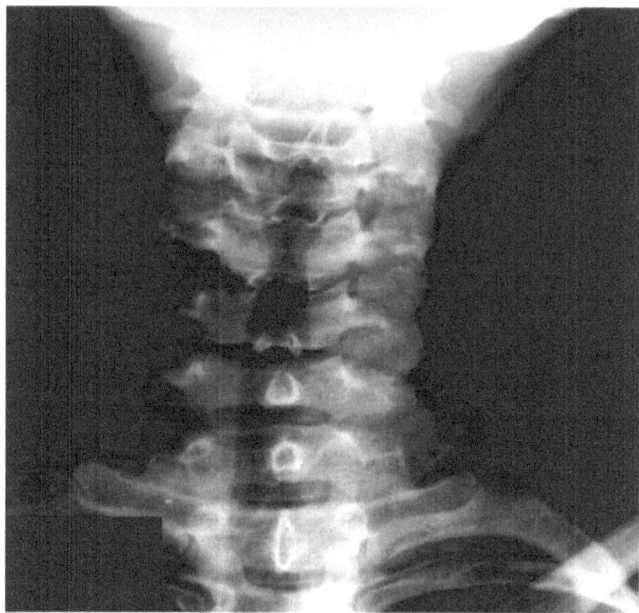

Figure 5.5 (a) A-P view.

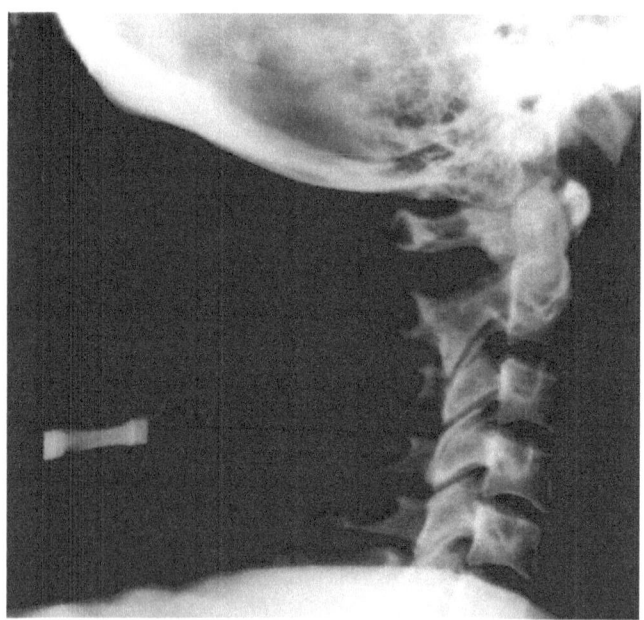

(b) Lateral view - this is an inadequate view, and requires a repeat with shoulders drawn down or a swimmer's view to show down to the C7-T1 junction.

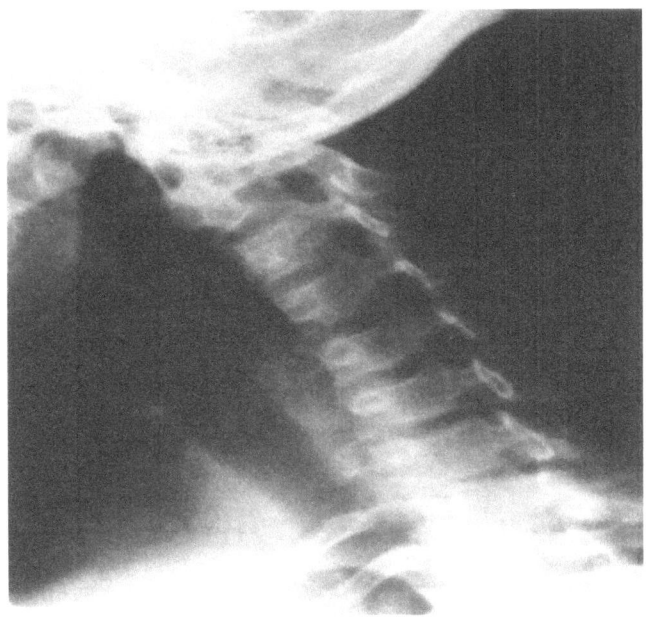

(c) Oblique view showing intervertebral foramina and facet joints.

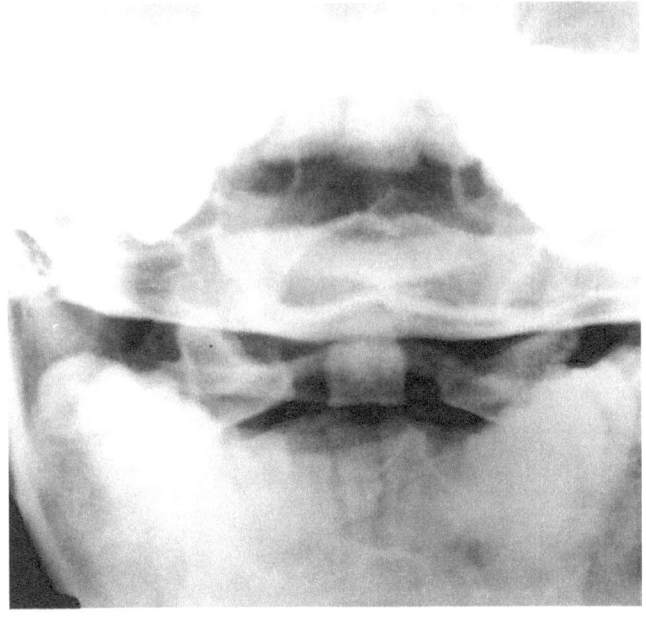

(d) Open mouth view showing odontoid process.

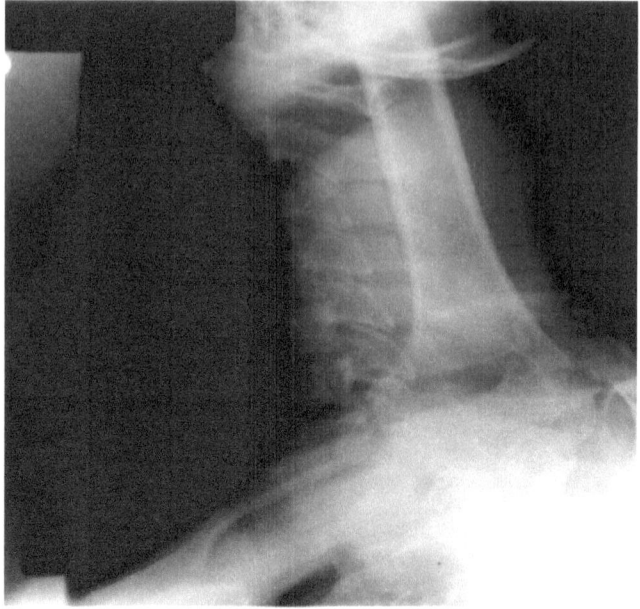

(e) Swimmer's view showing cervicothoracic junction.

Figure 5.5 (a-e) Series of normal cervical X-rays.

Stable fractures of the thoracolumbar spine

Wedge and compression fractures are usually due to flexion loading and are usually stable. There may be narrowing of the spinal canal if the vertebral body bursts backwards. There may be an underlying osteoporosis in the elderly patient. Fractured transverse processes of the lumbar vertebrae may be associated with abdominal injury.

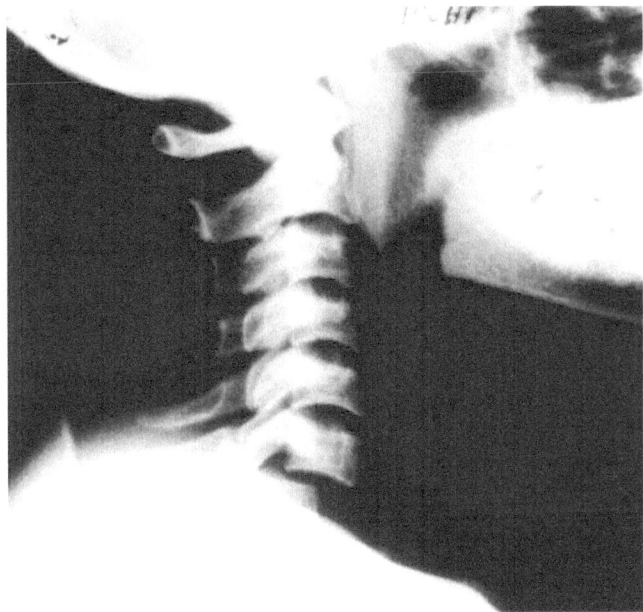

Figure 5.6 (a) Fracture dislocation of cervical spine at C6- 7. Note this is an inadequate film because the cervicothoracic junction is not shown. Unstable.

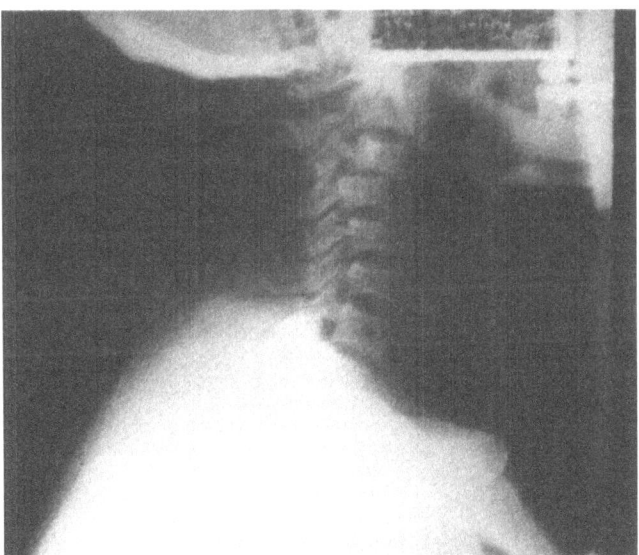

(b) Subluxation at C3- 4 with facet fracture C3. Unstable.

Figure 5.6 (a-b)

Table 5.3 Radiological signs of instability of the cervical spine.

Subluxation/dislocation >3.5 mm (Figure 5.6).

Greater than 11 degrees of angulation of one vertebra relative to the next.

Discontinuity at the posterior margins of the vertebrae.

Pedicles splayed or on different levels - compared with those above or below.

Spinous process out of line on the A-P view.

Burst fracture (multiple fragments) - minor is probably stable, major is unstable.

Facet fracture.

Unequal spaces between vertebrae and between spinous processes.

Facets out of alignment - locked facets may be present.

Unstable fractures of the thoracolumbar spine (see Figure 5.7, next page)

The most frequently affected site is around the thoracolumbar junction. This is probably due to the relative immobility of the thoracic spine compared with the lumbar spine. The fractures tend to be unstable:
1. Oblique fractures through the body.
2. Fracture dislocation with kyphosis more than 40° and some scoliosis.
   - Flexion-rotation: dislocation with a variable amount of rotation.
   - shear: anterior column fails at the annulus of the disc because of an extension load. It will be recognised by A-P dislocation on lateral film.
     • Flexion-distraction: Chance fractures: fractures of the lumbar spine due to seat belts, especially the lap belt variety. The axis of flexion is anterior to the anterior column. The radiographic

signs are a horizontal fracture through the transverse processes and pedicles extending for a variable distance through the body. The spinous process may be fractured or the spinous processes may be separated. May be associated with visceral injury including rupture of the duodenum.

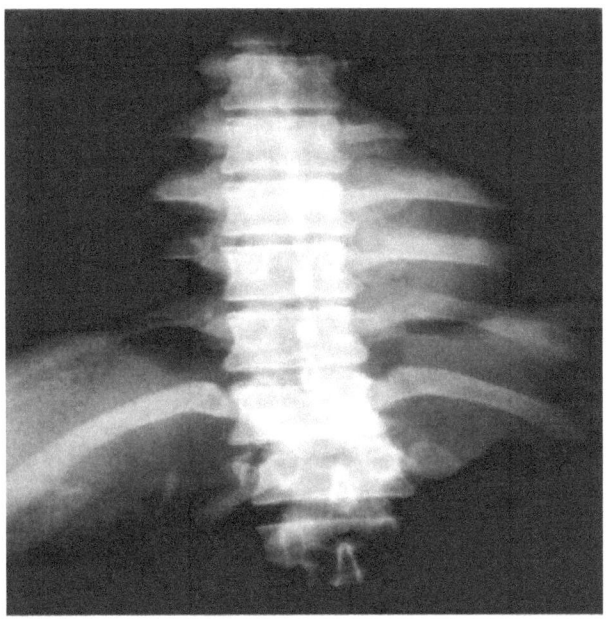

Figure 5.7 Fracture dislocation of thoracolumbar junction. Note the malalignment of vertebral bodies and pedicles.

Management (Table 5.4, next page)

Most spinal trauma in the developing world can be managed non-operatively, apart from skeletal traction (skull tongs or halo or Hoen's traction - see below) for the cervical fracture dislocation. There is an increasing trend in developed countries to early open reduction and internal fixation of unstable spinal injuries irrespective of the neurological status. This permits a rigid stabilisation of the bones, and early mobilisation of the patient, without concern about instability causing new or worsening neurological deficit, and diminishing the complications of prolonged immobilisation in bed. These procedures are not generally available in the developing world because of lack of surgical expertise and unavailability of expensive spinal fixation instrumentation. There is some evidence that for partial spinal cord injury that early surgical decompression and instrumented fusion using pedicle screws provides additional improvement to that which would have occurred naturally. Surgical decompression and stabilisation may also prevent further injury of the spinal cord.

An incomplete lesion may slowly improve over many months. Complete neurological deficit usually remains complete if it has been present more than 24 hours. Acute traumatic complete quadriplegia in the developing world is a disaster and palliative care is often provided until death occurs. Note also that spinal fractures will likely heal but ligamentous injury may not heal completely, thus causing late instability.

Table 5.4 The general management of the acute spinal cord injury

---

Frequent initial observations

Wide-bore nasogastric tube

Urinary catheter

i.v. fluids - the blood pressure will take a few days to come up

Enema after 5-7 days

Nil orally until bowel sounds

Regular pressure care

Inspection/documentation of pressure areas

(Soft foam or water bed mattress if available)

Log roll 2 hourly, log lift

Recent evidence-based guidelines on management of acute spinal cord injury include maintaining the MAP >85mm Hg. There is evidence that hypotension worsens the neurological recovery because of compromise of spinal cord perfusion. There is weak evidence that high dose methylprednisolone administered as a 24-hour infusion within the first 8 hours after injury improves motor recovery. So, this remains a treatment option. There is also a risk of increasing septic complications with this therapy which should be considered.

Anticoagulant thromboprophylaxis such as subcutaneous low molecular weight heparin is recommended to commence within 72 hours of injury.

REFERENCES AND FURTHER READING:

- Fehlings MG, Wilson JR, Tetreault LA, et al. A clinical practice guideline for the management of patients with acute spinal cord injury: recommendations on the use of Methylprednisolone Sodium Succinate. Global Spine Journal. 2017;7(3S):203S-211S.
- Fehlings MG, Tetreault LA, Aarabi B, et al. A clinical practice guideline for the management of patients with acute spinal cord injury: recommendations on the type and timing of anticoagulant thromboprophylaxis. Global Spine Journal. 2017;7(3S):212S-220S.
- O'Toole JE, Kaiser MG, Anderson PA, et al. Congress of neurological surgeons systematic review and evidence-based guidelines on the evaluation and treatment of patients with thoracolumbar spine trauma: executive summary. Neurosurgery. 2019;84(1):2-6.
- doi.org/10.1093/neuros/nyy394.
- Yue JK, Winkler EA, Rick JW, et al. Update on critical care for acute spinal cord injury in the setting of polytrauma. Neurosurgery Focus. 2017;43(5):E19.
- doi: 10.3171/2017.7.FOCUS17396.

Practice point

Maintain the MAP > 85mm Hg in a patient with acute spinal cord injury. Ischaemia of the cord will worsen neurological recovery.

Practice point

Do not assume a deficit is complete if you have not checked for sacral sparing of sensation.

Cervical spine injury

The indications for neck immobilisation in a firm collar until a cervical spine injury has been excluded are:
- a significant head injury (about 10 percent of severe head injuries are associated with a cervical spine injury),
- the mechanism of the injury suggests a possible cervical spine injury,
- neck pain following injury,
- abnormal neurological signs.

Uncontrolled movement may convert a partial spinal cord injury into total injury, or produce neurological deficit. Therefore, correct and assiduous immobilisation techniques are essential. In-line traction is used when the patient is rolled or the airway is manipulated. The chin is held with one hand, the occiput is held with the other hand and gentle traction is applied.

A collar is applied early in the treatment of a trauma case where there could be a spine injury present. A rolled towel, sheet or blanket and safety pins can be used as a temporary collar with sandbags at either side of the neck for added security.

A rigid collar can be made from cut out and padded cardboard or plastic cut to shape. When moving the patient, use a log roll and log lift with four people. The patient is transported in a supine position.

Management decisions

1. Stable injury - apply a collar.

2. Unstable injury - place the patient in skeletal traction when the patient is resuscitated.

3. If status uncertain - traction one week and if there is no neurological improvement - no advantage in continuing - apply a collar.

4. Burst fracture - with no neurological signs - traction 6 weeks, collar 12 weeks.

Skeletal traction

Indications for skeletal traction:

1. Unstable fracture/dislocation of the cervical spine with or without partial spinal cord injury,
2. complete spinal cord injury with a prospect of improvement.
3. If there is clearly complete quadriplegia which will be permanent - skeletal traction is not applied.
4. Skeletal traction is usually applied for 6 weeks then a cervical collar or cuirass (plaster or plastic jacket covering the occiput, chin, neck and chest) is applied for 6 weeks.

Methods of skeletal traction:

1. **Gardner-Wells** traction (skull 'tongs') (Figure 5.8, next page) (also see Figure 11.12, page 571 and Figure 11.36, page 626).
2. **Hoen's** traction (see Figure 11.13, page 572).
3. **Halo** traction.

A metal halo can be simply constructed in a metal workshop with four sharp-pointed screws passed through the frame with locking bolts at the junction of the screw with the frame and ropes and a pulley system assembled. The traction is applied in a straight line. A pull of 5-15 kg is initially applied, depending on body size and degree of muscle spasm and the level of the injury (see Table 5.5, next page). To reduce a fracture dislocation 15 kg may be needed initially but later only 3- 5 kg are needed to maintain the traction. Less traction is required for injuries higher up the cervical spine. The head of the bed is raised on blocks so that the body weight applies countertraction. The weights are strung over a pulley attached to the head of the bed. If there is a dislocation repeat the X-ray within 4 hours and check for reduction. Add weight 1- 2 kg at a time until check X-rays show the spine is reduced. Try to achieve reduction in the first 12 hours because the longer the period of oedema, pain and muscle spasm, the harder it will be to achieve reduction. Once 2-3 days have passed, reduction may not be possible although sometimes the dislocation is reduced between 7-10 days when the oedema subsides.

If the fracture re-displaces when the weight is lowered, then the weight is replaced and these patients may require a fusion procedure. After 2-3 weeks the traction is reduced to approximately 3-5 kg, and weekly X-rays obtained. After 6 weeks the traction is replaced with cuirass or a halo-thoracic brace (Figure 5.9, page 235). Repeated X-rays involve considerable effort in the average developing world hospital. Increasing weight could also be applied in theatre with an image intensifier used to confirm reduction.

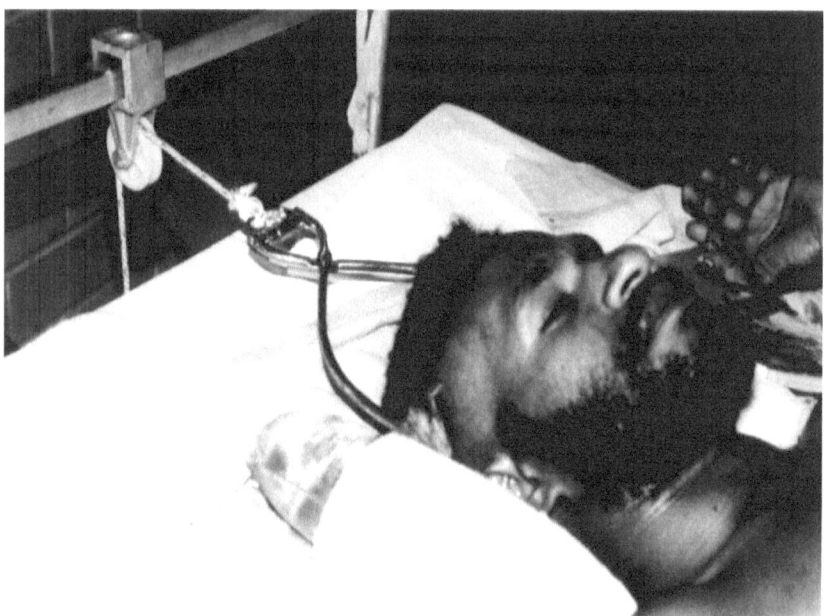

Figure 5.8 Patient with fracture dislocation of cervical spine with skull tongs applied, having skeletal traction, and with sandbags either side of the neck. This patient was injured playing rugby and was quadriplegic with movement at the shoulders and elbow flexion preserved.

Table 5.5 Approximate traction requirement according to level of injury.

C1	2.5-5 KG
C2	3-5 KG
C3	4-7 KG
C4-5	5-10 KG
C5-6	7-15 KG

233

Classification and management of cervical spine injuries

C1 (atlas) Atlas fracture

Mechanism: compression on top of head (axial loading).

The posterior arch, lateral mass or blow out fractures of the ring of the atlas (Jefferson fracture) do not usually present to hospital with spinal cord injury because when they do, they are fatal. Such fractures of the atlas should be treated as unstable fractures although they can be managed in a rigid collar for 6 weeks.

C2 (axis)

Odontoid subluxation may occur because of injury to the transverse ligament which attaches the odontoid to the anterior arch of C1 (the atlas). Injury often occurs without spinal cord injury because the spinal canal has room for displacement. Steel's rule of three states: one-third of the space within the spinal canal is occupied by the odontoid (C2), one third by the spinal cord, and one third is vacant. This helps to determine how much room there is for the spinal cord.

Odontoid (dens) fractures (Figure 5.10)

Mechanism: impact to front of skull which gives rise to sudden extension.

- Type I - a rare fracture of the tip or body of the odontoid (usually stable).
- Type II - fracture of the base of the odontoid (unstable).
- Type III - extend into the body of the axis (unstable).

The odontoid has an epiphysis until the age of 6 years and this epiphysis may appear to be a fracture. There is normally no neurological deficit because the spinal canal is wide and spinal cord transection is incompatible with life. These fractures are treated by skeletal traction. However, if the fracture is in a reasonable position and there is no neurological deficit, a cuirass or a halo-thoracic brace maybe applied until bony union occurs, but this treatment is not as reliable as traction. (Internal fixation with a screw(s) applied through an anterior approach is now available in specialist centres and avoids the need for cervical traction.

234

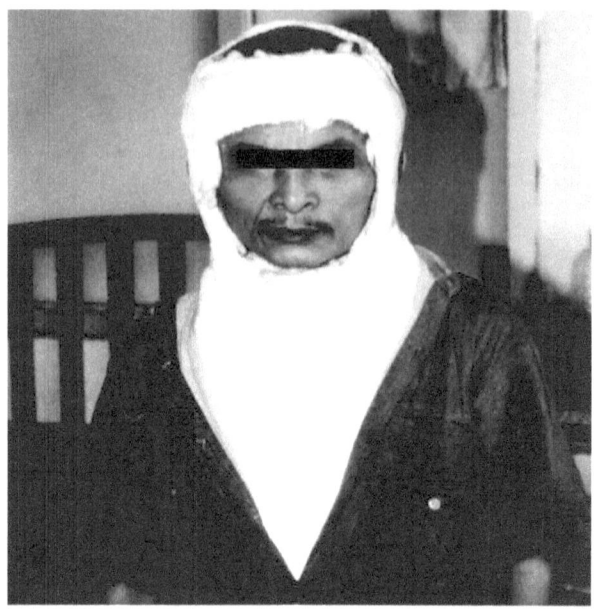

(a) Application of plaster cervicothoracic cuirass in Vietnam in the early 1980's.

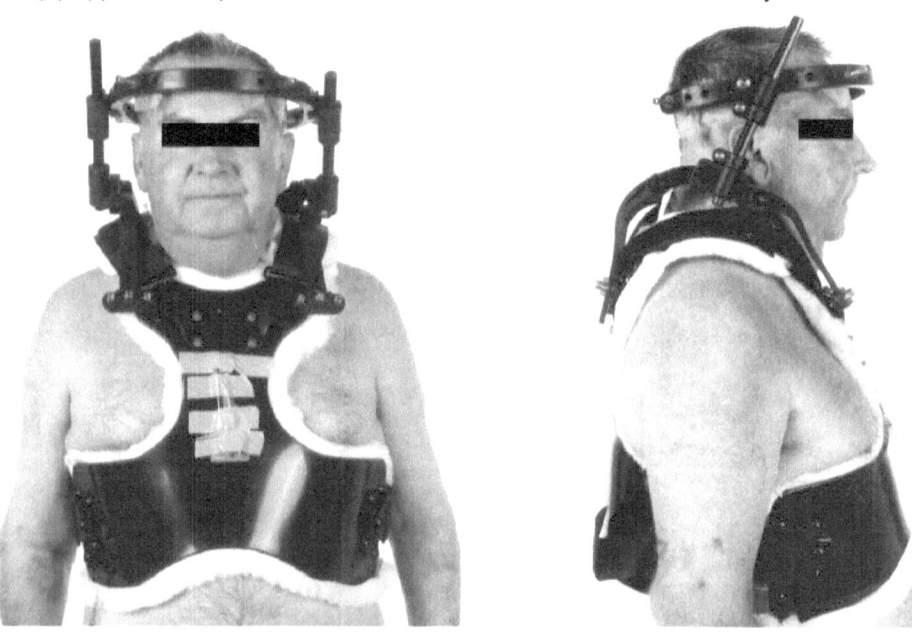

(b) An alternative to the cuirass is the application of a halothoracic brace which is used in the developed world, following major cervical fusion procedures.

Figure 5.9 (a-b) Immobilisation of the cervical spine in the ambulant patient.

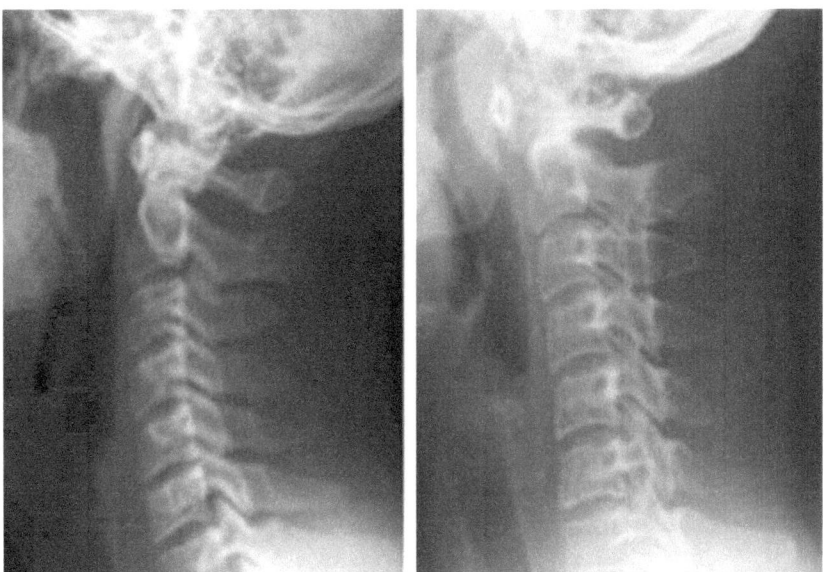

Figure 5.10 (a) Lateral cervical radiograph. Normal alignment of C1 and C2.

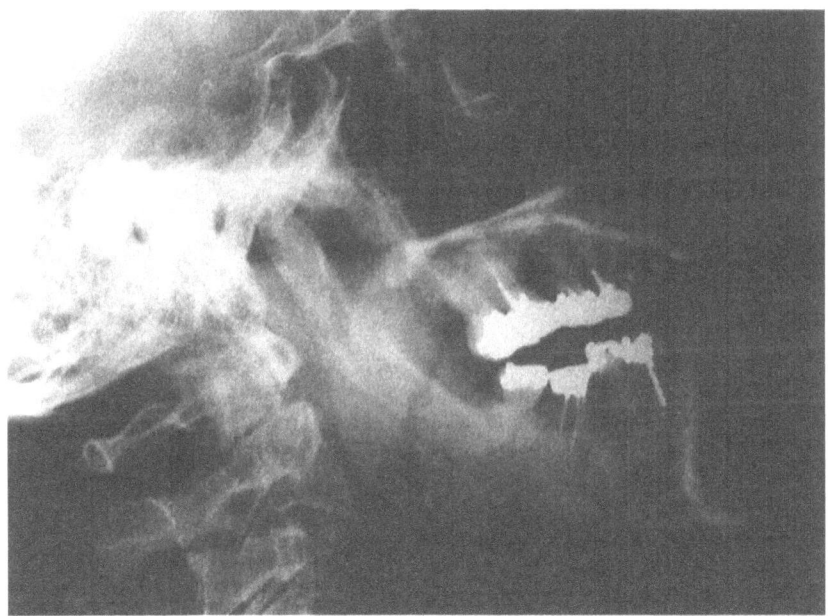

(b) Lateral cervical radiograph. Fractured base of the odontoid process (dens) with atlanto-axial subluxation. Note the distance between the anterior arch of the atlas (CI) and the C2 Body. The dens has fractured off the C2 body and is not clearly seen.

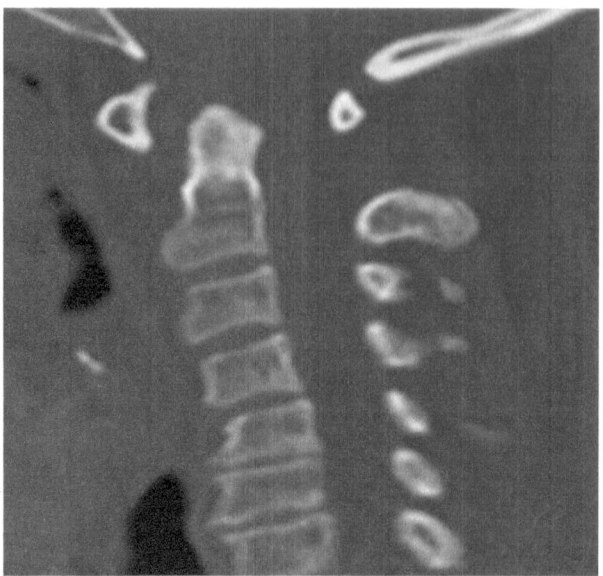

(c) Different patient from a and b. Lateral radiograph showing a fracture at the base of the dens with atlanto -axial subluxation of several mm. Note the loss of alignment of the dens with the body of C2.

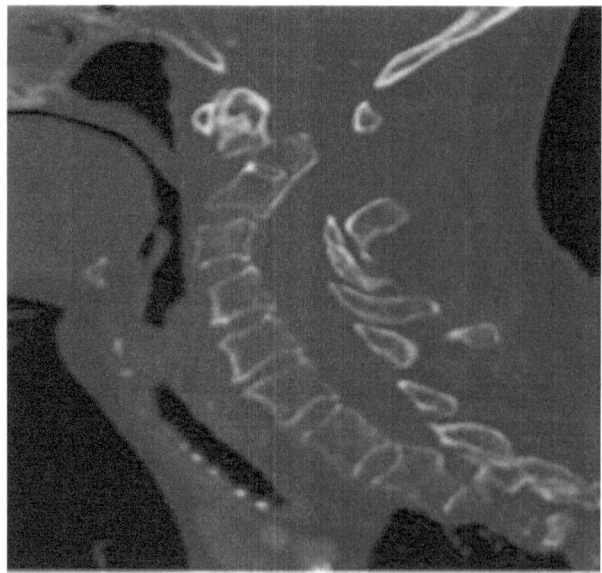

(d) Different patient from a to c. CT scan sagittal reconstruction (bone windows) showing separation between the anterior arch of the atlas and the odontoid process. This is atlanto-axial subluxation due to ligament rupture.

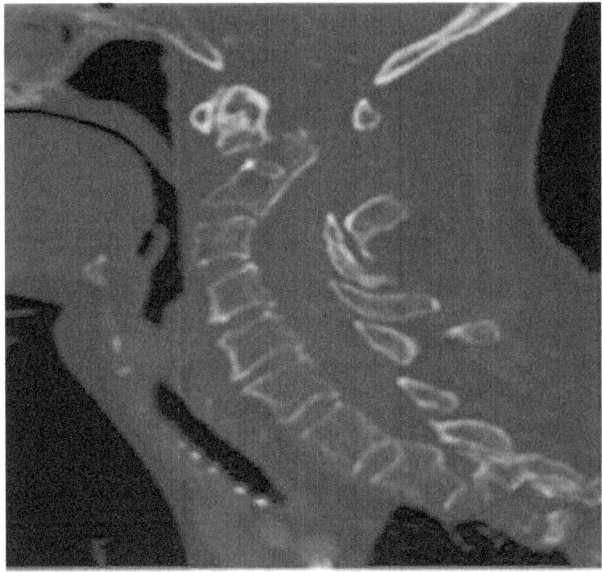

(e) Different patient from d. CT scan sagittal reconstruction (bone windows) showing a fractured odontoid process with gross displacement & angulation.

Figure 5.10 (a-e) Fracture of the odontoid process (dens) with resultant atlanto-axial subluxation.

Atlanto-axial instability

This is a ligamentous injury causing subluxation. Pain, stiffness and possibly torticollis are the manifestations. Neurological deficit is rare at presentation. It is a potentially unstable fracture and should be treated with traction and stability should be assessed after the 6-12 weeks of axial traction. Atlantoaxial fusion with a sublaminar wire loop and bone grafts.

Hangman's fracture

A hangman's fracture is a bilateral fracture through the isthmus of the pedicle of C2 (the pars interarticularis), i.e. involves the posterior elements of C2. The mechanism of injury is usually a motor vehicle or diving accident resulting in extension and axial loading although flexion can cause more severe grades of injury. Most of these patients are neurologically intact. True hanging will produce the fracture by hyperextension and distraction.

Most hangman's fractures result in minor degrees of displacement of C2 on C3 and are stable if managed in a collar for 12 weeks. The collar should preferably have chin and occiput support - SOMI (suboccipito-mental immobilisation) e.g. Philadelphia collar. More than 90 per cent will heal this way. Cervical traction is contraindicated. The few unstable fractures following a period of immobilisation or those with gross displacement judged unstable initially require open reduction and internal fixation with a C2-C3 fusion.

Fractures of C3 to C7 (Sub-axial cervical spine)

These fractures can be classified as anterior column or posterior column injuries and stable or unstable.

1. **Anterior column.** Consists of vertebral body, anterior longitudinal ligament, and disc.
   a. **wedge fracture** - usually stable if amount of compression is less than 25 percent of height of vertebra.
   b. **burst fracture** - fragments may burst backwards into the spinal canal. Potentially unstable.
   c. **tear drop fracture** - results from hyperextension and is unstable. There is a small fragment of bone (tear drop) at the anterior inferior edge of the vertebral body with subluxation of the vertebra backwards on the vertebra below. There is often a vertical fracture line seen on the A-P X-ray which exits through the disc and an anterior or lateral wedging of the vertebral body. The facet joints may be disrupted (seen on the oblique views) and the adjacent disc space narrowed indicating disc disruption. There will also be prevertebral soft tissue swelling.
   d. **disc disruption** - narrowed disc space on lateral x-ray. Often associated with bony injury, e.g. tear drop fracture.
   e. The anterior longitudinal ligament (ALL) is torn with a small bone fragment attached. This is a simple avulsion fracture which must be distinguished from the teardrop fracture. It is usually stable.

2. **Posterior column.** Consists of spinous process, lamina, pedicle and ligaments (supraspinous, interspinous and ligamentum flavum).
   a. **Spinous process avulsion** - extension or hyperextension injury - stable.
   b. **Facet fractures and dislocations.** Severe flexion injuries may result in locked facets.

- unilateral facet dislocation: caused by flexion and rotation. The patient is usually neurologically intact and the injury is usually stable. The oblique X-rays are helpful in diagnosis and CT, if available, is diagnostic.
- bilateral facet dislocation - bilateral locked facets. There is gross ligamentous and annulus disruption and usually a cervical cord and cervical root injury.

Cervical spine facet dislocation – unilateral and bilateral

Conservative treatment of facet dislocation may result in chronic neck pain, neck stiffness, and torticollis (Figure 5.11, below), which becomes very difficult to treat with late surgery because of chronic scarring around the injury site. These injuries particularly if bilateral, regarded as unstable. Early reduction by traction and manipulation (if the skill to perform is available) is indicated.

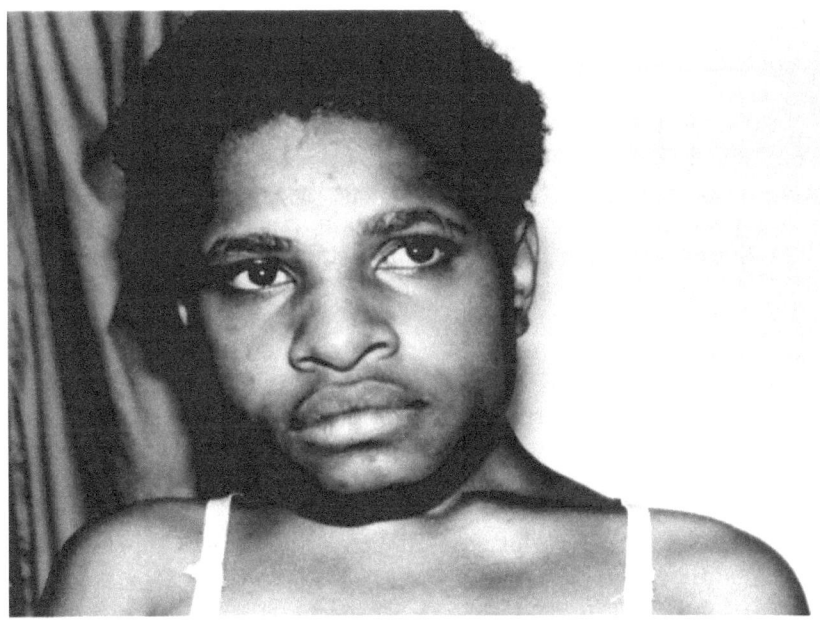

(a)

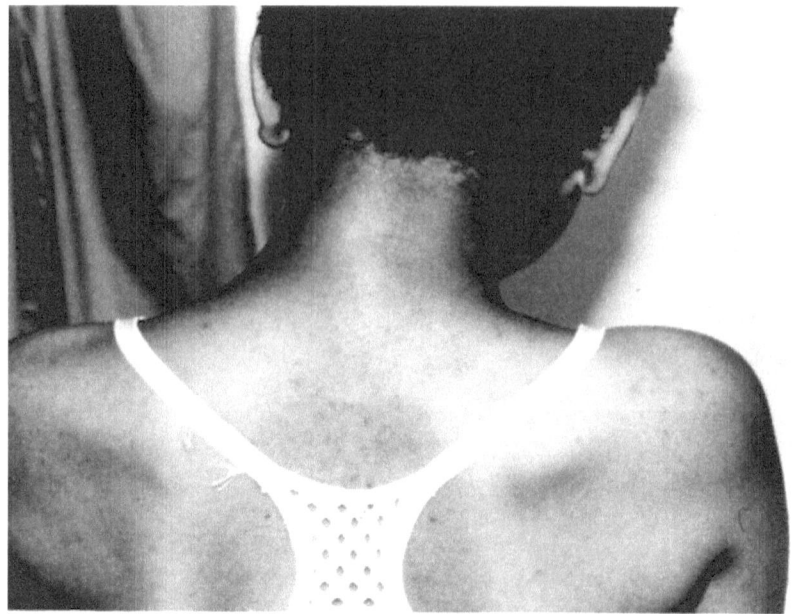

(b)

Figure 5.11 (a-b) Chronic torticollis due to untreated locked facets.

Start with 5-7 kg and add 2 kg every 15 minutes checking for neurological change. After 15 kg for 30 minutes - perform an X-ray - facets may begin to disengage but it may take longer. If no disengagement occurs, then leave on 15 kg traction for maximum of 12-24 hours and X-ray every 6-12 hours. When the articulating processes are disengaged, overriding is corrected, the distance between the pedicles is narrowed, reduce the weight and keep the neck in a straight line. After 6 weeks of traction, a cervical collar or cuirass is applied. At 3 months post injury, the collar/cuirass is removed and A-P, lateral and flexion/extension views X-rays are performed. If stable, then the collar stays off. If unstable (uncommon) - the patient may need referral to a neurosurgeon or orthopaedic surgeon for an operative reduction of the locked facets and fusion. This is a difficult operation and requires a surgeon experienced in cervical surgery.

Cervical hyperextension injury ('Porter's neck')

• Mechanism: occurs when people (usually females), carry loads on head and trip leading to hyperextension injury.

- May result in quadriparesis although there is usually a good prognosis. The patient can be treated with soft collar immobilisation.
- A hyperextension injury in an elderly patient with a degenerate cervical spine is more prone to neurological deficit because the hypertrophied ligamentum flavum buckles and compresses the spinal cord.
- Late cervical instability will require operative intervention to fuse the spine. This can often be achieved by a posterior approach.

Thoracolumbar spine injury

Thoracolumbar spine injury is common at the points of hyperflexion T7-8, T12-L1, L4-5. Unfortunately, spinal cord injury, if it occurs, is frequently complete because the spinal canal is narrowest in the thoracic region. If a wedge fracture occurs following a minor injury - suspect osteoporosis or an underlying malignancy. Wedge-compression fractures are usually stable. Up to 25 per cent loss of anterior vertebral height can be assumed to be stable. Greater than this and the patient should be treated symptomatically but closely followed up for signs of increasing kyphosis which would indicate instability. Burst fractures are usually unstable (60 percent have a neurological impairment).

Anterior decompression may be indicated, particularly if there is progressive neurological deterioration. Fracture dislocations are associated with greater than 75 percent complete neurological deficit.

Stable fracture

Six weeks of bed rest on a firm mattress, analgesics, and then mobilisation. In LMICs, the conservative management of stable thoracolumbar injuries is recommended.

Unstable - not paraplegic

In LMICs, the conservative management of unstable thoracolumbar injuries is undertaken unless the expertise and equipment are available to stabilise the spine and allow for early mobilisation. Rest in bed - 2 hourly turns. The patient can usually turn himself in bed after 3 weeks. After 6-10 weeks mobilise on crutches.

Unstable - paraplegic

Paraplegia care. Place foam under the fracture - this promotes a mild extension and also opposes the tendency to collapse. Mobilise after 6-8 weeks. Most of these fractures will unite in 6-8 weeks with bed rest. Malalignment is not a problem even with a complete cord lesion. The ongoing management and rehabilitation of the paraplegic patient is described in Chapter 12, page 638. Early posterior stabilisation with internal fixation and bone grafts may be indicated for the unstable thoracolumbar fracture dislocation, but only if the general condition of the patient allows it. Spinal cord or cauda equina compression by anterior haematoma and bony fragments from a bursting injury may be relieved by anterior decompression and instrumented fusion. In addition, open reduction and stabilisation of the thoraco-lumbar spine is indicated for those cases who do not respond to postural reduction with bed rest. These operations are not likely to be available in the developing world but permit early mobilisation in a wheelchair even if there is a complete cord lesion. However, the prognosis remains poor in complete cord lesions.

Practice point

Don't apply plaster jackets to paraplegics as this increases the risk of pressure sores.

Prognosis of spinal cord injury

There is a poor prognosis for neurological recovery if there is a complete deficit, however the prognosis is uncertain if there is a partial degree of function present. The prognosis will become much clearer after a few days and you should not be dogmatic about prognosis in this early period, however, if there is no perianal sensation, no toe flexion, and no rectal sphincter function at 24 hours post injury, there is a 90 percent chance of permanent paraplegia or quadriplegia.

SPINAL CORD COMPRESSION

Spinal cord compression causes partial or complete paralysis. The earlier the compression is relieved the greater the chances of recovery. The first sign of cord compression is usually lower limb weakness and inability to walk. Upper limb weakness may occur with lesions compressing the cervical spinal cord.

Clinical presentation

Cord compression has a variable rapidity of onset. The presentation depends on where and what proportion of the cord is compressed. Sensory, motor, visceral and autonomic function may be affected. The symptoms and signs vary according to the segment of the cord involved, the rate of expansion of the lesion and the site (anterior, posterior, lateral, extradural, intradural, extramedullary or intramedullary). Back and neck pain are discussed on page 203.

Gait or locomotor problems are discussed on page 437. There are three types of pain caused by spinal cord compression:
1. central spinal (bone and soft tissue) pain,
2. truncal radicular pain - intercostal and abdominal wall,
3. limb radicular pain.

Practice point

Thoracic back pain is never benign until proved otherwise. When pain is radicular, the greatest error is to assume that it is due to a degenerative facet joint or disc lesion and forget the possibility of retroperitoneal involvement of the lumbosacral plexus by neoplasm. Progressive, nocturnal root pain also suggests malignancy rather than the usual disc protrusion.

Case report

A 14-year-old girl presented with left sciatica without back pain. The pain was continuous and made worse on exertion. She complained of paraesthesiae in the foot. Her neurological examination was normal and she was diagnosed as having a prolapsed intervertebral disc. This is an unlikely diagnosis in a 14-year-old. A myelogram was carried out which was also normal. She was then referred for a CT scan which was also normal. A pelvic ultrasound demonstrated a 3 cm cystic mass on the lateral pelvic wall which was compressing roots of the sciatic nerve.

Case report

A 36-year-old woman had had an anterior resection for carcinoma of the rectum 4 years previously. She presented with numbness on the lateral side of her right foot and pain in the buttock radiating down the back of her right leg. An ultrasound showed right hydronephrosis and a plain X-ray showed erosion of the right sacrum. She had tumour recurrence. CT scanning confirmed the above findings and excluded a prolapsed intervertebral disc.

Practice point

The clinical hallmarks of spinal cord compression are pain, weakness or paralysis, sensory loss, and bladder and bowel dysfunction, with urinary retention and overflow.

Acute cord compression will produce a flaccid weakness but after a week or more, upper motor neuron signs will develop with spasticity, hyperreflexia and upgoing plantar responses. At the level of pathology, there may be a zone of hyperaesthesia, and below this level, hypoaesthesia or anaesthesia. There may be bladder distension, urinary dribbling, and a lax anal sphincter with evidence of faecal incontinence. The patient is likely to be having increasing difficulty walking and often there is a history that they have not been able to walk for days or even weeks. It is very easy to miss thoracic spinal cord compression as a diagnosis if the patient is resting in bed and the power of the lower limbs is not formally tested.

How to determine the cause

The main causes of spinal cord compression are:
1. **Trauma** (covered in the spinal trauma section on page 216).
2. **Infection** (covered in the spinal TB section, page 253): Other causes of spinal infection most commonly involve staphylococcal osteomyelitis, which causes pronounced continuous back pain and sometimes tenderness; swinging fever, vertebral collapse, epidural abscess and leukocytosis. If the patient is not responding to TB therapy and a compressive lesion affects the cord, an open drainage of the pus may be required, e.g. via costotransverse-ectomy.
3. Cases which are not typical of TB may be approached by the needle aspiration of the vertebral body under X-ray or CT guidance, with culture of the pus and institution of the appropriate antibiotics. Osteomyelitis of a lumbar vertebral body requires rest in bed and a 6-week course of parenteral antibiotics. Some immobilise the lumbar spine in a plaster of Paris jacket, but this should not be used if there is neurological deficit in the lower limbs, particularly with sensory loss, as pressure sores may result from the plaster jacket.
4. Malignant spinal cord compression is commonest in the thoracic region and the causes are metastatic malignancy of the breast, lung, prostate, myeloma, lymphoma, renal carcinoma and bowel carcinoma.

A classification of spinal cord compression based on the site of the pathology is presented in Table 5.6 on page 247.

Practice point

Patients with spinal cord compression may deteriorate neurologically following myelography due to a change of CSF pressure with CSF loss from the lumbar puncture site.

Practice point

The treatment of spinal cord compression is a surgical emergency.

Malignant spinal cord compression in children

In children less than 1-year old, metastatic malignancy in the spine is usually due to neuroblastoma, and in children older than 1 year of age, drop metastases occur from medulloblastoma or ependymoma in the posterior fossa. Burkitt's lymphoma causes extradural compression. Primary tumours of the spinal cord such as astrocytomas or ependymomas are uncommon and extramedullary intradural tumours such as schwannoma should also be considered, particularly in children with neurofibromatosis.

Table 5.6 Pathology of spinal cord compression.

Extradural

1. Infection

- Extradural abscesses which may spread from the bone, venous plexus, the lymphatics or by direct extension from the retroperitoneum
- Tuberculosis (Pott's disease page 237), which affects the vertebral body and the intervening disc

2. Tumour

- Primary bone tumours - rare

Table 5.6 *(Continued)*

- Secondaries to bone from breast, thyroid, prostate, kidney, lung
- Burkitt's lymphoma is quite common in children living in malaria-endemic zones.

3. Trauma

- Haematoma

- Bony fragments from a fracture or dislocation

4. Degenerative disease

- Osteoarthritis

- Disc degeneration

Intradural

Intramedullary

1. Tumour

Primary tumours of the spinal cord include the tumours of neuroepithelial tissue (astrocytoma, oligodendroglioma, ependymoma)

2. Cysts (neoplastic, syrinx)

3. Infections

- Schistosoma granuloma in spine

- Syphilitic gumma

- Tuberculosis

4. Arteriovenous malformations – rare

Extramedullary

1. Metastasis

2. Neurofibromatosis

3. Meningioma

4. Cysts (arachnoid, dermoid)

5. Arteriovenous malformation (rare)

Malignant spinal cord compression in adults

In adults' primary spinal tumours affect the:
- bone (myeloma, osteosarcoma, Ewing's sarcoma),
- dura (meningioma),
- nerve root (schwannoma or neurofibroma),
- spinal cord (astrocytoma, ependymoma). The myelogram should be able to distinguish between intramedullary, intradural, extramedullary and extradural compression (see Figure 5.12, below).

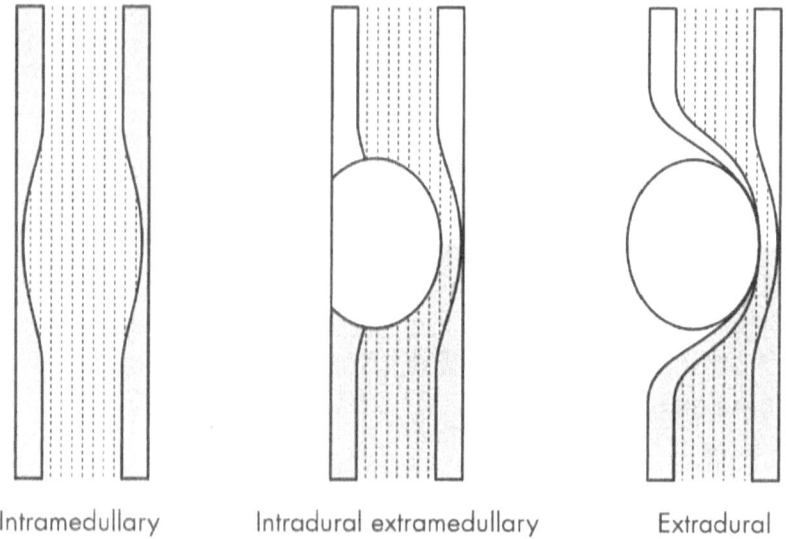

Intramedullary   Intradural extramedullary   Extradural

Figure 5.12 Diagrams demonstrating the three types of myelographic block. The dark shading represents the contrast agent injected from below.

In the developing countries, myelography is the definitive investigation of spinal cord compression and is best followed by CT if available. MRI has proved very useful in spinal cord compression because of the sagittal and axial images showing clearly which part of the cord is compressed and to what degree. It is also non-invasive. Myelography may only show the lower end of the block and if there is a total block, will not show the upper end, unless a separate cervical puncture is made with flow of contrast inferiorly to show the upper end of the block (Figure 5.13 (a), next page and Figure 5.13 (b), page 251).

Management of malignant spinal cord compression

Radiotherapy has been used as a primary treatment if the primary tumour is known and is highly radiosensitive, e.g. lymphoma and some cases of breast carcinoma. However, radiotherapy often produces swelling in the tumour and may worsen the neurological state, if it is given without surgical decompression. Steroids alone will not solve the problem. The surgical treatment of malignant spinal cord compression is very similar to that of the surgery for spinal TB (see page 253). If the primary disease is controlled, there are not multiple metastases, the patient is likely to live more than 6 months, and there has not been a complete neurological deficit for more than 24 hours (i.e. paraplegia or quadriplegia), it is worth decompressing the spine. The patient also should be judged medically fit enough to withstand a major spinal operation which may involve a thoracotomy.

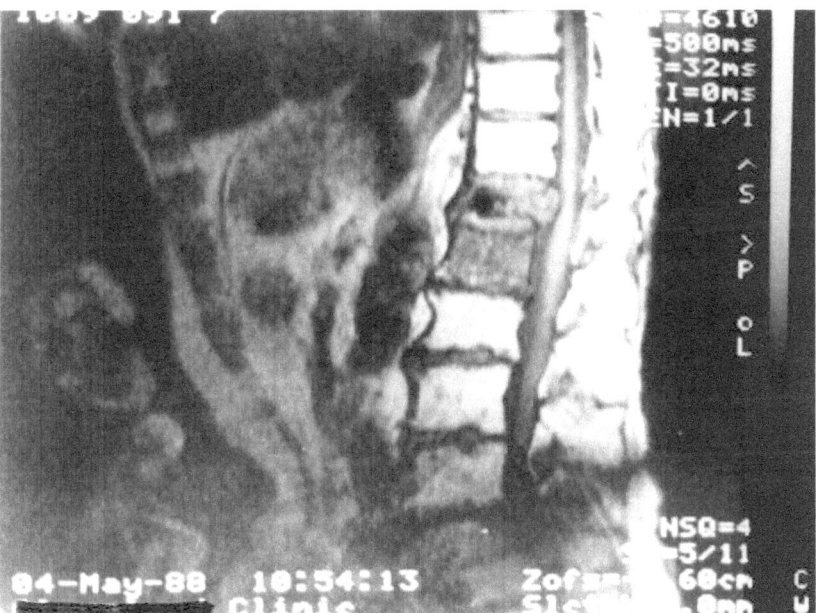

Figure 5.13 (a) Sagittal MR image showing breast carcinoma invading the thoracic spine with the collapse of a vertebral body and posterior growth of the tumour into the spinal canal with spinal cord compression.

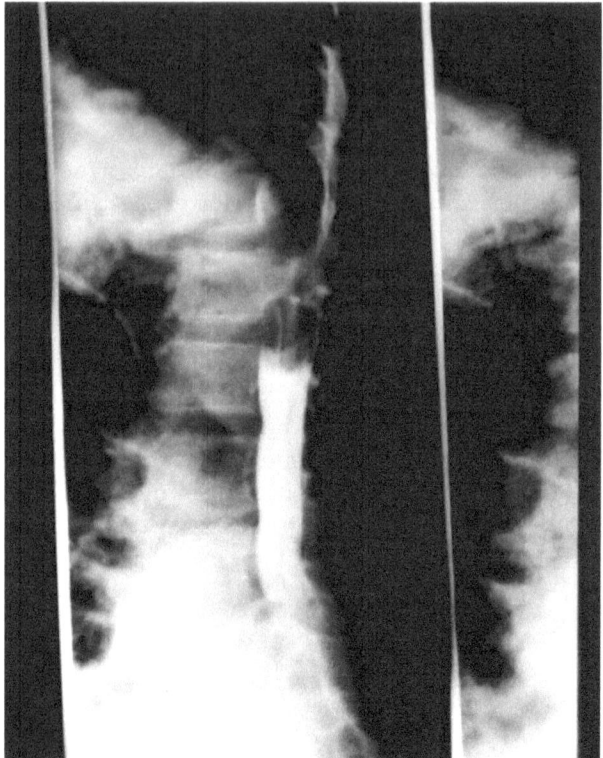

(b) Total block due to spinal cord ependymoma in the upper lumbar region. Note the meniscus of contrast curved downwards, which is the lower edge of the tumour.

Figure 5.13 (a-b)

You should determine from the myelogram whether the compression is mainly posterior or anterior and whether there is any destruction and collapse of vertebral bodies. If the compression is mainly anterior then either a costotransversectomy approach, or an anterior approach via thoracotomy or thoracolaparotomy to re-sect the involved vertebral bodies and reconstruct the spine is the best palliative treatment. A single spinal level can be reconstructed with K wires between the unaffected vertebral bodies and acrylic cement if available, otherwise rib grafts can be used, which can be impacted in position. Preferably, metallic constructs are needed to stabilise the bone grafts and adjacent spine, if the expertise and technology are available. However, in the developing world the costotransversectomy is probably the most suitable operation. When the tumour is mainly anterior to the spinal cord and a laminectomy alone is performed, poor results are often obtained because the spinal cord has not been adequately decompressed and increased spinal angulation may occur. For predominantly dorsal disease, a standard laminectomy approach is appropriate. Dexamethasone can be given to try and lessen the neurological deficit, or at least hasten recovery.

Once histology is obtained, postoperative radiotherapy and/or chemotherapy can be administered. If these are not available, the surgical decompression alone will have to suffice. It is far better for the patient with metastatic spinal disease to die having been mobile up until a short time before they died, rather than be paraplegic or quadriplegic and incontinent, for many weeks or months before dying. In HICs, the spine is internally fixed using pedicle screws in addition to the laminectomy and resection of tumour. This prevents further instability and angulation of the spine.

The medical management of malignant spinal cord compression is often nihilistic and defeatist, whereas with an adequate decompression and adequate control of pain, very good palliation will be obtained for many months. If the patient already has advanced malignancy with an uncontrolled primary and/or multiple metastasis or is likely to die within the next few months, then they should not be subjected to major spinal surgery.

SPINAL TUBERCULOSIS

John E. Jellis

Extrapulmonary tuberculosis (TB) accounts for 25-30 percent of tuberculosis in the tropics. Bone and joint TB accounts for about 5 percent of the extrapulmonary total and spinal TB comprises about 50 percent of this. Spinal TB is often the second commonest spinal problem encountered, spinal trauma being the most common. The incidence of TB is increasing in many tropical countries due to a breakdown in TB control programmes and a rise in the incidence of HIV. In sub-Saharan Africa about 50 per cent of TB sufferers are also HIV positive.

Clinical presentation

The main symptom of spinal tuberculosis is a dull aching pain related to the affected vertebra. The pain is constant but aggravated by exercise. Irritation of nerve roots adjacent to the disease may cause girdle pain around the rib cage or pain and paraesthesia in the limbs. General malaise, tiredness, loss of weight and night sweats are other common symptoms. Symptoms and signs of tuberculosis involving other body systems (pulmonary, lymphatic, elementary or renal) may accompany or precede spinal disease, while those of HIV disease (rashes, especially herpes zoster, weight loss, fevers, diarrhoea and oral thrush) may be present.

A history of close TB contact is often present, especially in children and close relatives may have died of the disease. Most patients with spinal tuberculosis have an obvious gibbus by the time of presentation. Vertebral body destruction produces an angular kyphosis or prominence of the spinous process of processes of the affected vertebrae. The patient will usually be underweight. There may be signs of lymphadenopathy or pulmonary tuberculosis or tuberculosis of a major joint. A tuberculous abscess may show itself by a general fullness of the neck in cervical disease. Rarely posterior swelling accompanies thoracic disease. Signs of a psoas abscess (flexion deformity with painful loss of hip extension and a fullness above the pelvic rim) quite commonly accompany lumbar disease and the abscess may extend distal to the inguinal ligament, presenting as

253

a fluctuant mass in the groin. Quadriparesis or paraparesis may already be present at the time of presentation.

The human immunodeficiency virus specifically attacks those cells, the tissue macrophages and the thymic (CD4) lymphocytes that constitute the body's defence against tuberculosis. The two diseases are therefore synergistic and, in many tropical countries, there is a dual epidemic of HIV and tuberculosis. In Zambia, adult patients with spinal tuberculosis are often HIV positive and tuberculosis is the most virulent of the opportunistic infections encountered in HIV disease. Although tuberculosis may be acquired early in the course of HIV infection, signs of HIV disease (generalised lymphadenopathy, weight loss and skin rashes) are often evident.

Investigations

Classically the diagnosis of spinal tuberculosis was made from the history, clinical examination and haematological investigations (a relative lymphocytosis and high erythrocyte sedimentation rate (ESR)) combined with a radiological appearance of the spinal lesion. This is still the case but the position has been complicated by HIV disease. Tuberculin skin tests (Mantoux or Heaf) are often confusing in their interpretation, especially where infantile inoculation with BCG is practised and HIV is rife. Other tests for tuberculosis such as the polymerase chain reaction test (PCR) and bacteriophage replication are currently only used as research tools. Spinal tuberculosis produces a moderate leucocytosis with more than half of the cells being lymphocytes. In an HIV positive patient however, the total lymphocyte count may be normal or even low. The ESR is usually raised (60-200 mm per hour) in spinal tuberculosis but is also raised in HIV disease and other spinal infections.

The radiographic signs of spinal tuberculosis are usually of erosion of two adjacent vertebra with collapse of the intervening disc (Figure 5.14). A paraspinal abscess may develop, which is seen on a lateral radiograph of the cervical spine as an increased distance (normal of less than 1.5 cm) between the vertebral bodies and the tracheal air shadow (Figure 5.15). In the thoracic region a paraspinal abscess appears as a fusiform swelling in the A-P projection (Figure 5.16). Loss of the psoas shadow and a slight concave scoliosis may indicate a psoas abscess on that side. These paraspinal abscesses can also be clearly demarcated by ultrasonic scanning. An intravenous pyelogram may also show deviation of the ureter (Figure 5.17, page 257).

Tuberculosis is a great mimic and can give rise to a variety of appearances including the collapse of a single vertebra, which is more typically due to a tumour deposit, trauma or an eosinophilic granuloma. Tuberculosis can also involve the posterior elements of the vertebra. Computed tomography (CT) scan clearly demonstrates the extent of the bony pathology and has shown that the incidence of involvement of the pedicles and laminae is greater than suspected from plain radiographs alone. Magnetic resonance (MR) imaging has proved a useful tool (where available) for the further elucidation of spinal lesions. The spinal cord as well as abscesses and granulation tissue can be clearly visualised and the response to treatment can be followed.

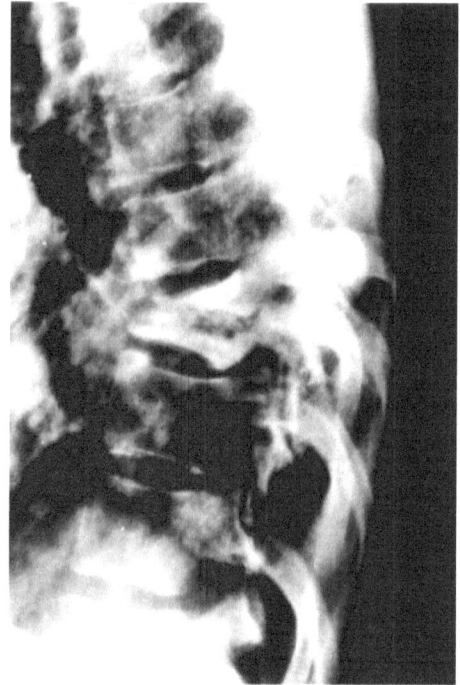

Figure 5.14 Lateral radiograph of the thoracic spine showing tuberculous destruction of adjacent portions of the bodies of two vertebrae and the intervening disc.

Spinal problems

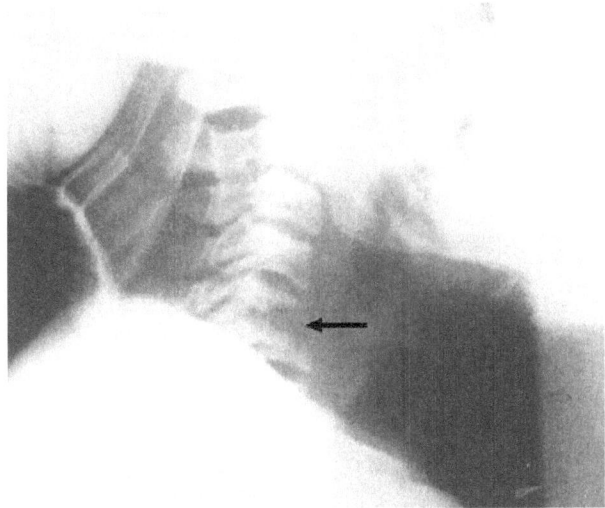

Figure 5.15 Lateral radiograph of the cervical spine in which tuberculosis is affecting the fifth and sixth cervical vertebrae (horizontal arrow). The intervertebral disc has been destroyed and a pre-spinal abscess has increased the distance between the front of the spine and the tracheal shadow.

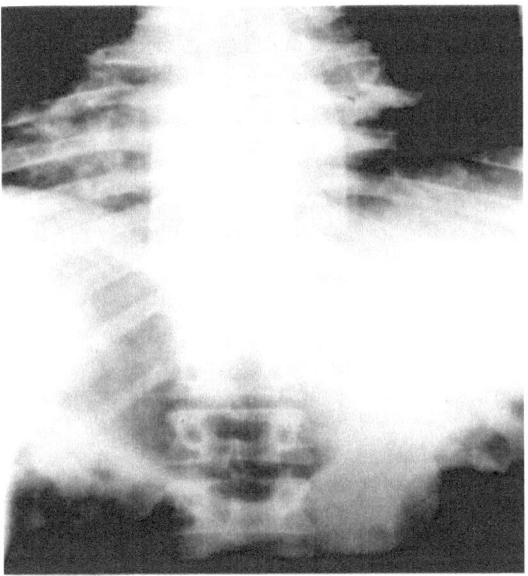

Figure 5.16 Anteroposterior radiograph of the thoracolumbar spine of a patient with tuberculosis. A large paravertebral abscess is present.

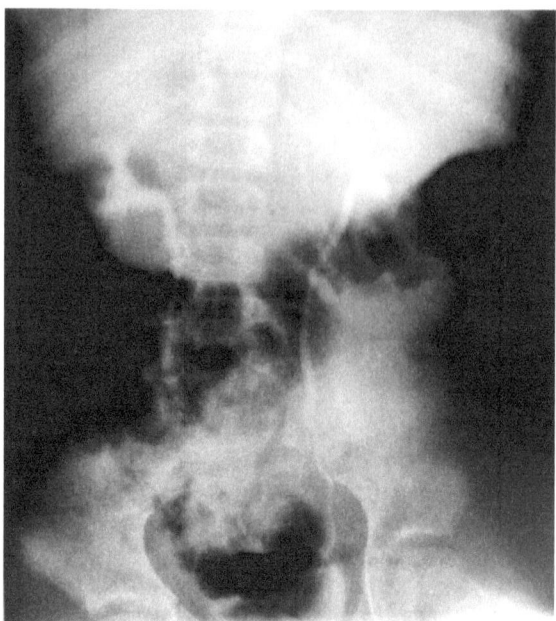

Figure 5.17 Intravenous pyelogram (IVP) showing displacement of the left ureter due to psoas abscess. This 7-year-old girl presented with an irritable hip with a fixed flexion deformity at the hip, but no sign of an abscess at the groin. The plain films were not conclusive. The IVP confirmed the diagnosis and she settled rapidly with antituberculous therapy.

Most spinal tuberculosis is treated without the benefit of histological and bacteriological diagnosis. Where the response to chemotherapy is suboptimal the possible differential diagnosis of tumour deposits or other chronic granulomatous infections must be considered. Staphylococcal or salmonella osteomyelitis or discitis may be confused with tuberculosis but the history in those conditions is usually shorter and the symptoms more severe, despite the similarity of the early radiological appearances. In some areas of the tropics, brucellosis may enter the differential diagnosis. Although pus may be obtained by a wide-bore needle aspiration from a cold abscess or at operation, the number of tubercle bacilli in a spinal lesion is relatively small and direct culture on Lowenstein-Jensen medium may need to be supplemented by animal inoculation. Routine open spinal biopsy is not · justified but when the diagnosis remains in doubt trephine needle biopsy guided by fluoroscopy is a valuable tool.

Open biopsy is a major procedure and is rarely justified unless performed in the course of surgery for other indications such as the relief of paraplegia.

The typical granuloma of tuberculosis is diagnostic especially if acid-fast bacilli can be demonstrated in the lesion by Ziehl-Neelsen staining. There are now rapid diagnostic Polymerase Chain Reaction (PCR) diagnostic cartridge-based tests available which perform nucleic acid amplification. Their accuracy depends on the numbers of TB organisms in the specimen. A spinal or CSF specimen may return a negative result but this does not exclude TB as the cause.

Pott's paraplegia (spinal tuberculosis with neurological signs)

Neurological complications regularly accompany spinal tuberculosis especially in disease of the thoracic spine. The pressure of pus, sequestra of bone or disc and granulation tissue may all cause a spastic paraparesis by pressure on the spinal cord. Rarely cord infarction may occur. In the early stages, hyperreflexia and spasticity are the main signs to be replaced by a flaccid paralysis as cord damage increases. The prognosis of Pott's paraplegia is comparatively good, especially if anti-tuberculous drug therapy can be supplemented by surgical anterior decompression of the cord. Late Pott's paraplegia is the term used for paraplegia occurring years after a tuberculous spinal lesion has been treated and supposedly cured. Recurrence of the disease is now common, especially in patients with HIV disease, and paraplegia may occur from any of the causes listed above.

Case report

A 50-year-old man was referred to the visiting neurosurgeon because of increasing difficulty walking. As a young man he had spinal tuberculosis with paraplegia but had regained the use of his limbs. On examination he had a gross forward stoop due to a 70° gibbus in the lower lumbar spine. His sensation was intact but he had weakness, hypertonicity, hyperreflexia and clonus in both lower limbs. He had late Pott's paraplegia due to an increasing angle of kyphosis and gradual collapse of the spine. Surgery for this case would have been extremely hazardous and he was recommended to wear corsets and remain mobile. This strategy has proved successful for the last 5 years and he has not particularly deteriorated.

Case report *(Continued)*

The visiting neurosurgeon, not having seen him previously and in the absence of a documented neurological examination was also left to wonder how much of his signs might have been residual from his bout of active tuberculosis (Figure 5.18 (a), below).

Another form of late Pott's paraplegia occurs after childhood spinal tuberculosis in which several growth plates have been destroyed anteriorly while the posterior elements remain unaffected (Figure 5.18, below). The tuberculous infection has been 'cured' but even if fusion of the affected vertebral bodies has occurred, failure of growth anteriorly increases the kyphosis and the cord becomes stretched over the internal gibbus which is the angulated posterior surface of the vertebral bodies. Symptoms and signs of spastic paraparesis arise from oedema and gliosis of the spinal cord and usually occur at or soon after the pubertal growth spurt. Treatment consists of the difficult surgical resection of the internal gibbus which usually consists of sclerotic bone. Once access to the spinal canal has been obtained anteriorly above and below the apex of the lesion the bone is gradually removed taking every precaution to prevent further damage to the stretched spinal cord. The spine requires reconstruction and fusion.

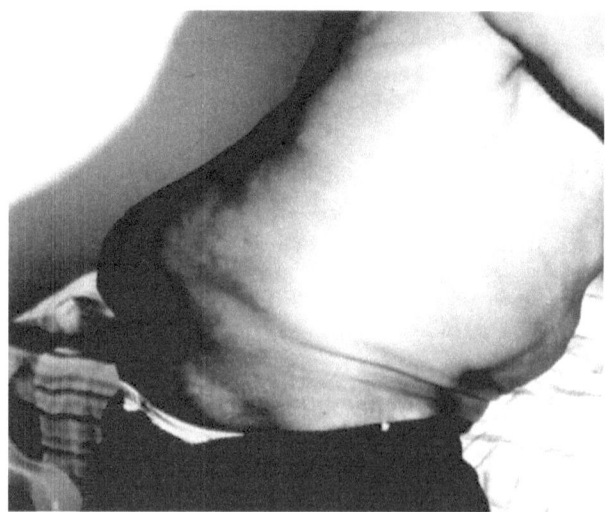

(a) Man with lumbar spinal gibbus due to chronic tuberculosis.

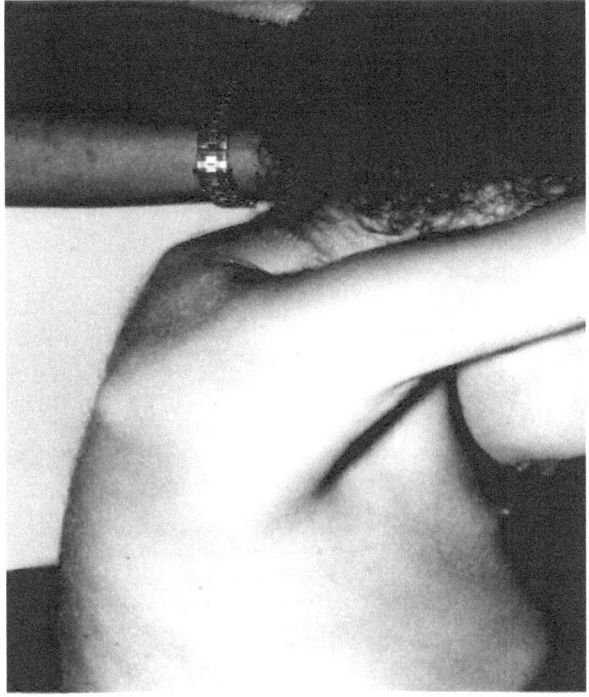

(b) Child with cervical gibbus due to vertebral collapse and destruction following tuberculosis infection.

Figure 5.18 (a-b)

Treatment

Antituberculous drugs

For many years the mainstay of treatment has been bed rest, good food and antituberculous drugs. Some patients have been treated as ambulant outpatients. It has been shown that no supports, plaster jackets or plaster casts improve the overall prognosis or lessen the eventual deformity. Until recently, treatment consisted of a combination of isoniazid 300 mg daily and thioacetazone 150 mg daily for 2 years supplemented by streptomycin 1 g daily for the first 2 or 3 months of treatment. This was a relatively cheap regimen with high patient compliance. As HIV disease became prevalent there was a corresponding rise in the incidence of drug reactions. Serious reactions occurred especially to thioacetazone which carried a 3 per cent incidence of fatal Stevens-Johnson syndrome. Streptomycin also became an expensive drug by virtue of the expense of the syringes, needles and personnel needed for administration. Patients are now commenced on a four-drug regime of rifampicin, isoniazid, pyrazinamide and ethambutol for 2 months continuing with three of these drugs for a further 9 months. Anti-tuberculous and anti-retroviral regimens are constantly being updated and readers should make themselves familiar with the appropriate hospital and/or national guidelines.

Case report

A 30-year-old woman was admitted with lower back pain for 3 months. She had developed weakness in her lower limbs over the preceding 3 weeks and was now almost unable to stand. She had been treated in the clinic with analgesics and anti-inflammatories. On examination of her lower thoracic spine she had a gibbus and she was hyperreflexic in her lower limbs with up going plantars and brisk knee and ankle jerks. Sensation was intact. An X-ray of her thoracolumbar spine showed three diseased vertebrae with collapse of the intervening disc spaces. A myelogram was not performed. She was put on bed rest and commenced on antituberculous therapy. After 4 weeks her motor function of her lower limbs improved. After 9 months of treatment she was neurologically normal.

The role of surgery (see Figure 5.19, page 263)

The late 20th Century Medical Research Council (MRC) trials clearly demonstrated that surgery has little role in spinal tuberculosis without neurological symptoms. When neurological signs are present the most practical treatment where there is no spinal surgeon is bed rest and chemotherapy for 4 weeks. At this stage a decision must be made according to the clinical progress as to whether or not surgery should continue to be withheld. Those whose paraplegia deteriorates or who fail to show any sign of improvement may benefit from anterolateral decompression of the tuberculous process and interbody spinal fusion (The Hong Kong procedure).

This procedure has the advantage of also arresting progression of kyphosis which may become increasingly problematic for the patient in later years, restricting chest expansion, or pressing on the spinal cord. The Hong Kong procedure is a major operation and is only applicable in centres that have the orthopaedic/neurosurgical and anaesthetic skills available for major spinal surgery. More recently, the Kalaphong operation has been used to simultaneously clear the area of disease, fuse the spine with living rib graft and perform a posterior fusion after correction of the kyphosis. Pressure from a cold abscess can be relieved by costotransversectomy, which does not destabilise the spine (see Chapter 11, page 577). This should be considered in patients with rapidly deteriorating neurological signs and it is an operation which can be performed by a general surgeon. A laminectomy is certainly to be discouraged because having lost anterior stability, posterior instability would be disastrous.

Case report

An 8-year-old child presented with acute paraplegia over a few days. In actual fact she had been complaining of back pain and difficulty in walking for about 3 weeks but the parents thought this was because she had fallen out of a mango tree. She had an auntie and an uncle who were being treated for tuberculosis. A chest X-ray showed a paraspinal abscess in the mid-thoracic region. No CT scanner was available.

An urgent myelogram was performed which showed a block at T6, similar to the one in Figure 5.20, page 264. She was started on antituberculous therapy and a surgeon was consulted. Because of the risk of compression of the cord's blood supply by the cold abscess a costotransversectomy was carried out. This drained 50 ml of pus. Two weeks later her neurological signs started to improve. However, the best procedure for cases with deteriorating neurological signs or not responding to medical treatment is still the Hong Kong procedure.

Treatment of Spinal Tuberculosis

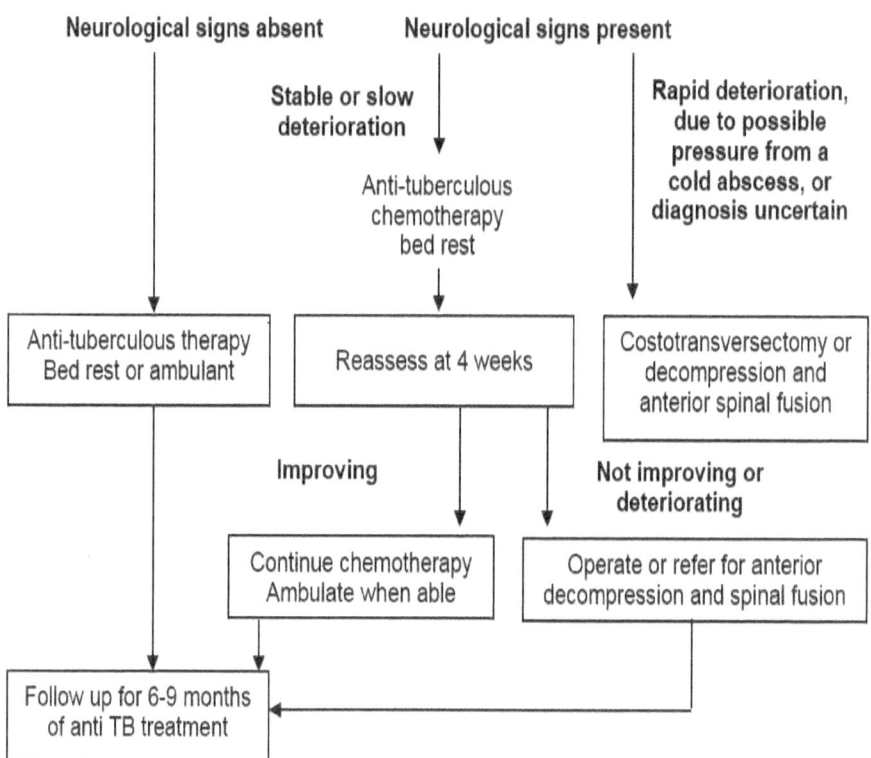

Figure 5.19 Decision algorithm for the treatment of spinal tuberculosis.

In the case where a patient does not improve on 4 weeks of antituberculous treatment and it is impossible to refer to a surgeon who can eradicate tuberculosis and decompress the spinal canal through the Hong Kong procedure or costotransversectomy, we advise persevering with medical treatment alone. MRC trial from Korea showed that tuberculosis can be 'cured' by drug therapy in 77 per cent of cases, but it is likely that neurological improvement will only occur in those cases where embarrassment of the spinal cord was due to either pus or granulation tissue rather than mechanical pressure.

Most patients with neurological deficits respond quite quickly after anterior decompression and fusion but a few with very long-standing disease and particularly those who are HIV positive take some months to recover and some never recover completely, often being left with spastic paraparesis. After successful medical therapy alone further deterioration in the spine may occur. Complete bony fusion occurs in only 44 per cent, vertebral body height is lost and the angle of kyphosis increases by over 30° from a mean of 40° in a fifth of the patients.

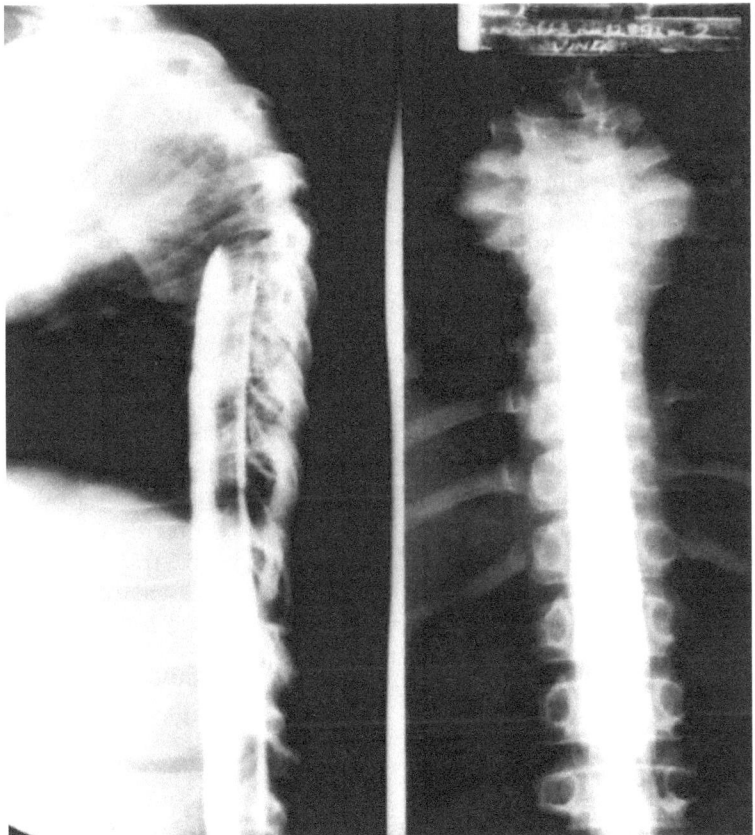

Figure 5.20 Tuberculosis causing an upper thoracic complete myelographic block.

The influence of HIV infection on treatment

The advent of HIV has considerable altered our attitude to such major surgery. HIV-positive patients, particularly those with clinical signs of HIV disease have a high incidence of complications after major surgery especially thoracotomy. If an HIV-positive patient is suffering from Pott's paraplegia and is not improving on drug treatment alone, his immune competence should be assessed and the risks of surgery discussed. Even without anti-retroviral therapy HIV-positive patients with spinal tuberculosis may live for years. Those surviving the complications of major surgery do improve neurologically but recovery is often slower than in HIV-negative patients. The clinical classification of HIV disease suggested by the World Health Organization puts all patients with extrapulmonary tuberculosis into Stage 4 of the disease along with those with frank AIDS and the AIDS-related complex, Kaposi's sarcoma, lymphomas and lethal opportunistic infections. While HIV is primarily a sexually transmitted disease, tuberculosis is acquired by inhalation or ingestion.

A patient may acquire tuberculosis during the early months of HIV infection or a tuberculous patient may become HIV positive later. We feel that it is important to assess, both clinically and haematologically (by lymphocyte counts or CD4 cell counts), the immune status of the patient before discussing the probable outcome of surgery and obtaining informed consent. Preliminary results of our research in patients with bone and joint tuberculosis and HIV disease suggests that the prognosis depends very much on the state of HIV reached before therapy is started. Before anti-retroviral therapy was introduced in sub-Saharan Africa, the mean survival time for HIV positive patients with pulmonary TB was about 22 months. Anti-retroviral therapy combined with compliance and drug availability offers an opportunity of maintaining HIV infection in remission almost indefinitely.

SCOLIOSIS

John E. Jellis

Although there are many causes of scoliosis, any of which may occur in tropical countries, the major types of scoliosis seen result from congenital malformations, neuromuscular weakness (usually following poliomyelitis) or are idiopathic. Scoliosis from trauma, neurofibromatosis or other causes is rare.

Scoliosis due to congenital malformation

Congenital lesions seem more ˉcommon in the tropics because of the high birth rate and the population demographics in LMICs where a high proportion of the population is under 15 years of age. The main congenital lesions causing scoliosis are failure of segmentation (unilateral fusion bars) and the presence of one or more hemivertebrae. The infant is usually presented during the first year of life because the mother has noticed a spinal deformity or the deformity may be discovered during examination for some other congenital anomaly such as talipes equinovarus.

It should be remembered that congenital lesions are often multiple and the other major body systems especially the renal system should be thoroughly checked before major surgery is embarked upon. As long as there is no neurological deficit, the child can be treated expectantly and the progress assessed both clinically and by repeated radiological examinations at 6ˉmonthly intervals.

Neurological problems are rare in congenital scoliosis as opposed to the situation in congenital kyphosis or myelomeningocele. If present, neurological abnormalities are usually due to other coˉexistent spinal dysraphisms such as diastematomyelia (split spinal cord with a bony or cartilaginous bar between the two cords which causes tethering (see Chapter 4, page 195) or to a tethered filum terminale. Chiari malformation and syringomyelia may also cause secondary scoliosis (page 297). Quite frequently there is more than one area of congenital malformation, so the whole spine should be examined radiologically. Sometimes multiple lesions occur on both right and left sides and may roughly balance each other to minimise the deformity.

A single hemivertebra or short fusion segment is usually well compensated for if it occurs in the thoracic or upper lumbar spine but may cause a severe spinal/pelvic tilt if low in the lumbar spine. Thus, the actual geometry of the lesion may give some idea of the prognosis and alert the surgeon to the need for early intervention. Once the child is standing and walking, axial loading of the spine increases and any abnormal angulation is likely to progress more rapidly. From 2 years of age, all radiographic determinations of scoliosis should be taken standing so that measurement of the scoliosis (the Cobb angle - Figure 5.21, below) can be as accurate as possible. If the deformity is rapidly increasing, surgical intervention is indicated.

Early surgery, at about 2-3 years age, is aimed at destroying the extra growth plates on the convexity of the curve, whether this is due to hemivertebrae or to a fusion bar on the concavity. Unfortunately, posterior fusion is often inadequate and an anterior procedure with excision of the intervertebral discs over the apex of the curve is also required. Any form of internal or external fixation seems unnecessary at this stage.

In the older child developing severe angulation, combined anterior and posterior fusion with internal fixation using Harrington compression rods or sublaminar wiring to Luque rods or a Hartshill rectangle, may be needed to arrest further angulation. If the angulation is already severe, especially if it is low in the lumbar spine, or if there is neurological deterioration, combined anterior and posterior operations may be necessary to excise the hemivertebra and decompress the spinal cord.

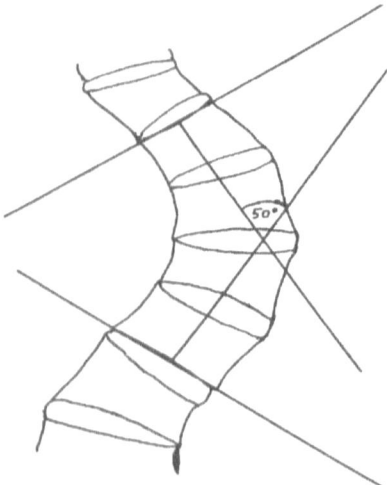

Figure 5.21 Cobb's spinal angle for scoliosis measurement.

Paralytic scoliosis

In a child weakened by poliomyelitis, spinal muscle atrophy or other neurological problem, the advent of scoliosis is a very considerable increase in disability. A curvature in the thoracic region will give an unsightly rib hump but more importantly it will severely reduce the child's respiratory capacity. Children with lower limb disabilities already use an increased amount of energy for locomotion and a decreased vital capacity will limit their activity considerably. They become critically ill if they develop respiratory tract infections because they have little or no respiratory reserve.

Lastly, if the curve involves the lumbar spine as it usually does, the child may be unable to sit without using his arms and hands to hold himself up. A child already immobilised by lower limb weakness then becomes incapable of using his upper limbs while sitting and is unable to use his hands or even feed himself. In times past, external braces, jackets and corsets have been recommended for this sort of problem. The results were very poor because they were cumbersome or often very difficult to fit. They cause ulceration at pressure points and further reduced the child's vital capacity. With modern methods of spinal internal fixation, it is possible to fuse long lengths of the spine soundly, without the need for external braces. The internal fixation is strong enough to allow sitting within a couple of days of surgery. The major complications of such surgery are those of blood loss and respiratory inefficiency. The respiratory musculature will usually be weak.

The vital capacity will be low and will be further reduced by the effects of surgery and blood transfusion on the lungs. Some patients will need to have respirator assisted ventilation for a few days after surgery with careful monitoring of haemoglobin level and for chest infection. With adequate precautions however, such surgery can be very successful. Figure 5.22, next page shows a teenager with post-polio paralysis who could not sit unsupported. An anterior lumbar fusion (Dwyer fixation) was performed as a first stage to straightening the major lumbar curve. At a second stage, 3 weeks later, a posterior Harrington procedure extended the fusion into the thoracic spine with little additional straightening of the rather stiff thoracic curve. Ten years later, the patient works from a wheelchair managing an orthopaedic appliance workshop.

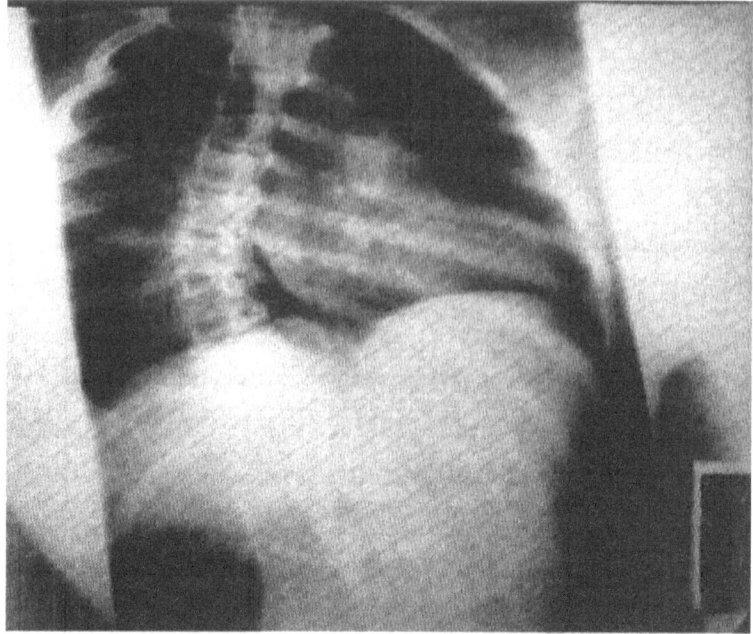

Figure 5.22 Scoliosis of the thoracolumbar spine.

In children with severe mobility problems, it is important to avoid fusing the lumbar spine to the pelvis. Such fusion will prevent the child swinging from a wheelchair to bed or other similar activities.

Idiopathic scoliosis

In tropical countries, idiopathic scoliosis seems less common than in developed nations. The infantile and juvenile forms are rare. Adolescent idiopathic scoliosis seems much less common among disadvantaged populations than elsewhere. There is a lot of evidence that the well-nourished (perhaps over-nourished?) populations of Europe and America are getting progressively taller while under-nourished populations remain of short stature. In Zambia we find that almost all children seen with adolescent idiopathic scoliosis come from well-to-do families and the disease is very rarely seen in children from the lower socioeconomic levels. One is forced to the conclusion that adolescent idiopathic scoliosis is due to rapid spinal elongation around the pubertal growth spurt and that this is maximal in those families eating a high protein, high fat, western-type diet. The treatment of idiopathic scoliosis in the tropics does not differ from the treatment elsewhere. Braces, jackets and other supports are cumbersome and of limited effect unless they strongly distract or compress, but then the complication risk will become unacceptable high. They are poorly tolerated in hot and humid climates.

An adolescent with a curvature approaching 50° Cobb angle should be offered a posterior instrumented fusion to stop further deterioration. For those with curves ranging from 60° to 90° prior shortening by anterior discectomy is advised to prevent stretching the spinal cord. Curvatures of over 90° need a two-stage wedge resection of the spine if straightening is to be achieved. In a single-stage procedure, the surgeon should be conservative in attempting to gain correction and certainly not exceed the straightening that can be shown possible on a preoperative A-P radiograph taken with manipulative straightening of the curve. Iatrogenic paraplegia is a disaster to be avoided at all costs. The equipment for intraoperative neuromonitoring to minimise the risk of iatrogenic neurological deficits may not be available in LMICs. An alternative that relies on a good anaesthetist and much patience, is a wake-up test to be performed after the fixation is in place. Ankle clonus can be demonstrated as the depth of anaesthesia is lightened at the end of an operation and recently it has been suggested that the presence of ankle clonus during a wake-up test is a positive indication of spinal cord function.

If clonus remains absent any distraction or straightening of the spine should be reduced. If this test proves reliable in the local setting, it can be valuable for spinal cord monitoring during scoliosis surgery.[48]

Cosmetic considerations

In most instances it is not the lateral bending of the spine that is noticed and complained of by the patient or parents but the rib hump caused by the rotational component of the deformity. A little time explaining the cause and natural history of the deformity will be well spent because after an initial fusion, the spine will not be straight nor will the rib hump have changed. If time and the condition of the patient allow, the rib hump can be reduced at initial surgery by excising the posterior segments of the affected ribs. This provides extra bone for the fusion mass but it is difficult to excise the relevant sections of rib lying behind the rib hump without penetrating the parietal pleura and thus opening the chest. Especially if the patient

[48]Hoppenfeld S, Gross A, Andrews C, Lonner B. The ankle clonus test for assessment of the integrity of the spinal cord during operations for scoliosis. Journal of Bone and Joint Surgery: American Orthopaedic Association. 1997;79(2):208-212.

is to have respirator-assisted ventilation after surgery, an underwater seal chest drain should be left in place. Alternatively, the rib hump may be removed by thoracoplasty at a second procedure. Patients are often very grateful for this. The vital capacity of the chest is not further reduced by such excision.

Although the workload of general and paediatric orthopaedic surgery in LMICs is high and orthopaedic surgeons are few, scoliosis surgery is a rewarding interest for those undertaking other forms of spinal surgery. The techniques however, especially in Europe and America, are complicated and the equipment and implants expensive. Even if a surgeon is experienced in the operative treatment of spinal trauma and tuberculosis, a visit to a scoliosis specialist would be of value. Of even more value, is to invite that scoliosis specialist to operate in your operating theatre where the methods can be taught and safely adapted to local circumstances. This should be done at the outset, before lots of expensive equipment and implants are purchased which may never be used. Under these circumstances, scoliosis surgery is a challenging but safe proposition in LMICs.

MANAGEMENT OF PROLAPSED INTERVERTEBRAL DISC AND OTHER PROBLEMS

Lower back pain (lumbago)

Most patients with acute back pain will improve with a period of limiting activity. If possible, a patient with back pain should not be confined to bed unless pain makes it impossible for them to remain mobile. Trials have shown that patients with lower back pain do better if they remain active. Traction also does not benefit patients with acute back pain. Exercises designed to strengthen the abdominal and paraspinal muscles, improve posture and mobility (e.g. hyperextension exercises providing symptoms are not aggravated by hyperextension) form part of the general management of back pain.

Advice about lifting, avoidance of stressing the back and sleeping on a mattress on the floor or a board under a mattress should be given. The patient should be encouraged to remain active. Beware of patients with a large emotional or psychological component to their back pain. Operating on back pain makes some patients worse and carries a risk of permanent nerve root damage or instability. Also beware of those who wish to avoid work or magnify their complaints to boost claims for compensation.

Lumbar canal stenosis (see Figure 5.23, next page)

Lumbar canal stenosis (LCS) arises from degenerative changes in the lumbar spine which cause a narrowing of the central canal but also a narrowing of the lateral recess on each side of the canal in which the exiting nerve roots pass to their foramina. The cause of the narrowing is a combination of facet joint hypertrophy (osteophytes and ligamentous hypertrophy), disc bulging and hypertrophied ligamentum flavum. There may also be a congenital element to the canal stenosis which predisposes the individual to becoming symptomatic.

Lumbar canal stenosis usually presents in the 60s and 70s. The symptoms are low back pain and aching in the buttocks and lower limbs, on exertion or after prolonged standing. The individual must stop and have a rest when the cramps in the legs become intolerable. The walking distance gradually diminishes and the history is similar to vascular claudication, except that there is no evidence of vascular disease in the lower limbs, and thus the condition is called **neurogenic claudication**. On examination, there may be some stiffness of the lumbar spine, but the only neurological abnormality is usually a loss of ankle reflexes.

Plain CT scan is the best diagnostic test, and shows the pathology of canal stenosis clearly. The treatment is lumbar laminectomy with excision of the hypertrophied ligament and trimming of the facet joints (see Chapter 11, page 573). 'Burnt out' TB of the thoracolumbar spine may produce a similar clinical picture, particularly if the spine is kyphotic (see case report on page 258 of a 50-year-old male). Thoracic canal stenosis due to degenerative causes is uncommon.

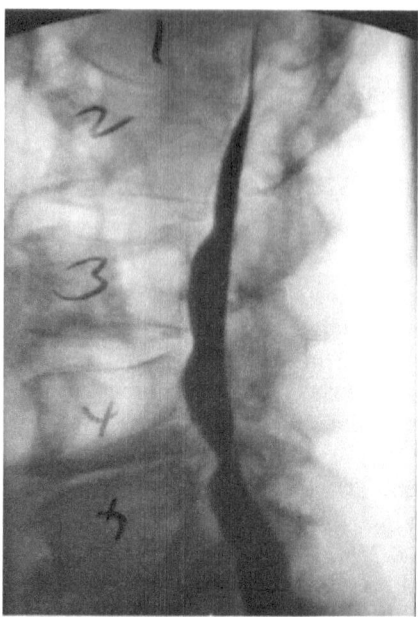

Figure 5.23 (a) Myelogram showing multiple hourglass deformities of lumbar canal stenosis.

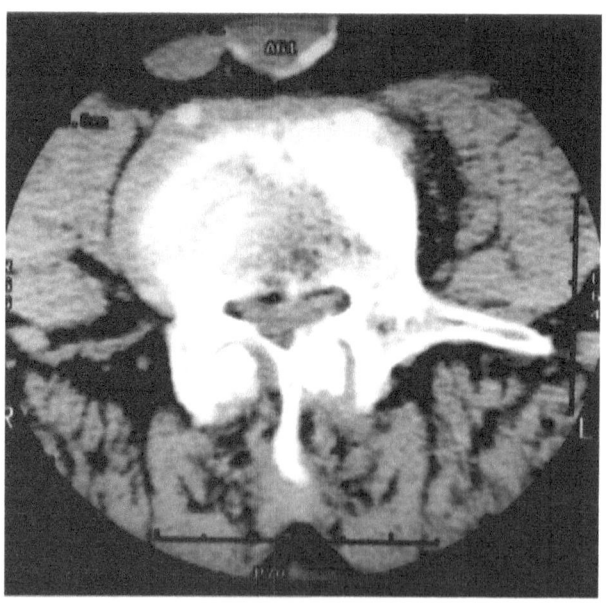

(b) Narrow trefoil pattern of lumbar canal stenosis with tight lateral recess on both sides and narrow A-P diameter due to bony encroachment and ligamentous hypertrophy on axial CT. Note the lack of contrast in the canal.

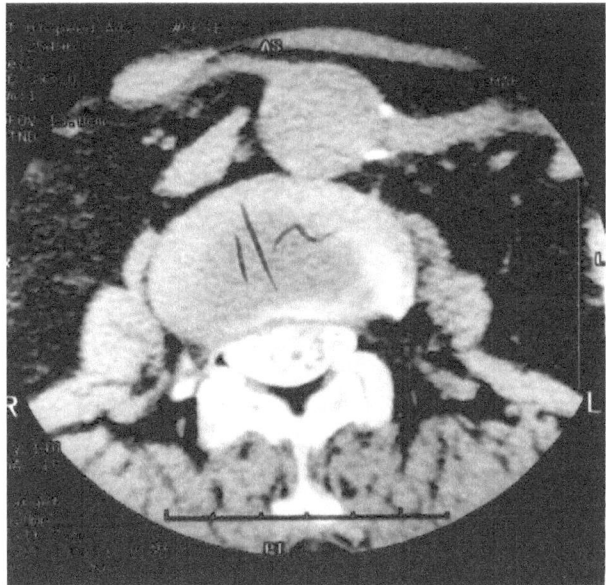

(c) Normal spinal canal on CT myelogram axial scan.

Figure 5.23 (a-c) Lumbar canal stenosis.

The achondroplastic dwarf has congenital spinal canal stenosis and this may progress to symptomatic lumbar canal stenosis with neurogenic claudication in the teens and require laminectomy.

Lumbar spondylolisthesis

There is a slip of between adjacent lumbar vertebrae. This is nearly always L4-5 or L5-S1. The usual cause is either a congenital or post-traumatic spondylolysis which is a discontinuity in the bone between the two articular processes of the vertebra (the pars interarticularis) which may be bridged by fibrous tissue. It is less commonly secondary to TB or neoplasm. This defect can be seen on the oblique lumbar X-rays. Minor degrees of slip can be managed conservatively with a back brace and analgesics. If the slip is progressive or severe and there is nerve root compression, then a wide dorsal decompression may be indicated which includes excision of the facet joints, insertion of pedicle screws, and rods which join the pedicle screws, and bone grafts. This is a major spinal fusion procedure, and would need specialist care. Surgical decompression alone is not enough to relieve the problem and may result in increased slippage.

Prolapsed intervertebral disc

Patients with a proven intervertebral disc prolapse may require surgery. The natural history of low back pain and sciatica is for improvement although relapses are common.

Clinical trials have shown after 4 years there is no difference between groups of patients treated by discectomy or conservatively. Therefore, surgery should be reserved for the following:
1. Absolute indications
   • spinal cord or cauda equina compression
   • persistent or deteriorating neurological signs
2. Relative indications
   • intolerable pain
   • severe postural tilt and pain
   • Persistent pain or neurological signs, which restrict ability to work or perform household or recreational activities

Patients who are operated on for the relative indications listed above improve more rapidly after surgical treatment but their long-term results are not be significantly better than those who do not have surgery.

Case report

A 50-year-old active ex-footballer experienced severe pain in his left buttock, thigh and calf and was referred by his GP for a venogram, which was normal. The calf was not swollen and he had good foot pulses. He was unable to stand straight, walking with his spine flexed. His ankle jerk was diminished and dorsiflexion of the foot was weaker than the unaffected side. There was diminished sensation on the dorsum of his foot and the lateral calf. The pain in his calf was aggravated by straight leg raising.

Lesson: *the diagnosis was a prolapsed L4-5 intervertebral disc, which was later confirmed on an MRI scan. He presented with sciatica which was much more painful than his back. The patient was treated expectantly for ten weeks but failed to improve so underwent laminectomy and discectomy. Within six months he had resumed full activities including swimming and running.*

Lumbar disc prolapse (Figure 5.24, next page)

Lumbar disc prolapse is a common problem and is a cause of lumbar back pain and discogenic pain which may radiate to the buttock and upper thigh. The disc prolapse may occur spontaneously or following physical exertion. A true sciatica radiates down the back of the thigh, leg and sometimes into the foot and toes. It may be associated with paraesthesia in the distribution of the pain.

Coughing or straining usually aggravate the pain and straight leg raising and Lasegue's stretch tests are positive. The relevant nerve root is being compressed by a posterolateral disc prolapse or rupture. Compression of the upper lumbar roots causes anterior thigh pain and the femoral stretch test may be positive. Note that a so-called far lateral disc prolapse will cause compression of the nerve root belonging to the pedicle above the disc, e.g. the L4-5 disc compresses the L4 nerve root in this situation, whereas the common posterolateral disc prolapse at L4-5 will compress the nerve root crossing the disc to reach the pedicle below the disc, which is the L5 nerve root. A central lumbar disc prolapse if large enough, will cause cauda equina compression or rarely, conus compression, at L1-2. These patients will present with bilateral sciatica and sphincter involvement. Decompression in this case is a surgical emergency.

The operation is best performed posteriorly as described in the operative surgery section. For standard posterolateral disc prolapse, a period of conservative treatment is reasonable, as many cases will improve. If the patient is no better in ten days with bed rest and strong analgesics, and there are neurological signs of nerve root compression persisting, it may be appropriate to consider a discectomy. The crucial features in deciding to operate are the degree of pain and suffering, and the degree of neurological deficit. A plain X-ray will not show a ruptured disc. It may show some narrowing and degenerative changes at the relevant disc space. The definitive investigation is a lumbar myelogram which will clearly show if any nerve root is being compressed. CT scan following the myelogram is of added benefit, and will clearly show the pathology in the axial projection with contrast in the intradural compartment (Figure 5.24, next page).

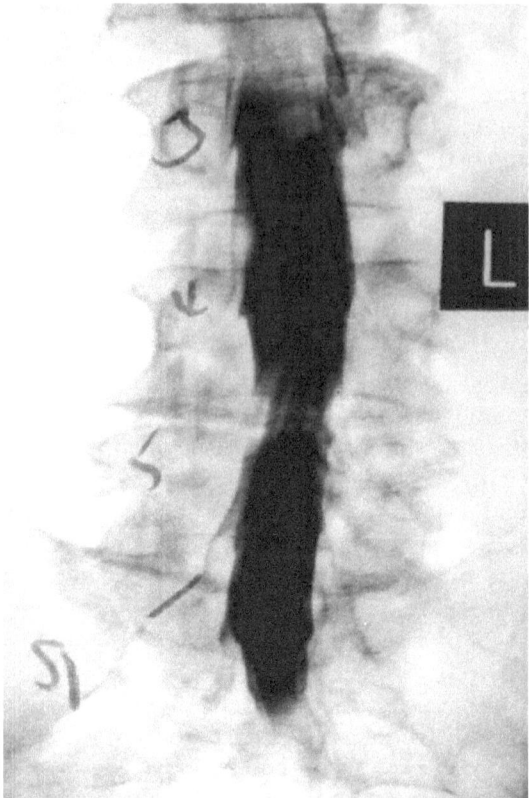

Figure 5.24 (a) Myelogram showing L5 nerve root cut off on the right side due to posterolateral disc prolapse.

Magnetic resonance imaging (MRI) is an alternative to myelography/CT and is not invasive. In the developing-world setting, myelography alone may have to be the standard investigation, which is quite satisfactory. In HIC, MR is usually the definitive imaging performed. Myelography is rarely performed. For recurrent sciatica after surgery, MRI is very helpful because it can distinguish between scarring and recurrent disc prolapse, by using the contrast agent gadolinium which gives enhancement of scar tissue, but does not enhance disc material. Plain CT alone is not very helpful unless the resolution is very clear, and disc prolapse is very significant. It is far better to perform myelography followed by CT if the latter is available.

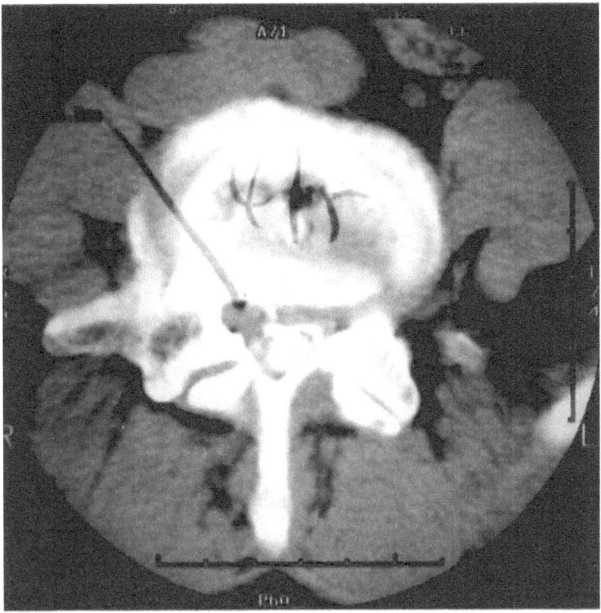

(b) Axial CT showing posterolateral disc prolapse at L4-5.

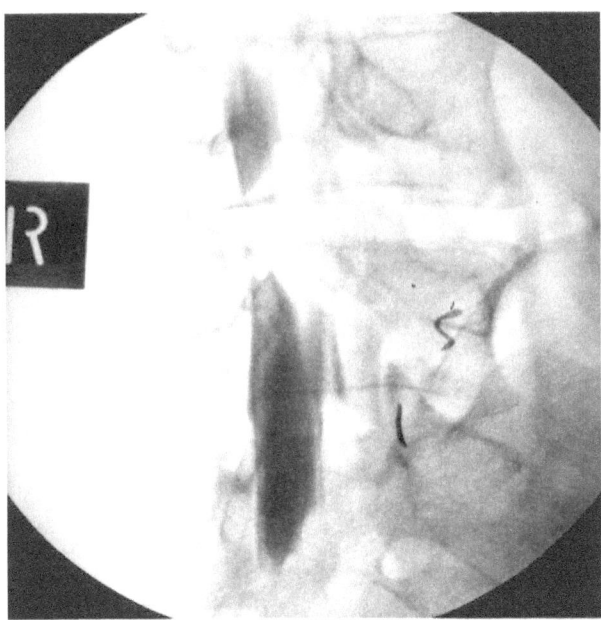

(c) Myelogram showing almost complete block at L4-5 due to a large central disc prolapse.

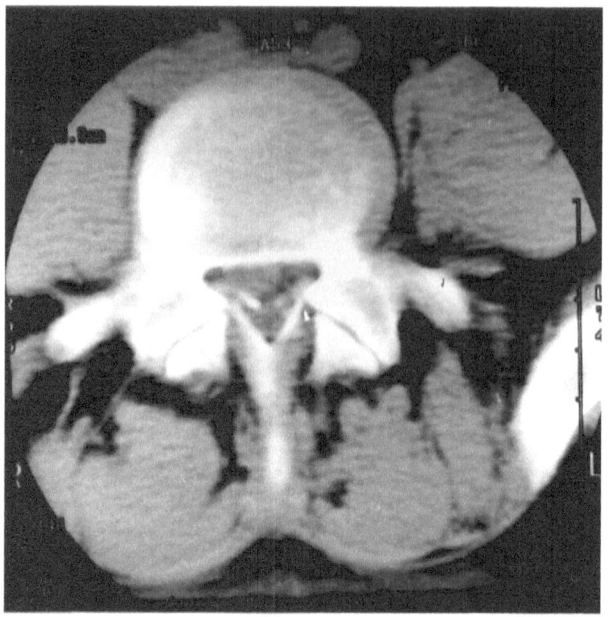

(d) CT scan showing large central disc prolapse at the L4-5 level, with severe compression of the dural sac. The intradural contrast is white. Urgent decompression was performed.

Figure 5.24 (a-d) Lumbar disc prolapse.

Practice point

Do not operate on the basis of X-ray findings alone, and there must be a good correlation between the clinical and the imaging findings, otherwise the patient should not be having an operation for a prolapsed intervertebral disc.

The operation of discectomy is described in Chapter 11 (page 573). There is no evidence that adding a fusion to the discectomy is any better than discectomy alone, although this is a somewhat controversial point. Excellent results can certainly be obtained by discectomy alone. Note also that sequestrated (free) disc fragments do not return to the disc space with conservative management or manipulation. They will remain outside the canal and will remain a source of compression to the adjacent nerve root. These are usually associated with large disc prolapses or prolapse which has extended well away from the disc space, although this is not invariable. Essentially if the pain is not improving with conservative management and there is evidence of nerve root compression, then surgery is indicated.

Cervical disc prolapse (Figure 5.25, next page)

Central cervical disc prolapse causes cord compression and is described below in the section on cervical myelopathy. Posterolateral cervical disc prolapse compresses the adjacent cervical nerve root, causing arm pain (brachialgia) which is usually a lancinating severe pain, passing down the entire arm and often into the fingers, associated with paraesthesiae in the distribution of the pain. The history and the neurological signs will usually identify the offending disc. The commonest levels to prolapse are C6-7, followed by C5-6, followed by C7-T1. These will compress the C7, C6, and C8 nerve roots respectively (see Figure 2.11, page 30).

The disc prolapse may occur spontaneously or after physical exertion. There may also be an element of central neck pain. The pain in the arm is often so severe as to require admission to hospital and opiate analgesics. The initial treatment should be conservative, with rest, placing the neck in a collar and non-steroidal anti-inflammatory drugs if available, as well as standard analgesics. Many cases will settle with conservative management, however after 10 days, if there is a failure to settle, or persistent or advancing neurological signs, decompression of the affected nerve root may be indicated. The investigation of choice in LMIC is the cervical myelogram followed by CT. The cervical myelogram alone will suffice, if CT is not available. MRI of the cervical spine is now the investigation of choice in HIC.

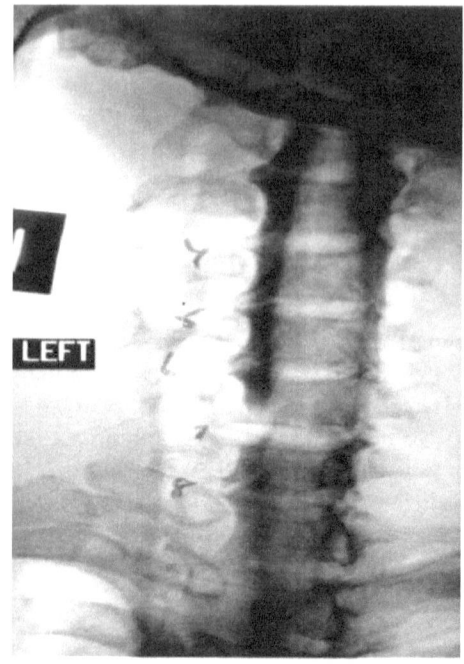

Figure 5.25 (a) Cervical myelogram showing left C7 nerve root cut off.

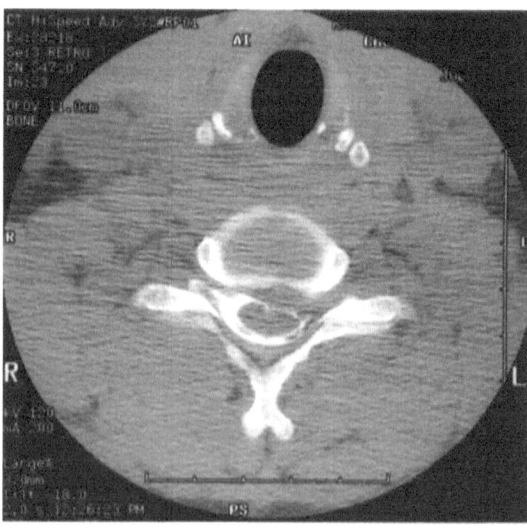

(b) Axial CT showing posterolateral disc prolapse at C6-7, displacement of the dural sac, and compression of the adjacent left C7 nerve root, with a lack of contrast within the nerve root sheath.

Figure 5.25 (a-b) Cervical disc prolapse.

Operative surgery of cervical disc prolapse

In LMIC settings, decompression is best done by a foraminotomy, which involves a hemi-laminectomy approach at the appropriate level. The patient is best placed in a prone position with the head fixed in the three-pin headrest. If this is unavailable the patient can be placed in a lateral position, with the head resting on a horseshoe ring, at the appropriate level. The head of the table is elevated to reduce venous pressure and bleeding. The correct spinal segment is identified at operation by placing a needle at the relevant interspinous level and performing a lateral X-ray on the table or using the image intensifier, if available. A more reliable method is to count down with the finger from the spinous process of C2, downwards. The C2 spinous process can readily be distinguished from the arch of the atlas (without a spinous process) above it. This requires a more extended incision to be able to pass the finger down from above.

The paraspinal muscles are reflected in a subperiosteal plane off the affected side only. The operation is very similar to the lumbar discectomy exposure, except that it is in the neck. The hemilaminectomy (interlaminar approach) at the relevant level is extended out laterally to include the facet joint and the exposed ligamentum flavum is excised. The power tool with a cutting 'match-head' burr, and the angled bone punches of varying sizes are recommended. The lateral edge of the dura and the axilla of the relevant cervical root are exposed. The root is decompressed laterally. There are often large epidural veins around the nerve root, which will require bipolar coagulation and Surgicel.

It is often impossible to retrieve the disc from in front of the nerve root without retraction and damage to the nerve root. If there are sequestrated fragments it may be possible to lift them out gently from beneath the nerve root, using a blunt dissector such as a Watson-Cheyne, however, most cases will improve with the dorsal decompression alone. If there is a large soft disc component, this may be better decompressed via an anterior approach with an anterior cervical discectomy and fusion. However, this requires neurosurgical or orthopaedic expertise and is not recommended for the beginner. The results of decompressing a nerve root after cervical disc rupture are excellent for relief of pain and improvement of neurological signs, provided the operation is done soon enough, before irreversible nerve root or spinal cord damage has developed.

Practice point

Make sure that when you operate on the spine you have identified the correct side and the correct spinal level. Intraoperative imaging may prove helpful.

Cervical spondylosis

Cervical spondylosis is a degenerative osteoarthritis affecting the cervical spine. It affects about half the population over 50 years but only about 20 percent develop symptoms. Younger people may be affected after neck injury either in a generalised way or specifically at the level of previous trauma. The pathology is multifactorial and includes osteophytes, disc bulging, and ligament hypertrophy. This causes a progressive narrowing of the cervical intervertebral foramina compressing nerve roots, cervical radiculopathy and/or the cervical canal compressing the spinal cord - cervical myelopathy. Cervical myelopathy may develop when the canal diameter is less than 12 mm (normal 17±5 mm). Instability may develop in long-standing cases and contribute to the neural impingement.

Cervical spondylosis causes chronic neck pain, which may radiate to the shoulders or occiput. Pain radiating down the arm indicates a radiculopathy is present. The treatment of the spondylosis during periods of flare-up is rest in a soft cervical collar, simple analgesics, and non-steroidal anti-inflammatory drugs. Regular mobilising neck exercise is important, when the pain settles, to combat stiffness and recurrent pain. The indication for surgery is significant or progressive nerve root or spinal cord compromise, or less commonly, cervical instability. Surgery is not recommended for chronic neck pain unless accompanied by these complications.

Cervical myelopathy

Cervical myelopathy is usually an insidious and progressive problem due to spinal cord compression, which results in weakness and spasticity of the limbs, loss of manual dexterity, sensory loss in the periphery, particularly the hands, a shuffling unsteady gait, loss of balance, and frequent falls.

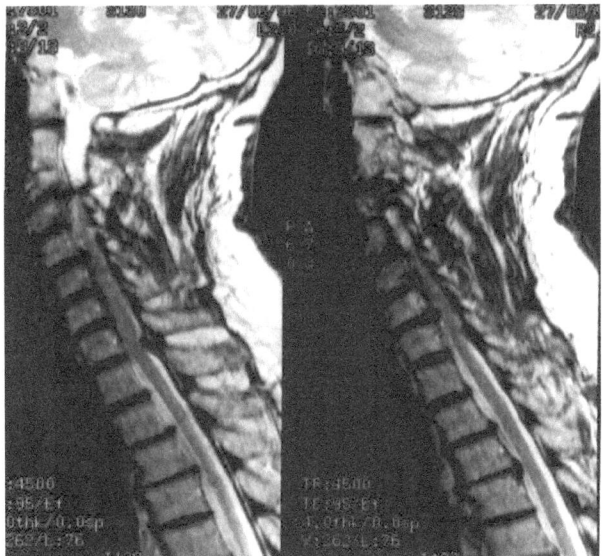

(a) A case of cervical myelopathy due to cervical spondylosis with a narrow cervical canal and hourglass deformities at C2-3 and C7-T1 on sagittal MR image. Note the lack of CSF around the spinal canal in the cervical canal.

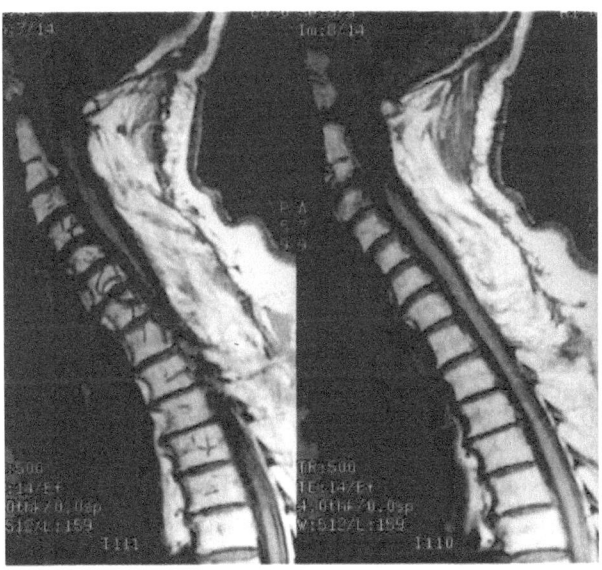

(b) Post decompression. The spinal cord has significantly more room. Unfortunately, the patient's myelopathy remained problematic, probably because of permanent damage in the spinal cord (myelomalacia).

Figure 5.26 (a-b)

Cervical myelopathy is due in younger adults to central cervical disc prolapse, and in the elderly is due to degenerative arthropathy in the cervical spine with a combination of facet joint hypertrophy, ligament hypertrophy, disc bulging, spondylolisthesis and repeated trauma to the cervical cord in a narrow canal. There may also be an element of cervical cord ischaemia. Neck pain may be a feature of the degenerative changes in the cervical spine (Figure 5.26, previous page).

Other less frequent causes are:
1. Craniocervical junction pathology, e.g. congenital disorders of the skull base - platybasia with the odontoid process protruding through the foramen magnum or rheumatoid arthritis with erosive destruction of the dens with an inflammatory mass (pannus) in its place.
2. Atlantoaxial subluxation - caused by trauma, or destructive arthropathy, eg. rheumatoid arthritis.

The treatment will depend on the cause:
1. Central disc prolapse will require an anterior cervical discectomy and interbody fusion.
2. Degenerative canal stenosis will require a cervical laminectomy over the affected segments, although if the compression is largely anterior, an anterior discectomy, osteophytectomy and interbody fusion will be required. This may be necessary in addition to a posterior decompression in severe cases.
3. Atlanto-axial instability will require an atlanto-axial fusion.
4. Craniocervical junction abnormalities require neurosurgical expertise which may involve trans-oral decompression of the craniocervical junction and possibly a dorsal decompression and fusion to prevent instability. This is sometimes done as a combined procedure under the one anaesthetic.

Mild myelopathy due to degenerative changes may respond to conservative treatment with immobilisation of the neck in a firm collar and non-steroidal anti-inflammatory drugs to lessen any acute inflammatory change. However, if there is already advanced myelopathy or a deteriorating neurological state, and investigations reveal significant cord compression, a decompressive procedure is indicated.

People with cervical myelopathy who acutely jar their neck in a fall could suffer much more severe damage to the cervical cord, and possibly quadriplegia. This is another reason for decompressive surgery when the compromise has reached the stage of loss of balance and falls.

Syringomyelia (Figure 5.27, below and Figure 5.28, page 288)

Syringomyelia is a slowly progressive and insidious condition with a dilatation of the central canal of the spinal cord. **Communicating syringomyelia or hydromyelia** extends down the spinal cord from the medulla /cord junction (obex level) and is associated with pathology at the craniocervical junction such as cerebellar ectopia (Chiari malformation), or chronic adhesive arachnoiditis and the pathogenesis is still debated.

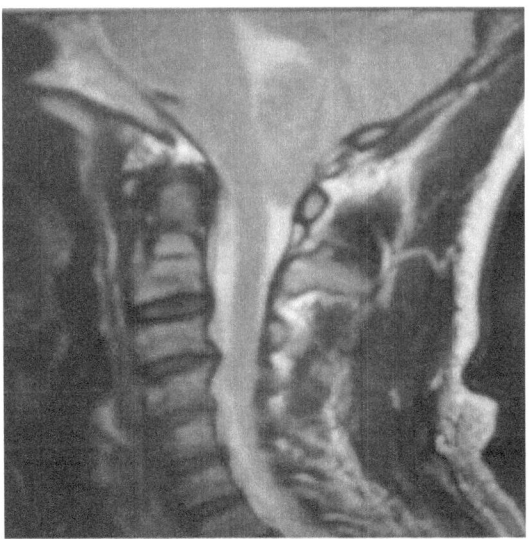

Figure 5.27 (a) Sagittal MR image showing Chiari I malformation with descent of the cerebellar tonsils down to the level of the posterior arch of C1 and a crowding of structures at the craniocervical junction. There is no cervical syrinx.

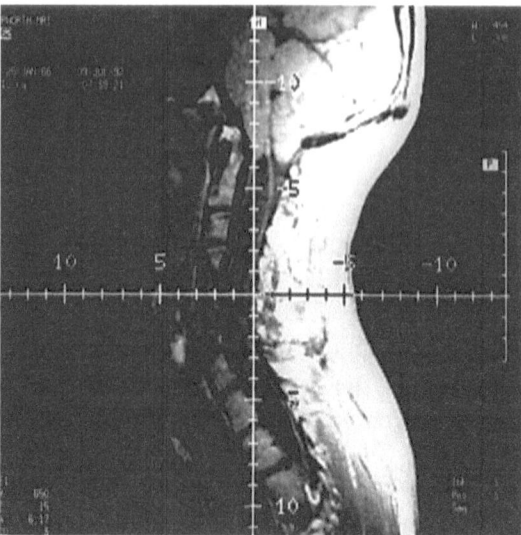

Figure 5.27 (b) Sagittal MR image showing Chiari I malformation with herniation of the tonsil below the level of the foramen magnum into the upper cervical canal. There is a large syrinx in the cervical cord, although it is not clearly defined.

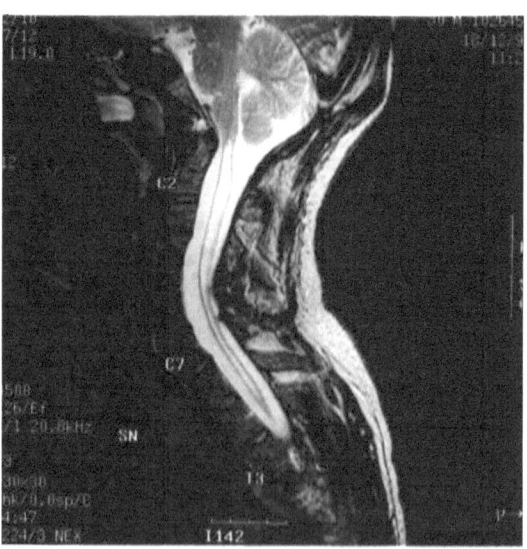

Figure 5.27 (c) Following craniocervical junction decompression, there is more room for the neural structures; however, the syrinx remains. Note the very thin layer of spinal cord (grey signal) with the large fluid collection occupying most of the volume of the cord (white signal).

Figure 5.27 (a-c) Chiari malformation and syringomyelia.

The clinical features are:

- chronic neck and occipital pain often aggravated by coughing or straining,
- cape-like sensory loss over the upper trunk,
- burning dysaesthesia in the extremities and in advanced cases with a loss of pain and temperature sensation and sparing light touch and joint position sense (dissociated sensory loss),
- neuropathic (Charcot's) joints and ulcers,
- lower motor neuron hand and arm weakness with muscle wasting,
- long tract signs in advanced cases,
- scoliosis or torticollis.

Non-communicating syringomyelia is an isolated fluid collection in the substance of the spinal cord and may be a delayed complication after complete spinal cord injury (incidence about 3 per cent), or develop adjacent to an intrinsic spinal cord tumour. Symptoms may develop more acutely in the case of posttraumatic syringomyelia, e.g. after coughing. (Figure 5.28, below).

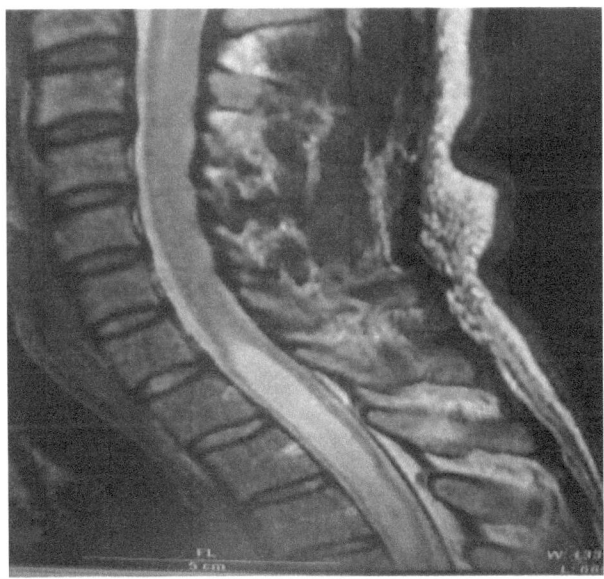

Figure 5.28 Sagittal MR image showing non-communicating syringomyelia with a syrinx in the upper thoracic spinal cord.

CT of the spine is performed in LMIC. Myelography may be difficult to interpret. MR is the preferred imaging modality if available. The treatment of communicating syringomyelia requires craniocervical decompression for a craniocervical junction disorders, and a syrinx to subarachnoid or pleural or peritoneal shunt if the decompression procedure fails to relieve the syrinx. The treatment of non-communicating syringomyelia may also require a shunting procedure. These operations require neurosurgical expertise.

Space occupying lesions and tumours

SPACE OCCUPYING LESIONS

J.V. Rosenfeld & J.K.A. Clezy

Space occupying lesions (SOL) (or mass lesions) are a relatively common diagnostic and management problem in LMICs. Whereas the diagnosis is much easier to make with the aid of computed tomography (CT) or magnetic resonance imaging (MRI), the clinician without these facilities must rely heavily on clinical skills to diagnose a SOL.

Clinical presentation

The presentation involves combinations of raised intracranial pressure (ICP) (which includes impaired conscious state), epilepsy and focal neurological signs.

History

Raised intracranial pressure (ICP)

Raised ICP in the older child and adult presents with headache which is often prolonged, generalised, worse in the mornings on awakening, and sometimes unremitting in advanced cases. It tends to progressively worsen over a period of weeks if the lesion remains untreated. There is often nausea and repeated vomiting. Projectile vomiting may occur without warning or underlying nausea.

The clinical features of raised ICP in young children and infants are listed in Table 4.2, page 144.

Epilepsy

The epilepsy may be focal or generalised (grand mal). It is the commencement of the focal seizure that is so important for defining the origin of the seizure activity. The focal epilepsy involves one part of the body and is called Jacksonian (after the famous 19th century English neurologist John Hughlings Jackson) when it commences in one area, e.g. a hand or a foot, then marches up the limb and may become secondarily generalised. Partial seizures of temporal lobe origin (complex partial seizures) may start with an olfactory or visual aura then involve staring and automatic repetitive movements such as lip smacking.

Table 6.1 Causes of space occupying lesions in the brain.

Slow onset
Neoplasms
Brain tumour - primary or secondary
Trauma
Chronic subdural haematoma
Abscess complicating penetrating injury
Infections
Tuberculoma
Brain abscess: secondary to sinus or ear disease, or open fracture
Complications of HIV: toxoplasmosis, non-Hodgkin's lymphoma
Fungal infections: aspergillus, coccidioidomycosis, blastomycosis
Cryptococcoma (cryptococcal abscess): single or multiple lesions
Other parasitic infestations: cysticercosis (Taenia solium), hydatid disease (Echinococcus granulosus), toxocara, sparganosis
Rapid onset
Vascular
Intracerebral haematoma or infarction
Arteriovenous malformation*
Infection
Brain abscess (pyogenic) often secondary to sinusitis or mastoiditis

Note: with arteriovenous malformation rupture causes an acute intracerebral haematoma but a slow onset is also possible if the lesion steals blood from adjacent eloquent brain (esp. the sensori-motor areas).

The onset of epilepsy in adult life is widely believed to be a common presentation of cerebral tumours, but in fact no more than 10 or 15 percent of such cases of epilepsy will be found to have a tumour. The combination of epilepsy and headache is much more sinister.

Headache

Headache alone in an adult, without abnormal neurological findings, will rarely be due to tumour. On the other hand, chronic headache in a child should never be disregarded. Tumour headache is typically worse in the morning, perhaps because of nocturnal hypercarbia. It will be made worse by coughing or straining, but benign headache sometimes also has these features.

Neck stiffness

A history of neck and back stiffness should also be sought before proceeding to general examination. Neck stiffness may be due to cerebellar tonsillar herniation (also possibly due to infection or blood in the subarachnoid space). Neck tilt and stiffness may form part of the presentation of children with posterior fossa tumours.

Case report

A 3-year-old girl was referred from a provincial hospital with a diagnosis of 'atlantoaxial subluxation'. She had in fact been sick for some months, suffering from headache, neck pain, impaired gait and incontinence. On examination she was irritable, and held her neck in a stiff, flexed posture. She was unable to walk and had bilateral papilloedema. A clinical diagnosis of posterior fossa tumour was made and a ventriculogram was planned but not carried out because of X-ray failure. The parents agreed to exploration. First a ventricular drain was inserted via the occipital horn of the lateral ventricle and then the posterior fossa was opened. The dura was tense and the cisterna magna was opened to drain CSF and relieve pressure.

Case report *(Continued)*

A cerebellar tumour was found in the left hemisphere and was debulked. There was no cystic component. Histology later showed an astrocytoma. The child made an excellent postoperative recovery. The child regained the ability to walk and began to behave normally.

Note: *Cerebellar hemisphere astrocytomas may have an excellent prognosis particularly if there is a cyst with a mural nodule and the nodule is removed. This makes exploration of the posterior fossa well worthwhile and once the cerebellum is decompressed only 10 percent of children will need permanent shunting.*

Other symptoms

Even educated patients may be quite unaware of quite gross loss of visual acuity, unilateral deafness, and mild degrees of limb weakness, although diplopia is usually mentioned when present. Subtle mental changes, as seen in some frontal lobe tumours, may be remarked upon by relatives, but the patient will be unaware of them. Acromegalic patients may come complaining of joint pains or nasal mucous discharge, being unaware of the slow skeletal and soft tissue changes developing in them.

Examination

The intracranial localisation of focal neurological signs is described in Chapter 2, page 42. An assessment of cranial nerve function including olfaction and vision, sensorimotor function, cerebellar function including balance and gait, higher mental function and endocrine disturbance are all necessary. Don't forget to examine the ears, nose, throat and scalp. Impaired conscious state may be due non-specifically to raised ICP or to direct involvement or distortion of the deep cerebral structures or the brain stem. It may vary from lethargy and drowsiness to coma, with unilateral or bilateral third nerve palsies, indicative of coning.

Mental state

Examination should commence with assessment of the mental state by whatever parameters are appropriate. The common tests of memory, numeracy and spatial discrimination used in the West will be unsuitable in most cases. Examiners must devise their own tests, perhaps using local historical and current events and activities of political figures to assess memory and alertness, and sham buying and selling with local currency to assess numeracy. (See the section on Mental Status Examination in Chapter 2, page 19).

Cranial nerves

The cranial nerves can be tested in a couple of minutes, with practice. Patients with chronic raised ICP may have unilateral or bilateral sixth nerve palsy, of no localising value, which is due to stretching of the sixth nerve as a result of brain stem displacement. Less commonly the tumour directly affects the sixth nerve. Other cranial nerve palsies may be of diagnostic help. If the patient is fully alert, examination of the visual fields by confrontation is usually quite accurate, although a perimeter is essential for serial records (as in the follow-up of pituitary tumour surgery).

Optic fundi

There are many causes of headache, and many causes of vomiting. If the optic fundi are not inspected as part of general medical examination, the vital sign of papilloedema will be missed, and intracranial masses will go undiagnosed. Papilloedema is a cardinal sign of raised ICP and will be missed if the fundi are not examined with an ophthalmoscope (see page 25). Papilloedema will not usually be present before the fusion of the cranial sutures (below the age of 2 years). Consecutive optic atrophy occurs following longstanding papilloedema, when there has been permanent loss of axons in the optic nerve head. The disc appears white with a crisp margin. **Foster-Kennedy syndrome** is optic atrophy on one side, and occurs when there is a compressive lesion directly on one optic nerve (classically an inner sphenoidal wing meningioma), and raised ICP causing papilloedema on the other side.

The skull

The skull itself should be examined: are there signs of acromegaly; is there the tell-tale unilateral exophthalmos and expansion of the temporal fossa seen in some sphenoidal ridge meningiomas; or bossing of the calvarium over an underlying meningioma? Sometimes these findings are quite subtle.

Motor and sensory system

Posture and gait may have already been observed informally, but these findings should always be reviewed and recorded. The motor system is then assessed with regard to tone, power, reflexes and coordination. Examination of the sensory system then follows, with particular attention being paid to light touch and its localisation.

General examination

In view of the frequency of otogenic abscess, the tympanic membranes must always be inspected. Examination of the skin occasionally provides findings suggestive of one or other uncommon neurocutaneous syndromes such a neurofibromatosis. Finally, in view of the fact that intracranial metastases occur, all systems of the body need review.

How to determine the cause

The epidemiology and known disease patterns in the geographic region are clearly relevant in determining the cause of the SOL. Tuberculoma is the commonest cause of SOL in endemic regions, particularly if there are multiple lesions. However, our experience in the South Pacific is that brain tumours are still the commonest cause despite the prevalence of tropical infections. Brain abscesses (pyogenic) are often secondary to sinusitis or mastoiditis. The history and examination should point to sinus or mastoid infection and there may be changes on plain X-rays. Orbital cellulitis (page 357) may be present if the patient has fronto-ethmoiditis. Enlargement of the abscess or increasing brain oedema may cause rapid deterioration.

Table 6.1 on page 291 shows the common causes of SOL in the tropics. Posterior fossa tumours in children present with headache and ataxia, often slowly progressive over many months. Tilting of the head is due to differential stretching of the dura with cerebellar tonsillar herniation, but is not a certain lateralising sign. An astrocytoma in the cerebellar hemisphere may produce clear ipsilateral cerebellar signs, but in the vermis it may not be clinically distinguishable from ependymoma or medulloblastoma. These latter two tumours usually have a shorter history, and nystagmus will be gross and bilateral. If the brainstem or basal cisterns may be involved and there may be lower cranial nerve palsies, which may be partial and subtle, as well as long tract signs. In both children and adults, consideration of the length and evolution of the history and the examination findings will often allow the site of the lesion to be diagnosed with some accuracy. Even so, proof of this is essential before any operation is undertaken.

Investigations (Table 6.2)

Plain skull X-rays are well worthwhile. Pineal calcification, so helpful in the West, is usually absent, but there may be the copper beating and posterior clinoid erosion of chronic raised ICP. In meningioma there may be prominent vascular markings, or hyperostosis related to the underlying tumour. In oligodendroglioma, craniopharyngioma and occasionally in tuberculoma, there will be calcification. Most pituitary tumours will have gross enlargement of the sella, and the changes of acromegaly will often be striking. In suspected eighth nerve tumour a good basal view of the skull will demonstrate widening of the internal auditory meatus. In children and young people there will be spreading of sutures, with thinning of the occipital bone in many posterior fossa tumours. Finally, evidence of chronic middle ear sepsis will often be visible, and will raise the question of brain abscess.

Table 6.2 Investigations for the suspected space occupying lesion.

---

1. Skull X-ray (SXR): look for skull erosion, or hyperostosis, intracranial calcification, copper beating, pineal shift, the shape of the pituitary fossa, the density of the dorsum sellae, the aeration of the sinuses and the mastoid air cells.

2. Ultrasound in the infant whose fontanelles are not yet closed (Figure 2.15, page 50)

Table 6.2 *(Continued)*

3. CT or MRI scan if available
4. Pneumoencephalogram / ventriculography in the absence of CT
5. Cerebral angiogram in the absence of CT
6. Mantoux
7. Cryptococcal antibodies
8. General medical investigations including full blood examination, blood film for malaria parasites or trypanosomes, erythrocyte sedimentation rate (ESR), electrolytes, chest X-ray and HIV serology.

Lumbar puncture should never be done in a patient with a suspected intracranial tumour. The absence of papilloedema by no means makes it safe, and patients with normal fundi have coned on the point of the needle.

Practice point

Do not perform a lumbar puncture if there are signs of raised ICP, particularly papilloedema, because the setting up of a differential pressure between the head and spine may induce coning which may be fatal. If a patient is coning following a lumbar puncture, the rapid insertion of a ventricular drain may reverse the process.

If otogenic brain abscess is ruled out clinically, and there is nothing to point to a meningioma, pituitary tumour or craniopharyngioma, the next question is: has this patient a tuberculoma? If CT facilities are available, and the radiologist is familiar with its appearances, a tuberculoma ought to be more confidently diagnosed. Otherwise, in patients without critically raised, ICP our practice has been to perform a Mantoux test, and immediately commence standard therapy for tuberculosis while awaiting the result, which will usually be strongly positive. This trial of treatment must never include steroids, which will reduce the ICP regardless of the correct diagnosis, and therefore only cause confusion. Careful re-examination of cases of tuberculoma on treatment will almost always show convincing evidence of improvement over the course of 3 weeks, except in some rare instances where liquefaction of the lesion has occurred. Such cases may require localisation and excision of the tuberculoma as an emergency. In practice, only a small minority of tuberculomas are removed, and then only because improvement on a trial of treatment is minimal or doubtful.

If abscess, tuberculoma and acromegaly have been effectively ruled out, the next step is to localise the lesion radiologically. For much of his career Dr Harvey Cushing, the father of modern neurosurgery, operated on the basis of the history and the neurological signs, but even he occasionally opened the wrong side of the head. Dr Walter Dandy introduced air ventriculography, having already noted and published a paper on the diagnostic value of air under the diaphragm seen on X-rays of cases of perforated peptic ulcer. Where CT facilities do not exist, air or contrast ventriculography will usually be the investigation of choice (see example in Figure 6.1, next page. Properly performed under local anaesthesia, ventriculography is a very safe procedure, and is described separately (Chapter 2, page 53). An anatomical diagnosis having been made; craniotomy should be performed forthwith.

For supratentorial lesions, carotid angiography can still be a valuable procedure. Although some may perform direct puncture angiograms under local anaesthesia, the neurosurgeon performing this investigation will usually prefer a general anaesthetic. If direct puncture fails, a cutdown is entirely justifiable.

Meningiomas have a characteristic tumour blush in late films, and high-grade gliomas have a plethora of irregular small vessels visible. Tuberculomas and abscesses will show no more than displacement of normal vasculature around the mass, which appears as something of a black hole, but even slow-growing tumours should show some pathological vessels. These may be sparse except on films of high quality. The differential diagnosis includes many other neurological problems, which may cause some of the same signs and symptoms. The following should be considered:

1. Basal meningitis - especially TB (see Chapter 7, page 350)
2. Communicating hydrocephalus (see Chapter 4, page 158)
3. Pseudotumour cerebri (benign intracranial hypertension) (see Chapter 9, page 464)
4. Encephalitis (see Chapter 7, page 363)
5. Cerebral malaria (see Chapter 7, page 348)
6. Sickle cell crisis (see Chapter 8, page 424)

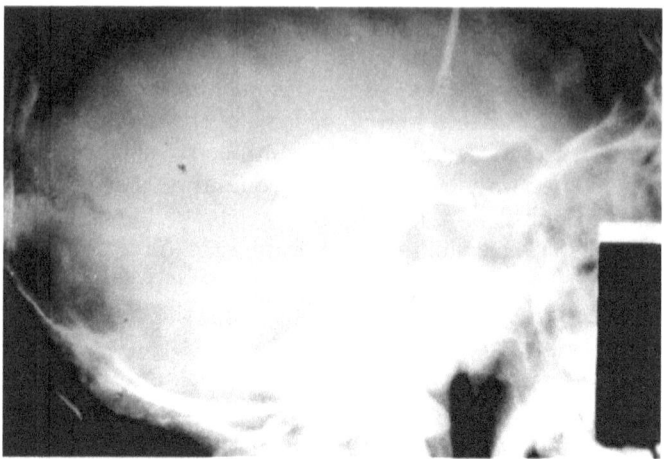

Figure 6.1 Contrast ventriculogram showing ventricular catheter passing down to third ventricle with contrast in the third ventricle and then contrast entering the aqueduct and fourth ventricle, but the fourth ventricle is compressed forwards by a posterior fossa mass and is the thin linear strip of contrast in the posterior fossa.

Management of the space occupying lesion

In the absence of definitive investigations, you need to have some idea of your local patterns of pathology, in particular which infections listed above are common and may cause space occupying lesions. You need to determine the speed of onset of symptoms and consider seriously a diagnosis of chronic subdural haematoma which is potentially curable by surgical evacuation. A history of trauma may not always be given, particularly if it is some weeks since the injury or if the patient was drunk, is an alcoholic or elderly. A cerebral angiogram in the A-P projection is useful to diagnose a chronic subdural haematoma if CT is unavailable. The cortical vessels are displaced away from the inner table of the skull and there is medial displacement of the main branches.

Practice point

Always consider the possibility of chronic subdural haematoma. The prognosis is excellent if it is evacuated early.

Without CT, you may not know whether the lesion is single or multiple. Multiple lesions would suggest tuberculosis, cryptococcosis or metastases. If you are missing metastases by treating blindly for tuberculoma it will probably not affect the outcome much. But you want to avoid treating a chronic subdural haematoma as a tuberculoma.

Case report

A 60-year-old man presented to the physicians with headache and a deteriorating conscious level over a few days. He had slightly unequal pupils but no papilloedema. There was no neck stiffness and he had no focal neurological signs. His malaria slide was negative, his blood glucose was normal and he had a clear lumbar puncture. Skull X-rays were normal. On further questioning he had been involved in a motor vehicle accident 2 months previously. In the absence of other diagnostic facilities, the family were consulted and it was agreed to perform diagnostic burr holes. A large chronic subdural haematoma was evacuated and the patient made an uneventful recovery.

Slow onset pathology

If chronic subdural haematoma is excluded and the exact cause of the SOL is not apparent because CT scanning or angiography is not available the patient should be initially treated with anti-TB chemotherapy. Failure to improve within 2-3 weeks is an indication to begin steroid therapy (dexamethasone) on the assumption the patient has a neoplasm. Empirical treatment for cryptococcosis (amphotericin B and flucytosine, Chapter 7, page 367) should only be given if cryptococcal antibody titres in the CSF are high (CSF 1:8 dilution). If lumbar puncture is contraindicated cryptococcal titres in the serum can be used. Cryptococcosis can cause bilateral blindness. Unilateral blindness suggests some other cause. If cysticercosis is endemic, and the X-rays are suggestive, a course of albendazole and/or praziquantel should be tried.[49]

---

[49]*Diagnosis and Treatment of Neurocysticercosis: 2017 Clinical Practice Guidelines by the Infectious Diseases Society of America (IDSA) and the American Society of Tropical Medicine and Hygiene (ASTMH). 2018;98(4):945–966.*

The diagnosis and treatment of neurocysticercosis depends on whether there is evidence of elevated ICP. In patients with untreated hydrocephalus or diffuse cerebral edema, clinical practice guidelines recommend management of elevated intracranial pressure alone and not antiparasitic treatment. The management of patients with diffuse cerebral edema should be anti-inflammatory therapy such as corticosteroids, whereas hydrocephalus usually requires a surgical approach. In the absence of elevated intracranial pressure, we recommend the use of antiparasitic drugs. For example, albendazole (15 mg/kg/day) combined with praziquantel (50 mg/kg/day) for 10–14 days rather than albendazole monotherapy for patients with more than two viable parenchymal cysticerci. Ventriculography (Chapter 2, page 53) may define the position and extent of a lesion. Consider burr hole aspiration and/or biopsy of the suspected pathology or full craniotomy, particularly if the lesion is close to the surface and if the general surgeon has had some neurosurgical experience. Some tumours are cystic and relatively benign and the patient may do well with a cyst decompression. The use of steroids should be delayed until the antibiotics have had a chance to act otherwise it becomes confusing to assess which drug is working. Steroids will significantly reduce oedema around a tumour, abscess or tuberculoma, but beware of using steroid alone if infection is still a possibility, because the infection may advance further due to the immunosuppressive effect of the steroid.

Rapid onset pathology

If infective, treat as bacterial meningitis or cerebral malaria. The patient is likely to have impaired consciousness and, in the absence of papilloedema, a lumbar puncture is indicated to exclude meningitis and subarachnoid haemorrhage. If haemorrhagic usually manage conservatively in the tropical countries. CT Angiogram, if available, may show the cause. A suspected deep-seated brain abscess can be treated by burr hole and aspiration. An abscess associated with frontoethmoid sinusitis requires frontoethmoidectomy and drainage of the subdural or brain abscess. Mastoidectomy with additional temporal and occipital burr holes to aspirate the temporal lobe and cerebellum may be indicated for brain abscess complicating mastoiditis (See Chapter 11, page 600).

Chapter Six

INTRACRANIAL TUMOURS

J.K.A. Clezy & J. V. Rosenfeld

Intracranial tumours occurring in LMICs tend to present late, with headache (typically unrelenting, worse in the morning and getting progressively worse), vomiting (often without nausea), and papilloedema. The incidence of the various intracranial masses differs from that seen in the developed countries.

Abscess and tuberculoma are so common in the tropics that they need to be considered in every case of presumed intracranial tumour. In adults, two-thirds of tumours are supratentorial, whereas in children approximately half are infratentorial. Although the incurability of many intracranial tumours casts a gloom over neurosurgical endeavour, some lesions such as meningiomas, pituitary tumours, schwannomas and some low-grade gliomas, are well worth removing. Unfortunately, many tumours present late with the tumour having grown to a large size making resection more challenging, or in some patients, impossible.

The aim of management is to prolong useful life, any surgery ought to avoid making the patient worse. There is little to be gained by excising a large eloquent area of the brain, leaving the patient hemiplegic and aphasic. Similarly, there is little point in performing any other procedure that has no chance of doing any good, except in the occasional case where the patient or his family insists on a tissue diagnosis, when burr hole biopsy may be justified. The occasional neurosurgeon will need truly expert anaesthesia, and should make sure that cerebral oedema is minimised by the use of mannitol and/or steroids, the latter given for at least 24 hours before the operation. Dexamethasone 8mg b.d. or prednisolone 25 mg t.d.s. may be used. The operating microscope is standard equipment in modern neurosurgical theatres, but the generalist performing occasional neurosurgery is unlikely to be skilled in its use, even if he has access to such instrumentation. Much useful work can still be done with the naked eye and good illumination.

Classification of intracranial tumours

The detailed World Health Organization classification of intracranial mass lesions is abbreviated in Table 6.3 (below) to cover the great majority of tumours.

Table 6.3 Classification of intracranial tumours (adapted from WHO).

---

1. **Tumours of neuroepithelial tissue**

    - Astrocytoma (various grades, grade I being the least aggressive)

    - Oligodendroglioma

    - Ependymoma

    - Medulloblastoma

2. **Tumours of nerve sheath cells**

    - Schwannoma (eighth nerve, rarely fifth nerve)

3. **Meningeal tumours**

    - Meningioma

4. **Anterior pituitary tumours**

    - Functional

    - Non-functional (null cell)

5. **Tumour-like lesions**

    - Craniopharyngioma

6. **Pineal region tumours**

7. **Metastatic tumours (lung, breast, colon, melanoma, many others)**

Tumours of neuroepithelial tissue

Astrocytoma (20-30 percent of intracranial tumours)

In the West, the commonest single brain tumour is the highly malignant **glioblastoma multiforme** (about 50 percent of astrocytomas), a rapidly growing, anaplastic and highly cellular astrocytoma with areas of haemorrhage and necrosis (see Figure 6.2 (a), page 306). It tends to be a tumour of later life, typically occurring after the age of 50, and this may account for it being rather uncommon in the tropics, where better differentiated astrocytomas are more usual. Even with aggressive surgical excision and radiotherapy survival is usually 6-12 months. Some patients live up to 2 years and there are rare survivors beyond this. Aggressive surgical excision, chemotherapy, radiotherapy and immunotherapy are improving survival but unfortunately these options are not readily accessible in the developing countries. Astrocytomas occur in the cerebral hemispheres, merging imperceptibly with normal brain tissue (see Figure 6.2 (b), page 307). Well-differentiated (grade 1 and 2) astrocytomas are firm and pale and some are cystic with a mural nodule (ie the nodule is in the cyst wall). Wide excision of grade 1 and 2 lesions may allow good survival for many years.

The **anaplastic astrocytoma** are grade 3 on a four-tiered scale, do not have histological evidence of necrosis, but have a poorer prognosis than grade 1 and 2 tumours. Astrocytomas tend to recur as higher-grade lesions, with rapid deterioration towards the end. In adults' higher grade astrocytomas are rarely curable. Astrocytomas usually present with symptoms of raised intracranial pressure (ICP), often with little in the way of obvious localising signs.

Epilepsy sometimes occurs, and may or may not have localising features. Careful examination may reveal mild motor signs, or visual field defects in tumours involving the temporal, parietal or occipital lobes. Tumours in the frontal lobe may present with vague personality changes or apathy. Any patient with signs of raised ICP and apparent mental changes may be assumed to have a frontal lesion unless there are clear signs indicating another area of the brain.

Case report

A 35-year-old public servant, was brought to hospital because he had had a seizure. He could not say why he had come, and denied symptoms until questioned directly, when he admitted headache of uncertain duration. His wife stated that this had been present for 2 months. His performance at work was said to have deteriorated, and he had been increasingly irritable with her and with the children. On examination he was lying curled up in bed, and co-operated poorly. He would answer questions, but could not describe his work. He could name a wristwatch, and its band, but not the hands or the winder. His neck was slightly stiff.

His pupils were equal and reactive. Bilateral papilloedema was present. Visual field examination was unsatisfactory, but was thought to be normal. There was a mild right spastic hemiparesis, more obvious in the face and hand than in the leg. Gait was unsteady, of no particular type, and he required assistance. Examination of the eardrums was normal.

Skull X-ray was normal, apart from doubtful thinning of the posterior clinoid processes. The Mantoux test was negative. Ventriculography, performed through biparietal burr holes, showed a large left mid-frontal mass, with midline shift.

Left frontal craniotomy revealed a tight brain with flattened sulci, and yellowish discoloration of the cortex. Incision of the brain exposed a soft partly cystic mass, which was macroscopically excised, together with the frontal pole. He was temporarily aphasic, and the hemiparesis was worse for a few days, but he left hospital well, on phenytoin 300 mg daily in a single dose.

The pathology report described the lesion as an astrocytoma grade II. The man returned with regrowth of the tumour 7 months later, complaining of recurrent headache. He obtained some palliation from oral steroids (prednisolone 75 mg daily) and was able to go home, dying a few weeks later.

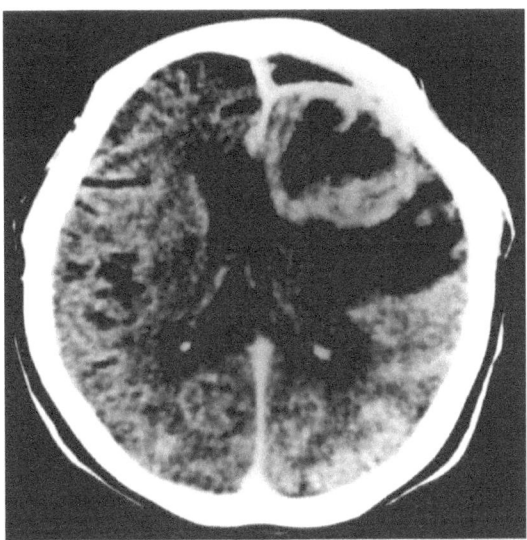

Figure 6.2 (a) i CT scan with contrast showing a large irregular rounded tumour in the right frontal region, with a thick enhancing rim and a low-density centre, representing tumour necrosis. The low-density periphery around the enhancement is oedema. Note the compression of the ventricular system.

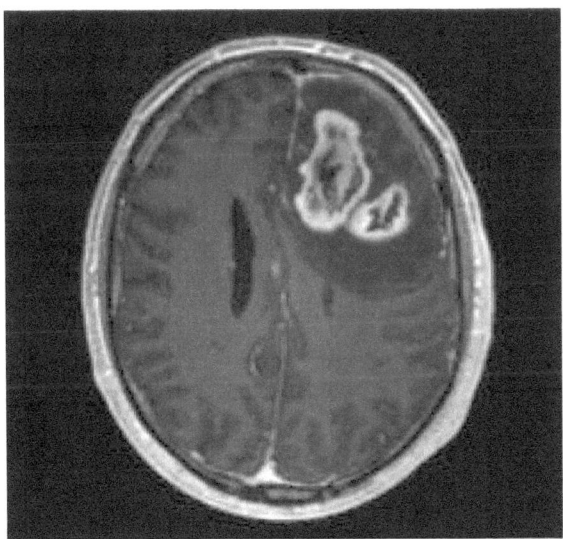

(a) ii MRI scan with contrast showing a left frontal glioblastoma with surrounding oedema. There is clearer definition of the tumour on MRI compared with CT scan.

Space occupying lesions and tumours

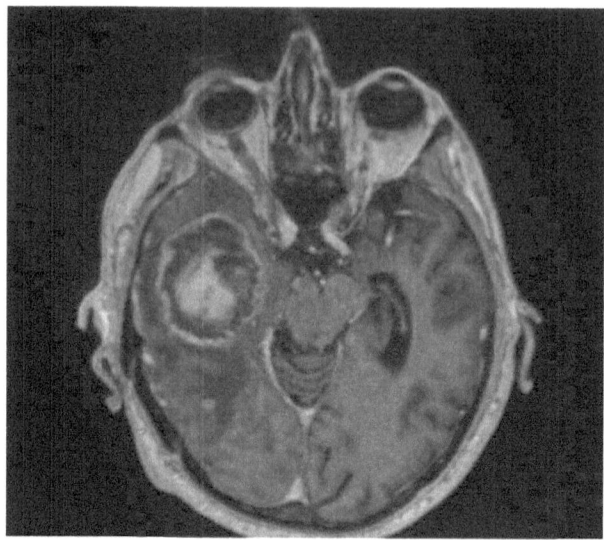

(a) iii MRI scan showing a right temporal glioblastoma with surrounding oedema. Note the uncal herniation with compression of the midbrain.

(a) i-iii Glioblastoma multiforme.

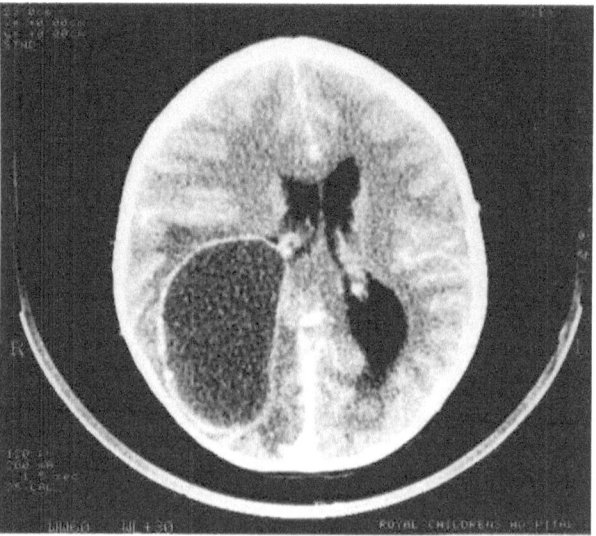

(b) CT scan showing a low-grade astrocytoma of the right cerebral hemisphere in a child presenting with headaches, vomiting and poor vision. The tumour consists of a thin rim of enhancing tissue with a low-density cystic centre.

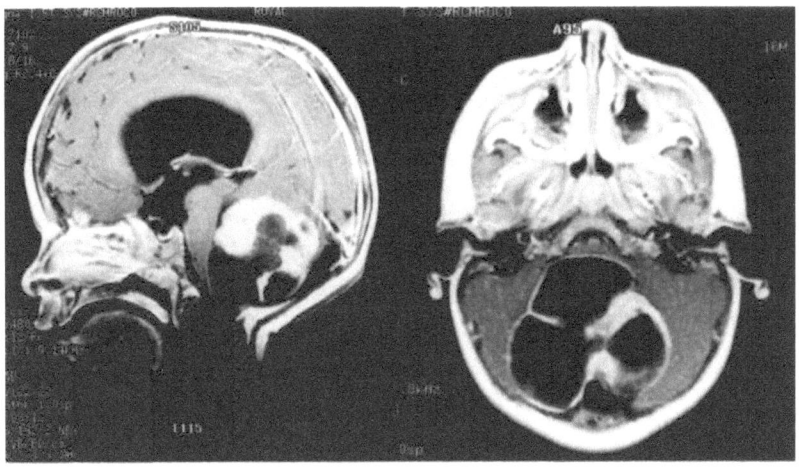

(c) i   **(c) ii**

(c) i-ii Cerebellar astrocytoma. Low grade. This large cystic and solid tumour is seen on MR scan, in axial and sagittal images and was excised completely.

Figure 6.2 (a-c) Astrocytoma.

In children, astrocytomas most often occur in the cerebellar hemispheres or in the brain stem. **Cerebellar astrocytomas** present with headache, vomiting, ataxia and head tilt, with some neck stiffness. Limb ataxia may be quite gross on the affected side. These tumours may be largely cystic, with a small solid component which has a particular benign histological character called pilocytic because the elongated astrocytes are packed in parallel and resemble hairs. The patient is often cured if this **mural nodule** of tumour is resected completely. The solid cerebellar astrocytomas of children are usually more aggressive but the children do well following excision (Figure 6.2 (c), above and Figure 6.3, page 310). **Brain stem astrocytomas** of childhood are usually malignant, are surgically inaccessible, and produce a confusing mixture of bilateral multiple cranial nerve palsies (often incomplete) and long tract signs, often of rapid onset over a few days to weeks. Hydrocephalus does not usually occur until late. Radiotherapy in children more than 2-3 years of age offers some palliation but progressive deterioration and death usually occurs within a few months. **Optic chiasm/hypothalamic gliomas** cause progressive visual loss in children, often indicate a central form of neurofibromatosis, and behave in a very indolent manner compatible with long term survival.

Oligodendroglioma

Oligodendroglioma (10 percent of the intracranial tumours) seems to be commoner in the tropics than in the West. It is usually a slow growing well circumscribed tumour of adulthood. Focal epilepsy is more common than in other gliomas. This may occur long before headache is much of a problem. It is a cellular tumour, with darkly staining nuclei and clear cytoplasm. Fine calcification is common and may be seen on the plain skull radiograph. If wide excision is possible, long survival may be achieved, but usually this tumour eventually recurs as a high-grade astrocytoma.

Ependymoma

Ependymoma seems to be rarer in the tropics than elsewhere, but this may reflect diagnostic failure. It is largely a tumour of children, arising most commonly in the floor of the fourth ventricle, which it usually infiltrates, causing early obstruction to CSF flow, with signs of raised ICP more obvious than those of cerebellar dysfunction. Ataxia affects the trunk more obviously than the limbs. The mass ranges from quite pale to red in colour, and looks rather like coral, but is soft and vascular. Perivascular rosettes of tumour cells are seen in histological sections. This tumour tends to grow out of the fourth ventricular outlets into the basal cisterns and envelops the lower cranial nerves and the upper cervical cord. In those cases where complete macroscopic removal is possible, the addition of radiotherapy may result in long-term survival. This includes the entire neuraxis (brain and spinal canal), as the ependymoma is notorious for seeding within the CSF spaces. However, there is now a trend to spare the young child's spine from irradiation if there has been a complete excision of the posterior fossa tumour. Ependymomas may also occur in the lateral or third ventricular region.

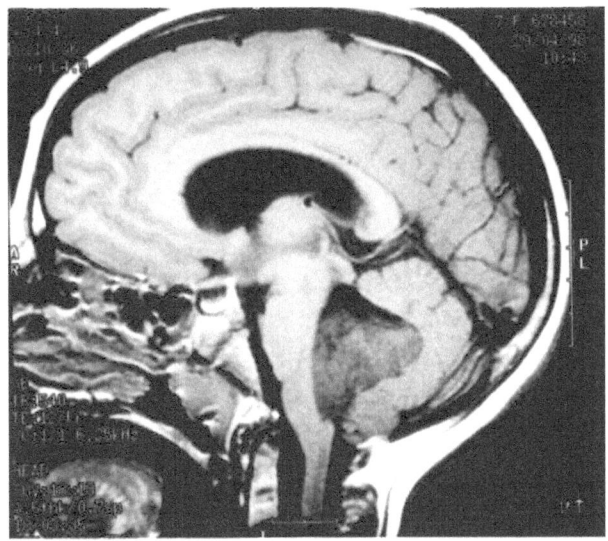

(a)

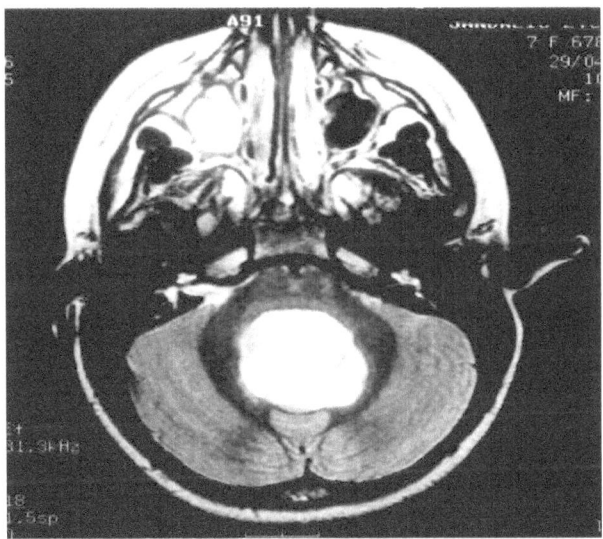

(b)

Figure 6.3 (a-b) MR scan showing a large midline cerebellar vermis tumour filling the fourth ventricle and compressing the brain stem. This is seen well on the sagittal image. The differential diagnosis is medulloblastoma or ependymoma. Both are malignant tumours.

Medulloblastoma

Medulloblastoma is also rarely diagnosed in the tropics, although it makes up a third of posterior fossa tumours seen in paediatric neurosurgical practice elsewhere. It presents much as does the ependymoma but the presenting symptoms are usually of short duration. Almost all arise in the vermis of the cerebellum, where they are soft purplish masses at surgery. Histologically, densely packed sheets of round anaplastic lymphocyte-like cells are seen, forming something like the rosettes of the ependymoma, but without their clear perivascular organisation. They ate highly malignant, regularly seeding throughout the CSF pathways. Surgery alone is of little benefit, but where radiotherapy is available treatment of the entire neuraxis results in many cures. Various chemotherapeutic regimes are providing some additional improvement in long-term results. There is up to 70 to 80 percent 5-year survival but it is around 60% in patients where the pattern of disease indicates a more aggressive tumour (Figure 6.3, previous page). Chemotherapy and radiotherapy are important adjuvant therapies for patients with brain tumours. The most common chemotherapy drugs for brain tumours in adults are:

- temozolamide
- procabazine
- carmustine (BCNU)
- lomustine (CCNU)
- vincristine

Radiotherapy has major effects on the growing brain and spine in young children. Therefore, children less than 3 years old usually have chemotherapy instead of radiotherapy if they have:

- primitive neuroectodermal tumour (PNET)
- ependymoma
- medulloblastoma
- high grade glioma

The most common chemotherapy drugs in children are:

- cyclophosphamide
- vincristine
- cisplatin
- etoposide
- carboplatin
- high dose methotrexate

Once the child is over 3 years old, they can have radiotherapy. However, for some types of brain tumours in children, chemotherapy treatment is very effective and radiotherapy can be avoided. Stereotactic focussed radiotherapy (Radiosurgery) is now available in HIC and provides higher doses of radiotherapy focussed on the tumour. This reduces the dose to the surrounding normal brain.

Tumours of nerve cell sheaths

Schwannoma (10 percent of intracranial tumours)

This is a slow-growing, well-encapsulated yellowish tumour, most commonly eighth nerve, where it originates on the vestibular division within the internal auditory meatus, which it expands at an early stage. The alternative common name for this tumour is the **acoustic neuroma** (Figure 6.4, next page). The first symptom will often be tinnitus, which may be present before the patient notices that he is deaf in one ear. Despite the mass being far lateral in the cerebellopontine angle, limb ataxia may not be obvious to the patient, but falling over while walking in the dark draws attention to truncal ataxia. By the time the patient presents he may have headache, vomiting, papilloedema, widespread unilateral cranial nerve involvement, cerebellar and long tract signs.

Until the advent of the operating microscope, removal of these cerebellopontine angle tumours usually resulted in destruction of the facial nerve, which is stretched over and adherent to the deep surface. In such cases there is always enough fifth nerve damage to cause at least temporary corneal anaesthesia.

Just as in leprosy, the combination of facial paralysis and corneal anaesthesia will result in early and rapid corneal ulceration unless measures are taken to avoid it - lateral tarsorrhaphy and the use of glasses to keep wind and dust out of the eye.

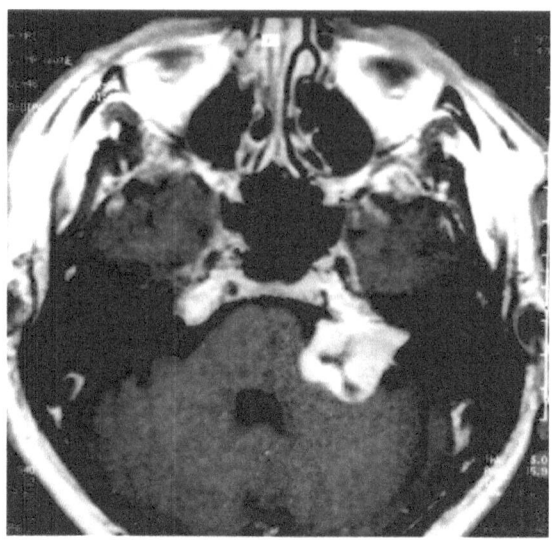

Figure 6.4 MRI scan showing left cerebellopontine angle tumour. Acoustic schwannoma. Note the tumour passing through the internal acoustic meatus into the temporal bone. Note also the distortion of the adjacent brain stem and fourth ventricle.

Case report

A young woman had been unwell for 2 years, and complained of headache, double vision and staggering gait. She denied tinnitus or deafness. She had a stiff neck, normal pupils, gross papilloedema, bilateral sixth nerve palsies and mild nystagmus to the left. Fields were normal to confrontation. Corneal reflexes were absent bilaterally. There was a partial left lower motor neuron facial palsy, and nerve deafness on the left. The palate moved asymmetrically, and the gag reflex was doubtful. She was hoarse. Power, tone and reflexes were (surprisingly) normal in the limbs, apart from a possible right Babinski. There was slight left cerebellar incoordination. Skull X-ray showed gross erosion of the left internal auditory meatus.

An eighth tumour was diagnosed, and with the patient lying in the park bench position a left parietal burr hole was made to allow a 5 Fr feeding tube to be placed in the greatly dilated lateral ventricle, decompressing it.

313

Case report *(Continued)*

A left paramedian exposure of the posterior fossa revealed a large gritty mass extending from above the tentorium to the foramen magnum, and covered by a thin crescent of cerebellar hemisphere. The tumour was gutted and removed with care to avoid pressure on the brainstem or damage to its vessels.

She awoke with complete facial palsy, and inability to swallow, so nasogastric feeding was required. After some days she pulled this out, and discovered that she could swallow if she drank through a straw while lying on her right side. Good swallowing eventually returned. Care of the cornea with eye ointment meant that the intended tarsorrhaphy was not required. Corneal sensation returned.

Gait was poor for several weeks, due to increased cerebellar incoordination, she was eventually able to leave hospital walking with the aid of a stick.

In well-equipped neurosurgery centres where there is a combined otological/neurosurgical approach to acoustic neuromas, there is preservation of the facial nerve in most cases and the preservation of some hearing in the small to medium sized tumours. A large acoustic schwannoma can be sub-totally excised by debulking from the centre of the tumour outward and preserving the capsule to avoid damaging the cranial nerves and brainstem. This technique is suitable for the non-neurosurgeon and may give years of palliation. Although this schwannoma is a tumour of later life, some patients with von Recklinghausen's neurofibromatosis develop eighth nerve tumours at an early age, and these are frequently bilateral. Signs of von Recklinghausen's disease may be minimal.

Schwannomas also occur on the fifth nerve, but these are very uncommon. Neurofibromatosis type 1 (NF-1) (von Recklinghausen's disease) is due to an autosomal dominant mutation crossing all racial, ethnic and national boundaries. It is one of the most common mutations in humans and has a prevalence of about 1 in 3000. The gene is located on chromosome 17. NF-2 is also known as bilateral acoustic neurofibro-matosis, has a prevalence of less than 1 in 50 000, and the responsible gene is located on chromosome 22 with loss of a tumour suppressor gene being the main problem. Spinal schwannomas represent about 30 percent of extramedullary, intradural tumours of the spinal cord. Sometimes they present with acute spinal cord compression. They affect the dorsal roots and may sometimes have a dumb-bell shape, with an intradural and extradural component. The latter may extend through the intradural foramen and enlarge in the paraspinal tissues.

Case report

A 23-year-old woman with neurofibromatosis presented with a 6-month history of progressive lower limb weakness and anterior thigh pain. On examination she had multiple cutaneous neurofibromas and café-au-lait spots. She had bilateral upgoing plantar reflexes and the knee jerk (but not the ankle) was hyperreflexic. A chest X- ray revealed a 3 cm paraspinal mass on the right and left side at T6 and spinal X-rays showed a loss of the interpedicular distance (T4-6), loss of the T6 pedicle and enlargement of the TS/6 intervertebral foramen. A myelogram showed a complete block at T6. Soon after admission she developed complete paraplegia and incontinence of urine. Dexamethasone was given and an emergency laminectomy was performed.

An extramedullary neurofibroma was cleared from the spinal canal and a thoracotomy was required to excise the paraspinal component. She made a complete neurological recovery.

Lesson*: Rapid deterioration or acute onset paraplegia is a surgical emergency. Patients with neurofibromatosis may have schwannomas of the dorsal roots.*

Tumours of the meninges

Meningioma (20-30 percent of intracranial tumours) (Figure 6.5, next page). This slow-growing tumour is almost always histologically benign, and therefore in theory ought to be curable, but if there is any spread into the adjacent venous sinuses or the cavernous sinus, recurrence will occur, and a late recurrence may also result from a field change in the adjacent dura. Meningiomas arise from the arachnoid layer. Some 90 per cent of them are supratentorial, 20 per cent are parasagittal, about 20 per cent occur over the convexity, and another 20 per cent (or more) occur in relation to the sphenoidal wing.

315

Less common are tumours in the olfactory groove on the floor of the anterior fossa (where they may be bilateral), or in the suprasellar region. Occasionally they are found in the cerebellopontine angle, on the tentorium, or attached to the dura near the foramen magnum. Some 5-9 percent of meningiomas are multiple and this figure increases following cranial irradiation. Rarely, meningiomas occur directly beneath the scars of old scalp wounds, and there has long been a belief, often challenged, that at least some of these tumours are post-traumatic in origin. Meningiomas are very uncommon in children. Great vascularity and involvement of venous sinuses (which it often invades) or cavernous sinus and internal carotid artery provide a surgical challenge.

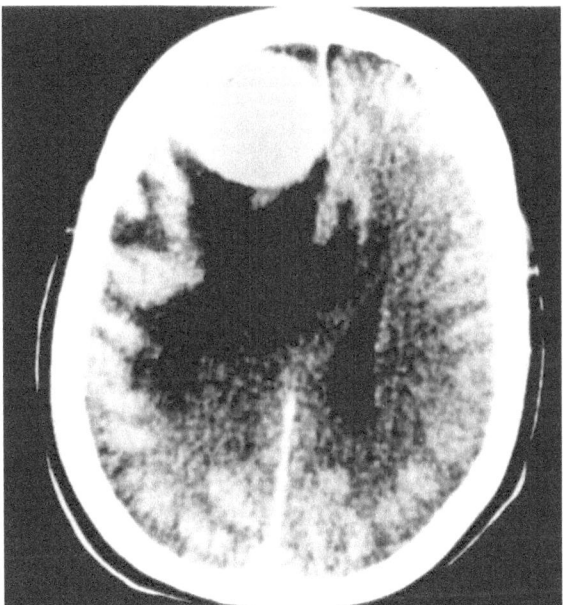

Figure 6.5 (a) CT scan showing large round right frontal meningioma with gross surrounding oedema, and ventricular compression. The lesion enhances vividly.

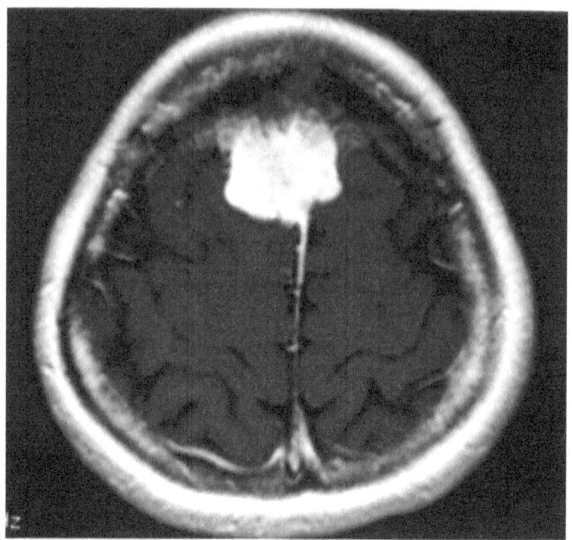

(b) i

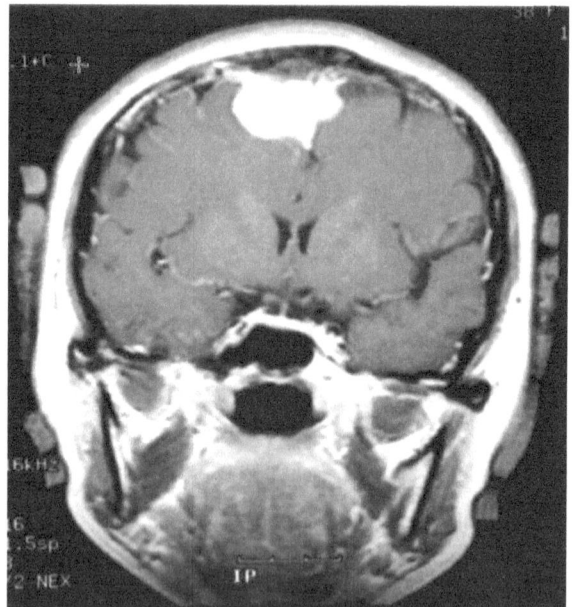

(b) ii

(b) i-ii MR scan showing midline parasagittal meningioma near the vertex involving the sagittal sinus and displacing the posterior frontal lobe on each side (right greater than left). This lesion was excised completely. The obstructed sagittal sinus was demonstrated on preoperative MR venography.

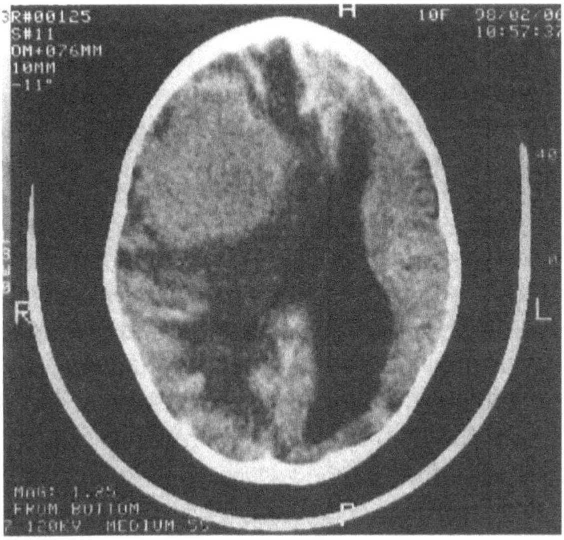

(c) Presumed large right frontal meningioma with gross surrounding oedema and ventricular compression. The large base of the tumour along the convexity of the skull is in favour of meningioma, i.e. an extrinsic brain tumour as opposed to a purely intrinsic tumour. The CT is not completely reliable for making this distinction but MR is more accurate.

Figure 6.5 (a-c) Meningioma.

Meningiomas present with headache and/or epilepsy, which is frequently focal. They are usually quite large by the time they are diagnosed, and local pressure effects will be found on careful examination, allowing fairly exact clinical localisation in many cases. There is often a skull hyperostosis which is palpable overlying the tumour and an enostosis at the central origin of the tumour, both of which may be seen on a skull radiograph. These tumours are pale pink, with a finely nodular surface, a fleshy consistency with fibrous septae and are clearly demarcated from the surrounding brain, which is pushed aside and deformed by the rumour. The degree of cellularity varies, with the characteristic concentric calcified psammoma bodies being seen in many cases. They attach to the dura, and frequently invade the adjacent bone. The major blood supply is from meningeal vessels, whose large size produces correspondingly obvious markings on skull radiographs.

Case report

An elderly man was brought to hospital having had a fit the previous day. He denied previous symptoms, but had had headache since the fit. On examination the only abnormality was spastic weakness of the right leg, with obvious foot drop. Relatives now stated that there had been some difficulty with gait for weeks or months. Skull X-ray showed dense sclerosis in the left parasagittal area in front of the motor strip, with a large middle meningeal groove in the bone. Left carotid angiogram revealed the characteristic tumour blush of a meningioma. The superior sagittal sinus could not be seen clearly at this point, but the films were less than perfect. After receiving dexamethasone 8mg b.d. for 2 days the patient was taken to theatre and craniotomy was performed, which exposed a small meningioma adherent to dura, which was opened leaving a 2 cm piece of dura attached to the tumour.

The tumour was gutted with diathermy and removed completely with the adjacent dura, except for a tiny sliver of tumour along the sagittal sinus, which did not seem to be invaded. This area was thoroughly diathermied and then covered with a little patch of pericranium. The dural defect was repaired with temporalis fascia and the craniotomy closed. After a week the foot drop was recovering, and the patient was discharged on phenytoin 300 mg daily.

Meningiomas ought always be removed, as completely as possible. Cerebral oedema can be a serious problem, either immediately following the ventriculogram or angiogram, or postoperatively. Steroid use is particularly important, and the operation itself must be carried out with the absolute minimum of brain retraction. Ideally, the tumour is gutted with the diathermy and allowed to fall away from the surrounding brain. Convexity and some other tumours may be removed completely, but those invading the sagittal sinus, surrounding the carotid bifurcation or invading the greater wing of the sphenoid rarely can be, and will therefore inevitably recur. Reoperation after some years is well worth while, and is not necessarily more difficult than the original procedure.

Pituitary tumours

Pituitary tumours comprise about 5-10 percent of brain tumours and may cause debilitating and eventually fatal endocrinopathies and blindness if untreated. Young adults are most commonly affected. The general surgeon, if capable of performing a craniotomy, may prevent blindness and other disability in those with pituitary tumours. If the general surgeon cannot do the procedure an attempt should be made to refer the patient. Most prolactinomas can be managed with medication alone (see below). There is often a delay in diagnosis of pituitary tumours because the patient does not recognise that vision is being lost, or that the body shape is changing, or in the case of the non-secretory type of tumour, the patient and doctor may not notice the subtle signs of hypopituitarism. All these patients should be managed in association with the physicians.

Anatomy of the pituitary fossa

The pituitary gland is a round 7-10 mm diameter structure attached to the hypothalamus by a pituitary stalk. It resides in the sella turcica surrounded by sella dura and a variable subarachnoid space antero- superiorly. It is covered over to a variable degree by a shelf of dura called the diaphragma sellae.

Relations (see Figure 2.3, page 10)

- Superior: diaphragma, optic chiasm, hypothalamus, third ventricle.
- Inferior - sphenoid sinus.
- Posterior: dorsum sellae, clivus, prepontine cistern, basilar artery, brainstem.
- Lateral: cavernous sinus, carotid artery, cranial nerves- 3, 4, 6.

The adenohypophysis (anterior pituitary)

Secretes thyroid secreting hormone (TSH), adrenocorticotrophic hormone (ACTH), prolactin, human growth hormone (HGH).

The neurohypophysis (posterior pituitary)

Secretes antidiuretic hormone (ADH) (the hormone directing concentration of urine in the distal tubule of the kidney), and oxytocin (the hormone of the lactation reflex).

Basic physiology

Control of anterior pituitary hormones is by the secretion of releasing hormones from the hypothalamus. They reach the pituitary via the hypothalamo-pituitary portal circulation. The posterior pituitary hormones are released directly from axon terminals in the stalk and neurohypophysis. These neurons originate in the hypothalamus.

Pathology

The hypersecretory syndromes are Cushing's disease (ACTH), acromegaly (HGH, and often there is hyperprolactinaemia as well), gigantism (HGH), and prolactinoma (prolactin). Other hypersecretory disorders are rare. Nonsecretory (null cell adenoma) comprises about 25 percent of pituitary adenomas. **Microadenomas** are small discrete tumours several millimetres in size which are confined to the pituitary gland, whereas **macroadenomas** cause an enlargement of the entire gland. **Invasive macroadenomas** extend outside the confines of the sella and invade surrounding structures. **Hyperplasia** is a diffuse pathological change common in Cushing's disease. The larger tumours may compress or destroy the normal pituitary gland causing general hypopituitarism in addition to the hypersecretory effect of one of the syndromes.

Pattern of growth and effect on surrounding structures

The tumour may extend or invade laterally into the cavernous sinuses. It may erode the bony floor and anterior wall of the sella and extend into the sphenoid sinus. Superior extension will compress the optic chiasm and sometimes the optic nerves and hypothalamus. Large tumours may compress the third ventricle causing hydrocephalus. Posterior extension is uncommon but may proceed over the dorsum sellae into the posterior fossa. Destruction of the dorsum sellae and clivus may occur with invasive adenomas.

Clinical presentation

The clinical features of pituitary tumours are the endocrinopathy, headache, and optic chiasmal compression. Acromegaly is usually obvious when it is thought of, but patients rarely complain of it directly.

The prolactinoma, so commonly seen in the West in infertility clinics, where women present with varying degrees of amenorrhoea and galactorrhoea, is less often recognised in the tropics. Headache may be due to stretching of the dura over the sella, or in more advanced cases it may be due to grossly raised ICP from pressure on the floor of the third ventricle, obstruction of the foramina of Munro and hydrocephalus. Obvious bitemporal visual field defects are common, and may be quite asymmetrical.

Central vision is preserved for a long time, and an illiterate patient may function quite well with advanced signs that may be missed unless each field is tested separately. Non-functional tumours present as slow-onset hypopituitarism, mostly in elderly men. These are usually chromophobe on histology (relatively non-staining with haematoxylin and eosin). It is likely that many of these tumours are never diagnosed, the slow decline of the host being interpreted as a natural process.

Endocrine effects

Prolactinomas present with weight gain, amenorrhoea, infertility, male and female galactorrhoea, impotence and general lethargy. Some features of acromegaly and Cushing's disease are listed in Table 6.4 but a full description is beyond the scope of this book. The features of general hypopituitarism are loss of facial and pubic hair, thinning of the hair, a pallid complexion, and a general lethargy and often impotence.

Table 6.4 Clinical features of acromegaly, Cushing's disease and prolactinomas.

Cushing's disease (ACTH)	Acromegaly (HGH)	Prolactinomas
Moon face	Protrusion and growth of jaw	Galactorrhoea
Buffalo hump	Overgrowth of hands and feet	Loss of libido
Abdominal striae	Cardiomyopathy	Infertility
Hypertension	Hypertension	Amenorrhoea
Diabetes mellitus	Diabetes mellitus	Impotence in men
Serum cortisol raised	Growth hormone: 5-1000 ng/ml	Growth hormone: 20-200 ng/ml
Dexamethasone suppression test	Glucose suppression test IGF 1 level elevated	Prolactin: > 5-10 times normal

24-hour urinary free cortisol elevated

Normal range serum growth hormone	Normal range serum prolactin
< 5 ng/ml - (basal morning)	Premenopausal, non-lactating female: 4-20 ng/ml
	Male or postmenopausal female: 0-15 ng/ml

ACTH, adrenocorticotrophic hormone; HGH, human growth hormone;
IGF, insulin-like growth factor

Local pressure effects

- **Visual failure** due to compression on optic nerves and chiasm. Usually a bitemporal hemianopia.
- **Headache** may occur with large tumours particularly if the third ventricle is being compressed by the tumour and secondary hydrocephalus is developing.

Effects of invasion

Pituitary apoplexy is the clinical presentation of a pituitary tumour that is undergoing haemorrhagic necrosis. The patient presents acutely with acute severe headache, visual failure, bilateral cranial nerve palsies (combinations of 3, 4 and 6), sometimes meningism due to subarachnoid haemorrhage, and confusion or impaired conscious state.

CSF rhinorrhoea may occur with invasion of the sphenoid sinus.

Investigations

A skull X-ray is a very helpful investigation for the diagnosis of pituitary tumours in the developing world. The sella is expanded (see Figure 6.6 (a), next page), but not if it is a microadenoma, and there may be some erosion of the surrounding sphenoid bone with an invasive adenoma. CT scan-direct coronal images are the best projection to demonstrate the pituitary tumour (see Figure 6.6 (b), page 326). (MRI provides the definitive imaging when available). Visual fields should be recorded by an ophthalmologist if possible. Biochemistry of hormones may be difficult to obtain in many LMICs. Serum often has to be sent away to a reference laboratory or even overseas. In a prolactinoma, prolactin levels will be raised and if the diagnosis is in doubt, thyrotropin releasing hormone (TRH) stimulation may help. The normal pituitary gland secretes prolactin in response to TRH but if there is a prolactinoma this ability to increase the secretion is usually lost.

Prolactin levels may also be raised in patients with other tumours or lesions compressing the pituitary stalk hence the value of a TRH stimulation test. In cases of suspected Cushing's disease serum cortisol levels may be increased and also in a 24-hour urine sample. Cortisol secretion is raised by stress, depression and some psychotropic drugs but this increase can be blocked by dexamethasone. A dexamethasone suppression test can be used to confirm the presence of an adenoma. In acromegaly, growth hormone levels are raised and glucose administration cannot reduce the levels to normal. Retrograde venous catheterisation of the inferior petrosal vein to distinguish between ACTH levels in the cavernous sinus and the systemic circulation is possible but the technology and skills will not be available in LMICs. A raised ACTH level in the inferior petrosal vein is diagnostic of a corticotrophin secreting pituitary adenoma.

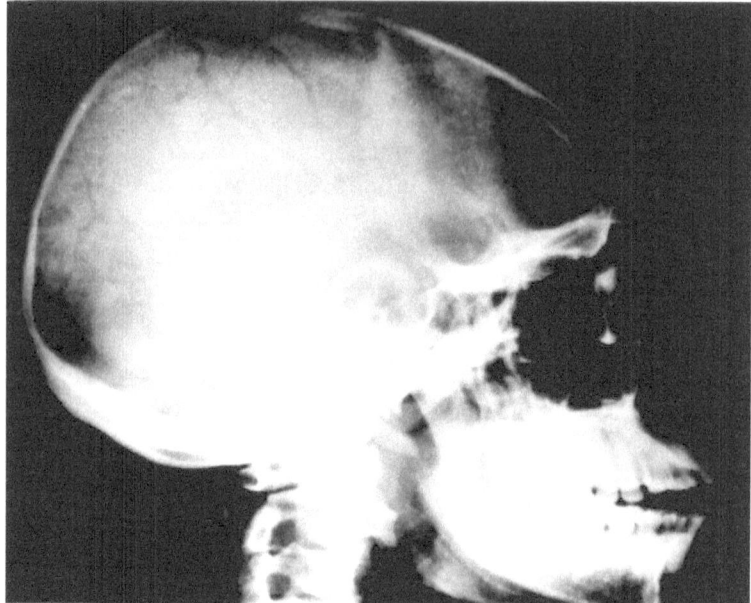

Figure 6.6 (a) i

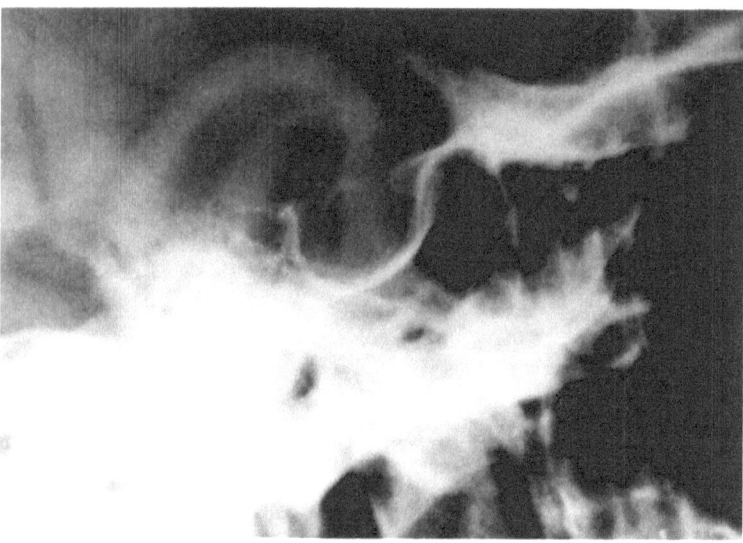

(a) ii

(a) i-ii Lateral skull X-ray showing enlarged pituitary fossa with erosion and truncation of the dorsum sellae. This patient had clinical acromegaly.

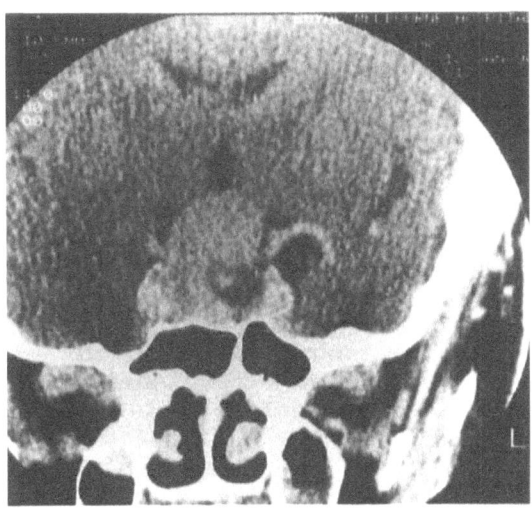

(b) Direct coronal CT scan showing large pituitary tumour with suprasellar extension involving the third ventricle. Null cell non-secretory pituitary adenoma. This tumour was removed via a transsphenoidal approach and the patient received postoperative radiotherapy. The patient has remained recurrence free for over 5 years. Direct coronal cuts on CT tend to be grainy compared with Axial slices.

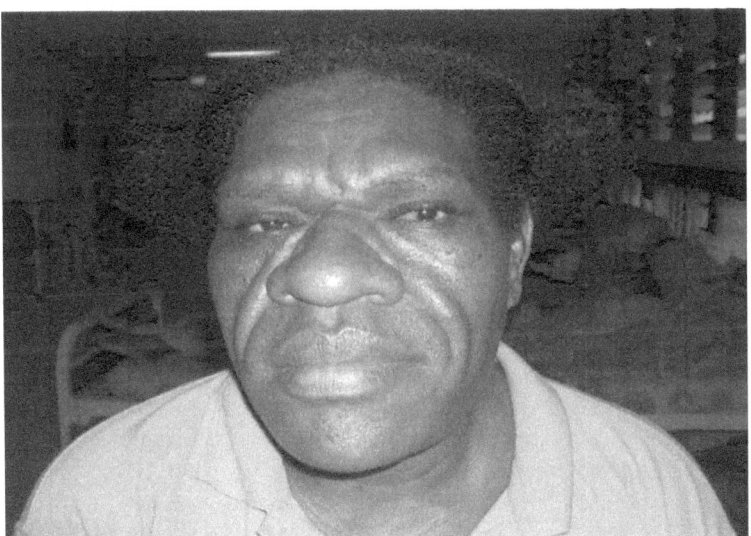

(c) A young female with gross features of acromegaly. She has coarse oily thickened skin, prominent cheek bones (malar), prominent supraorbital ridges, an enlarged mandible, a large broad nose and large lips. A large tongue (Macroglossia) is not seen in this photograph is another feature.

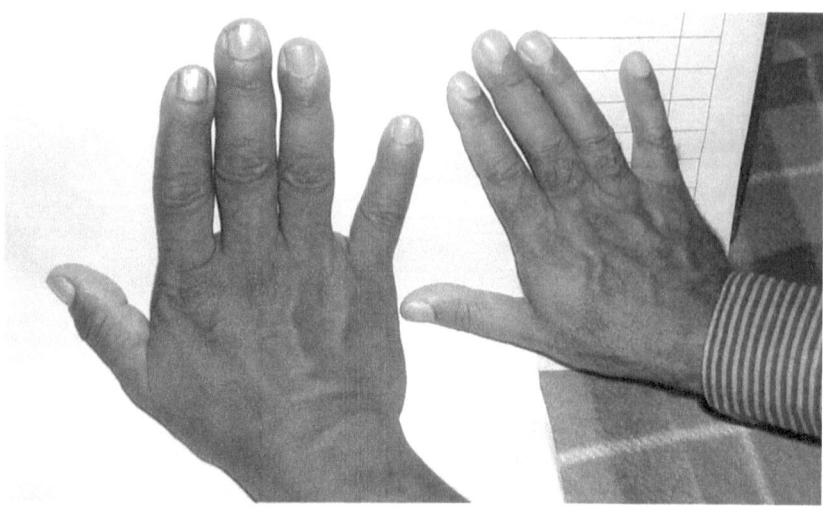

(d) The same patient as in (c) has a large hand compared to the male doctor's hand. She also has enlarged feet.

Figure 6.6 (a-d) Pituitary tumour.

Treatment

Wherever possible, a physician or endocrinologist should be involved in the investigation and management of pituitary tumours.

Medical therapy

The prolactinomas respond to bromocriptine medication (dose 2-10 mg per day), and usually shrink in size significantly. Cabergoline is an alternative. Optic chiasm compression is often totally relieved. However, the disease is not cured and the drug must be continued indefinitely. The drug may be poorly tolerated causing nausea and vomiting. The progress of the tumour can be followed clinically and by repeated prolactin estimations. The other pituitary tumours generally respond poorly to medical therapy. If prolactin levels are unavailable and it is possible that the tumour is a prolactinoma, a trial of bromocriptine is reasonable. If the patient lives a long way from medical care, it may be preferable to decompress the tumour surgically and preserve their eyesight, particularly if the supply of bromocriptine is unreliable or non-existent. Intravenous steroid replacement will be required for any patient having a pituitary operation. It can be commenced intraoperatively.

Surgery

1. **Craniotomy.** Pituitary tumours of the size that present in the tropics are best dealt with by normal craniotomy, although this is now rare in the West, where transsphenoidal removal is standard. A frontotemporal craniotomy on the side most convenient to the operator (right for right handers) allows approach along the sphenoidal ridge. A catheter in the frontal horn allows temporary drainage of CSF, and gentle retraction of the brain exposes the basal cisterns. If the arachnoid is opened, large quantities of CSF can be sucked away, exposing the anterior clinoid process, then the optic nerve, until finally the smooth bulging pituitary mass comes into view. This is then opened with diathermy. The contents are then sucked out. There always seems to be some normal pituitary in the recesses of the cavity, and this remains, so that postoperative hypopituitarism is not a problem. Transfrontal craniotomy with elevation of the frontal lobe is described in greater detail in the operative surgery section. Pituitary apoplexy will also require urgent exploration and decompression of the tumour by the transfrontal approach.
2. **Trans-sphenoidal hypophysectomy.** This is now the method of choice in neurosurgery centres for pituitary surgery. The approach is usually transnasal using nasal endoscopy. Most pituitary tumours can be removed via this route with a lower risk of serious morbidity for the patient compared with transcranial approaches. It does however require special surgical training, special instruments and a good quality image intensifier, none of which are available in many parts of the tropics.
3. **Complications of surgery.** Specific complications related to pituitary surgery are:
   a. Postoperative intracranial bleeding from the pituitary fossa which requires re-exploration. It usually manifests as deteriorating vision after surgery. Regular checks on the vision following surgery are thus essential. Counting fingers is a crude but useful method in the early postoperative period.
   b. Diabetes insipidus is usually transient and is treated by fluid replacement (5 percent dextrose) to avoid dehydration and pre-renal renal failure. Desmopressin intranasally or intravenously is the definitive therapy if available.
   c. CSF rhinorrhoea is unlikely after a transcranial approach.
   d. Addisonian crisis with cardiovascular collapse is avoided if steroid replacement therapy is given (100 mg hydrocortisone i.v. 6-hourly, then oral prednisolone 15-30 mg orally daily in divided doses).

4. **Postoperative replacement therapy.** Once the tumour has been removed, the patient may require long-term hormone replacement especially cortisone acetate and thyroxine, which are both relatively inexpensive.

Case report

A young nulliparous Enga woman from the Highlands of Papua New Guinea came with severe headache, deteriorating eyesight, amenorrhoea of uncertain duration, and galactorrhoea for 7 years. She blamed all this on the contraceptive pill. On examination she had gross signs of acromegaly, with enormous hands and feet, a big tongue, and thick facial features. Pupils were large and reacted slowly. Vision in the right eye was down to hand movement only, but she could count fingers to a metre with the left eye. Temporal and upper nasal fields were lost, readily demonstrable on confrontation. Skull X-ray showed the changes of acromegaly, and an enormous pituitary fossa. A liberal left frontotemporal craniotomy, with an approach to the sella along the sphenoidal ridge, revealed a left optic nerve flattened and stretched over a bluish mass. This was aspirated with a fine needle, and proved not to be an aneurysm. The cyst was opened with diathermy. Its soft contents went down the sucker.

The whole pituitary fossa was gently curetted out. Slight ooze of blood from the fossa was controlled by little pledgets of Oxycel, and hydrogen peroxide. The craniotomy was closed with a thin glove-rubber drain down to the sella; the drain was pulled out after 24 hours. The patient went home free of headache, but with no obvious improvement in eyesight.

Radiotherapy

Radiotherapy is indicated for an invasive tumour. There will be residual tumour in the cavernous sinuses, but this treatment will usually not be available or feasible if imaging is not available to follow the progress of the tumour.

Tumour-like lesions

Craniopharyngioma is a slow-growing tumour arising from squamous epithelium in Rathke's pouch remnants, usually in the immediate suprasellar region (Figure 6.7, below). It is more common in children and young people than in adults. It consists of cysts filled with material resembling sump oil, and irregularly calcified solid components. Compression of the pituitary, the hypothalamus and the optic pathways results in growth retardation, hypopituitarism and visual field defects. The mass is usually situated asymmetrically, often behind the optic chiasm rather than beneath it, and such cases may have homonymous hemianopia.

Large tumours cause hydrocephalus by bulging up into the third ventricle just as pituitary tumours do, and headache is therefore a common symptom. Despite its benign histological status these are dangerous tumours, often being densely adherent to surrounding structures, making successful complete removal very difficult. This tumour provides a major technical challenge in paediatric neurosurgical practice.

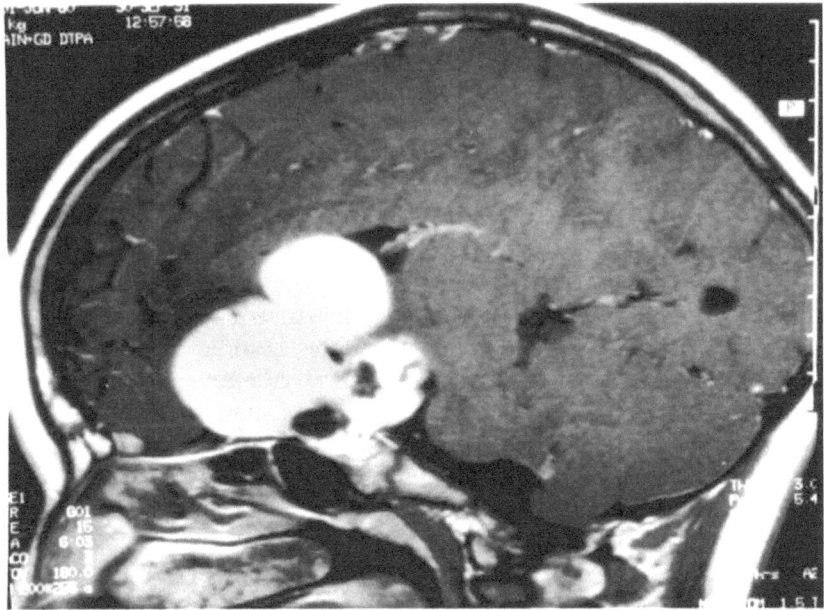

Figure 6.7 Craniopharyngioma.

Sagittal MR image showing multicystic sellar and suprasellar tumour filling the third ventricle and compressing the adjacent frontal lobe and brain stem. This tumour was completely excised at craniotomy.

Pineal region tumours

Pineal tumours comprise 0.4-0.9 per cent of intracranial neoplasms, but in Japan intracranial germ cell tumours account for 3.1 per cent of all primary brain tumours. There is a wide range of pathology affecting the pineal region. The incidence of germ cell tumours is about 0.2 per 100 000 population, and the incidence of pineal cell tumours (pinealoma) is about 0.01 per 100 000. Pineal tumours present variably with headaches, nausea, vomiting, blurred vision, diplopia, altered mental state, ataxia, drowsiness or rarely, precocious puberty. The germ cell tumour may spread to involve the neurohypophysis (posterior pituitary) and presents with diabetes insipidus, amenorrhoea, growth retardation or visual impairment. Diabetes insipidus may occur with a pineal mass alone. On examination, there may be papilloedema, Parinaud's syndrome and other ocular movement disorders, e.g. fourth nerve palsy, enlarged head in an infant with bulging anterior fontanelle, and long tract signs. Involvement of the cerebral hemisphere may result in a hemiparesis or epilepsy.

There may be a mixed clinical picture if tumour is present in the pineal and neurohypophysial or suprasellar locations (Figure 6.8, next page). The two main options are biopsy or craniotomy and excision, followed by adjuvant therapy for the malignant tumours. There is controversy relating to these choices, firstly because of the problem of a sampling error occurring if there is a biopsy alone. The pineal germinoma is an exquisitely radiosensitive tumour. The surgeon's judgement of a uniform tumour having the typical appearance of a germinoma based on the radiological appearance, resulting in a biopsy showing germinoma, may have missed a small component of malignant germ cell tumour which is radioresistant and requires chemotherapy in addition to the standard radiotherapy. About 20-37 per cent of pineal germ cell tumours contain mixed elements, and 27 per cent of pinealomas contain mixed elements. The alternative and preferred approach is to excise the tumour aggressively to achieve maximal debulking followed by the appropriate adjuvant therapy, which varies according to the pathology.

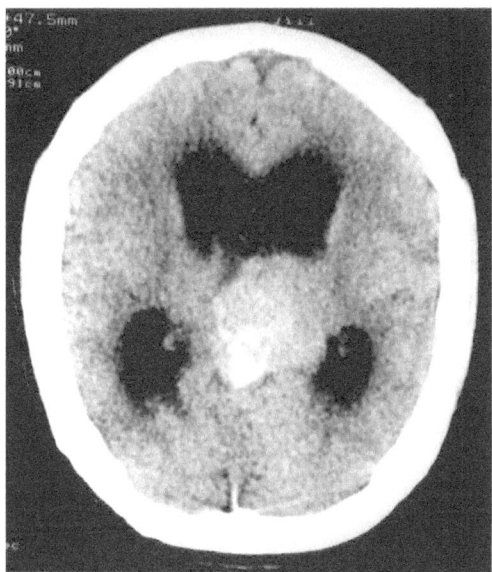

Figure 6.8 (a) Axial CT scan showing pineal region mass with irregular enhancement and obstruction of the third ventricle with lateral ventricle dilatation. The tumour histology was germinoma.

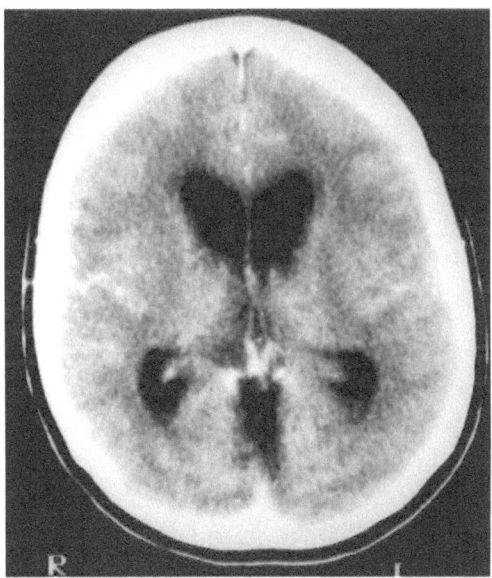

(b) Axial CT scan post removal of the tumour with reduction in ventricular size. The patient was treated with radiotherapy and has done well for over 10 years. He is regarded as being cured.

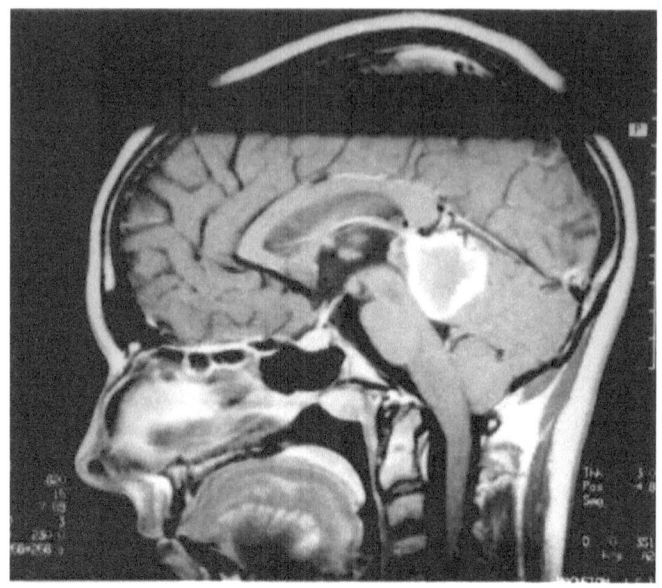

(c) i

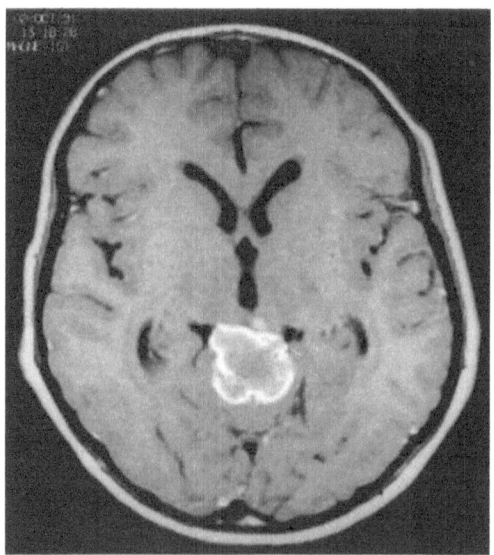

(c) ii

(c) i-ii Large pineal mass on axial and sagittal MR with enhancing wall. Astrocytoma on histology. The tumour was completely excised macroscopically.

Figure 6.8 (a-c) Pineal tumour.

Between 36 percent and 50 percent of pineal tumours are benign and are encapsulated and resectable, or are radioresistant, so that excision of these tumours is also preferable to biopsy as the primary therapy. This prevents unnecessary irradiation of the brain, which pertains particularly to the child's brain. There is also evidence that extensive surgical debulking may improve the response to adjuvant therapy, and may improve the survival rate compared with partial removal or biopsy, although this latter conclusion must be interpreted cautiously because of bias in the selection of cases.

Metastatic tumours

Metastatic tumours may occur anywhere in the brain, and sometimes present before the primary tumour. They are often multiple. The onset of headache may be sudden, suggesting a bleed into necrotic tumour. Some patients present with focal epilepsy (Figure 6.9, next page).

Surgery

Removal of a single metastasis, when this can be done safely (frontal pole or cerebellar hemisphere, for example) is often well worthwhile if the patient is otherwise in good condition, although cure is rare. Metastases may not be recognised as such until they have been removed. They are usually well demarcated from surrounding brain, giving a false impression of complete removal.

Radiotherapy

Stereotactic radiotherapy (Radiosurgery) is often used in HIC to treat selected metastases up to 3 cm diameter which may avoid the need for surgical excision. Multiple metastases (usually less than 3) may also treated by radiosurgery to each metastasis. There is a trend away from whole brain radiotherapy because of the cognitive side effects but if radiosurgery is unavailable it may still be used. Open surgery is preferred in some cases, particularly larger metastases and selected metastases in the posterior fossa.

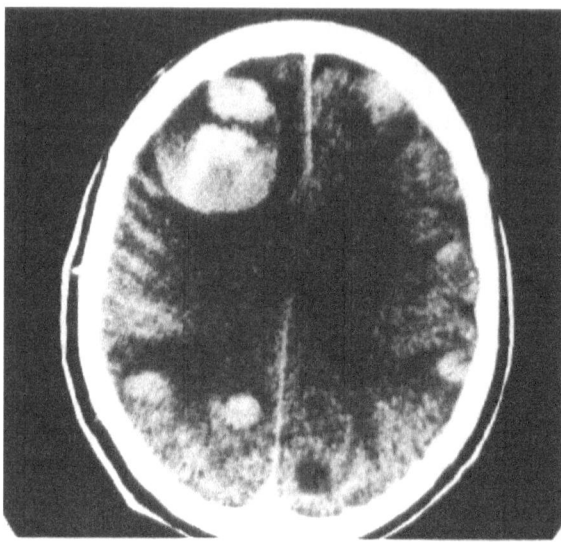

Figure 6.9 Metastatic brain tumour. Note the multiple round enhancing deposits of tumour scattered throughout the hemispheres. The primary tumour in this case was melanoma.

Steroids

Dexamethasone (12-20 mg daily in two to three divided doses) reduces brain oedema and often results in dramatic, if temporary, improvement in the patient's symptoms. Side-effects are the usual ones of steroids such as weight gain, Cushingoid appearance, development of diabetes, susceptibility to peptic ulceration or infection but there is also a valuable tendency to improve the mood.

TUMOURS OF THE SCALP AND CRANIUM

Tumours of the scalp may arise from any of the structures, skin, fascia, fat, sweat gland, muscle, blood vessel or nerves. A detailed approach is beyond the scope of this book. The general approach is to examine the lesion, the remaining scalp and the regional lymph nodes. Consider the possibility of a dermoid cyst or an encephalocele. Take an X-ray to exclude invasion of the skull. If there is no invasion, perform an excision biopsy, with a margin of at least 1 cm if malignancy is strongly suspected. Lesions expected to be benign can

335

be excised with a 2-5 mm margin. A malignant melanoma will require a wider excision (2-5 cm) once the diagnosis is confirmed. Closure may require a scalp rotation flap. If the lesion is huge or fixed (as is the case with angiosarcomas) a fine needle aspiration or incisional biopsy can be performed. The different tumours that may be encountered are listed in Table 6.5, below.

Practice point

Beware that the midline scalp lump could be an encephalocele or a dermoid cyst with intracranial extension.

Intracranial dermoid/epidermoid cysts may occur without any external connection (see Figure 6.10, next page). Malignant primary tumours of the scalp or skull which are confined and have not metastasised or invaded the underlying brain are best excised en bloc, i.e. the tumour, surrounding normal scalp, pericranium and underlying involved skull and sometimes dura are excised as a single specimen. The depth of invasion is determined by skull X-ray but CT, if available, may show how much intracranial extension is present. The resultant surgical defect is closed in layers paying particular attention to achieving watertight dural closure. The scalp defect is closed using scalp flaps as described in Chapter 11 on page 540. A delayed cranioplasty may be performed to replace the missing skull bone. This aggressive treatment gives the patient the best chance of long-term survival and may be particularly applicable in younger patients with sarcomas. Unfortunately, these lesions are often too advanced in LMICs to enable any surgery, and palliative care must be provided (see Figure 6.11, page 338).

Table 6.5 Tumours of the scalp and cranium.

Tumours of skin

Benign naevus, keratosis, papilloma, inclusion dermoid, wart

Sebaceous cyst

Basal cell carcinoma (locally invasive)

Squamous cell carcinoma (especially albinos, Caucasians and depigmented scars)

Table 6.5 *(Continued)*

Malignant melanoma (rare in pigmented skin on the scalp)

Tumours of fat
Lipoma
Liposarcoma

Tumours of muscle and fascia
Fibroma and fibrosarcoma
Myoma and myosarcoma

Tumours of blood vessels
Haemangioma
Angiosarcoma

Tumours of nerve and nerve sheaths
Neuroma
Schwannoma

Tumours of the cranium
Primary bone tumours such as osteosarcoma, myeloma, chordoma
Secondary bone tumours, especially breast, thyroid, lung, renal and prostate

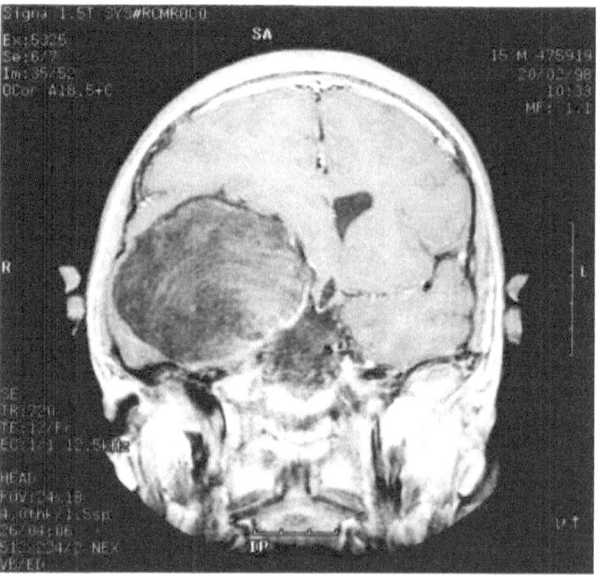

Figure 6.10

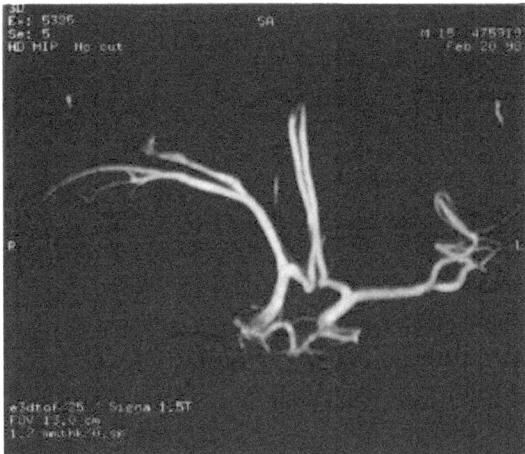

Figure 6.10 Intracranial epidermoid cyst occupying the entire right middle Iossa and compressing the frontal and temporal lobes on coronal MR. The displacement of the middle cerebral artery upwards and inwards can be seen on the MR angiogram. Note the layering of keratin in the tumour.

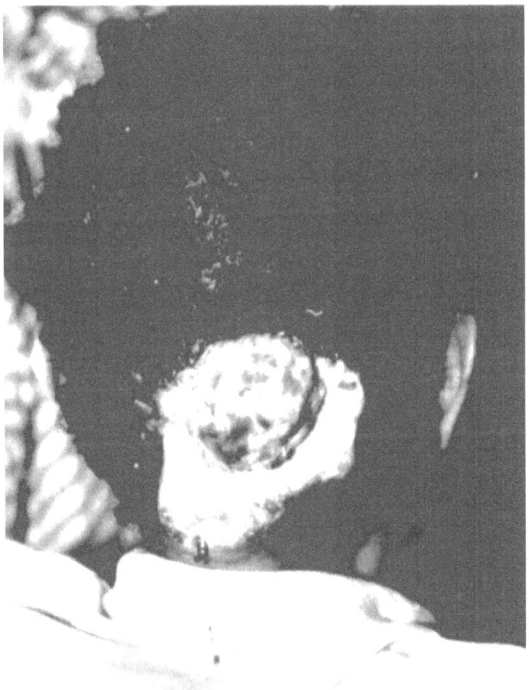

Figure 6.11 Advanced squamous cell carcinoma of the occipital scalp in a middle-aged Papua New Guinean woman. There was bone and presumed brain invasion. Management was conservative and palliative.

Practice point

Meningiomas may invade the skull causing a bony swelling (exostosis) which may have an overlying bruit: These tumours are extremely vascular and the size and extent of the intracranial component must be determined before surgery. The surgeon should be prepared for major blood loss.

There are many different types of primary tumour that affect the skull, but a detailed description is beyond the scope of this book. In the advanced centres, malignant primary skull tumours, such as osteosarcoma and chordoma, may require biopsy and debulking followed by adjuvant radiotherapy and in some cases chemotherapy. Chondrosarcoma may grow slowly and in some cases be completely removed with good long-term results.

Chordoma is a primitive highly malignant tumour, which is believed to arise from the primitive embryonic notochordal remnant. It particularly affects the base of the skull in the sphenoid/clivus region and the sacrum. It should be aggressively excised and irradiated although recurrence rates are high. Isolated histiocytosis of the skull occurs in children and can be cured by excision, but multiple skeletal and sometimes visceral deposits of histiocytosis require chemotherapy.

Metastatic tumours to the skull are not uncommon and arise most commonly from metastatic carcinoma of the breast, lung, prostate, thyroid and multiple myeloma (Figure 6.12, next page). Breast and prostatic metastases may be sclerotic in type rather than lytic.

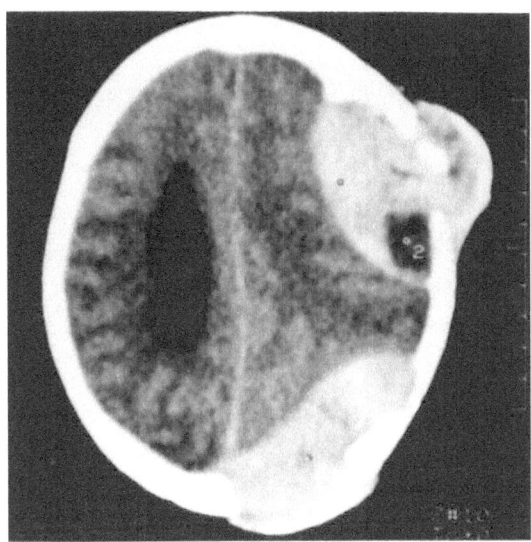

Figure 6.12 Axial CT scan showing two large erosive skull lesions with intracranial and extracranial extension. Secondary carcinoma of the thyroid.

Haemangioma of the scalp, face & neck (Table 6.6, below)

Haemangiomas are vascular tumours with rapid endothelial proliferation over several weeks to months followed by a slow period of involution over 5-10 years. They have an incidence of 1-2 per cent in infants and about 30 per cent are present at birth as a pale or telangiectatic area, and most of the remainder develop in the first month. Superficial haemangiomas are lobulated, clearly demarcated and bright red. The deeper haemangiomas have a blue colour.

Table 6.6 Classification of vascular lesions of the scalp, face and neck.

Haemangioma	Strawberry naevus
Vascular malformation	
Capillary	Port-wine naevus
Venous	Cavernous haemangioma
Lymphatic	Lymphangioma, cystic hygroma
Arterial	

The indications for treatment of haemangiomas are restricted to the following:

1. Lesions interfering with vital functions, e.g. eyelids, lips, nares, larynx, airway.
2. Ulcerated lesions, especially involving the eyelids, nares, lips or pinnae.
3. Large lesions associated with high output cardiac failure.
4. Large facial lesions that distort the facial features.
5. Pedunculated lesions.

Oral prednisolone may hasten the resolution of the haemangioma if given in the early proliferative phase. The course is 4-6 weeks but is not given after 20 weeks of age. Surgery is usually reserved for correction of deformity in the involutional phase. Other treatments that have been used are laser therapy for the ulceration, intralesional corticosteroid and alpha interferon therapy.

Practice point

Most haemangiomas require no treatment.

In contrast to the haemangiomas, the cutaneous vascular malformations are structural anomalies, present at birth, do not involve cell proliferation, and do not regress, i.e. are static lesions. The port-wine capillary naevus in the distribution of the trigeminal nerve (usually the forehead and upper face), is a feature of the Sturge-Weber syndrome, and may indicate underlying cortical involvement with the haemangioma and results in chronic epilepsy.

Angiosarcoma of the scalp

Angiosarcoma is a rare tumour of the scalp and is a vascular tumour of endothelial origin. There are single or multiple violaceous or bluish nodules or papules which may ulcerate and bleed. The differential diagnosis is Kaposi's sarcoma and amelanotic melanoma. There is rapid subdermal spread to involve large areas of scalp and it may spread to the face. Distant metastases to cervical lymph nodes, liver and lung are common. There is a poor chance of survival but if the lesion is seen and treated early with wide excision and clear histological margins obtained on all sides the outcome may be better.

TUMOURS OF THE ORBIT

The orbit is bounded inferiorly by the roof of the maxillary sinus, laterally by the zygoma, frontal bone and greater wing of sphenoid, superiorly by the floor of the anterior cranial fossa, and medially by the lateral wall of the ethmoid and sphenoid sinuses.

Table 6.7 Tumours of the orbit.

1. Retina: retinoblastoma and melanoma.
2. Optic nerve: glioma - usually benign (pilocytic) astrocytoma, neurofibroma/schwannoma
3. Optic nerve sheath: meningioma. This may extend intracranially through the optic foramen or be part of an intracranial meningioma spreading distally into the orbit
4. Metastases: breast and lung in adults; neuroblastoma, Ewing's sarcoma and leukaemia in children.
5. Paranasal sinus: carcinoma
6. Bony wall: osteoma
7. Lacrimal gland: pleomorphic adenoma or carcinoma, lymphoma, e.g. Burkitt's lymphoma
8. Connective tissue: rhabdomyosarcoma.
9. Non-neoplastic lesions: cavernous haemangioma/lymphangioma; paranasal sinus mucocele; exophthalmos due to thyrotoxicosis, sarcoidosis, pseudo-tumour.

Pathology

Tumours may arise from the orbital contents themselves, or spread from adjacent structures. The pathology can be divided according to the various elements making up the orbit including the retina, optic nerve, sinus, lacrimal gland, and soft tissues (Table 6.7, above).

Clinical presentation

The patient may present with proptosis, orbital pain, secondary lid swelling, diplopia, decreased visual acuity in the affected eye, or a palpable mass in the orbit (Figure 6.13 (a), next page and Figure 6.13 (b), page 344 and Figure 6.14, page 346). A vascular lesion may have an associated bruit, and cause pulsation of the eye. Inspection of the face from above may allow the detection of a mild proptosis, when the two sides are compared.

Investigations

X-ray of the orbit may reveal bony erosion, dilation of the optic foramen (optic nerve tumour) and possibly calcification in a retinoblastoma or lacrimal tumour. CT scan if available, is helpful to show the position of the tumour (Figure 6.13 (c), page 345 and Figure 6.14, page 346).

Management

A large orbital mass may require a needle biopsy to define the pathology before further therapy is planned. Benign tumours can be excised except for benign optic nerve or nerve sheath tumours, which are usually managed conservatively. Intracranial meningiomas with orbital spread require debulking. The malignant tumours may require debulking or biopsy and radiotherapy.

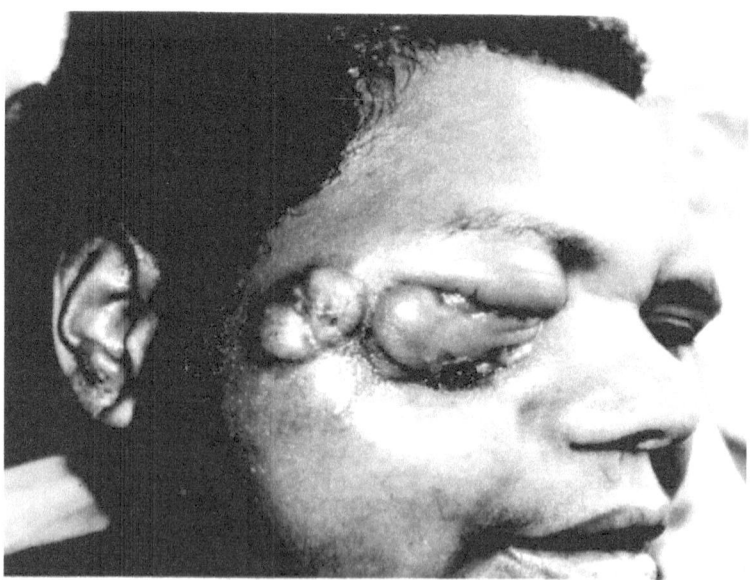

Figure 6.13 (a) Malignancy of the right orbit in a middle-aged woman. Presumed carcinoma secondary to maxillary sinus disease. Palliative care provided.

343

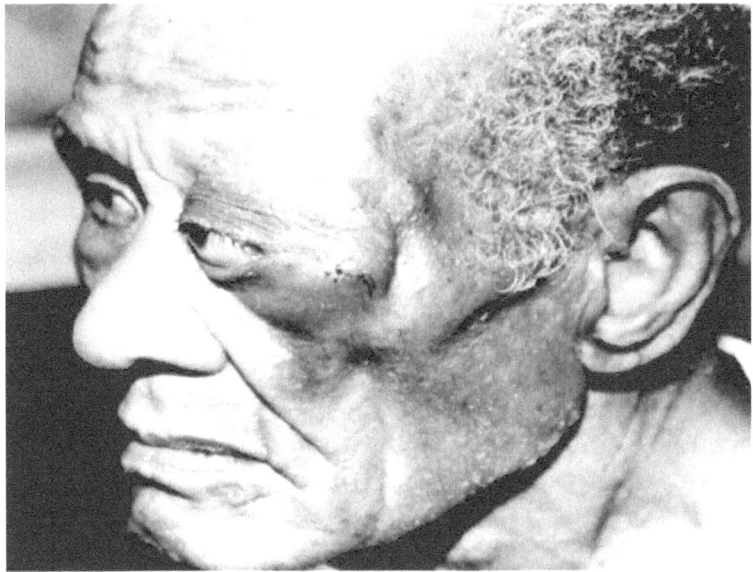

(b) Left orbital tumour in an elderly man causing proptosis and blindness in the left eye. Pathology undetermined. Palliative care provided.

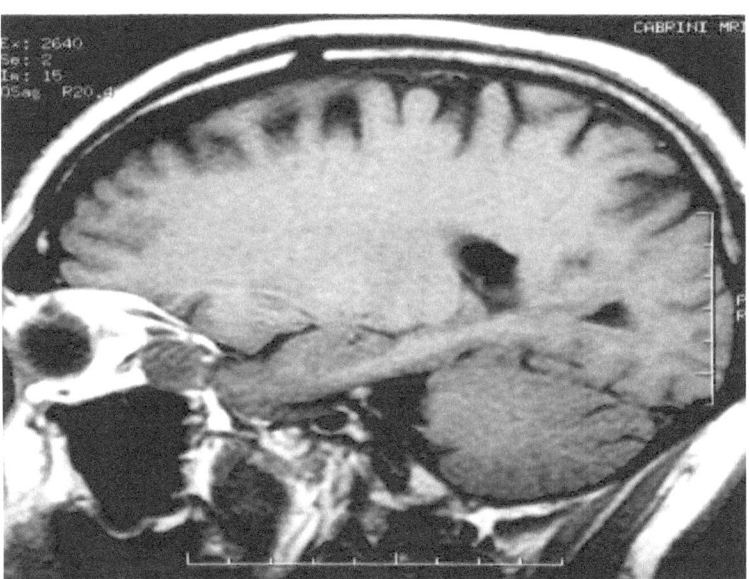

(c) i

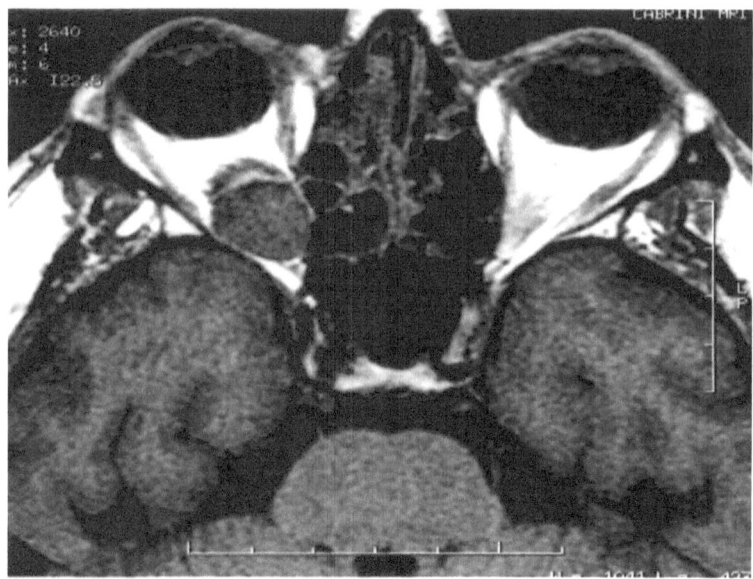

(c) ii

(c) i-ii Axial and sagittal MR image showing right orbital apex round tumour. Cavernous angioma.

Figure 6.13 (a-c) Tumours of the orbit.

Note the relationship in Figure 6.13, above of the tumour to the ocular muscles, placing it in an extraconal position, i.e. outside the muscle cone and not involving the optic nerve. This tumour was approached via a medial orbitotomy, transethmoidal approach to remove it from below. The patient was a middle-aged man who presented with vague headaches and the tumour was picked up incidentally on a CT scan.

Lymphomas may require chemotherapy. If the biopsy shows inflammatory tissue, the condition is a pseudotumour or orbital granuloma and may respond to high dose steroids. If a paranasal sinus carcinoma invades through the orbital fascia and a radical en-bloc excision is being performed, the orbital contents will require exenteration.

The **operative approaches** to the orbit are:
1. Transfrontal: through the roof of the orbit, via a frontal craniotomy.
2. The lateral orbitotomy approach.
3. The medial orbitotomy can be partly transethmoidal, if necessary.

It is possible for thyroid endocrinopathy to result in a unilateral exophthalmos without abnormal thyroxine levels. If the disease progresses, with corneal ulceration, papilloedema and loss of vision, decompressing the walls of the orbit may improve the visual outcome.

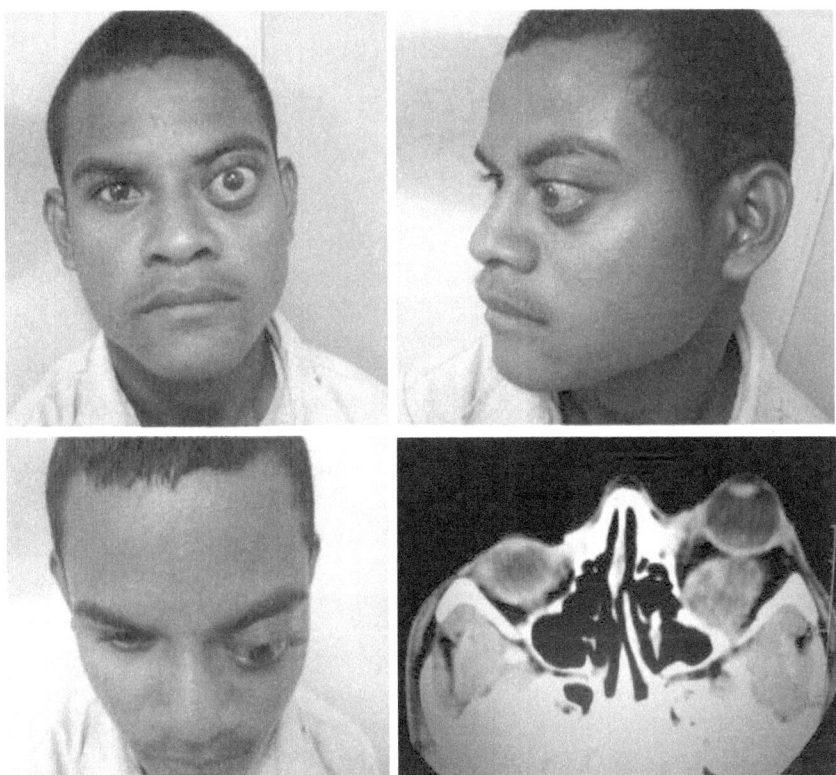

Figure 6.14 Young man with gross proptosis of the left eye seen on frontal, side view and from above.

CT axial scan shows a large tumour posterior to the left eye. It is probably a meningioma of the optic nerve sheath.

Infection

INTRODUCTION AND DEFINITIONS

Infection and trauma are the two commonest problems affecting the nervous system in the tropics and many LMICs. Infection is defined as invasion and destruction of tissues by microorganisms. For the purpose of this chapter worm infestation is included alongside bacteria, fungi, viruses, protozoans and prions as infective agents. Infection may be the primary cause of neurological disease (e.g. tuberculoma) or complicate some other neuropathology, trauma or operative procedure (e.g. intracranial abscess complicating skull base fractures, penetrating brain injuries, or sinusitis). Patients with immunodeficiency are prone to develop opportunistic infections which may affect the nervous system.

Ventriculoperitoneal shunts and other catheters may act as a site of entry for bacteria to the central nervous system. There are many infectious diseases causing neurological complications. Those with particular surgical relevance are discussed below but this chapter is not intended to be exhaustive. Many infections, particularly those causing peripheral neuropathy, myelopathy, meningitis or encephalitis, will not come to surgery but still need to be considered in the differential diagnosis of a neurological problem. The geography and epidemiology of infection also need to be considered, not only where the patient lives, but also where they have lived previously or travelled recently. Any history of contact with infectious diseases such as tuberculosis is also relevant. The investigation and medical management of neurological infections are not covered in detail because they are more appropriately covered in tropical medicine textbooks.

However, the basic principles of investigation and management are outlined. Acute infection tends to present with fever, leukocytosis and rapid development of clinical signs. Chronic infection may develop insidiously, even years after the primary infection, or as a recrudescence of previously quiescent disease.

Infection

The onset and duration of illness are important aspects in the history that will help determine whether a patient has acute or chronic infection.

Table 7.1 Clinical manifestations of common neurological infections.

Presentation	Infection	Possible investigations
Intracranial manifestations of infection		
Meningitis	Bacteria	LP
	Tuberculosis	LP, CT scan
	Cryptococcccus	CT scan
	Viral	Ventriculogram
Altered consciousness and coma	Bacterial meningitis Cryptococcal meningitis	LP
	Cerebral malaria	Blood film
	Encephalitis	
	Trypanosomiasis	
	Opportunistic infections	
Space occupying lesion*	Cerebral abscess	CT scan, angiogram
	Tuberculoma	CT scan, angiogram
	Hydatid cysts	CT scan, angiogram
	Gnathostomiasis	Blood count
	Sparganosis	Antibodies
	Cysticercosis	Skull X-ray, CT scan
	Cryptococcoma	CT, antibodies
	Toxocara	
Blindness Stroke	Cryptococcal meningitis Focal infective lesions	LP, serology
	Trypanosomiasis	
	Emboli from:	
	Bacterial endocarditis	
	Mycotic aneurysm	
	Cardiomyopathy (Chagas)	
	Gnathostomiasis	
	TB meningitis	
	Cysticercosis	

Table 7.1 *(Continued)*

Presentation	Infection	Possible investigations
Ataxia and gait disorders	Cerebellar infections Spongiform encephalopathy	CT scan, LP EEG, Brain biopsy?
Spinal and peripheral nerve manifestations of infection		
Paraplegia and spinal cord compression	Tuberculosis	Spine X-ray
	Intradural abscess	Myelogram
	Extradural abscess	CT, MRI, Biopsy, culture
Myelitis	Syphilis - tabes dorsalis HTLVI	VDRL Serology
	Schistosomiasis	Biopsy
	Paragonomiasis	
	Gnathostomiasis	
	Hydatid	
	Brucellosis	
	HIV	
Lower motor neuron signs	Guillain-Barre syndrome	
	Poliomyelitis	
Peripheral neuropathy	Leprosy	Nerve biopsy
	HIV	HIV serology

The different clinical problems are listed together with appropriate investigations (Table 7.1). Some infections are also discussed in the appropriate chapters relating to these clinical problems. For example, tuberculosis of the spine is discussed in Chapter 5, page 253.

SPACE OCCUPYING LESIONS AND BRAIN ABSCESSES

J.V. Rosenfeld, J.K.A. Clezy & D.A.K. Watters

The clinical presentation of a patient with a space occupying lesion (SOL) is discussed in Chapter 6, page 290. The actual signs are dependent on the site of the infection. The site of origin may be far removed from the central nervous system as in osteomyelitis or the SOL may result from direct spread from an adjacent septic focus as in abscesses complicating sinusitis, mastoiditis or an open fracture.

Tuberculoma

An important cause of the space occupying lesion and epilepsy in the tropics is the tuberculoma. There may be focal neurological signs and the tuberculomas are usually multiple. There has not usually been any episode of tuberculous meningitis. As discussed in the SOL section of Chapter 6, page 299, if CT is unavailable, a suspected tuberculoma should be treated medically.

The indications for surgery, assuming the skills are available and the lesion is accessible, are persisting SOL without diagnosis, lack of response to antituberculous therapy, and progressive neurological deterioration despite the medical therapy. The CT appearance of tuberculoma is non-specific with varying density, levels of calcification, cystic character and degrees of enhancement. It may resemble a typical ring enhancing pyogenic abscess.

Case report *(Figure 7.1 (a), next page)*

A 20-year-old man presented with convulsions. On examination he had a left sided weakness but all muscle groups could still oppose gravity (Grade 4). Skull X-rays were normal. CT scan showed a frontal lobe SOL with ring enhancement (Figure 7.1a). The patient was treated with antituberculous chemotherapy for 4 weeks without improvement. Craniotomy was then performed to excise the tumour, which proved to be a tuberculoma. **Note:** *Many tuberculomas would respond to anti-TB therapy and this should always be the first line of treatment.*

Case Report *(Figure 7.1 (b), next page)*

A young woman presented with new onset of seizures and her CT scan showed a right frontal enhancing lesion with surrounding oedema. This was presumed to be a tuberculoma and she was successfully treated with anti-TB therapy and anti-seizure medication.

Brain abscess

Brain abscess is not uncommon in the tropics, often presents late and has a high mortality, particularly if no surgery is undertaken. The microbiological flora within the abscess is usually mixed and includes anaerobes. The abscess is secondary to sepsis elsewhere. William Macewen (1848-1924) was a neurosurgical pioneer whose landmark publications dealt almost entirely with abscesses secondary to middle ear disease. Middle ear infections remain the commonest cause where ENT services are sparse. The causes are as follows:

- otitic (90 percent temporal lobe, 10 percent cerebellar),
- from nasal sinus sepsis (frontal lobe),
- secondary to skull trauma (open wound or compound fracture),
- metastatic (lung sepsis, osteomyelitis, dental sepsis).

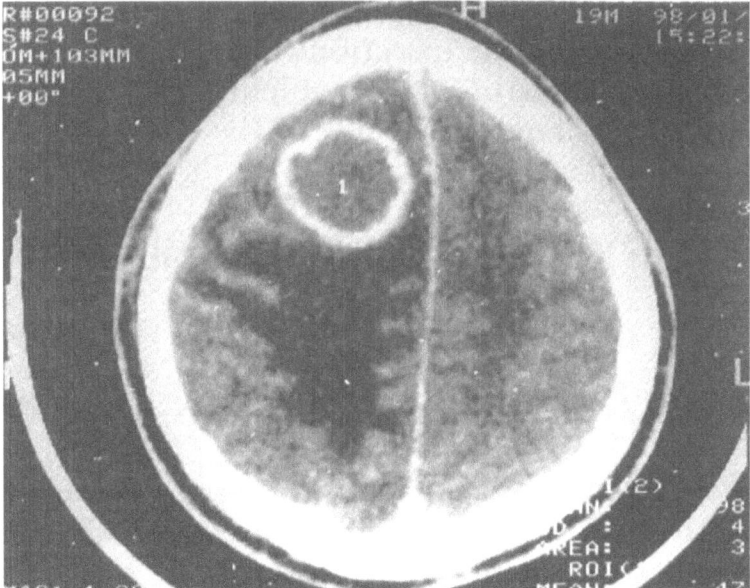

Figure 7.1 (a) CT scan showing space occupying lesion. Right frontal ring enhancing lesion with surrounding oedema. Diagnosis: tuberculoma.

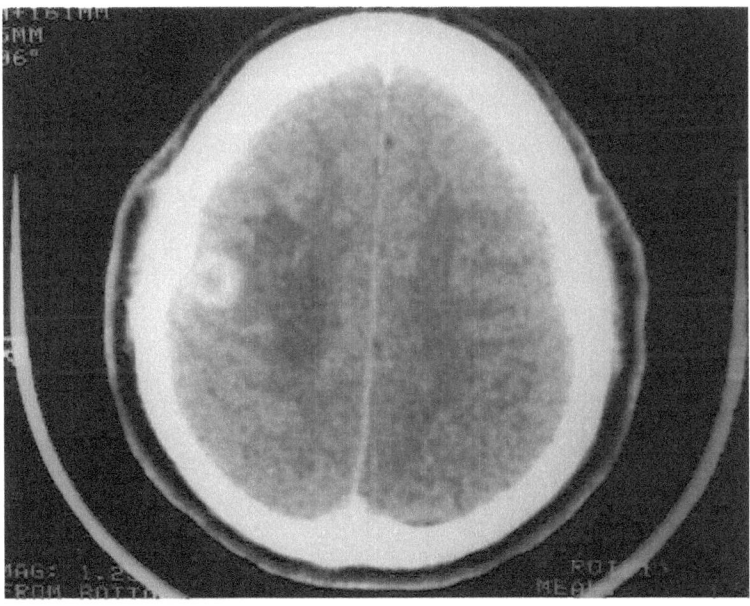

(b) CT scan showing a right posterior frontal enhancing lesion with surrounding oedema. This was presumed to be a tuberculoma.

Figure 7.1 (a-b)

352

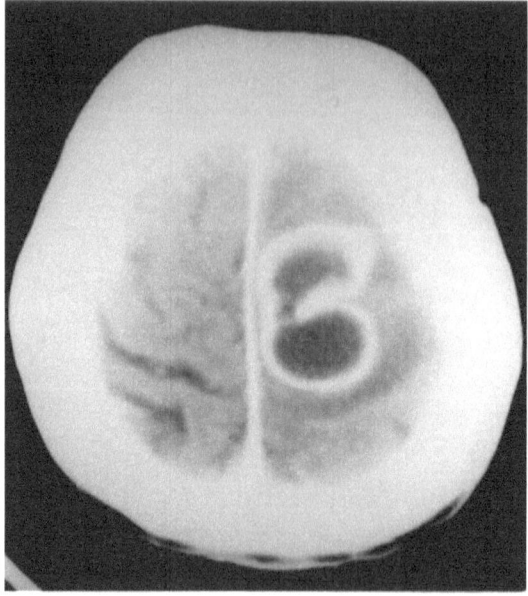

(a) CT scan with contrast showing single multiloculated brain abscess in an immunosuppressed patient.

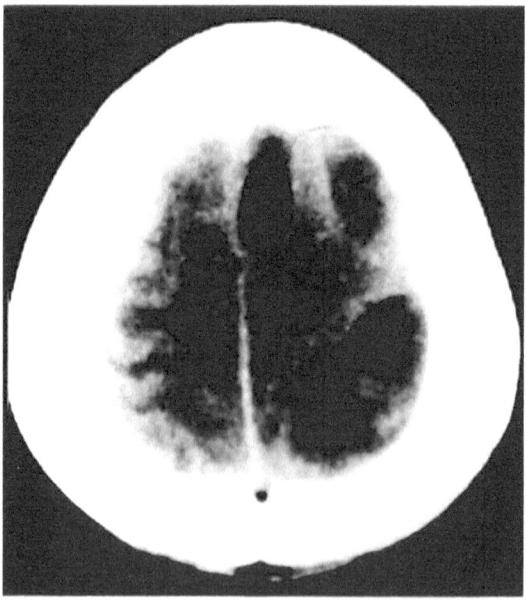

(b) CT scan without contrast showing multiple brain abscesses.

Figure 7.2 (a-b)

Clinical presentation

Fever and leucocytosis are common but may be absent if the abscess is chronic. Headache and vomiting are symptoms of raised ICP and occur especially when oedema develops around the abscess. Altered conscious state may develop with irritability initially followed by confusion, lethargy, drowsiness or coma. Papilloedema is variable. It is important to perform a thorough neurological examination to detect focal signs. Focal seizures may also indicate the site of pathology. The diagnosis should be suspected, if these problems are present 10 days or more after an acute infection. The differential diagnosis is cerebral tumour, encephalitis, tuberculous meningitis, and trypanosomiasis in endemic areas. A brain abscess may present with fever, lethargy and headache without focal signs. Bilateral abscess may be present with only unilateral signs, or multiple unilateral abscesses may be present. Meningitis (haemophilus, pneumococcus, meningococcus) may be secondary to a ruptured brain abscess. Any neurosurgical procedure may be complicated by a brain abscess. There is a significant recurrence rate of brain abscess.

Investigation

Lumbar puncture is contraindicated if there is raised intracranial pressure as the patient may cone. Convulsions, focal signs and papilloedema are contraindications to lumbar puncture. The radiological investigations, where CT is unavailable, are cerebral angiography and ventriculography, which are complementary. The angiogram should be tried first as it may allow the localisation of the abscess without the need for the more invasive ventriculogram.

Presentation and management of specific abscesses

Otitic brain abscesses

Clinical presentation: Otitic abscesses occur in patients with chronic middle ear sepsis, often when prolonged discharge has recently ceased. The patient presents with increasing headache for days or weeks. Some fever is usual. The mastoid may be tender, and mild long tract signs are usually present. Papilloedema is common.

Neck stiffness, if present, is not as marked as in meningitis. In temporal abscesses a visual field defect may be present, but patients are rarely co-operative enough for this to be detectable. Nystagmus may or may not be detectable in cerebellar cases. Plain films of the skull show signs of chronic ear sepsis, best seen in the Towne's view. Sometimes a large cavity in the temporal bone indicates a cholesteatoma.

Management: If a temporal lobe abscess is confidently diagnosed clinically it may be drained via a burr hole immediately above the ear (see Chapter 11, page 509). The abscess has a firm wall, and is just under the surface of the brain. Thick pus flows through the needle, and should be aspirated as completely as possible. Macewen recognised that one puncture was inadequate, and used tubes of decalcified chicken bone as drains, apparently with success. Nowadays repeated aspiration, rather than open drainage, is standard. Aspiration may be required every 2 or 3 days for a week or so. Assessment of the need to re-drain may be simpler if a little contrast material is instilled into the cavity. Repeated drainage usually cures these abscesses, and their excision is rarely necessary. Antibiotic (gentamicin) may also be instilled following aspiration. If there is any doubt about the diagnosis, imaging is required. In the absence of CT or MRI, angiography is ideal, demonstrating a large avascular area in the temporal lobe, but in small children this will be a problem outside special centres, and ventriculography may be preferable. An otitic abscess will recur months or years later unless the source of infection in the mastoid is dealt with. It is appropriate to proceed directly from the first drainage of the brain abscess to a mastoidectomy, which is described in Chapter 11, page 604. Chronic mastoiditis may also cause lateral sinus (transverse or sigmoid) thrombosis with its complications of otitic hydrocephalus, septicaemia or metastatic abscess. The condition is described in Chapter 8 on page 422.

Case report

A 13-year-old female was a passenger involved in a motor vehicle accident in which she sustained a compound depressed parietal fracture which was elevated and repaired uneventfully although she had some cognitive and behavioural problems. A fractured base of skull passing through the left petrous bone was noted but as there was no CSF leak, this was managed conservatively.

Case report *(Continued)*

Two years later she complained of increasingly severe headaches over several months, and was repeatedly vomiting and losing weight. She became comatose one night and was brought to the emergency department and was noted to have fixed dilated pupils. A CT scan was performed and showed a large left temporal lobe ring enhancing lesion with severe mass effect (Figure 7.3, below), and she was taken immediately to the operating theatre for craniotomy and drainage of the abscess. Despite this, she died. Do not ignore the symptoms of raised intracranial pressure.

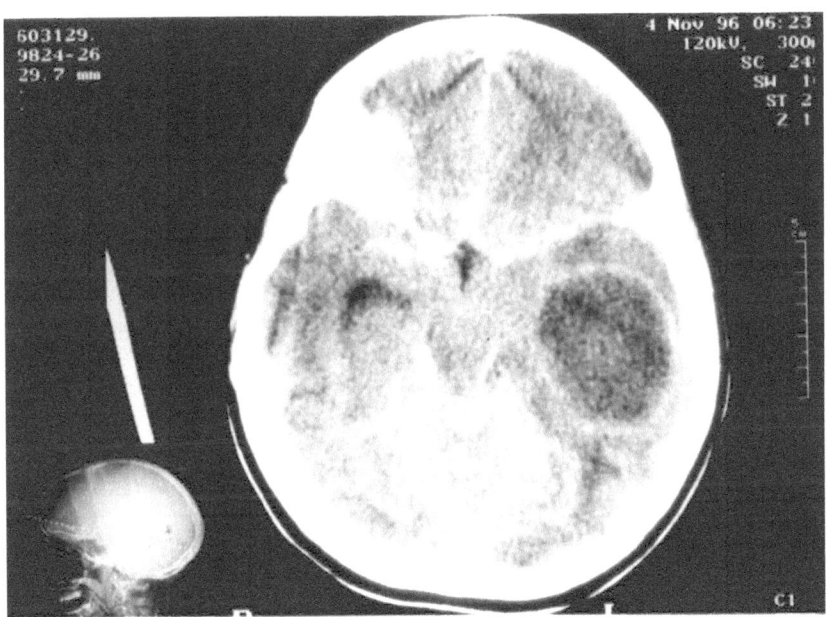

Figure 7.3 CT scan showing large left temporal lobe abscess occurring 2 years following a skull base fracture involving the left petrous temporal bone (see case report).

Abscesses complicating frontal sinusitis

Abscess due to nasal sinus disease usually originates from the frontal sinus, which will be opaque on X-ray. There may be orbital cellulitis (Figure 7.4, next page). Epidural empyema followed by subdural empyema and frontal lobe abscess are potential life-threatening complications. As well as drainage of a subdural empyema or brain abscess the cause needs treatment, and properly needs ENT specialist management. A frontoethmoidectomy will be required to clear the primary site of infection.

Orbital cellulitis

Clinical presentation: This condition usually occurs in children and presents with erythema of the eyelids and their surrounds, and lid swelling in a febrile, unwell child. The lid swelling frequently prevents eye opening. When the lids are separated with a lid retractor, there may be limitation of eye movement and proptosis (Figure 7.4, next page).

These two signs indicate spread of the infection into the orbit rather than preseptal or periorbital cellulitis where the infection lies in front of the orbital fascia. Proptosis may be severe enough to result in corneal exposure. Orbital cellulitis is frequently associated with infection in the adjacent sinuses. Bilateral orbital cellulitis may be associated with cavernous sinus thrombosis.

Management: Take the condition very seriously: admit and investigate. Intravenous antibiotics such as penicillin and chloramphenicol or penicillin and flucloxacillin, or a third-generation cephalosporin. Plain X-ray will show an opaque sinus. CT scan is very helpful to identify pus collections, and sinus pathology. Orbital abscess or sinus collections require drainage. Delay in diagnosis and treatment may result in death or permanent loss of vision.

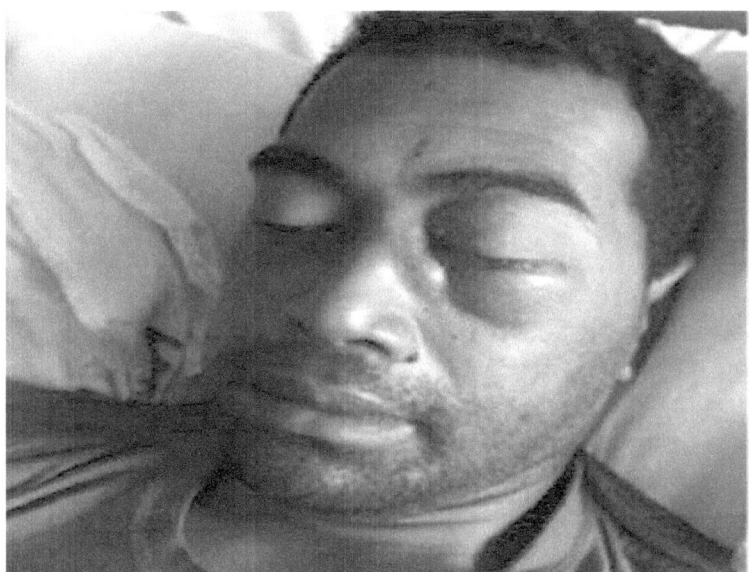

Figure 7.4 (a)

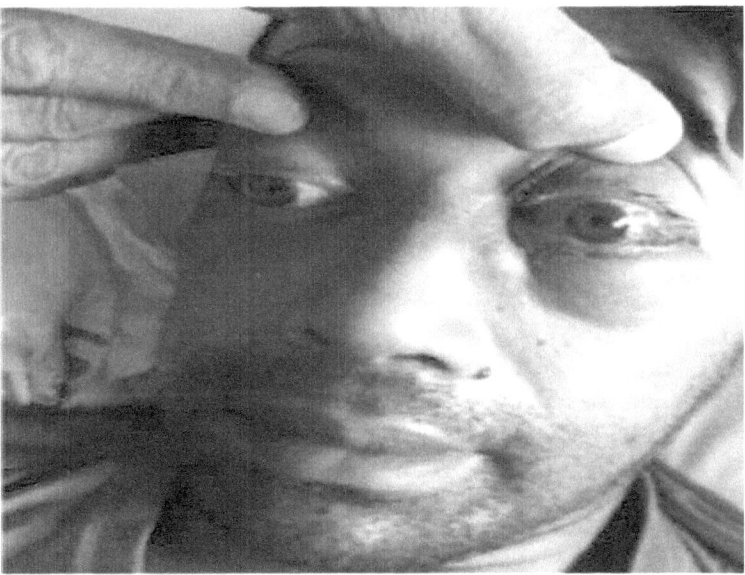

(b)

Figure 7.4 (a-b) Orbital cellulitis due to fronto-ethmoid sinusitis. The frontoethmoid region is markedly swollen in addition to the periorbital tissues. On opening the eyelids there is marked chemosis and proptosis.

Case report

An 18-year-old woman was admitted with fever, confusion and unilateral orbital cellulitis to a mission hospital. She was treated with intravenous antibiotics but made no progress. Plain X-rays showed an opaque frontal sinus. Over a weekend she continued to deteriorate and a visiting ENT surgeon was contacted for advice. He advised drainage of the sinus and she was booked for surgery. This was delayed by a further day because the patient was so sick. Under anaesthesia, 6 days after admission she coned and died. Her frontal lobe abscess had been growing during the period of delay.

Lesson: *consider a subdural empyema or frontal lobe abscess in patients with orbital cellulitis. This condition needs radical and prompt surgery. A frontal burr hole and drainage of the abscess would have saved her. The mission doctor could have done this and arranged a frontoethmoidectomy with an ENT surgeon later. The ENT surgeon's advice was inadequate because he only advised drainage of the sinus.*

Frontal epidural abscess

An epidural collection of pus posterior to a frontal sinusitis may result in scalp and eyelid swelling in the region, continual headache, fever and signs of meningism. The pus may collect over the orbital roof (Figure 74, previous page). Complications of an untreated epidural abscess are cerebral abscess, subdural empyema, meningitis and osteomyelitis of the frontal bone with secondary scalp swelling which is due to oedema and often subgaleal pus collection (**Pott's puffy tumour**). This tender lump may occur at a distance from the frontal sinus (Figure 7.5, next page). Osteomyelitis of the skull may also complicate middle ear infection. The epidural collection may be difficult to diagnose without a CT. If there is no CT, the infected sinus needs to be drained and the epidural space in the vicinity inspected. The appropriate intravenous antibiotics are commenced. Any infected bone requires debridement and delayed cranioplasty.

Abscess complicating open fracture

Abscess secondary to compound fracture is remarkably uncommon, and usually means that foreign material has been left in the brain at the time of initial treatment. The cavity should therefore be explored carefully. Abscesses also occasionally follow lacerations without evidence of fracture. The injury may have been weeks before, and the abscess may therefore be found unexpectedly.

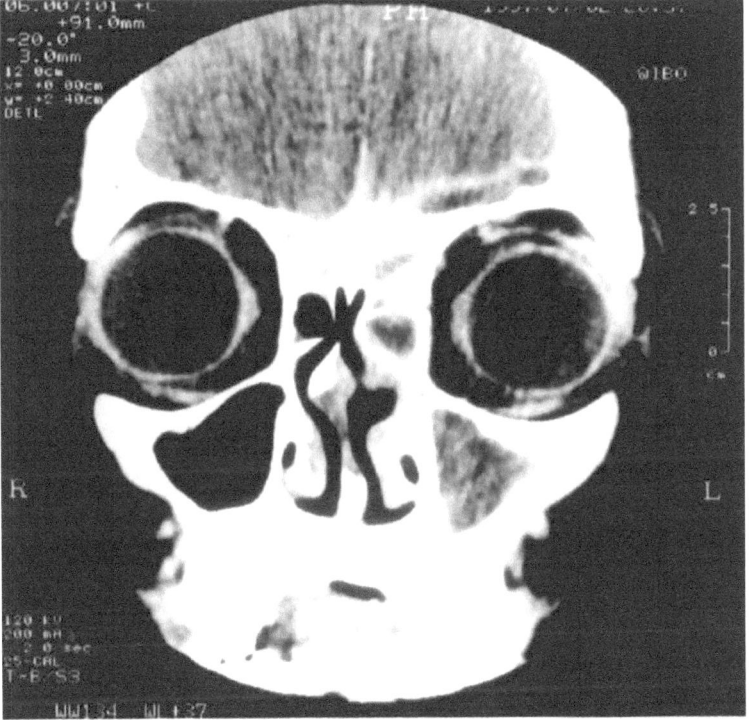

Figure 7.5 CT scan showing supraorbital epidural abscess secondary to frontal sinusitis.

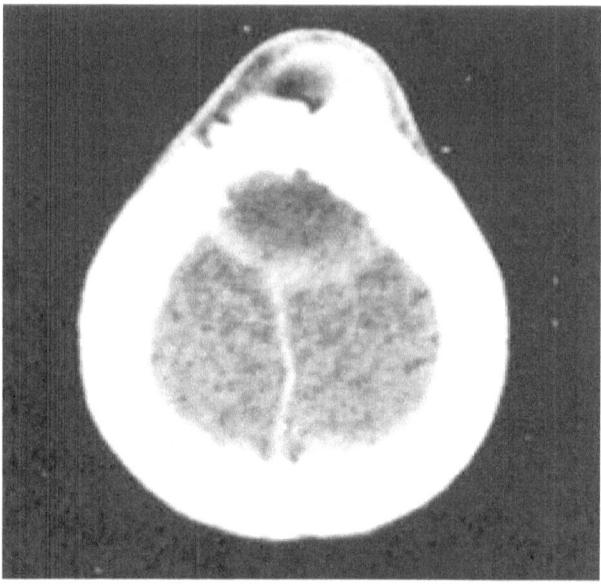

(a)

(b)

Figure 7.6 (a-b) CT scan showing osteomyelitis of the frontal bone with subgaleal and epidural abscess. Note the gross scalp swelling which is in the mid-frontal region. This was secondary to frontal sinusitis, and represents a Pott's puffy tumour.

Case report

A young woman presented with severe headache and papilloedema, and stated that her husband had stabbed her in the back of the head 4 weeks previously. The wound had been sutured at the aid post. There was a short, soundly healed laceration on the occiput. Apart from some neck stiffness no other abnormality as was detected. Carotid angiography suggested a paucity of veins in the left occipital lobe. A burr hole disclosed an occipital abscess which was drained twice, with apparent cure.

Metastatic abscess

Metastatic abscess may occur anywhere in the brain, but most commonly in middle cerebral territory. It is sometimes of a dumbbell shape or loculated, so that apparently satisfactory drainage produces a poor clinical response, perhaps with persistent severe headache, or dilated pupil failing to return to normal. Where CT facilities are available there should be no confusion, but otherwise the imaging studies should be carefully reassessed, repeated or extended. This is the situation in which emergency craniotomy to allow excision of the whole abscess complex is sometimes required. The known abscess is exposed, its wall is carefully dissected out, and this leads to the second half of the dumb-bell.

Chapter Seven

MENINGITIS AND ENCEPHALITIS

John D. Vince

Meningitis is an inflammation of the meninges as a result of infection with bacteria, viruses, fungi or protozoa. Secondary infection may spread to the meninges from open skull fractures, sinusitis, or middle ear infections. Among the commonest bacteria are *Neisseria meningitidis*, *Haemophilus influenzae* and *Streptococcus pneumoniae*. Viral meningitis is usually due to enteroviruses, or mumps. Subacute meningitis may be due to tuberculosis or cryptococcal infection.

Listeria monocytogenes and *Cryptococcus neoformans* (var. *neoformans*) may occur in immune deficient patients. Meningism is the sign of meningeal irritation but without infection, such as may occur with subarachnoid haemorrhage. Encephalitis is diffuse infection of the brain with an altered conscious level. The commonest organisms are rabies, trypanosomiasis, post infectious (mumps, measles, chicken pox, rubella and cytomegalovirus), herpes simplex, and arboviruses often specific to a particular geographic area (e.g. Japanese B encephalitis). In HIV infection, toxoplasma encephalitis is not uncommon, although few centres have CT facilities for diagnosis.

Clinical recognition

The typical signs are fever, headache, neck stiffness and altered consciousness. Neck stiffness may be obvious or difficult to detect and may be accompanied by Kernig's or Brudzinski's signs*[50] in 50 percent of adult cases. Neck stiffness may be absent in the very young, the very old or the very ill. Cranial nerve palsies, fits and focal cerebral signs occur in no more than 30 percent of cases. Papilloedema is rare in meningitis, occurring in less than 1 percent. It is important to consider the diagnosis in all patients with unexplained fever, headache, neck stiffness or altered consciousness. The diagnosis

---

[50]*Kernig's sign is a sign of meningism: the patient is supine; the thigh is flexed and the leg is extended. It will be very stiff.*
Brudzinski's sign: passive flexion of the neck causes flexion of the legs, or flexion of one leg causes similar movement of the other leg.

363

cannot be confirmed without a lumbar puncture, which should be performed in every case unless there is papilloedema or the patient is critically ill. Failure to perform a lumbar puncture is a common cause of treatment delay or misdiagnosis in the tropics.

Practice point

Any patient who has been noted to have neck stiffness, unexplained fever or altered consciousness should have a lumbar puncture, providing there is no papilloedema and the patient is not critically ill.

Practice point

Do not wait for the results of the lumbar puncture to start antibiotics because meningitis may be fulminating and cause death within a few hours if untreated.

Management

Patients with cloudy CSF or polymorphs on microscopy should be started empirically on intravenous antibiotics while the results of culture are awaited. Third generation cephalosporins (cefotaxime or ceftriaxone) if available are the antibiotics of choice. In their absence chloramphenicol or high dose penicillin or amoxycillin (or ampicillin) can be used Note that gentamicin does not cross the blood-brain barrier readily but is recommended for *Listeria monocytogenes* and Enterobacteriaceae infection.

Once the type of meningitis is determined by the laboratory the treatment can be altered. The treatment of tuberculous and cryptococcal meningitis is discussed on page 367. Antibiotic therapy is recommended for at least 10 days for *H. influenzae* and *N. meningitidis* and 14-21 days for other bacterial infections depending on the organism and the response of the patient. Cryptococcal infection requires 6 weeks of antifungal therapy. If the patient fails to improve or deteriorates consider the development of an intracerebral abscess, or undiagnosed coexistent malaria. A repeat LP should be performed to allow the CSF to be re-examined for other organisms. The development of raised intracranial pressure and coma should be treated as described on page 431.

Tuberculous meningitis

Tuberculous meningitis occurs following the acute haematogenous phase from a primary focus in the lungs or lymph nodes. It must be treated early as there is a high mortality and morbidity if treatment is delayed. The disease presents at a variety of different stages.

1. **Early course** - insidious onset with a low-grade fever, vomiting, apathy, drowsiness alternating with irritability, headache in older children and adults. At this stage there may be no neck rigidity.

2. **Intermediate stage** - after 1-2 weeks - meningism, photophobia, focal neurological signs - such as cranial nerve palsy, hemiparesis. On fundoscopy there may be papilloedema or, rarely, choroid tubercles.

3. **Late stage** - coma with decerebrate rigidity. Multiple permanent neurological deficits if patients survive.

There may be a florid inflammatory reaction with basal arachnoiditis resulting in secondary hydrocephalus (acquired, communicating hydrocephalus). The CSF (Table 7.2, next page) shows a pleocytosis of 15-50 cells/mm^3, but may be several hundred in the acute phase, with a predominance of lymphocytes. The protein is usually > 1 g/100 ml, glucose is low, and the acid-fast bacilli may be detected in the CSF. The availability of PCR technology in the form of GeneExpert testing can confirm the diagnosis within a matter of hours. A **chronic tuberculous meningitis** may develop and includes hydrocephalus, cranial nerve palsies and arteritis.

Table 7.2 Laboratory diagnosis of meningitis.

Investigation	Pyogenic	Viral	Other
Blood	Polymorphs	Lymphocytes	Lymphocytes in TB
Culture	Useful	No	No
Antigens	Useful	May be useful	No
CSF			
Appearances	Turbid or purulent	Clear	Clear
Cells	Polymorphs	Lymphocytes	Lymphocytes in TB
Organisms	Gram stain or culture	Special culture	India ink stain for Cryptococcus; culture for TB PCR(GeneExpert) for TB
Antigens	For negative Gram stain: Polymerase chain reaction (PCR) for meningoccus	No	For cryptococcus
Biochemistry			
Glucose	Low	Normal	Low in TB
Chloride	Norman	Normal	Low
Protein	Raised	Raised	Raised

A lymphocyte predominance in the CSF may occur in bacterial meningitis in about 10% of cases, particularly in neonates with Gram negative meningitis, and in Listeria monocytogenes meningitis.

The principles of treatment are similar to those for other forms of tuberculosis. Multiple drugs are necessary to prevent emergence of resistance. First line agents are isoniazid, rifampicin, pyrazinamide, ethambutol and streptomycin. Corticosteroids may improve the condition of patients with severe cerebral oedema or focal neurological signs.

Cryptococcal meningitis

Cryptococcus neoformans is an encapsulated fungus and a cause of meningitis and encephalitis or brain abscess (cryptococcoma) in the tropics. There are two subspecies, var. *gattii* which affects immune competent patients and var. *neoformans* which is prevalent worldwide and most frequently pathogenic in immune suppressed and HIV patients. It is sometimes transmitted from parrots and other birds' faeces (pigeon fancier's disease). The patient may present with bilateral blindness but this is more common with var. *gattii* infection than var. *neoformans.*

The mortality untreated is very high. The higher incidence of blindness with var. *gattii* may be related to an immune reaction to the infection, which explains the higher incidence in the immune competent and the reduction by steroid therapy (see below). The diagnosis is made by microscopy of the CSF stained with Indian ink stain. If lumbar puncture is contraindicated because of raised intracranial pressure, serum cryptococcal titres greater than 1:8 dilution strongly suggest cryptococcal infection. A chest X-ray may reveal a mass (or rarely multiple) lesion of cryptococcus, typically in the lung apex but coexistent brain and chest masses are extremely rare.

Therapy is with intravenous amphotericin B (0.3-1 mg/kg/day) and flucytosine 150 mg/kg/day in divided doses) for at least 6 weeks. Corticosteroids may prevent or reduce visual loss (100-250 mg hydrocortisone daily).

Subdural effusion

This may complicate bacterial meningitis in infants. It presents during the second week with fever, irritability, vomiting and sometimes convulsions or increasing head size with a tense bulging anterior fontanelle. The diagnosis is made by a subdural tap, which is also therapeutic. A lumbar puncture needle is passed from the lateral edge of the fontanelle forwards and laterally, keeping close beneath the bone edge, aspirating on the withdrawal. The fluid should be sent for microbiological analysis.

PARALYSIS, SPINAL CORD DISORDERS AND PERIPHERAL NEUROPATHY

Spinal cord compression is discussed in detail in Chapter 5. The common infectious causes are tuberculosis and staphylococcal or other pyogenic abscesses. Tuberculosis is usually but not always extradural, and originates in the adjacent vertebrae and discs. Spinal tuberculosis is discussed in detail in Chapter 5, page 253. Pyogenic abscesses may be extradural, subdural or intramedullary and the most common organism to be implicated is *Staphylococcus aureus.* The prognosis for recovery is usually poor after pyogenic infections, but with tuberculosis over 70 per cent of cases can be expected to make a full neurological recovery. The differential diagnosis of paralysis includes many interesting infectious or tropical diseases. The list below is only a selection. The principle of diagnosis is to consider a wide range of possibilities and to provide ventilatory support if necessary. A full account of the presentation and management of these diseases is beyond the scope of this book. A brief description is given below and the reader should refer to textbooks of tropical or infectious diseases for further details.

Acute infectious polyneuritis (Guillain-Barré syndrome)

There is often a preceding mild upper respiratory infection or fever days or weeks earlier, occasionally following a recognised infection such as infectious mononucleosis. There is demyelination in the peripheral nerves, nerve roots and sometimes the anterior horn cells. The patient presents with a sudden onset of weakness, usually symmetrical, which ascends from the lower limbs and may lead to respiratory paralysis. Muscle tenderness and paraesthesia may occur but sensory symptoms are uncommon. There may be facial nerve involvement, and meningism may occur in children. The symptoms progress for 7-10 days before recovery occurs - which may be slow, over many months, and incomplete. There is no therapy in the developing world. Plasmapheresis has helped lessen the severity of the illness. The patient should be transferred to somewhere with facilities for ventilatory support in case the disease progresses to involve the intercostal and phrenic nerves.

Poliomyelitis

Polio is a viral infection of the gastrointestinal tract which spreads to cause meningitis and damages the anterior horn cells. It is usually more severe, and the onset of the paralysis is slower than Guillain-Barré; it is also less symmetrical and morepatchy. Polio results in a motor neuropathy with flaccid paralysis and preservation of sensation. Activity during the prodromal phase makes the eventual paralysis worse. There is no effective antiviral treatment for polio. The patient should rest to minimise eventual paralysis and if the intercostal muscles or brain stem is involved may need ventilatory support. During the illness and the recovery phase all affected joints should be put through their full range of movement to avoid contractures. The rehabilitation of a polio victim may involve organising aids such as a calliper, crutches or wheelchair. Tenotomies may be indicated in selected patients with contracture due to muscle imbalance.

Tick paralysis

A number of hard ticks (Family Ixodidae) can cause paralysis: *Dermacentor andersoni* (female - wood tick), *D. variabilis* (female - dog tick), *Amblyomma americanum* (nymph - lone star tick) and *A. maculatum* and *Ixodes holocyclus* (female). They live in domestic and wild animals. May attach to human skin for several days and may bite between hairs on the scalp. The toxin injected from the salivary gland of the gravid female may cause acute ascending bilateral flaccid paralysis, including respiratory depression. The diagnosis must be considered and the body searched for ticks. The tick should be removed with its mouth parts for a chance of recovery. Ether, spirit, tincture of iodine, or petrol should be applied to the tick which is then removed with forceps.

Lathyrism

Lathyrus sativus (grass pea or khesari) is a hardy crop, but when its seeds form more than one-third of the diet for 3-6 months, lathyrism occurs. There is an acute or subacute onset of muscle cramps, weakness and stiffness in the lower limbs with progression to paraplegia in some. The toxic agent is ß-oxalyl-L-α,ß-diaminopropionic acid (ODAP).

There is microgliosis in the anterior and lateral horns of the spinal cord, with degeneration of motor tracts.

Retropharyngeal abscess

A large retropharyngeal abscess may cause subluxation of the atlantoaxial joint with quadriparesis.

Spinal neurosyphilis

Absent ankle reflexes, loss of posterior column sensation in the lower limbs are the classical signs of tabes dorsalis. Argyll Robertson pupils, where the affected pupil is small and the two pupils are irregular and unequal, there is loss of reaction to light but the reaction to accommodation is preserved, are another characteristic sign of neurosyphilis. There may be Charcot joints (joints deformed and destroyed by lack of sensation) and neuropathic ulcers on the lower limbs. The serum and CSF should be screened for syphilis. Syphilis should always be considered, especially if the pupils are unequal. The patient will need effective penicillin therapy.

HTLV I and II

Human T cell leukaemia virus I is a retrovirus endemic in the Caribbean, Japan and some parts of West and Central Africa. It is a retroviral infection which is spread by sexual intercourse, blood transfusion or intravenous drug abuse. It is associated with tropical spastic paraparesis (HTLV associated myelopathy) and adult T cell leukaemia. Most people infected by the virus remain healthy with a lifetime risk of 2.5 per cent for leukaemia and 0.25 per cent for tropical spastic paraparesis. HTLV II is endemic in New Mexico (USA) and some Native Americans and may also very rarely cause chronic neurological disease.

Clinical manifestations of HTLV I

1. **HTLV-I Associated paraplegia (HAP) also called 'tropical spastic paraparesis' (TSP).** There is a slowly progressive spastic paraparesis usually beginning after the age of 30 but sometimes even after the age of 70. Associated bladder involvement and back and lower limb pain are common. There may be mild sensory signs.

The disease may arrest and the degree of disability varies considerably in the chronic stage. Myelography should be used to exclude a compressive lesion and often shows an atrophic cord in chronic cases.

2. **Peripheral neuropathies and myositis.** There is a mild sensorimotor neuropathy affecting the distal lower limbs.
3. Associated systemic symptoms such as **uveitis, lymphocytic alveolitis and sicca (Sjögren's) syndrome**.

Human immunodeficiency virus (HIV) infection

HIV infection may result in neuropathy and myelopathy. (See complete section on HIV, below).

Early: subacute and chronic idiopathic demyelinating neuropathies may develop during the period of clinical latency. The pathogenesis is usually autoimmune.

Late: vacuolar myelopathy (part of AIDS dementia complex).

Opportunistic infection with cytomegalovirus (CMV) may cause a subacute progressive polyradiculopathy by direct infection of the nerve roots. It presents with pain and ascends after first involving the lumbosacral roots. CSF pleocytosis with neutrophil predominance is found.

Spiders, scorpions, snakes and jellyfish

Bites from species with neurotoxic venom may present with rapid onset paralysis and ventilatory failure. It is important to be aware of which species live in your area and always consider the possibility of a bite in a case of unexplained paralysis. In many parts of the world including Papua New Guinea snake bite is the commonest reason for requiring ventilatory support. Examine the entire skin surface for signs of a bite. There may be little or no local reaction. Systemic symptoms may develop within minutes or hours after a bite or sting. Treatment involves admission for observation, ventilatory support when necessary, and appropriate antivenom if available.

Tetanus

Tetanus is characterised by muscle rigidity, spasms, sweating, hypersecretion and autonomic instability. Tetanospasmin and tetanolysin are the two toxins produced by Clostridium tetani, an obligate anaerobe. Non-immune individuals are at risk. The onset is 2-10 days, with head wounds presenting before foot wounds because the toxin has to travel along the nerves to the spinal cord and/or brain stem. The patient may present with inability to open his mouth (lockjaw) or difficulty in walking. In Zambia head wounds are the commonest wound to result in tetanus but any wound may result in tetanus, particularly dirty and deep ones.

The diagnosis is clinical. Anti-tetanus immunoglobulin may be beneficial even after symptoms have started and may be given intrathecally. The wound should be excised and left open. The treatment is to reduce muscle rigidity with diazepam, sedation with opiates which may reduce the autonomic instability, and maintain fluid balance. Beta blockers may be indicated for tachycardia. Patients should not be nursed in a darkened room and neglected.

They require monitoring, and intensive nursing care to avoid death from pneumonia. Ventilatory support and muscle relaxants may be needed for severe cases which comprise at least two-thirds of cases, and this respiratory support may need to be continued for several weeks, if the facility and resources are available.

Peripheral nerve disorders

Leprosy is discussed in Chapter 10 on page 494. HIV infection causing peripheral neuropathy is discussed in detail in the next section.

HIV INFECTION (AIDS)[51]

HIV causes the Acquired Immune Deficiency Disease (AIDS). AIDS was first recognised in 1981. At this time opportunistic infections were treated and supportive care provided. By 2017, there were 36.9 million HIV-infected people in the world. Since the

[51]Fauci AS, Marston H. Achieving an AIDS-free world: science and implementation. Lancet. 2013;382:1461-62.

Deeks SG, Lewin SF, Havlir DV. The end of AIDS: HIV infection as a chronic disease. Lancet. 2013;383: 1525-1533.

Fauci AS, Marston HD. Ending the HIV-AIDS pandemic - follow the science. New England Journal of Medicine. 2015;373:2197-2199.

beginning of the epidemic, more than 70 million people have been infected with the HIV virus and about 35 million people have died of HIV by 2017. By 2012, 9.7 million HIV-infected individuals worldwide were receiving antiretroviral therapy (ART). Combinations of various preventive measures were proving more effective. The ART is a lifelong treatment. As a result, 4.2 million deaths were averted in the preceding decade in developing low-income and middle-income countries. HIV infection has become a major scourge in the developing world.

Treatment of an HIV-infected individual with ART reduces the risk of HIV transmission to his or her sexual partner, and reduces community-level of HIV incidence. An effective HIV vaccine is awaited. Co-infection with tuberculosis and hepatitis B and C further complicates the course of those with HIV. AIDS-related illnesses are no longer the threat they once were. As ART treated individuals have survived longer, chronic comorbidities associated with HIV infection have emerged. These include atherosclerosis, some cancers, liver and kidney disease and neurocognitive problems. Cumulative toxic effects from exposure to antiretroviral drugs for decades may also cause metabolic disturbance and end-organ damage. This chronic comorbidity may affect healthy ageing putting stress on resource poor health systems. However, the benefits of therapy far outweigh the toxic effects of the therapy.

NEUROLOGICAL MANIFESTATIONS OF HIV INFECTION

The human immunodeficiency virus (HIV) type 1 and 2 are lentiviruses, which are a subfamily of the retroviruses. At least 40 percent of patients with HIV infection develop neurological manifestations at some stage in their disease and 80-90 percent of patients have neuropathological findings at autopsy. In the tropics, heterosexual transmission and transmission via infected needles or blood are playing an increasing role in spreading the disease, as opposed to homosexual activity. High rates of infection are present in certain groups in some parts of Africa, such as pregnant women (30 percent), and prostitutes (90 per cent). Tuberculosis is resurgent along with the HIV epidemic and the course of tuberculosis is often accelerated in patients with underlying HIV infection. Recrudescence of active tuberculosis may also indicate an underlying HIV infection.

The incidence of syphilis is also increased in the HIV infected population. The protean effects of the HIV virus on the nervous system are due to opportunistic infections, tumours and to the direct pathogenic effects of the virus. It is thus important that physicians working in the tropics consider underlying HIV infection in patients with neurological disorders. The neurological complications of HIV cause considerable morbidity and a significant mortality, but accurate and early diagnosis is important as many of these complications can be treated. Acute neurological manifestations may occur when patients first develop antibodies to HIV, usually within 3 months of exposure to the virus, and before the development of Acquired Immune Deficiency Disease (AIDS).

Early CNS infection is usually asymptomatic or causes mild symptoms like headache or meningism. More definite episodes of encephalitis, meningitis, myelopathy and neuropathy may occur. The acute encephalitis involves fever, mood change, alteration in level of consciousness and convulsions and usually improves significantly within one week. The neuropathy may manifest as a facial palsy or brachial plexopathy. Subacute or chronic presentations of neurological disorders may occur before the development of AIDS like aseptic meningitis, which may recur or become chronic, involve cranial nerves 7 and 8, and develop long tract signs. Other presentations are subacute encephalitis, mononeuritis multiplex, peripheral neuropathy, and vacuolar myelopathy.

The AIDS-dementia complex (ADC)

ADC is the commonest CNS complication of HIV infection, affecting one third to two-thirds of AIDS patients in industrialised countries. The WHO definition of ADC requires that opportunistic infection and malignancy have been excluded although this would be difficult to do in the tropics where diagnostic facilities are limited. Cytomegalovirus, herpes simplex virus, atypical mycobacteria, diffuse lymphoma, and rarely varicella zoster may also cause a subacute encephalitis. ADC generally only develops when there is severe immune deficiency.

- **Cause:** Due to a direct effect of HIV on the brain including the cytotoxic effects of an immune reaction to the virus.
- **Symptoms:** There are five stages of ADC: 0 (normality), 0.5 (equivocal, subclinical), 1 (mild), 2 (moderate), 3 (severe), 4 (end stage). ADC usually starts with subtle cognitive changes such as forgetfulness, loss of concentration, and deterioration in handwriting. There may also be a loss of balance, and leg

weakness. Lethargy, apathy and withdrawal may suggest a depressive illness. An acute confusional state is a less common presentation. An impairment of conscious state may also be due to a metabolic encephalopathy such as hepatic, renal or pulmonary impairment or be drug induced.

- **Examination:** Mental state testing reveals cognitive impairment, motor examination variably reveals ataxia, limb weakness, spasticity and a positive Babinski sign. Frontal lobe release reflexes such as the grasp and snout reflexes may also be present. Abnormal movements such as tremor, myoclonus and chorea may also develop.
- **Investigations:** CT scan shows cerebral atrophy with dilated ventricle and prominent sulci. CSF may show a mild lymphocytic pleocytosis with increased protein, or lowered glucose.
- **Course:** There may be a rapid decline over several weeks or months leading to severe dementia with the patient becoming bedridden and incontinent. The 6-month cumulative mortality of ADC is 67 per cent. Zidovudine may have therapeutic and prophylactic value in ADC.

Psychiatric manifestations

Psychiatric disturbance is common in the patients with ADC. This may manifest as anxiety, depression, psychosis, or mania. A secondary stress reaction to the illness and medication effects may contribute as well as the organic disease.

Meningitis

- **Cause:** *Cryptococcus neoformans* is the most common. Can be aseptic, or tuberculous.
- **Symptoms:** fatigue, fever, weight loss, headache, nausea, vomiting.
- **Signs:** photophobia, meningism, focal signs. The infection may involve other organs such as skin, lungs, eyes, and kidneys.
- **Diagnosis:** Lumbar puncture shows a pleocytosis, raised protein, lowered glucose a positive identification on Indian ink staining. CT is usually normal.
- **Therapy:** Cryptococcus is treated with amphotericin (see Chapter 7, page 367).

Cerebral space occupying lesions

These may be due to:

1. Opportunistic infections - toxoplasmosis (5-20 percent of AIDS patients), candidiasis, *Myco-bacterium tuberculosis*, cytomegalovirus (CMV).
2. Tumours - primary cerebral lymphoma.
   These develop only in the presence of severe immune deficiency.
   - **Clinical features:** Raised ICP and focal signs (often a hemiparesis).
   - Lethargy and confusion may be present for days or weeks.
   - **Investigation:** CT scan may show ring enhancing lesion(s).
   - **Therapy:** Toxoplasmosis can be treated with pyrimethamine and sulphadiazine or clindamycin (for those allergic to sulpha drugs). In the tropics, the treatment can be commenced when the clinical diagnosis is made, and usually patients will respond within a few days of starting the therapy. Prophylactic anticonvulsants should also be used because of the high risk of associated epilepsy.
   The prognosis of cerebral lymphoma is poor.

Progressive multifocal leukoencephalopathy (PML)

- **Cause:** Demyelination is caused by JC papova virus infection.
- **Clinical features:** Affects 2-5 percent of AIDS patients and presents with aphasia, blindness, ataxia, hemiparesis.
- **Investigation:** CT scan shows low density lesions without contrast enhancement.
- **Clinical course:** No treatment available. Usually inexorable decline to death.

Visual loss

- **Cause:** Cytomegalovirus retinitis is the most common.
- **Fundal examination:** Firstly, the vessels become irregular and narrower, then haemorrhages and exudates appear, and finally there is infarction of affected retina.
- **Course:** Untreated, the infection may progress to bilateral blindness. Toxoplasmosis chorioretinitis may also occur.

Myelopathy

- **Pathology:** Vacuolar myelopathy. Less commonly caused by varicella zoster myelitis or epidural or subdural lymphoma.
- **Cause:** Vacuolar myelopathy is probably due to the direct effect of HIV on the spinal cord.
- **Symptoms:** Paraesthesia, bilateral leg weakness. The leg weakness may be unilateral. Often associated with subacute encephalitis.
- **Signs:** Paraparesis with variable paraparesis, ataxia and sphincter involvement.

Peripheral neuropathy

Symptomatic neuropathy affects 5-10 percent of HIV infected patients. Most are due to autoimmune disease or the direct effect of HIV on the peripheral nerves.

The different types of neuropathy include:

1. **Inflammatory polyneuropathy** of the Guillain-Barré type in which there is mild to moderate motor deficit associated with fever, diarrhoea, rash, adenopathy and mononucleosis. It occurs at the time of seroconversion.
2. **Subacute multifocal neuropathy** is the commonest neuropathy of HIV occurring before the onset of cellular immunosuppression. There is a sensory and sensorimotor deficit in the lower limbs predominantly with paraesthesia and pain. The cranial nerves, especially the facial nerves may be affected. The reflexes are brisk and the Babinski sign may be present. Patients usually improve on steroids.
3. **Distal symmetrical polyneuropathy** or distal sensory polyneuropathy (DSPN) is the commonest occurring late in the course. There are burning foot pains with unpleasant dysaesthesia on skin contact. Motor involvement is usually minimal. It is often associated with subacute encephalitis.
4. **Dysautonomia.** Postural hypotension, sweating, paroxysmal hypertension, abnormal pupil reactions, and sphincter disturbances may occur in association with sensory neuropathy or separately.
5. **Cytomegalovirus (CMV) neuropathy** occurs in the late stage of immune system depression. CMV is the commonest viral infection in HIV (15-35 percent of patients). The peripheral neuropathy is associated with retinitis or with symptomatic infection of other

organs. It is treatable with ganciclovir or foscarnet. When a severe multifocal subacute sensorimotor neuropathy develops in an advanced HIV patient, specific treatment for CMV may be appropriate depending on the setting.

6. **Varicella zoster (shingles)** occurs in 10-15 percent of patients with HIV infection in the tropics and postherpetic neuralgia is common and often severe.

7. **Lymphoma** may infiltrate peripheral nerves or spinal roots and cause focal or multifocal nerve lesions.

Myopathy

Idiopathic inflammatory myopathy may occur in association with the peripheral neuropathy which further confuses the clinical picture. This leads to muscle cramps, muscle weakness and prominent muscle wasting. Steroids may be helpful. Staphylococcal myositis is a common complication of AIDS in the tropics.

Transient ischaemic attacks (TIAs) and strokes

TIAs and strokes are uncommon in children and adults with HIV infection. The course is often benign and the pathogenesis unclear.

Needle stick and scalpel injury

Surgeons wherever they are operating, should assume all patients potentially carry HIV and Hepatitis B and C and take all necessary precautions to avoid needle or scalpel injury during surgery. Continuous awareness and meticulous surgical technique in the handling of sharps is the best way to avoid the injury. For instance, all sharps should be handed by the instrument nurse or assistant in a separate bowl and the surgeon should place the used sharps back in this bowl.

The surgeon should avoid touching the sharp ends of fractured or partially drilled bone. Double gloving may afford some extra protection. If these injuries occur, the surgeon should immediately discard the gloves, unscrub and should wash the affected finger thoroughly in soap and water and betadine or an alternative antiseptic. The patient and the surgeon have blood taken to be tested for HIV antibody, Hepatitis B Surface antigen, and Hepatitis C antibody.

If the patient is HIV positive the surgeon should seek infectious disease consultation, commence ARV therapy as soon as practicable after the exposure and await retesting. The patient will need to be consented for the blood tests and the explanation given for them. Management of exposure to definite or possible

Hepatitis B depends on whether the surgeon has been previously vaccinated for Hepatitis B or been previously infected with it. When the surgeon has not been previously infected and is not immune, Hepatitis B immunoglobulin should be given within 72 hours of the injury. A hepatitis B vaccination should also be administered.

The risk of tetanus should also be assessed. The surgeon may require either tetanus immunoglobulin or a course of adult diphtheria and tetanus (ADT) or an ADT booster. The surgeon should ensure that the incident is clearly documented in the medical record.

SPECIFIC INFECTIONS

Cysticercosis

The commonest parasitic disease of the CNS.
- **Cause:** pork tapeworm - *Taenia solium*
- **Geographical distribution:** Latin America, Africa, Asia
- **Age:** rare in children
- **Incubation:** ± 5 years.
- **Cycle:** adult tapeworm - 2-3 metres length in human small intestine - pig eats ova or gravid worm segments - spread throughout the pig - human eats the infected pork or faecal oral contamination.
- **Spreads** through stomach to brain where the larval worm forms a fluid filled vesicle (with an invaginated scolex) (*Cysticercus cellulosae*) up to 20 mm. They degenerate over a number of years, calcify and incite an inflammatory reaction (Figure 7.7, next page). Multiple larger vesicles or inflammatory masses (Cysticercus racemosus) may develop in the ventricles, basal cisterns, spinal cord and nerve root. The disease may spread in the subarachnoid space and cause a meningoencephalitis. There may be recurrent clinical episodes over 2-5 years and then the disease subsides.

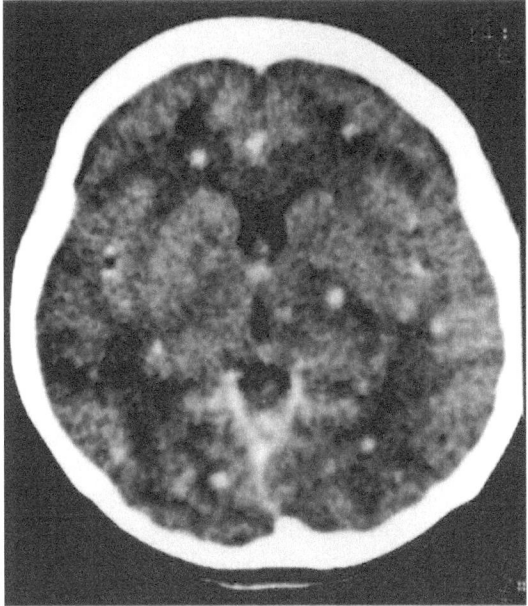

Figure 7.7 CT scan showing multiple calcified lesions, presumed to be cysticercosis and treated with praziquantel.

Clinical presentation

The clinical course varies from mild infection, which heals spontaneously, to sudden death after many years, or recurrent manifestations which result in a poor prognosis.

1. Raised ICP which may be due to hydrocephalus
2. Focal signs - especially related to basal cistern involvement, e.g.
   - optic chiasms/nerves - visual impairment
   - other cranial nerves
   - cerebellum
3. Epilepsy
4. Meningitis
5. Apoplectic: ? mimicking stroke
6. Psychiatric: mental disturbance. Confusional state - is the commonest
7. Spinal (5 percent) usually extramedullary
   - cervical commonest
   - rarely intramedullary

Investigation

- CSF antibodies
- Lymphocyte pleocytosis with eosinophils.
- Increased protein and IgG

Management

Medical

Praziquantel (50 mg/kg/day), and albendazole (15 mg/kg/day) kill viable cysticercus in the parenchyma and steroids are useful to limit the associated CSF inflammation.[52] Continue treatment for 10–14 days rather than albendazole monotherapy for patients with more than two viable parenchymal cysticerci. Patients with raised intracranial pressure should have this treated in the first instance before treatment with albendazole and praziquantel. Ventricular and subarachnoid cysticercosis are resistant to medication.

Surgery

- Treat the specific lesion causing the clinical problem.
- Indicated for progressive clinical deterioration.
- Excision is technically difficult when the lesion is in the basal cisterns because of adherence to surrounding structures.
- Hydrocephalus is treated with a ventriculoperitoneal shunt - revisions may be required.
- Endoscopic techniques are being increasingly utilised for loculated hydrocephalus, to fenestrate loculations, and drain the ventricles via a third ventriculostomy, which may avoid the need for a shunt.
- Laminectomy and excision of cysts is indicated for cord compression.

Signs outside the CNS

- Subcuticular cyst
- Tongue nodule

---

[52]*Diagnosis and Treatment of Neurocysticercosis: 2017 Clinical Practice Guidelines by the Infectious Diseases Society of America (IDSA) and the American Society of Tropical Medicine and Hygiene (ASTMH). 2018;98(4):945–966.*

Infection

- Ocular cysticercosis, which may cause sudden blindness
- Pseudohypertrophy of muscle
- Heart - arrhythmias; cardiac failure, heart block.

Schistosomiasis (Table 7.3, below)

- Trematode - *Schistosoma* spp.
- **Geographical distribution:** Africa, Middle and Far East, South America.
- **Definitive hosts:** mammals and birds.
- Intermediate hosts: snails.

Pathogenesis

- Worms (blood flukes) infest the liver, portal mesenteric veins, internal iliac and vesical veins. Eggs travel through to the spinal veins and reach the lower spinal cord.
- Eggs reach the brain via the pulmonary circulation
- Worms in the brain are rare and probably enter via the vertebral venous plexus.
- CNS involvement is uncommon. There is a host granulomatous reaction to the eggs.

Table 7.3 Distribution and pathology of schistosomiasis.

	Location	Involvement
Schistosoma mansoni	Africa, S. America, Caribbean, M. East	Spinal cord, brain, intestinal/hepatosplenic
Schistosoma japonicum	Asia	Brain, intestinal/hepatosplenic
Schistosoma haematobium	Africa	Spinal cord, urinary tract

Cerebral schistosomiasis manifestations

- Encephalitis, meningoencephalitis.
- Space occupying lesion.
- Chronic symptoms, raised ICP, epilepsy.

Diagnosis

- CSF pleocytosis, high eosinophils.
- Brain: CT - focal enhancing mass lesions, or parenchymal lucency ± oedema.
- Spine: CT myelogram/MRI.
- Stool: schistosome eggs.
- Rectal biopsy (*S. mansoni*): bladder biopsy.
- Urine microscopy.
- Anti: schistosomal antibodies.

Clinical course

- *S. japonicum* - praziquantel - good prognosis. Steroids are useful for acute inflammation.
- *S. mansoni I S. haematobium* - often silent infection, mass lesions uncommon. May cause epilepsy.

Spinal schistosomiasis

- **Age:** Usually 10-30 years. More common in males.

Pathology

- Transverse myelitis which may result in spinal cord necrosis
- Granulomatous mass(es) involving conus medullaris or cauda equina.
- T12-L1 is the commonest level of involvement.

Clinical features

Spinal schistosomiasis is a potential cause of non-traumatic paraplegia in endemic areas and may be acute in onset. It presents with myelopathy or radiculopathy.

The patient complains of:
- low back pain, which is burning, severe and may or may not radiate to the lower limbs,
- lower limb weakness, paraesthesiae,
- sphincter disturbance.
- Other clinical features include:
- urine - haematuria,

- bowel - blood/mucus/diarrhoea,
- skin papules, especially perineum,
- hepatosplenomegaly,
- fever, anorexia, malaise, sweating, lymphadenopathy.

Treatment

There is a good response to praziquantel in myelopathy. Steroids may prevent hypersensitivity reactions resulting from death of the adult worm, and improve neurological deficit. Surgery not usually required, although spinal decompression and biopsy via laminectomy may be indicated for rapid deterioration or acute paraplegia. It is not usually possible to remove the lesions.

Hydatid disease (cystic type)

- **Cause:** the larval form of *Echinococcus granulosus.*
- **Geographical distribution:** Middle East, North Africa, South America, Australia.
- **Definitive host:** dog
- **Intermediate host:** sheep
- **Spread: dog faeces** - infects humans especially children/young adults
- **Route of infection:** eggs breed in the small intestine and form unilocular cysts in the liver and lung. CNS involvement occurs with spread to the brain or spine in 1-22 per cent. Rarely myocardial embolisation to the brain occurs.
- Cerebral hydatidosis presents as a mass lesion. There may be secondary cysts.

Management

Aim to excise the cyst intact. Spilling contents spreads the infection by allowing daughter cysts to grow. The cyst is removed and hydrogen peroxide or 20 per cent saline can be used to sterilise a spill and should be used routinely following cyst excision. Formalin 10 per cent cottonoids can also be placed along the walls of the cyst cavity. The technique of using gentle warm saline hydrostatic pressure (irrigation) through a rubber or plastic catheter placed between the brain and the cyst will help expel it intact (Dowling's technique).

Alteration of the table to a 45° head down tilt will also help to expel it. Cottonoids are progressively placed between the cyst and the brain. The cyst will eventually float out on the saline and the cavity is then thoroughly irrigated to clear residual lamellae of the cuticle of the cyst. If the cyst is large - cyst puncture with evacuation of the contents and placing hypertonic saline 20 per cent, formalin 10 per cent, cetrimide or silver nitrate into the cyst, will sterilise any residuum. The shrunken cyst wall is then removed, taking care not to spill the residual content of the cyst. Albendazole/praziquantel are used as adjunctive treatment. Indications for medical therapy are:
1. Spillage of cyst contents intraoperatively.
2. Small to moderate sized cysts especially if multiple.

Alveolar hydatid disease

This is a second variety of hydatid disease and is caused by *Echinococcus multilocularis*. The cysts grow by exogenous proliferation because there is no restricting alveolar membrane and it therefore resembles a 'malignant' form of hydatid disease. It occasionally metastasizes to lung and brain. It is found in the northern hemisphere particularly N. America and Russia. It is not usually a tropical infection.

Brucellosis

- **Cause:** Species of Brucella, a non-motile coccobacillus spread to humans by contact with infected animals and milk.
- **Geography:** tropical and subtropical areas.
- **Nervous system involvement:** in 5 per cent of cases - this takes the form of an acute meningoencephalitis, a spastic or flaccid paraparesis due to spinal cord compression or myelo-radiculopathy, and hemiparesis and ataxia due to cerebral involvement.
- **Diagnosis:** blood or CSF culture is positive for Brucella. ELISA test on blood or CSF
- **Treatment:** rifampicin or tetracycline and streptomycin for 3 months.

Neurosyphilis

- **Cause:** the spirochaete *Treponema pallidum.*

- **Neurosyphilis** has been uncommon probably because latent syphilis has been treated by the widespread use of antibiotics to treat other infections. More recently there is an increasing incidence in association with HIV infection. Much of the structural damage of neurosyphilis is irreversible.
- The three types of tertiary syphilis are cardiovascular (80 per cent), gummatous (10 per cent), and neurovascular (10 per cent) which consists of **meningovascular** and **parenchymatous** types. There is a focal or diffuse obliterative endarteritis, which variably causes hemiparesis, neuropathy, severe headache, mental changes, convulsions, or acute optic neuritis. The oculomotor nerve is particularly affected resulting in the Argyll Robertson pupils which are small, irregular, fixed, accommodate and do not react, with synechiae (adhesions) at the edge of the iris.
- The two forms of parenchymatous neurosyphilis are tabetic and paretic. There is an absence of vascular lesions and a selectivity in distribution.

  1. **Tabes dorsalis.** The dorsal roots and dorsal spinal cord are affected causing pain, weakness and sensory loss below the affected level. 'Lightning pains', paraesthesiae of the lower limbs, ataxia, trophic foot ulcers, and Charcot neuropathic joints may develop.

  2. **General paresis** is a progressive dementia and may include focal or generalised seizures. Tabes dorsalis may also be present.
     - **Serology:** VDRL, FTA (fluorescent treponemal antibody test), TPHA (T. *pallidum* haemagglutinin assay).
     - **Treatment:** high dose penicillin.

American trypanosomiasis (Chagas' disease)

- **Cause:** *Trypanosoma cruzi* is transmitted by blood sucking insects of the Triatoma subfamily. The trypanosome from the insects' faeces penetrates skin abrasions, the conjunctiva or mucous membranes.
- **Geography:** Latin America. There are an estimated 20 million sufferers.
- **Presentation:** Initial acute inflammatory reaction with a skin lump (chagoma) and local lymphadenopathy. Unilateral orbital oedema (Romaña's sign) is common. The disease may remain asymptomatic for many years. The main neurological manifestation is an autonomic neuropathy affecting the heart with

chronic cardiomyopathy and arrhythmias, and the gastrointestinal tract with megacolon and megaoesophagus. Pulmonary or systemic embolism may develop due to breakup of intracardiac mural thrombosis. A stroke may result from embolism to intracranial vessels. Peripheral neuropathy is uncommon.
- **Treatment:** nifurtimox, benznidazole.

African trypanosomiasis (sleeping sickness)

- **Cause:** *Trypanosoma brucei gambiense* and *rhodesiense* transmitted by the various species of tsetse flies (genus Glossina).
- **Presentation:** CNS involvement may occur in weeks to months (*rhodesiense*), or months to years (*gambiense*) following the initial infection. There is insidious and gradual progression, initially with alteration in personality and behaviour, indifference, lethargy, meningoencephalitis picture with headache, meningism, and papilloedema, daytime somnolence, often with night time insomnia, choreiform movements, fasciculations, muscular rigidity, dysarthria, cerebellar ataxia, Parkinsonism (rigidity, tremor, shuffling gait), late seizures, mania, and euphoria. Finally, there is further mental deterioration, pruritus, wasting, somnolence and then coma, cardiac failure and death.
- **Diagnosis:** CSF increased white cells (predominantly mononuclear) and protein, CSF pressure and IgM. Blood and CSF culture. Serology.
- **Treatment:** Early stage - suramin, pentamidine. Later stage with CNS invasion melarsoprol, melarsonyl potassium, difluoromethy-lornithine (DFMO), nifurtimox.

Lyme disease

- **Cause:** *Borrelia burgdorferi* (a spirochaete) following a bite from the infected nymphal stage of the hard tick (genus Ixodes).
- **Geography:** Temperate climates.
- **Presentation:** Nervous system involvement includes meningitis, encephalitis, cranial neuropathy including ischaemic optic neuropathy, pseudotumour cerebri, acute transverse myelitis, radiculitis, neuropathy, progressive encephalomyelitis and late encephalopathy with memory loss and dementia.

Post malaria neurologic syndrome

This syndrome is uncommon and usually follows severe malaria. The incidence is 1.2 (range 0.7-1.8) per 1000 cases. The clinical presentation is an acute confusional state, psychosis, generalised convulsions, tremor, or delayed cerebellar syndrome. It occurs once the parasitaemia is cleared, is self-limiting (median duration 60 hours), and is associated with the use of oral mefloquine.

Paragonimiasis (lung fluke)

- **Cause:** *Paragonimus westermani* is the most common species. It is a lung fluke acquired by eating infected crustaceans.
- **Geography:** Asia, Africa, South America.
- **Presentation:** There is often a history of chronic bronchitis and haemoptysis. Flukes may migrate from the lung and reach any organ.
  Cysts, granulomas which may become calcified, or abscesses then form around the flukes or their eggs. Cerebral involvement with this fluke is relatively uncommon and usually affects children below 10 years and mostly males. The patient may present with a wide range of neurological disorders including epilepsy, encephalitis, meningitis, cerebral mass lesion especially affecting the temporal and occipital lobes due to migration through the jugular or carotid foramen at the base of the skull, focal neurological signs, progressive encephalopathy and ophthalmological signs. Death during an attack is not uncommon. Rarely spinal cord involvement presents as paraplegia or monoplegia.
- **Investigation:** CSF pleocytosis with a high eosinophil count.
- **Treatment:** praziquantel or bithionol.

Gnathostomiasis (eosinophilic myeloencephalitis)

- **Cause:** *Gnathostoma spinigerum*. A nematode. Host: dogs, cats, wild animals.
- **Geography:** Widespread - Asia, Africa, Middle East, America, Russia, Australia. Source of human infection: consuming raw or undercooked fish, or contaminated drinking water.

- **Neurologic manifestations:** the worm migrates along large nerve trunks into the CNS causing severe nerve root pain, followed by paraparesis, urinary retention or uncommonly quadriplegia. A stroke-like illness uncommonly occurs with sudden severe headache followed by coma. In endemic areas gnathostomiasis should be considered a cause of cerebral haemorrhage particularly in young people. Findings at necropsy are of multiple areas and tracks of haemorrhage and/or necrosis in the brain.
- **Investigation:** Peripheral blood eosinophilia is present - up to 90 per cent. CSF may be bloodstained or xanthochromic and usually cell count is below 500 per mm^3 with greater than 20 per cent eosinophilia.
- **Treatment:** surgical removal of the worm is required. Antihelminthics have not been effective.

Angiostrongyliasis (eosinophilic meningitis or meningoencephalitis)

- **Cause:** *Angiostrongylus cantonensis.* Helminth. Nematode. Rat lungworm.
- **Geography:** widely distributed throughout the tropics. Humans ingest infected molluscs or shrimp. The disease is generally benign and self-limiting, but may be severe and fatal. The presentation is severe headache (sudden or gradual onset). Nausea, vomiting, meningism in the early stages. Usually low-grade pyrexia. Sensory disturbance with hypersensitivity, and paraesthesiae over the trunk and limbs, and in severe cases limb weakness to paralysis and impaired conscious state to coma and death. The cranial nerves may be affected, particularly optic, facial, and abducens. Visual impairment, optic atrophy, periorbital oedema, diplopia, and visual field defects may occur.
- **Investigation:** CSF - raised pressure. Turbid. Pleocytosis with a high eosinophil count (25-75 per cent). Increased eosinophils in the peripheral blood (15-50 per cent).
- **Treatment:** expectant. Use of antihelminthics may result in clinical deterioration and death. The fatality rate is low (0.5-3 per cent).

Sparganosis

- **Cause:** infection with spargana, the second stage larvae of the tapeworm genus *Spirometra*. The tapeworms occur in domestic and wild carnivores. Frogs, other reptiles and mammals may be intermediate hosts. Humans are infected from contaminated drinking water, or ingesting the spargana in the intermediate host or from poultices prepared from the frog. It is an uncommon infection.
- **Geographical distribution:** South-East Asia (Thailand, Japan, Vietnam), N. America, E. Africa.
- **Presenting symptoms:**
  - subcutaneous nodule,
  - conjunctivitis, periorbital oedema,
  - brain/spinal cord granuloma.
- **Treatment:** excision, and praziquantel.

Toxocariasis

- **Cause:** The helminths *Toxocara canis* and *T. cati*. Humans are infected with the embryonated eggs of dog and cat ascarids. The larvae then migrate to liver, lung, brain, and eye.
- **Geography:** worldwide distribution.
- **Presentation:** in many cases infection is asymptomatic. Eye involvement (ocular larva migrans) is uncommon but causes poor or absent unilateral vision, squint, retinal scar, vitreous haze, and cataract. Involvement of the lung (patchy pneumonitis), liver (hepatomegaly) or brain is called visceral larva migrans. Cerebral infection causes encephalitis, epilepsy and calcified lesions in the chronic stage. Peripheral blood eosinophilia is common in active infection.
- **Treatment:** none in asymptomatic cases. Diethylcarbamazine or thiabendazole for symptomatic cases and prevents further damage.

Aspergillosis

The fungal genus *Aspergillus* causes opportunistic infection in the immunocompromised host and occurs in temperate and tropical climates. **Invasive paranasal *Aspergillus* granuloma** is a slowly progressive infection, which may involve the orbit and brain. It is particularly seen in Africa and the Middle East and is usually caused by *A. flavus*. The X-rays show a mass in the ethmoid or maxillary sinus with bony erosion.

The treatment is aggressive surgical excision and long-term itraconazole. An aspergilloma without granuloma formation may also occur in the paranasal sinuses. The second CNS manifestation is the isolated and often multiple **cerebral abscesses** which require aggressive excision and itraconazole or intrathecal amphotericin. *Aspergillus* cerebral abscess has a high mortality despite aggressive therapy.

Blastomycosis

Blastomycosis is a systemic fungal disease caused by *Blastomyces dermatitidis*. It occurs in the USA, Africa, India and the Middle East. It enters the respiratory tract and dissemination is usually seen in the tropics and in the immunocompromised host. The spread is to skin where it causes granulomas, ulcers and crusted plaque lesions, and to the bones where vertebral involvement may cause **spinal cord compression.**

Mucormycosis

Mucormycosis occurs in the tropics and in temperate climates and is uncommon. It is a rapidly progressive infection affecting the paranasal sinuses, orbit and lungs and is caused by the fungal genera *Absidia, Rhizopus and Rhizomucor*. It rapidly spreads intracranially and invades the brain. The mortality is high and it requires aggressive early surgical debridement and amphotericin B. It particularly affects diabetics and the immunocompromised host.

Amoebiasis

The parasitic protozoan *Entamoeba histolytica* is estimated to cause infection in 480 million people worldwide and is a consequence of unsanitary living conditions and contaminated water supply. Most colonised individuals are asymptomatic with the organism living as an intestinal commensal. About 10 per cent develop disease in the colon (dysentery), and in the liver (abscess). **Cerebral amoebiasis** is uncommon (1.2-2.5 percent of patients with amoebiasis at autopsy) and is often sudden in onset presenting as a meningoencephalitis on a background of amoebic dysentery or liver abscess.

Focal neurological signs may be present. It is difficult to diagnose and, if suspected, may require a brain biopsy, with direct microscopy of the wet preparation. Lumbar puncture is non-specific. CT scan may show diffuse low-density areas or ring enhancing lesions. Intravenous metronidazole and chloroquine and evacuation or excision of abscesses are used to treat invasive amoebiasis.

Primary amoebic meningoencephalitis is an uncommon infection and is due to the free-living amoebae *Naegleria* and *Acanthamoeba*. It may be contracted while swimming in contaminated water and may present as an acute meningitis or a subacute or chronic granulomatous meningoencephalitis or cerebral abscess. *Naegleria* may enter via the olfactory apparatus. *Naegleria* may be seen in the CSF along with a pyogenic reaction. Amphotericin is used for the acute form and flucytosine or sulfamethazine for the chronic form. The prognosis is poor because the diagnosis is usually late.

Melioidosis

Melioidosis is an infection which occurs in Northern Australia and SouthEast Asia and is caused by Burkholderia pseudomallei (formerly Pseudomonas pseudomallei). It particularly affects immune compromised individuals such as diabetics, alcoholics, the malnourished and those on steroid therapy. It is a rare cause of soft tissue, lung and visceral abscesses but infection may develop anywhere so that it has occasionally been reported to cause brain abscess, encephalitis, or Guillain-Barré type syndrome. The presentation is often occult and not dramatic. Isolation requires selective media and the use of broth pre-enrichment for culture as serology in endemic areas may only be an indication of previous exposure. After appropriate treatment of the presenting problem (e.g. drainage of a brain abscess) 14 days of ceftazidime therapy is indicated followed by maintenance therapy with oral co-trimoxazole or doxycycline for 3 months.

Subacute sclerosing panencephalitis (SSPE)

Subacute sclerosing panencephalitis (SSPE) is an invariably fatal degenerative condition of the central nervous system which predominantly affects children and young adolescents. It is associated with measles virus infection, and possibly linked to certain strains of the virus. Before the introduction of measles vaccination, the incidence in the USA was estimated to be around 0.6/million in the under 20 age group. Considerably higher incidences have been reported from the tropics and Papua New Guinea has had the highest incidences (56 per million under 20-year-old in 1991). The clinical picture develops months or years after measles infection. The earliest sign is of changes in the child's behaviour and social and academic performance. A state of dementia gradually develops and there is usually insidious, progressive deterioration although temporary remission of symptoms does occur. Symmetrical hypertonicity and myoclonic jerks are common. Cerebellar ataxia and hypotonia may also occur. Inability to feed and coma finally develop. Death occurs within 1-2 years. The clinical features are highly characteristic, but the diagnosis can be confirmed by detecting elevated levels of antibody to measles virus in both serum and CSF (CSF antibodies being synthesised within the CNS). EEG, if available, may demonstrate characteristic but not specific changes of 'suppressive-burst episodes'. CT scan and MR may be initially normal but later show cortical atrophy with ventricular enlargement. The differential diagnosis includes tuberculous and cryptococcal meningitis, other degenerative diseases and neoplasm. There is no specific treatment. Some success has been claimed for slowing progression of disease with inosiplex, interferon alpha and cimetidine. Supportive treatment includes control of convulsions with benzodiazepines, nutritional support, nursing care and family support. In areas where tuberculosis is common, it is reasonable, pending a definite diagnosis, to start treatment for tuberculous meningitis. Vaccination against measles greatly reduces the risk.

Prion infections and spongiform encephalopathies

Consider in the differential diagnosis of incoordination, memory loss and dementia where all other diagnoses have been excluded. Spongiform encephalopathies were first recognised in sheep in the 1700s and include, in animals, scrapie (sheep), bovine spongiform encephalopathy (BSE - mad cow disease) and transmissible mink encephalopathy (TME). The diseases are transmissible between and within certain species and have reached notoriety because of BSE being transmitted through contaminated British beef to humans, causing a new variant of **Creutzfeldt-Jakob disease** (CJD).

The classical form of CJD was described separately by two German doctors, Creutzfeldt and Jakob, in 1920 and 1921, and occurs as a sporadic mutation in the order of 1 case in a million. An inherited spongiform encephalopathy in humans is Gerstmann-Sträussler-Scheinker disease. In the Fore region of Papua New Guinea ritual cannibalism of dead relatives in the 1950s and 1960s (presumably previously) resulted in a spongiform encephalopathy 'kuru' being transmitted to women and children who ate the brains of their relatives. Incubation takes some years before the onset of symptoms. The infectious agent for spongiform encephalopathies was originally thought to be a 'slow' virus but now is more likely to be a protein or **prion**. The name Prion means 'proteinaceous infectious particle'.

They are resistant to inactivation by most procedures that modify nucleic acids, including standard sterilisation procedures. Steam autoclaving for one hour at 132°C will inactivate prions. Immersion in 1N sodium hypochlorite (household bleach) undiluted or up to 1:10 (0.5 per cent) for one hour is partially effective only. Spongiform encephalopathies should be considered in the differential diagnosis of neurological signs and memory loss. The diagnosis of CJD is best made clinically including imaging, EEG, and LP, or by brain biopsy at autopsy which will stain for prion protein but not for Alzheimer's amyloid. MRI is the most useful diagnostic modality.

Lumbar puncture for cell count, 14-3-3 protein, S100B protein is of limited value. The usual practice in developed nations is that if one is performing a brain biopsy where there is a risk of CJD, then the instruments and all the drapes are discarded at the end of the procedure. This avoids any chance of transmission to future patients. We advise that in the developing world the diagnosis of suspected CJD be made clinically and that a biopsy would not be indicated where instruments are scarce.

The surgeon, nursing staff and pathologist are potentially at risk of contracting the disease if brain material is inadvertently squirted into the eye or a needle stick injury occurs. CJD is invariably fatal and is characterised by a rapidly progressive dementia, ataxia and myoclonus. Death usually occurs within a year of the onset of symptoms. The characteristic EEG finding is that of bilateral sharp waves (0.5-2 per second). There is no specific treatment or cure for spongiform encephalopathy.

Vascular disorders

BASIC ANATOMY

Figure 8.1 (below) and Figures 8.2 and 8.3 on the next page.

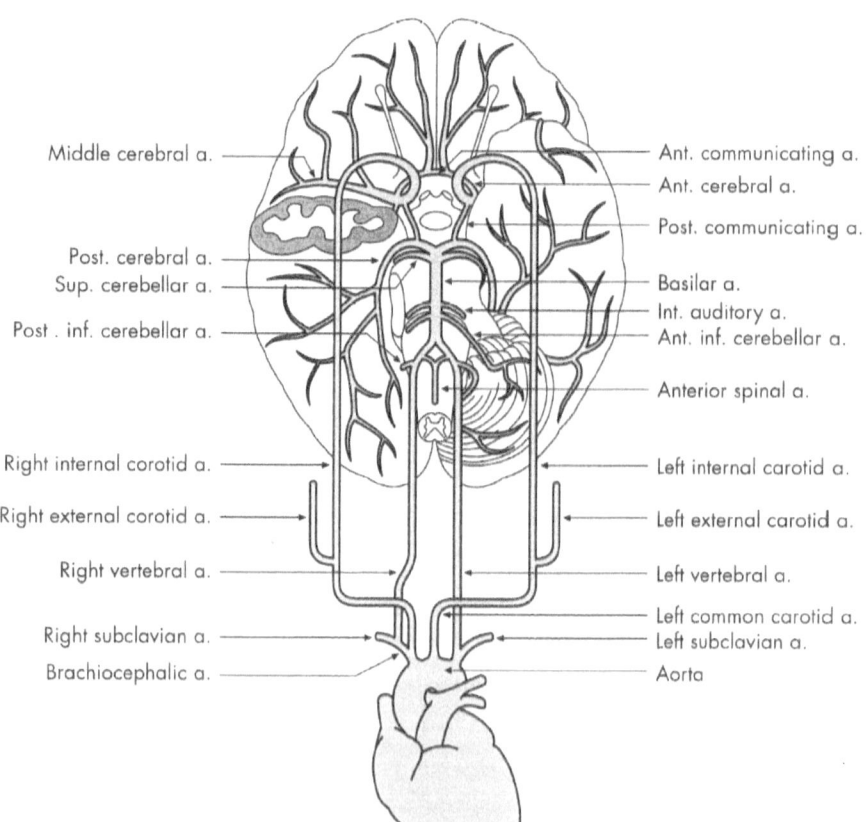

Figure 8.1 The arterial supply of the brain.

Vascular disorders

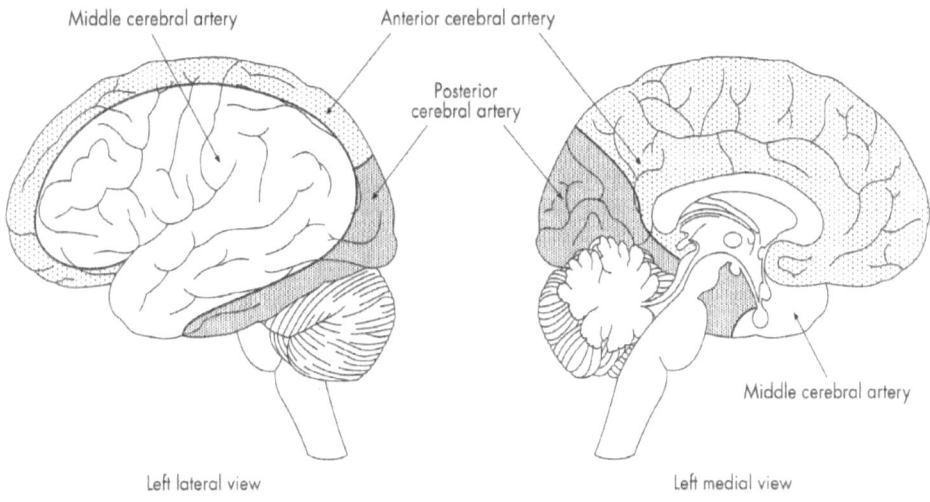

Figure 8.2 The arterial territories of the cerebral cortex.

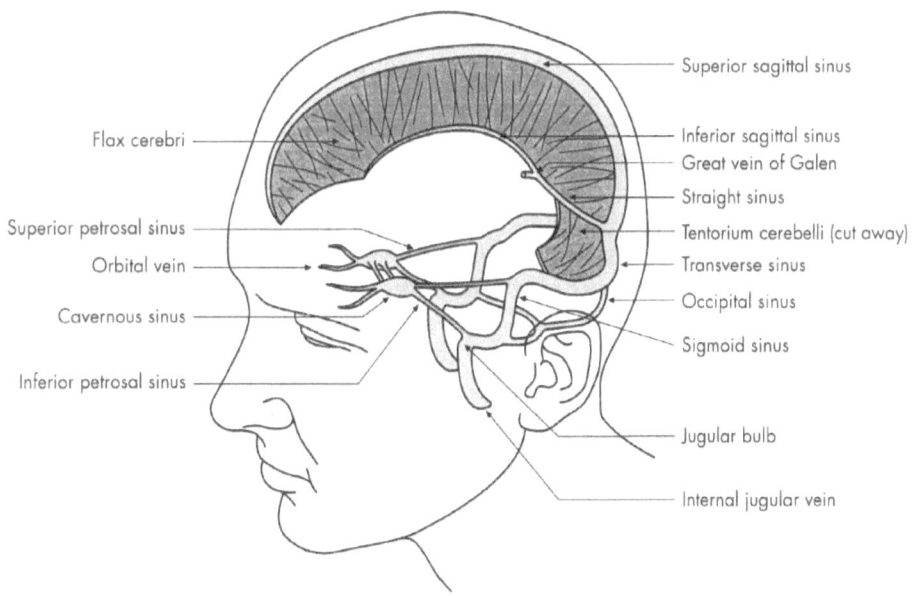

Figure 8.3 The main venous drainage of the brain.

Chapter Eight

STROKE

A stroke is a sudden neurological deficit caused by a vascular event affecting the brain, or rarely the spinal cord. It may cause sudden coma, focal neurological deficit such as hemiplegia, or rapid death. The two main causes are occlusion of a blood vessel by thrombus or embolus causing an ischaemic stroke, or rupture of a blood vessel or aneurysm to cause an intracerebral, subdural or subarachnoid haemorrhagic stroke. The global burden of disease study have reported marked increases in mortality and years lived with disability due to the various types of stroke (ischaemic and haemorrhagic) between 1990 and 2017. Over 6 million of the 56 million annual global deaths now occur as a result of stroke.

The risk factors for stroke are increasing age, hypertension, heart disease, diabetes, smoking, alcohol and polycythaemia. Smoking rates remain high in many LMICs. As life expectancy improves there is often increasing adoption of Western diets and a more sedentary lifestyle which are associated with the prevalence of hypertension, diabetes, atherosclerosis, myocardial ischaemia, and cerebrovascular disease. Stroke will therefore become an increasing problem in the developing world. The prevalence of hypertension has markedly increased in LMICs in recent decades.[53]

Non-communicable diseases have overtaken communicable diseases in global prevalence, with cardiovascular disease the number one cause of mortality. Cerebrovascular accident is the third leading cause of death, and this also holds true in many LMICs. The higher the blood pressure, the greater risk of hypertension related morbidity and mortality. There is generally a low awareness of risk, with limited access to treatment and affordability of control of hypertension in LMICs. Complications of hypertension have continued to increase. More public education on risk factors resulting from lifestyle and dietary change is required as well as regular health checks that include the measurement of blood pressure. 140/100 mmHg is proposed as an appropriate level to treat hypertension though national protocols vary.

---

[53]GBD 2017 Disease incidence and prevalence collaborators. Global, regional, and national incidence, prevalence, and years lived with disability for 354 diseases and injuries for 195 countries and territories, 1990–2017: a systematic analysis for the Global Burden of Disease Study 2017. Lancet. 2018;392:1789–1858.
https://www.thelancet.com/journals/lancet/article/PIIS0140-6736(18)32279-7/fulltext

Diagnosis

Computed tomography (CT) and magnetic resonance imaging (MRI) have revolutionised the management of these conditions, allowing more rapid decision making and early treatment for some strokes. Cerebral angiography (best done with digital subtraction) is also still a mainstay of investigation, although the quality of CT angiography (CTA) and MR angiography (MRA), CT perfusion studies and functional MRI (fMRI) demonstrating cerebral blood flow enable prompt decision making around interventional treatment and have largely superseded standard digital subtraction angiography in HICs. There has been a realisation in well-resourced health systems that stroke is a medical emergency just as is an acute myocardial infarct, and that early aggressive therapy improves outcome. Many HICs have introduced stoke team responses for patients presenting as an emergency.

Management

The management of stroke in the LMIC may be limited by resources available for diagnosis and treatment despite stroke becoming such a common emergency presentation. The unavailability of diagnostic imaging in many parts of the world hampers the management considerably. The indications for surgery are discussed for all of the vascular problems, but it is anticipated that in the developing world, the management of many of the conditions discussed in this chapter will of necessity be limited or conservative.

Space occupying lesions such as chronic subdural haematoma, abscess, tuberculoma and tumour may present with hemiplegia but the onset of hemiplegia is usually gradual. A history of head injury in the preceding 3 months and a gradual onset should prompt exploratory burr holes where CT scanning is unavailable. Those who could have either a subarachnoid haemorrhage or meningitis should have a lumbar puncture. In the absence of papilloedema a lumbar puncture is usually safe. If CT scanning is available, we recommend a scan for those patients with gradual hemiplegia, whether or not associated with altered consciousness. For patients with typical vaso-occlusive or haemorrhagic stroke of sudden onset, CT scanning is helpful to obtain a diagnosis and to establish the extent of the pathology.

Whether surgery is offered or performed will depend on the surgical expertise at hand, whether surgery could help, what the likely outcome will be, the patient and/or family expectations and the ability of the health system or the family to care for the patient if the survives with a severe neurological impairment. The patient with a gross neurological deficit who is 'saved' following a stroke, will remain disabled and require tremendous support from the family and prolonged rehabilitation to optimise the outcome. None of these services and supports may be available, thus defeating the purpose of aggressive management. The surgeon and physician in the developing world should be familiar with the various causes of stroke, decide which patients can be treated locally, and what the prognosis is likely to be, or which patients should be transferred to a more specialised centre, if that is feasible.

Ischaemic stroke (cerebral infarction)

The commonest cause of cerebral ischaemic events is atheromatous carotid stenosis at the carotid bifurcation in the neck or vertebrobasilar atheroma. It is thought that small emboli (platelet and atheromatous debris) travel upstream or temporary hypoperfusion occurs compromising the cerebral circulation. In the mildest form the patient experiences **transient ischaemic attacks (TIAs)**. The patient will complain of transient loss of vision in one eye like a curtain going down (**amaurosis fugax**) or a transient limb weakness or paraesthesia with the anterior circulation affected, or dizziness, vertigo, tinnitus and ataxia if it is the posterior circulation which is affected (vertebrobasilar ischaemia).

The symptoms usually reverse after a few minutes to an hour but may last up to 24 hours. Neurological deficit persisting beyond this time is a completed stroke. There may be a bruit in the neck, and uncommonly cholesterol emboli are seen in the fundal vessels. TIAs are a warning sign of a more serious stroke to follow. The risk of stroke after a TIA is about 5·10 percent per year compared with 1 percent in a control population. Medical therapy with aspirin and antiplatelet agents may be indicated following consultation with a physician, but a significant carotid stenosis may require a carotid endarterectomy. Thrombosis of an already narrowed carotid may occur suddenly and cause a major cerebral infarct with total hemiplegia. Carotid endarterectomy is not performed once an infarct has become established because there is a high risk of secondary haemorrhage. The performance of carotid endarterectomy requires specific vascular surgical training and experience in order to minimise postoperative stroke risk to acceptable levels. In HICs carotid stenting is an alternative to endarterectomy. Vertebrobasilar ischaemia is usually managed medically.

Haemorrhagic infarction develops when there is secondary haemorrhage within an infarct. Atheromatous intracranial cerebrovascular occlusive disease is often present with the extracranial disease and may complicate the decision making with respect to the extent of vascular surgery required. Chronic hypertension and vascular disease may cause narrowing and occlusion of arteries at the base of the brain (perforator disease), resulting in small (0.5 cm) deep, round, discrete **lacunar infarcts**. In advanced cases this may lead to cerebral atrophy and dementia.

The management of a carotid bruit

Carotid bruits are detected by auscultation. They usually indicate stenosis. Aneurysms of the carotid are rare but may develop due to atherosclerosis or, more rarely, they are false (pseudo-) aneurysms secondary to trauma or infection.

Three clinical presentations occur:
1. asymptomatic,
2. symptomatic with TIAs or other mild symptoms,
3. finding in a patient with a hemiplegia.

Where there is a skilled vascular surgeon, multicentre trials have shown an advantage to prophylactic treatment of patients with asymptomatic bruits, who have a 70 per cent or more occlusion of one carotid. However, if it is not easy to refer a patient to a vascular surgeon, there is probably little advantage in performing an endarterectomy on an asymptomatic patient. Carotid stenting is another option in HIC.

In the developing world where the patient is being managed by a general surgeon or physician, it may be better to restrict endarterectomy to symptomatic patients. The advantages of stroke prevention surgery may not outweigh the risks unless the patient already suffers from TIAs. With carotid false aneurysms or large arteriovenous fistulae following trauma, the carotid can normally be safely ligated in a young patient without neurological deficit. However, it is always preferable to repair the artery if possible and to use a shunt during the period of carotid clamping.

Cerebral embolism

Cerebral embolism is an uncommon cause of stroke. The main sources of cerebral emboli are:

- atrial fibrillation,
- bacterial endocarditis,
- cardiomyopathy,
- post-myocardial infarction,
- cardiac myxomas,
- septal defect with paradoxical embolism.

Many of these conditions are treatable and may require anticoagulation.

Haemorrhagic stroke

Hypertensive intracerebral haemorrhage

Chronic hypertension may cause rupture of small central perforators and lead to deep and often large intracerebral haemorrhages in the region of the basal ganglia and the internal capsule; the so-called **capsuloganglionic haemorrhage** (Figure 8.4,). There is usually a sudden development of a dense contralateral hemiplegia, and on the right side there are often also problems of apraxia and disorientation, whereas left side there are often dysphasias with complete aphasia in some cases. The indications for removal of these haematomas is controversial and depends on the patient's age and general health, previous level of independence, social supports, the adequacy of the rehabilitation services, the likely degree of permanent deficit, the patient's and family's wishes, and the neurological state of the patient. The main indication for evacuation is a progressive deterioration in the patient's conscious state. It must be emphasised that surgical evacuation of the haematoma usually will not alter the degree of focal neurological deficit. When the patient is coning due to raised intracranial pressure, surgical evacuation of the haematoma may be a life-saving procedure. However conservative management is appropriate if the patient is stable or improving, or is already deeply unconscious with a severe neurological deficit and a large haematoma. This recommendation is the likely approach to management in a well-equipped, modern referral centre. Surgery for patients with haemorrhagic stroke would not normally be attempted by a generalist in the tropics.

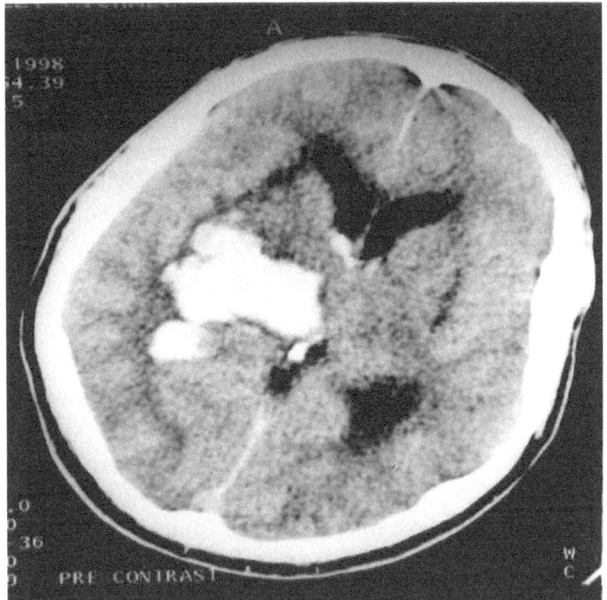

Figure 8.4 Hypertensive intracerebral capsuloganglionic haemorrhage. There is extensive haemorrhage in the right internal capsule, thalamus and the adjacent white matter.

Lobar haemorrhage

Lobar haemorrhage is a haemorrhage in the subcortical white matter of the cerebral hemisphere and is much less common than capsuloganglionic haemorrhage. It may be due to an underlying structural lesion or relate to a degenerative disease of the brain called **amyloid angiopathy**, which is associated with dementia. The haemorrhages may be recurrent, multiple or bilateral.

Cerebellar haemorrhage

Cerebellar haemorrhage occurs usually due to hypertension and is much less common than supratentorial hypertensive haemorrhage. Aneurysm and arteriovenous malformation rupture are also possible causes. The cerebellar haemorrhage is very dangerous because of the direct brainstem pressure, which may depress the vital functions and secondly, because of obstructive hydrocephalus due to fourth ventricle compression.

Hence, there is an urgency to remove these haematomas, particularly if the patient is deteriorating. Provided the patient is not deeply comatose with fixed dilated pupils, satisfactory recovery can be obtained, although there may be permanent cerebellar ataxia. This posterior fossa surgery is technically more demanding than surgery for cerebral haemorrhage and would not normally be attempted by a generalist in the tropics. Other causes of spontaneous intracerebral haematomas are rupture of an arteriovenous malformation, intracranial aneurysm, or vessels in a cerebral tumour, e.g. melanoma metastases.

Bleeding diathesis

It should not be forgotten that patients with a bleeding diathesis due to a clotting disorder may develop spontaneous intracerebral haemorrhages. Patients on anticoagulant drugs such as warfarin or other oral anticoagulant drugs (eg apixaban, rivaroxaban etc) are also at risk of intracranial haemorrhage, particularly following head trauma. This is often a subdural haematoma but there may be intracerebral haemorrhages.

SUBARACHNOID HAEMORRHAGE

Subarachnoid haemorrhage (SAH) due to rupture of a cerebral aneurysm is a complex and dangerous disease and is best managed under the care of a consultant neurosurgeon. Aneurysm rupture is commonest in the age range 40-60 years. The incidence of SAH is increasing throughout the world. From clinical and autopsy studies about 2-5 percent of the population may harbour asymptomatic aneurysms. The non-traumatic causes are listed in Table 8.1, next page. Head trauma may also cause subarachnoid haemorrhage.

Presentation

A sudden severe headache is a subarachnoid haemorrhage until proven otherwise. The patient presents with a sudden explosive headache that is totally out of character from any headache previously experienced. There may have been some premonitory less severe headaches over the preceding few weeks which probably represent minor leaks from the aneurysm ('herald bleeds'). There may be associated nausea, vomiting, epileptic fits, photophobia, meningism (neck stiffness), ± fever, focal signs, ± fundal haemorrhages, and an impaired conscious state. Take particular note as to whether a third nerve palsy is present because this may indicate an aneurysm arising from the internal carotid (posterior communicating artery) or the upper basilar/posterior cerebral artery complex. Some patients will be rendered immediately unconscious by the bleed, with varying degrees of awakening.

Table 8.1 Non-traumatic causes of subarachnoid haemorrhage.

Cerebral aneurysm	70%
Arteriovenous malformation	10%
Undiscovered	15%
Other	5%
Spinal AVM	
Tumour	
Bleeding diathesis	

Grading

There are several grading systems in use which help to categorise the severity of the subarachnoid haemorrhage.

The Hunt and Hess grading system is one example:
- **Grade 1** Asymptomatic or minimal headache and neck stiffness
- **Grade 2** Moderate to severe headache and neck stiffness. No neurological deficit.
- **Grade 3** Drowsy, confused or mild focal deficit.
- **Grade 4** Depressed conscious state, moderate to severe hemiparesis.
- **Grade 5** Deep coma. Decerebrate rigidity. Moribund.

The World Federation of Neurosurgical Societies SAH grade may also be used (Table 8.2, next page).

Table 8.2 World Federation of Neurosurgical Societies (WFNS) Subarachnoid haemorrhage (SAH) grade.

WFNS grade	GCS score	Major focal deficit*
0§	-	-
1	15	Absent
2	13-14	Absent
3	13-14	Present
4	7-12	Present or absent
5	3-6	Present or absent

WFNS, World Federation of Neurosurgical Societies; GCS, Glasgow Coma Scale.
* aphasia and/or hemiparesis or hemiplegia; § intact aneurysm
This scale uses the Glasgow Coma Scale to evaluate the level of consciousness, and uses the presence or absence of major focal neurologic deficit to distinguish grade 2 from grade 3. Young children may be non-verbal, requiring modification of the coma scale for evaluation.

Pathology of aneurysms

Berry aneurysms occur at arterial branch points close to the circle of Willis. Overall 85 per cent occur on the anterior circle of Willis. Multiple aneurysms occur in 15 percent of cases. Congenital or berry cerebral aneurysms are saccular and arise from a weakness in the muscular coat and the internal elastic lamina of the cerebral arteries at branch points on or close to the circle of Willis.

There are hereditary factors and hypertension and smoking are aggravating factors. Aneurysms tend to progressively grow in size and become a risk for rupture once they reach a size of 5 mm. Aneurysms 2.5 cm or greater in diameter are called giant aneurysms. Fusiform aneurysms may develop in cerebral vessels affected by atheroma.

Management

When to do an LP?

In the absence of CT scanning, a lumbar puncture is the most important investigation. This will help to exclude meningitis. Providing there is no papilloedema present an LP is safe. A malaria slide will also help to exclude cerebral malaria. When CT scanning is available it becomes the first line investigation and will reveal blood in the subarachnoid space in about 80 per cent of cases (Figure 8.5, below). CT may also show intracerebral haemorrhage and the aneurysm may show as a white round lesion when intravenous contrast is used. Early hydrocephalus may also be identified. A lumbar puncture is then performed when the CT scan is negative and reveals evenly blood-stained CSF and the presence of xanthochromia (a yellow supernatant from CSF spun in a centrifuge) beyond 6-8 hours from the bleed. Angiography is the definitive means of showing the aneurysm. This is now done with CT angiogram. Depending on the complexity of the aneurysm, a DSA may also be performed. This will usually involve transfer of the patient to a neurosurgeon (Figure 8.6, page 409).

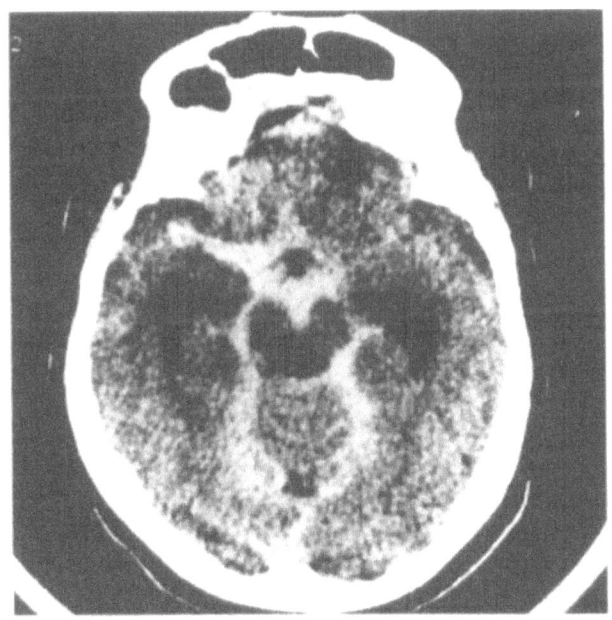

(a)

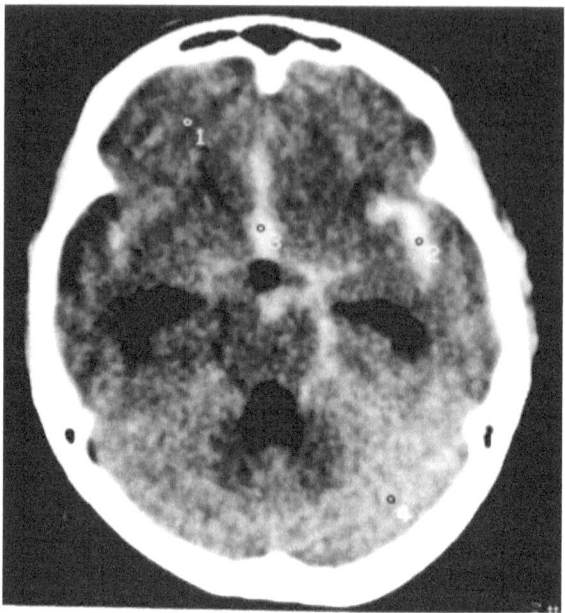

(b)

Figure 8.5 (a-b) Two examples of extensive subarachnoid haemorrhage in the basal cisterns and sylvian fissure.

When to transfer to a neurosurgeon?

Once the diagnosis is made the next difficult question is: Who should be referred? Many factors need to be taken into account, not least the possibility of transfer, the cost of transfer and ongoing treatment and the willingness of the patient and his or her relatives to make the journey. Then, the potential benefit needs to be considered. Discuss this with a neurosurgeon, but we would generally advise transfer of patients with Grade 1-3 SAH, and that transfer should be initiated as soon as practicable. The patient should be transferred on a stretcher, the blood pressure should be controlled if the patient is grossly hypertensive. Intravenous fluids (normal saline with KCl 20 mmol/l) are run at 120-140 ml/h for the first 24 hours and then gradually tapered to a maintenance level. A calcium channel blocker will help to lower the blood pressure (see below). Supplemental oxygen is administered if available. Light sedation with phenobarbital (phenobarbitone) may be helpful.

The risk of rebleeding

Without clipping, the risk of rebleeding is about 20 per cent in the first 2 weeks, 50 per cent in the first 6 weeks, then falls to 2·3 per cent per year. Half of the patients will die at the first rebleed. The risk of rupture of asymptomatic aneurysms is about 2·4 per cent per year.

The risk of vasospasm

Cerebral vasospasm occurs in about 30 percent of patients after SAH (and in up to 50 per cent of patients angiographically). About 25 percent of patients will suffer serious neurological morbidity or death due to the cerebral ischaemia. The effects of vasospasm peak at about 7·10 days after the haemorrhage and can be counteracted with hypervolaemic, hypertensive therapy with the use of calcium channel blocking drugs. This treatment becomes much safer once the aneurysm is clipped.

The potential benefit of surgery

The surgical clipping of aneurysms is technically challenging and requires a great deal of neurosurgical expertise to execute successfully. There is a trend for surgical clipping of the aneurysm within 24 hours of the bleed, which eliminates the risk of rebleeding and permits the aggressive prophylaxis and treatment of the vasospasm. Posterior circulation aneurysms are often left for longer until cerebral swelling settles.

The operation involves a craniotomy, often with resection of the adjacent skull base to minimise brain retraction, gentle fixed retraction on the brain, drainage of CSF, microdissection within the basal cisterns, exposure of the aneurysm, gaining proximal control of the feeding vessels, dissection of the neck of the aneurysm, and finally clipping of the neck sometimes with temporary occlusion of the feeding vessels to lessen the turgor of the aneurysm and thus prevent rupture of the aneurysm before the definitive clip is applied (Figure 8.7, page 413). An alternative to clipping is the interventional endovascular radiological techniques of the placement of a detachable metal coil in the aneurysm sac or a flow diverting stent placed at aneurysm origin. The coils induce thrombosis in the aneurysm.

The flow diverting stent reduces flow in the aneurysm so that it thromboses. The decision to coil or stent versus clip is complex but depends on the age of the patient, the type and size of aneurysm and the killset and experience of the specialists. In some centres many aneurysms are now being treated by interventional radiology rather than clipping. These coils are now favoured for aneurysms in the posterior circulation such as the basilar apex and also for carotid/ophthalmic aneurysms. This technology is expensive.

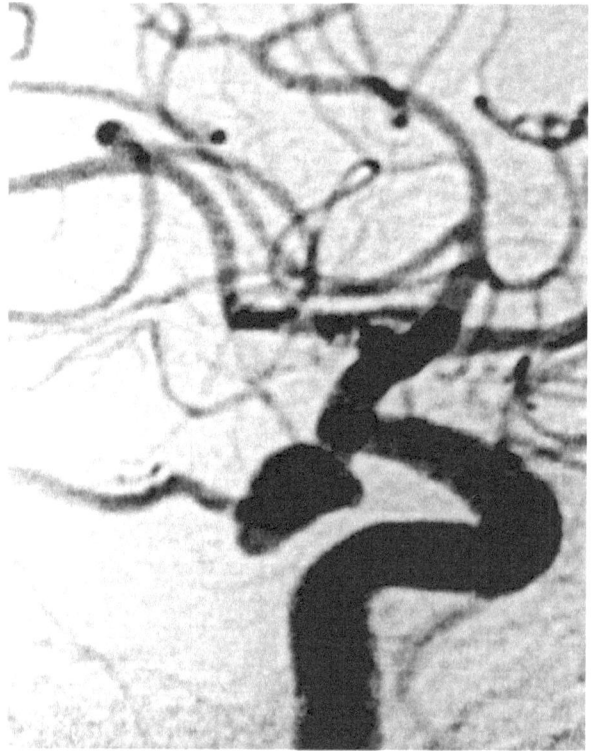

Figure 8.6 (a) Posterior communicating artery aneurysm. Carotid angiogram, lateral projection showing a large saccular posterior communicating artery (PCom) aneurysm arising at the point of origin of the PCom artery from the internal carotid artery. Note the posterior communicating artery is passing posterior to the aneurysm. It has passed from the ICA along the side wall of the aneurysm. It is in this case a large vessel and may be a foetal origin of the posterior cerebral artery (PCA) i.e. the first segment of the PCA is very small and the PCom A supplies most of the blood to the PCA on that side. This anatomical variation is estimated to occur in 20- 30% of people.

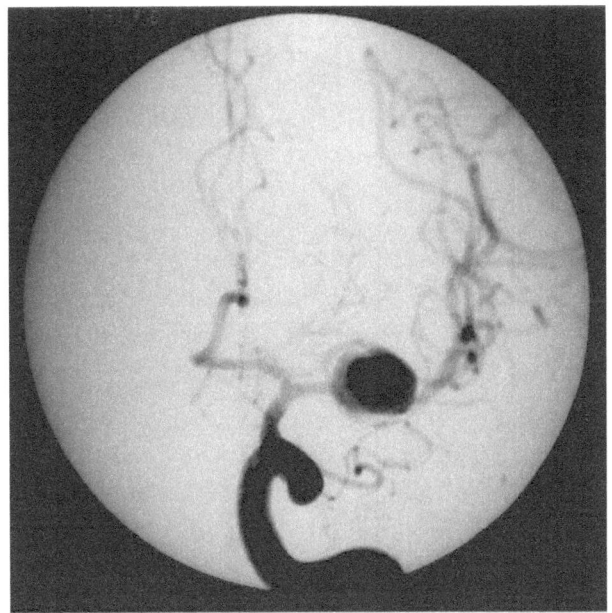

(b) i A-P view.

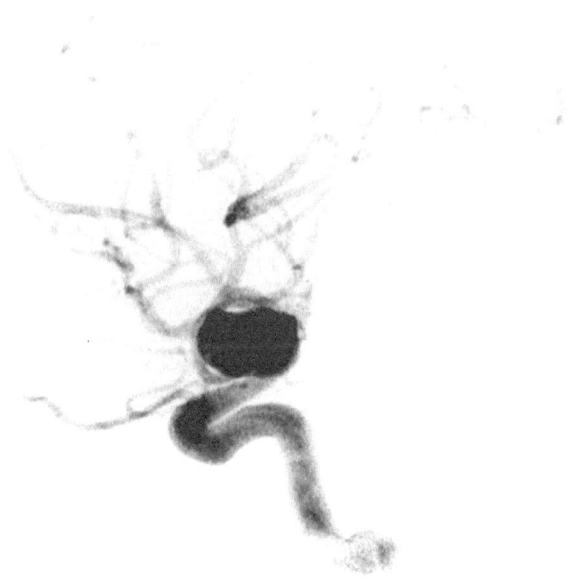

(b) ii Lateral view.

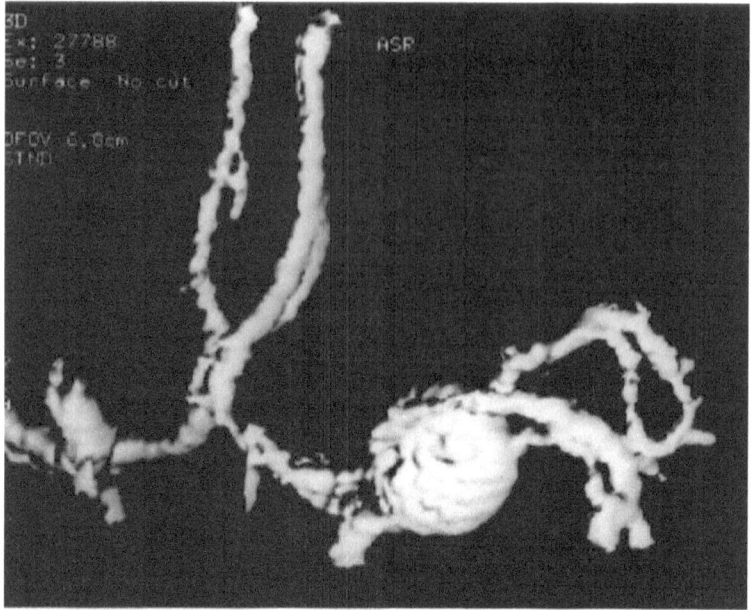

(b) iii Spiral CT angiogram.

(b) i-iii Giant left middle cerebral artery aneurysm.

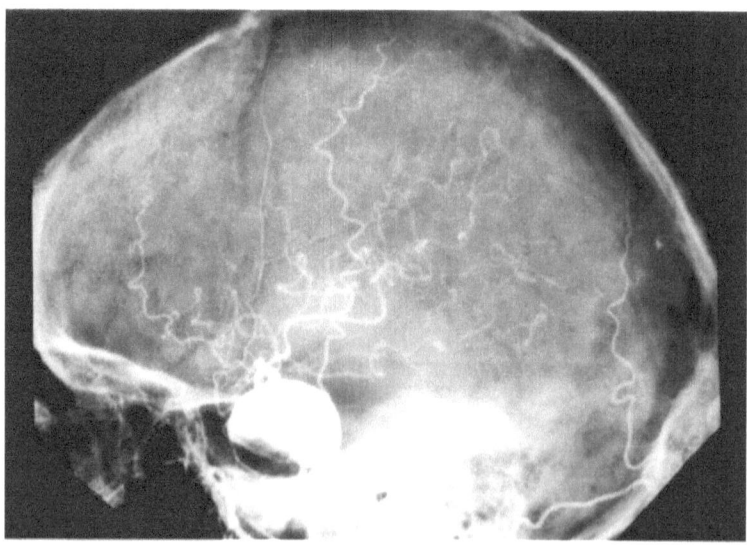

(c) i

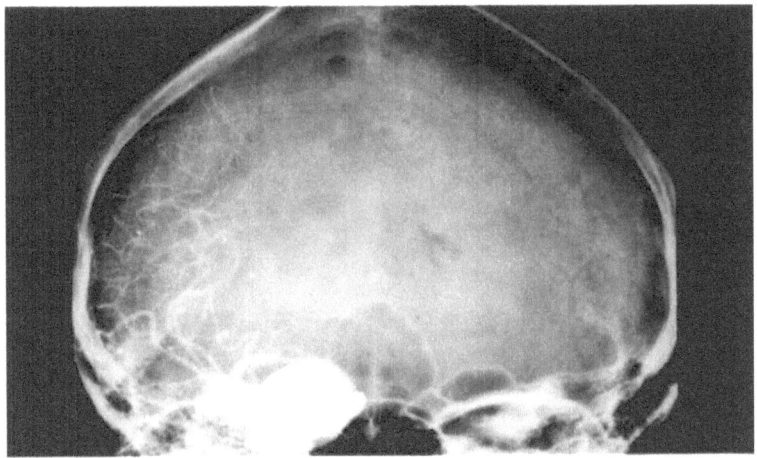

(c) ii

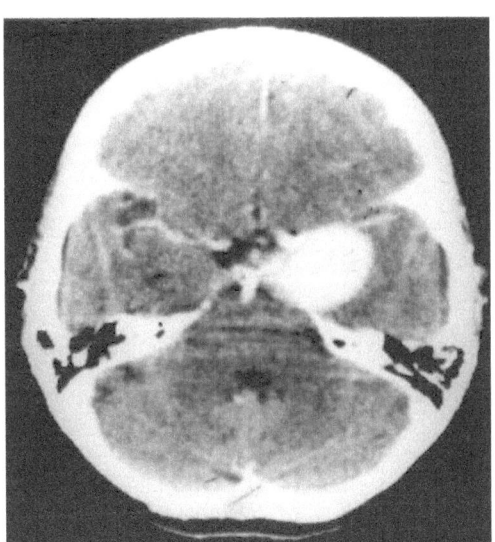

(c) iii

(c) i-ii Giant internal carotid artery aneurysm arising in the cavernous sinus and expanding laterally into the middle cranial fossa. These giant aneurysms present with chronic headache, facial pain and cranial nerve palsy. They may also eventually rupture. If they are purely intracavernous, this rupture would cause a carotid-cavernous fistula. The aneurysm can be treated with internal carotid ligation which gives partial protection although there is a risk of stroke from this procedure. *See also Reference: Little JR, Rosenfeld JV, Awad IA. Internal carotid artery occlusion for cavernous segment aneurysm. Neurosurg 1989; 25(3): 398-404.*

Figure 8.6 (a-c) Aneurysms.

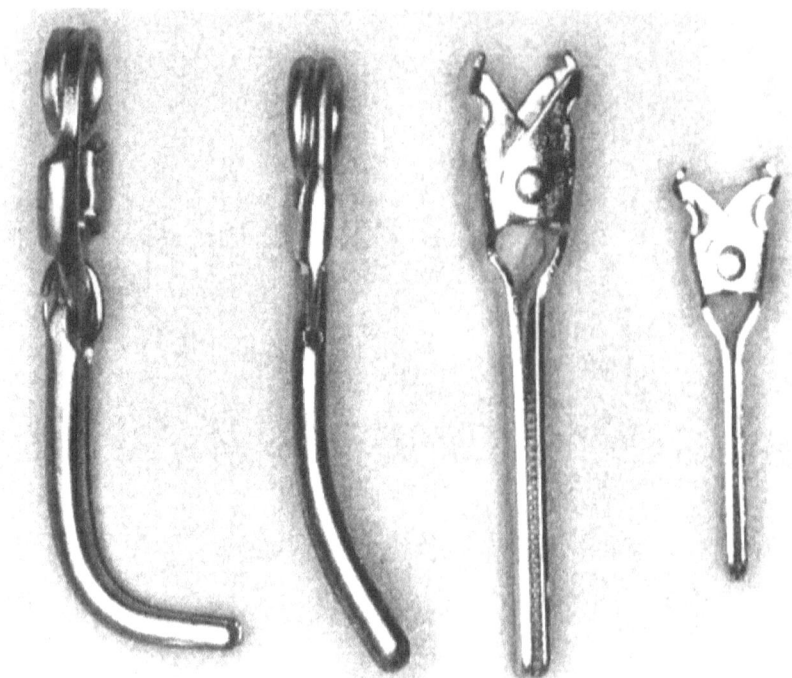

Figure 8.7 (a) Various aneurysm clips.

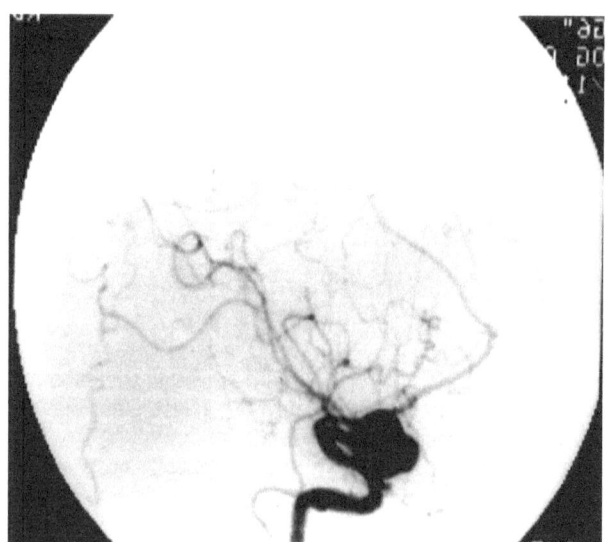

(b) i Internal carotid artery aneurysm before clipping.

Vascular disorders

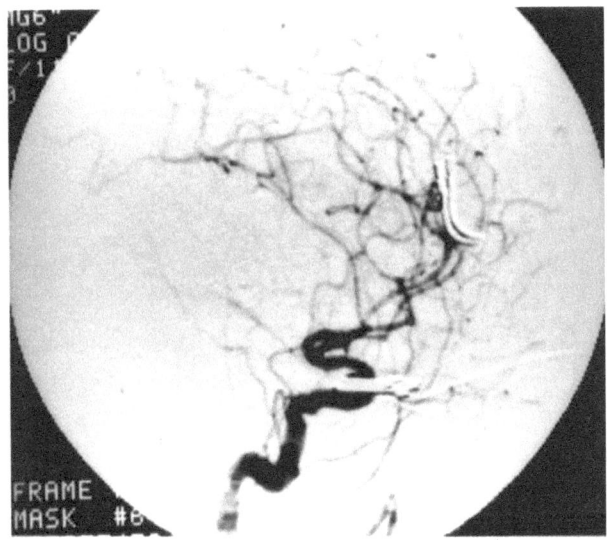

(b) ii Internal carotid artery aneurysm after clipping with complete control of the aneurysm. There are also two clips on a pericallosal artery aneurysm.

Figure 8.7 (a-b)

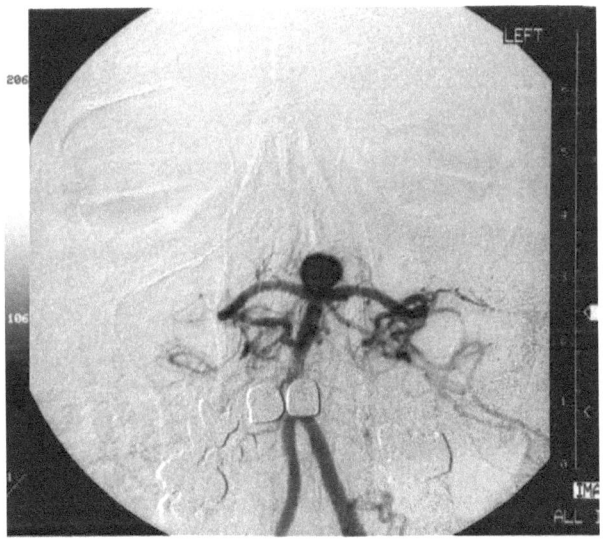

Figure 8.8 (a) A-P view.

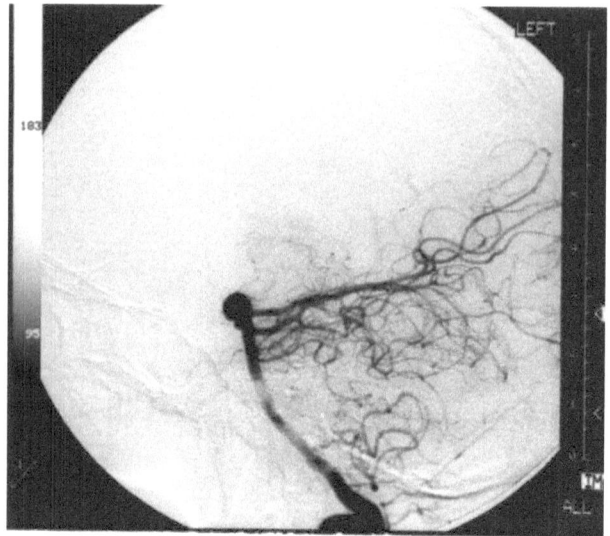

(b) Lateral view.

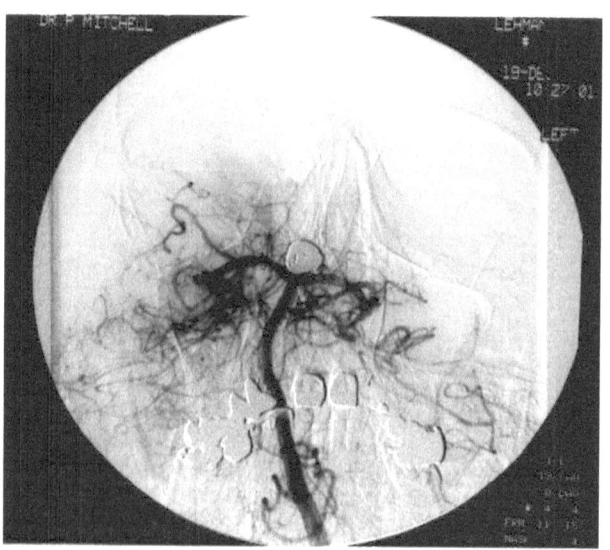

(c) Occluded with metal coil placed via the femoral artery.

Figure 8.8 (a-c) Basilar tip aneurysm.

When to use drugs?

If available, a **calcium channel blocking drug such as nimodipine** is administered. There is some evidence that calcium channel blockers improve the outcome but not mortality following SAH. Calcium channel blockers were thought to prevent vasospasm, but probably have a neuronal protective effect. The dose of nimodipine is 60 mg p.o., or nasogastric administration 4-hourly, initiated within 96 hours of the SAH and given for at least 14 consecutive days (some recommend 21 days). The dosage is halved for liver failure. An intravenous form is available but is more expensive. It is given as a continuous infusion via a central venous line. Side effects are hypotension (corrected with volume expansion), cardiac failure and pulmonary oedema. Aim for systolic blood pressure of 120-150 mmHg.

- ε-aminocaproic acid or cyclocaproic acid are **no longer used to prevent rebleeding** because the risk of ischaemic complications is too great.
  - **Anticonvulsants** (usually phenytoin) are administered to prevent epilepsy. Mild sedation, if required, is provided with phenobarbital (phenobarbitone). 30-60 mg p.a. or i.v. every 6 h.
- **Analgesic for headache**
- **Dexamethasone** may help the headache and neck stiffness, but is mostly used in the perioperative period to minimise cerebral oedema. Initial dose 4-6 mg every 6 h.
- **Stool softener** should be administered so there is no straining.
- H2 blockers have been used to prevent stress ulcers. Supplemental **oxygen** is administered.
- Intravenous fluids are described above. In addition, 500 ml of **albumin** or equivalent volume expander may be administered daily to try and minimise the risk of vasospasm.

Prognosis

10 to 15 percent of patients with SAH die before reaching medical care. This mortality will increase if there are delays to reach hospital. Patients with a higher clinical grade on presentation have a significantly worse prognosis. More aggressive medical and surgical therapy have improved outcomes from SAH but the overall mortality is still about 45% in some series. This poor overall outcome highlights the need to try and eliminate cerebral aneurysms before they rupture. Incidental and unsuspected cerebral aneurysms are in many cases amenable to surgical clipping or to interventional neuroradiological coiling.

Posttraumatic aneurysm

This is an uncommon condition, which presents as a sudden subarachnoid haemorrhage usually months after a blunt or penetrating head injury. The posttraumatic aneurysm is a false (pseudo-) aneurysm related to direct trauma of cerebral arteries in relation to relatively fixed and sharp-edged structures such as the falx cerebri. Thus, the anterior cerebral artery (pericallosal) is a common site. Alternatively, a cerebral artery may be traumatised directly following penetrating trauma and subsequently form a false aneurysm.

Therefore, any penetrating injury should be followed by a delayed cerebral angiogram (if available) at about one month after the trauma to detect any aneurysms, and plans should be made for elective clipping or excision. **Mycotic aneurysm** is a false aneurysm caused by a septic embolus usually from the vegetations of a bacterial endocarditis. The aneurysms usually occur on peripheral cerebral vessels (as opposed to berry aneurysms which occur close to the circle of Willis). They have a high risk of rupture and a high morbidity and mortality rate.

Arteriovenous malformation

The arteriovenous malformation (AVM) is a congenital lesion with abnormal communications between arteries and veins - multiple arteriovenous fistulas which form the **nidus**. There are often multiple large feeding arteries, and one or several large arterialised draining veins to a major venous sinus (Figure 8.8, page 414).

Clinical presentation

It is commonest in the first three decades of life. Rupture of the malformation causes intracerebral or less commonly, subarachnoid haemorrhage. An AVM rupture therefore causes a stroke with neurological deficit and depressed conscious state if the bleed is large enough. Other presentations include epilepsy (focal or general), chronic headache or migraine and progressive focal neurological deficit due to cerebral ischaemia surrounding the lesion.

Investigations

The AVM may be calcified and therefore visible on skull X-ray. A cerebral angiogram is vital for planning surgery, and if available, a CT scan and MRI are also indicated.

Management

Surgery may be indicated urgently to evacuate a haematoma. The AVM may be left *in situ* until further investigation is undertaken and the patient is more stable. Whether definitive resection of an AVM is undertaken depends on the size, site and venous drainage pattern of the lesion, the predicted risk of rupture of the lesion, the likely effect of that rupture and the experience and judgement of the surgeon.

Focused high dose radiotherapy (stereotactic radiosurgery) is another option for selected AVMs, particularly small deep lesions. For large lesions preoperative embolisation with glue may be an option to decrease the vascularity of the AVM, alternatively combinations of radiosurgery, embolisation and surgery are now being performed in some tertiary centres.

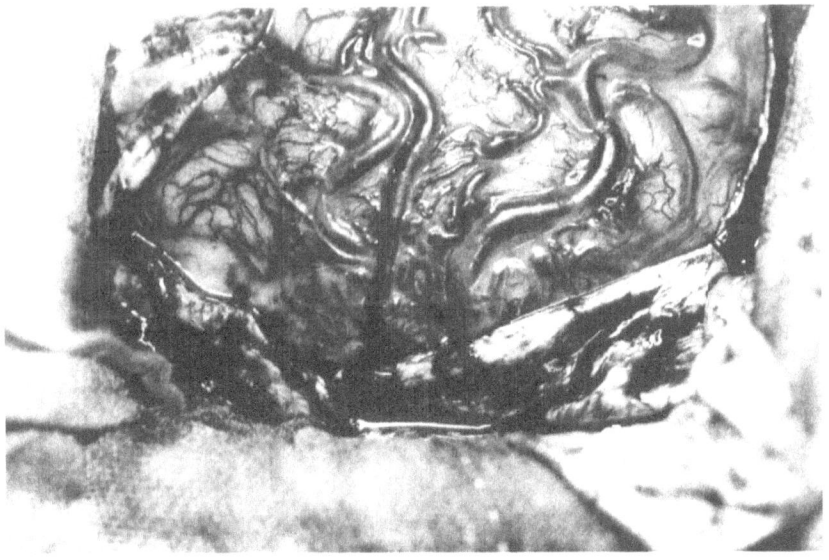

Figure 8.9 (a) The external appearance of the brain on exposure of an AVM. Note the multiple tortuous vessels of varying size on the surface.

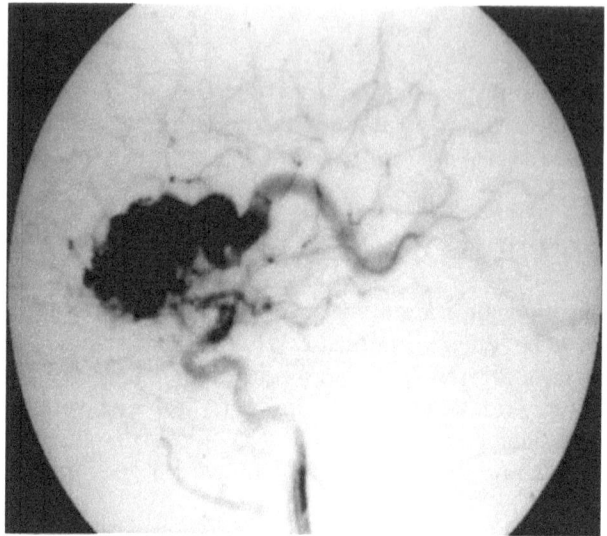

(b) Carotid angiogram showing a frontal lobe AVM with major carotid artery supply and a large draining vein passing posteriorly.

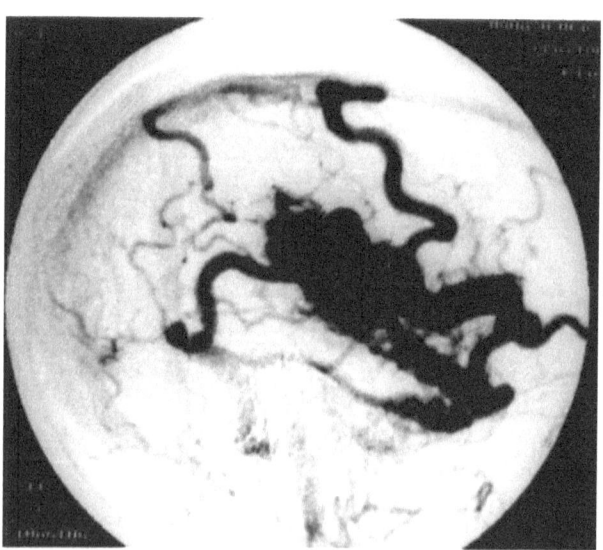

(c) Complex AVM showing multiple draining veins passing away from the lesion.

Figure 8.9 (a-c) Arteriovenous malformation (AVM).

Prognosis

The risk of haemorrhage in an unruptured AVM is approximately 2-3 per cent per year. The rebleed rate if the AVM remains *in situ* is 6 per cent in the first year and 2·3 per cent thereafter. The risk of death following an AVM haemorrhage is about 5 per cent which is much less than following aneurysm rupture. The AVM is cured when it is completely excised. It is unlikely the general surgeon in the tropics could beat the natural history of the condition, so if transfer to a neurosurgeon is not possible, we would advise the general surgeon to leave the lesion alone rather than try to operate on it inexpertly.

CEREBRAL THROMBOSIS

There are two main causes:
1. Extension of an inflammatory lesion to include the vessels in proximity. Suppurative otitis media and mastoiditis with transverse/sigmoid sinus involvement, osteomyelitis of the skull, cerebral abscess, tuberculoma or sepsis following trauma may all cause thrombosis in the adjacent sinus.
2. Dehydration, which causes increased blood viscosity.

Cavernous sinus thrombosis

Cavernous sinus thrombosis is a rare complication of facial, orbital, or middle ear/mastoid sepsis. Infection of the head and neck may involve the cavernous sinus via emissary veins. The superior ophthalmic vein communicates with the facial veins, the emissary veins from pharyngeal and pterygoid plexuses, emissary veins from the mastoid and auditory veins through the petrosal sinus, and cerebral and meningeal veins, all drain to the cavernous sinus. Infection around the face, especially around the eyes and nose, scalp infection, orbital cellulitis, sinusitis, pharyngitis, peritonsillar abscess, dental sepsis, otitis media, mastoiditis and occasionally remote sepsis, may be complicated by cavernous sinus thrombosis. The sinus involvement is often bilateral because of the inter-communications between the two sinuses.

The patient is severely ill and febrile, with marked periorbital pain and oedema, early proptosis and chemosis. Progressive ophthalmoplegia occurs. There is severe headache, rigors, oedema of the eyelids, proptosis, fixation of the eyeball, papilloedema with widespread retinal haemorrhages, chemosis and finally dilatation and paralysis of the pupil. Blood stained tears can occur.

There may be loss of vision. Delirium and depressed conscious state follow. The condition may become bilateral if there is rapid progression. If only the posterior part of the cavernous sinus is thrombosed, associated with pterygoid plexus infection or lateral sinus thrombosis, ophthalmoplegia may occur without the effects of deficient venous drainage from the eye. There is often a latent period of 5 days from the appearance of the primary lesion to the development of the cavernous sinus thrombosis. There is a high risk of blindness and death. The treatment is directed towards the primary site of sepsis. Use high dose, systemic antibiotics. Systemic anticoagulation should also be considered if the condition is progressive.

Sagittal sinus thrombosis

This is a rare condition in the West, but requires recognition in the developing world, where it is probably more common. The condition is difficult to diagnose in adults and may present variably with headache, vomiting, papilloedema, and increasing drowsiness. There may be a very high fever, convulsions, and pareses. The condition may be fulminating and result in rapid coma and death. Dilatation of the scalp veins occurs in infants, due to diploic veins transmitting the intracranial venous stasis. The fontanelle is full or tense. There may be oedema of the scalp over the mastoids and the occiput, and over the line of the affected sinus. Oedema of the upper eyelids may also occur. Spontaneous epistaxis is another indication of the raised venous pressure. The onset of unilateral convulsions, followed by hemiplegia, may represent the development of cerebral infarction.

Causes

1. **Dehydration.** Aseptic sinus thrombosis may complicate dehydration in infants and usually the middle three-fifths of the superior sagittal sinus is affected. The infant becomes drowsy, restless, with convulsions, bilateral paresis, vomiting, fever, and

meningism. The cerebrospinal fluid contains some red cells and is usually xanthochromic. The white cell count is normal with a preponderance of polymorphs. Some of these children have occult middle ear infection.

2. **Depressed fracture** of the vertex may occlude the superior sagittal sinus. This is occasionally a birth injury. Progressive venous thrombosis may occur and late benign intracranial hypertension may develop.
3. **General sepsis.** Venous sludging and hypercoagulability are aetiological factors.
4. **Sagittal sinus thrombosis** may rarely occur in the puerperal period.
5. **Polycythaemia.**
6. **Sickle cell crisis.**
7. Sagittal sinus thrombosis may also rarely complicate **cancer** or **inflammatory bowel disease.**

Management

Rehydration, antibiotics and anticoagulants are the mainstays of treatment, provided trauma is not the aetiology, in which case, anticoagulation is avoided. Surgical intervention to remove bony fragments from the sinus is hazardous, technically challenging, and is not recommended. Steroids probably do not alter the course. Anticoagulation may improve the outcome although there is a risk of cerebral haemorrhage. Use of thrombolytic agents, such as urokinase, infused topically within the sagittal sinus is a relatively new treatment, but requires specialist radiological facilities.

Prognosis

The condition has a high mortality. Infants who survive superior sagittal sinus thrombosis may develop cerebral atrophy with diffuse gliosis and a cerebral palsy picture.

Lateral (transverse or sigmoid) sinus thrombosis

Lateral (transverse) sinus thrombosis develops secondary to mastoiditis. The thrombus may become infected, leading to septic emboli, and (otitic) septicaemia. The patient has a swinging fever with rigors, leucocytosis, and sometimes tenderness over the ipsilateral jugular vein, and meningism.

During the intervening afebrile periods, the patient may look deceptively well. A sharp and high temperature peak (39-40°C) with a rigor occurring several days after a mastoidectomy is classical of a lateral sinus thrombosis. Venous congestion in the fundi or papilloedema, usually more marked on the side of the lesion, are often present and may indicate spread of thrombosis to the cavernous sinus, or the torcular and sagittal sinus, particularly if the patient is deteriorating. Cerebral oedema due to the obstructed venous drainage may cause headache, a depression of the conscious state, confusion and focal neurological signs, which may be difficult to distinguish from other septic complications of mastoiditis (see Chapter 11, page 600).

The **Tobey-Ayer** test can be done at the bedside and may help to diagnose this condition. A lumbar puncture is done with a manometer to measure CSF pressure. Compression of the contralateral jugular vein causes a rise in CSF pressure, whereas compression of the ipsilateral jugular vein produces no rise in the CSF pressure. Anomalies in the venous anatomy or bilateral infection may invalidate this test.

Blood cultures should also be done. Aspiration of the lateral sinus at mastoidectomy may produce a definitive diagnosis. Many patients with mastoiditis are already on antibiotics, which may dampen and confuse the clinical presentation of lateral sinus thrombosis. The ear condition appears to be responding, but the patient remains toxic and ill.

Treatment

Intravenous antibiotics are administered. A mastoidectomy is performed or reopened with exposure and examination of the sinus wall, which is often covered with characteristic granulations. These granulations or necrotic tissue may form a mass lesion and extrinsically compress the sinus. Removal of this tissue may restore the blood flow. If the sinus appears thrombosed, it is aspirated with a wide-bore needle passed a short distance. The experienced surgeon may be prepared to open the sinus, extract the thrombus and suture its wall using ribbon gauze at either end to control bleeding, but this is technically challenging. Rarely, if pyaemia continues, ligation of the internal jugular vein just above the junction with the common facial vein may be required. Anticoagulants are not usually given, because the risk of cerebral haemorrhage may increase.

Complications

1. **Otitic hydrocephalus** is an uncommon complication of lateral sinus thrombosis and presents with headache and papilloedema. A false localising sixth nerve palsy may also develop. Otitic hydrocephalus is a poor term because it usually represents a benign intracranial hypertension rather than a ventricular enlargement.
2. It is more common if the right lateral sinus is thrombosed because this sinus is the usually the dominant venous drainage of the brain. Repeated lumbar punctures may control the condition, but lumboperitoneal shunting will be required if it persists. Ventriculoperitoneal shunting is unsuitable because the ventricles are too small. Bitemporal decompression (craniectomy) is an alternative.
3. **Otitic septicaemia**.
4. **Systemic metastatic abscesses** may occur in poorly treated cases.
5. **Arteriovenous fistula**. The development of dural arteriovenous fistulas and malformations may be a long-term consequence of lateral sinus thrombosis.

Sickle cell disease

Sickle cell disease is an important cause of cerebral infarct in affected children and endemic areas. It is discussed below (page 429).

CEREBRAL VASCULITIS

Aetiology

- Basal meningitis - especially tuberculosis and syphilis.
- Systemic lupus erythematosis (SLE) and polyarteritis nodosa.
- Isolated CNS granulomatous angiitis (idiopathic).
- Drugs - heroin, cocaine and amphetamine abuse.
- Giant cell temporal arteritis.

Clinical presentation

Multifocal cerebral infarcts, epilepsy, focal neurological signs, headache, systemic signs, behavioural problems, depressed conscious state.

Giant cell temporal arteritis causes chronic headache (especially temporal), lethargy, and sometimes low-grade fever in elderly patients and may progress to ischaemic optic neuropathy, visual loss and cerebral infarcts if untreated. The affected scalp arteries may be thickened tender and non-pulsatile.

Investigation

- LP - increase in lymphocytes.
- Raised erythrocyte sedimentation rate (ESR).
- Cerebral angiogram - arteries have a beaded appearance.
- Brain or superficial temporal artery biopsy may be required for a definitive diagnosis in the aseptic cases.

Management

- Appropriate treatment for syphilis and tuberculosis.
- High dose steroids
- Sometimes immunosuppressants, e.g. cyclophosphamide, are used in severe autoimmune vasculitis.

CAROTID-CAVERNOUS FISTULA

Carotid-cavernous fistula is an uncommon but serious complication after head injury (and sometimes occurs spontaneously in elderly people). There is a fistula between the intracavernous carotid artery or its intracavernous branches and the cavernous sinus (Figure 8.10, next page). It usually follows a blunt injury fracturing the sphenoid bone, but may also complicate a penetrating injury. It is usually delayed in presentation to weeks or months after the injury. A unilateral pulsatile proptosis develops on the side of the fistula and may progress to visual failure.

The proptosis is reducible. There is chemosis (conjunctival oedema), and injection and arterialisation of the conjunctival vessels. The patient may hear the bruit in their head and it can also be heard with a stethoscope on the orbit or temple.

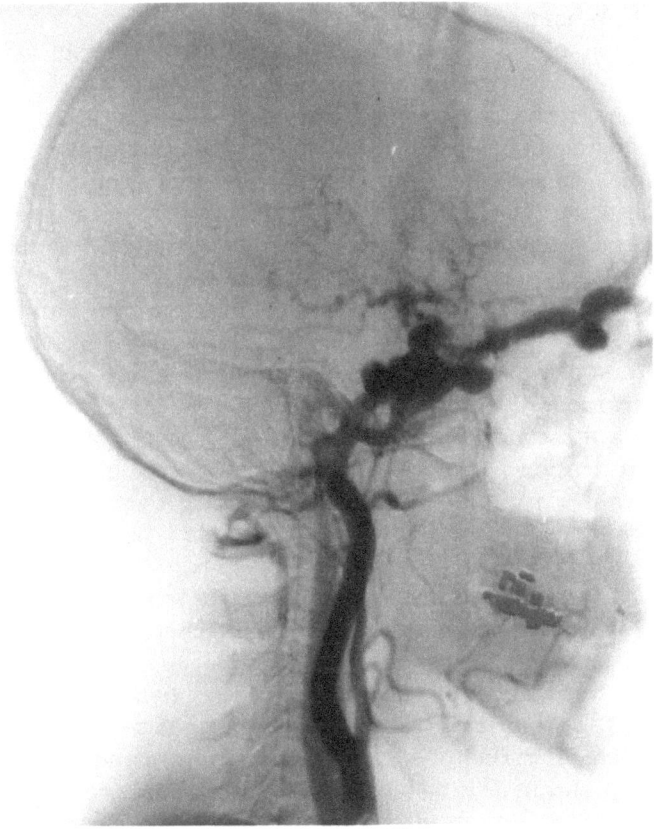

Figure 8.10 Carotid-cavernous fistula. Carotid angiogram showing dilated vessels in the vicinity of the cavernous sinus with retrograde filling of the ophthalmic vein and the internal jugular vein. The middle cerebral artery branches have also filled.

If left untreated, the other eye may be affected in the same way and the patient may gradually go blind. Small fistulae may eventually close spontaneously. Moderate to large fistulae are unlikely to close but may remain stable for a considerable time. The definitive management of persistent or progressive carotid-cavernous fistulae in advanced centres is to place a detachable balloon or metal coils in the fistula using interventional neuroradiological techniques. In low-resource settings it may be preferable to observe the patient, but if the condition is progressive or the vision is deteriorating on both sides, we recommend trapping of the fistula by ligation of the internal carotid artery, muscle embolisation of the fistula without intracranial exploration (described below). The muscle emboli are introduced into the internal carotid so that they pass upstream to occlude the fistula (Figure 8.11, next page).

Ligation of the supraclinoid carotid just after it leaves the cavernous sinus via a frontal craniotomy before the embolisation is the preferred technique because it prevents the muscle travelling too far and causing a stroke. However, this is difficult surgery because of the venous engorgement of the tissues and would require an experienced surgeon. Ligation of the internal carotid artery alone would usually not be enough to control the fistula because of the backflow from above.

Where transfer to a centre with interventional radiology is available, this is the best option. The procedure of muscle embolisation is preferably performed under local anaesthesia so that neurological complications can be detected immediately and reversed. Conversion to general anaesthesia may become necessary. The carotid bifurcation is exposed in the neck and the common internal and external carotid arteries encircled with loose ligatures. The cervical internal carotid artery is ligated, just distal to the bifurcation.

A 1 cm longitudinal incision is made above the ligature and a 3 mm diameter plastic tube containing the 3-5 cm muscle embolus with a small silver clip at each end is inserted into the artery, which is held in position by a ligature. A nylon ligature is tied to the end of the muscle graft so that it can be withdrawn if necessary. Saline is then gently injected into the tube by means of a syringe and this drives the embolus up the artery to block the fistula. The circulation of the retina should be protected through the external carotid collateral anastomoses if the ophthalmic artery is occluded. The position of the muscle can be checked with a lateral X-ray, because the two clips will be visible. The upper clip does not pass beyond the level of the anterior clinoid process otherwise the circulation to the hemisphere may be compromised. The bruit will disappear when the fistula is occluded, the nylon is cut and the arteriotomy closed.

Vascular disorders

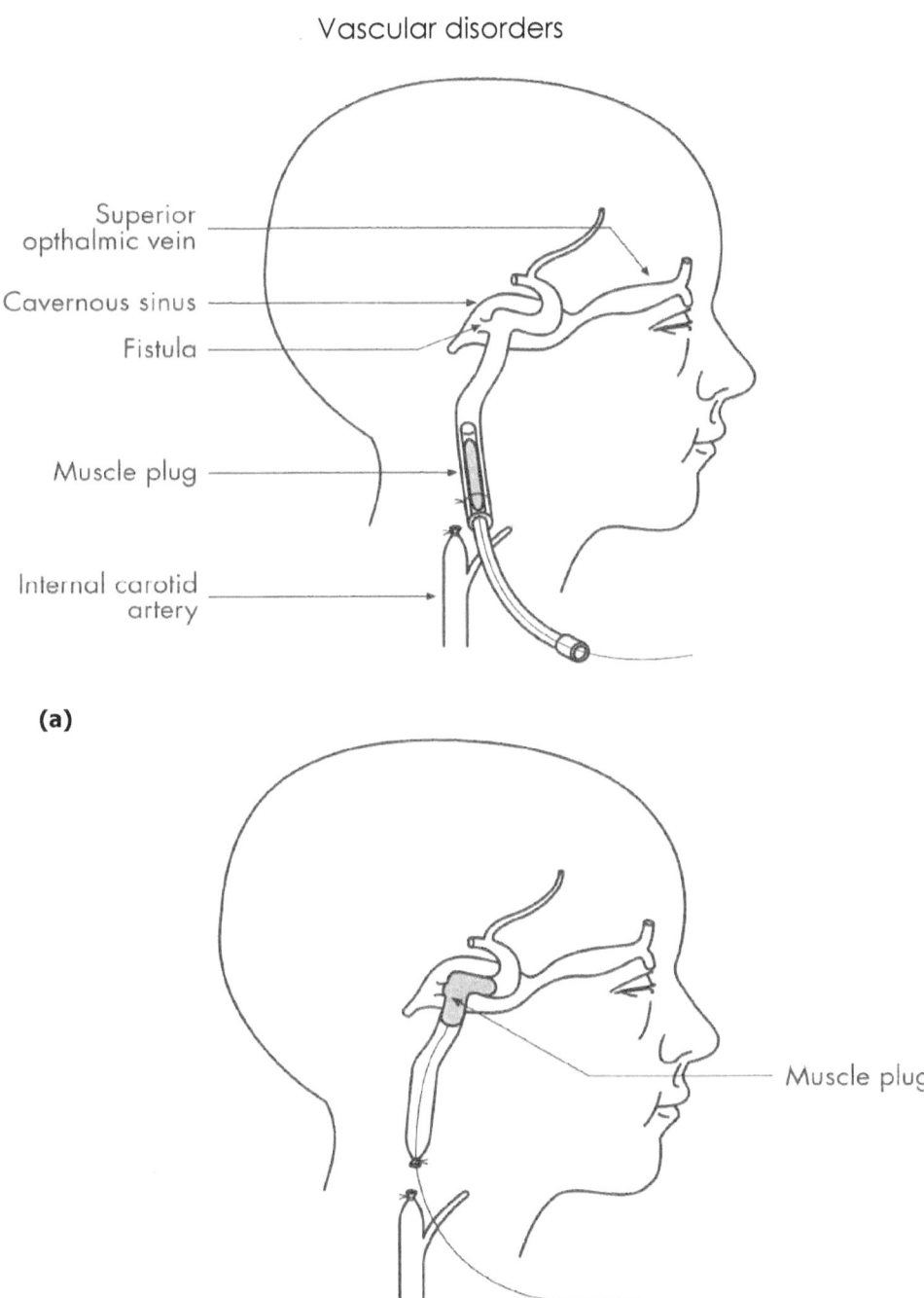

(a)

(b)

Figure 8.11 (a-b) The procedure of muscle embolisation of a carotid-cavernous fistula with ligation of the internal carotid artery.

A more reliable and controlled method is to place the patient under general anaesthesia, and prepare the neck in the same way as above, but to then proceed to a frontal craniotomy and expose the proximal internal carotid artery (ICA). The ICA is occluded with a clip, preferably proximal to the ophthalmic artery, but this may not be technically feasible. A silver Weck clip is satisfactory for the purpose. This craniotomy is technically challenging because of the vascular engorgement, hypervascularity and difficulties with access, and should only be attempted by an experienced intracranial surgeon.

SPINAL CORD STROKE

This is a rare problem but is a cause of a painful acute paraplegia in elderly patients without any compressive lesion on myelography. An infarction of the spinal cord develops and is due to a thrombosis of the anterior spinal artery on a background of generalised atherosclerosis. The management is conservative and the neurological deficit usually remains dense and permanent.

CEREBRAL INFARCT IN CHILDREN AND ADOLESCENTS

This is an uncommon problem which has many causes (Table 8.3, next page). The management is directed towards the underlying cause and ideally should involve a paediatrician.

Sickle cell disease

Sickle cell disease is an important cause of cerebral infarct in children and adolescents in endemic areas. The polymerisation of deoxygenated sickle cell haemoglobin (HbS) makes red blood cells less pliable and deforms some of them into a variety of interesting shapes. These cells may be prematurely destroyed or may block flow in the cerebral microcirculation. The clinical presentation is related to the effects either of haemolysis or blood vessel obstruction. Sickle crises may be provoked by hypoxia and infection.

Table 8.3 Causes of cerebral infarct in children.

Embolism

Cerebral vasculitis

Sickle cell disease

Migraine

Extracranial arterial dissection - spontaneous or post-traumatic

Fibromuscular dysplasia of the extracranial arteries

Mitral valve prolapse

Hypercoagulable states

Metabolic disorders

Moya-moya disease

Contraceptive pill in adolescent females

Moyamoya disease is a progressive occlusion of the basal intracranial arteries with secondary fine web of anastomotic vessels developing. The cause is unknown. The term moyamoya means puff of smoke in Japanese.

Children with sickle cell disease are prone to stroke (vaso-occlusion). It is most common around 6 years of age and affects about 8 per cent by the age of 14. Thereafter it is uncommon. Hemiplegia is the most frequent presentation and there is at least a 50 percent chance of recurrence within 3 years. Retinal ischaemia may precipitate proliferative sickle retinopathy, which may cause vitreous haemorrhage or retinal detachment.

Photocoagulation reduces the risk of vitreal haemorrhage but spontaneous autoinfarction may also occur and negate the effect of such treatment. Prevention of recurrent stroke can be attempted by chronic transfusion. Bone marrow transplantation is a viable option in patients with compatible siblings, but it is unavailable in the developing world.

Common clinical problems

COMA

Coma is a condition of subnormal consciousness. It is best measured objectively using the Glasgow Coma Scale (GCS) (see Table 2.2, page 18). Medical coma gradings, particularly, promoted for grading hepatic encephalopathy are less practical than the GCS, which can be applied to all types of coma. The aim of management in a patient with coma is to make a diagnosis and treat the potentially curable causes such as intracranial haematoma, malaria or meningitis. The cause of coma is often suspected from the history and by the performance of a few simple tests. In the absence of a CT or MRI scan approximately 20 percent of cases of non-traumatic coma remain undiagnosed. Figure 9.1, next page shows a diagnostic algorithm. The important investigations are a malaria film, blood glucose, serum electrolytes and lumbar puncture (in the absence of papilloedema). The causes of non-traumatic coma in the tropics depend on the local pattern of disease. Table 9.1, next page shows some of the common causes to be considered.

Specific management

The management is directed towards the specific cause and the management of medical causes of coma are beyond the scope of this book but can be found in general medical texts. The general care of the comatose patient is important and is outlined on the next page. It is essentially the same whatever the cause.

Common clinical problems

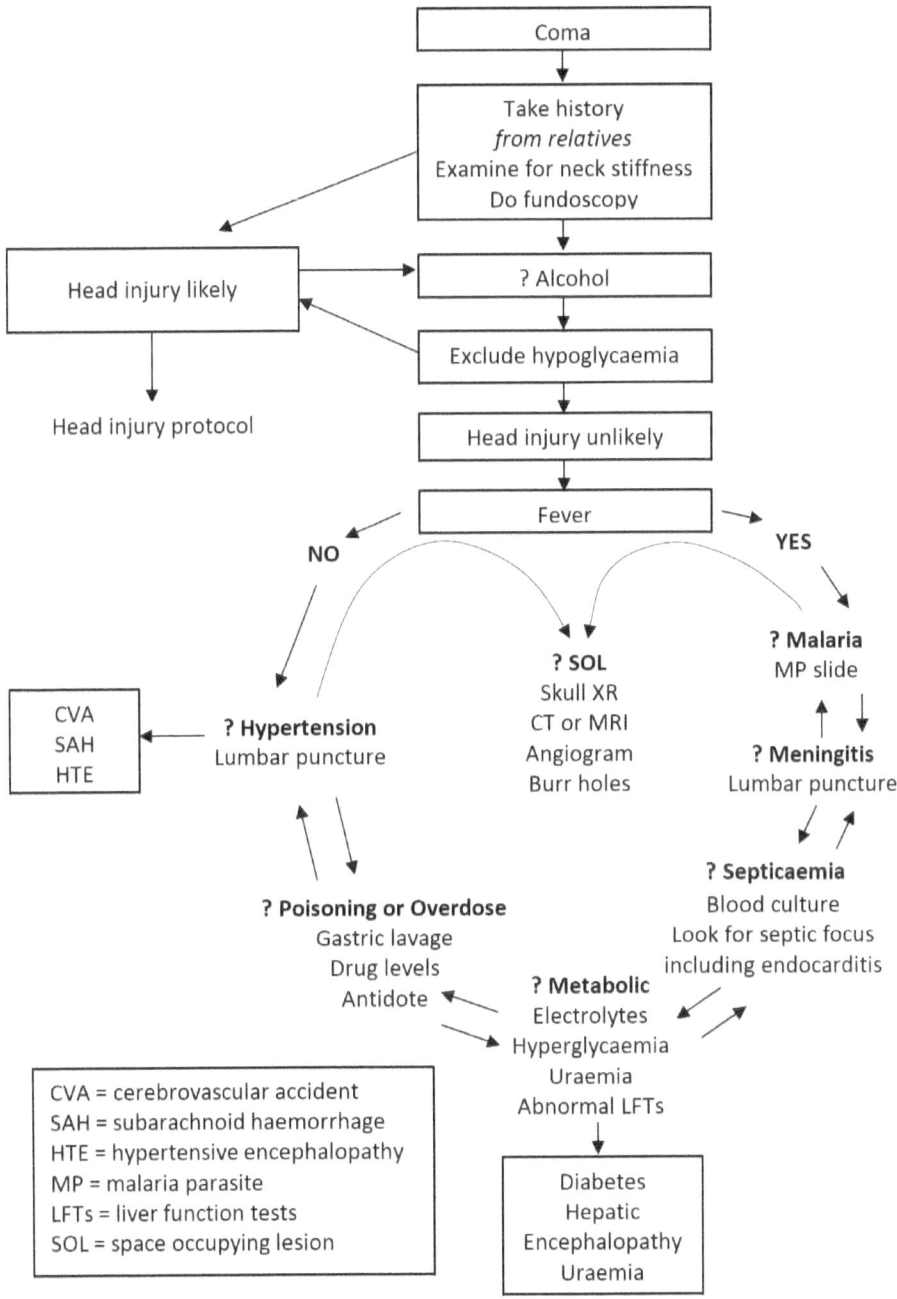

Figure 9.1 Diagnosis of non-traumatic coma in the tropics.

Table 9.1 Common causes of non-traumatic coma in the tropics.

Cerebral malaria

Meningitis

Cerebrovascular accident

Subarachnoid haemorrhage

Diabetes (ketoacidosis, hypoglycaemia)

Hepatic encephalopathy

Eclampsia

Poisoning

Chronic subdural haematoma

Space occupying lesion

Undiagnosed (up to 20%)

(Adapted from Sinclair JR, Watters DAK, and Bagshawe A, 1988).

General care of the comatose patient

This is covered in Chapter 3, Head injury.

Persistent vegetative state

Persistent vegetative state describes a comatose patient who has brain stem reflexes but no cortical function. The patient may open the eyes, grimace, have cycles of being asleep and awake and may be able to swallow and breathe spontaneously. However, there will be no awareness of what is happening around about. The diagnosis is made clinically although a CT scan may show a normal brainstem and cortical loss and abnormal basal ganglia. Patients are normally managed in hospital, in a nursing home or at home by dedicated carers.

The subject of the long-term management is emotive and has, in Western countries, attracted a lot of media attention. In the developing world, particularly those parts of the tropics where the readers of this text work, patients rarely survive in a persistent vegetative state. This is, at least in most cases, fortunate. The ethical issues that must be discussed for survivors include withholding antibiotic therapy for infections or withdrawing nutritional support, intravenous fluids for hydration or ventilatory support. Studies from the UK and USA suggest that the persistent vegetative state is sometimes misdiagnosed even by experts.

The chances of recovery are best after traumatic brain injury rather than after hypoxia for both children and adults.

However, the persistent vegetative state can probably be diagnosed confidently after 30 days following hypoxia or 60 days following head injury providing the patient is showing no signs of recovery (Figure 9.2, below).

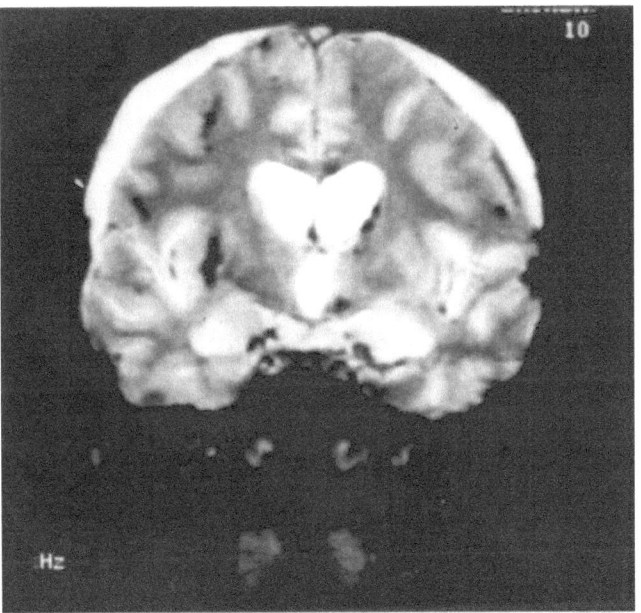

Figure 9.2 (a)

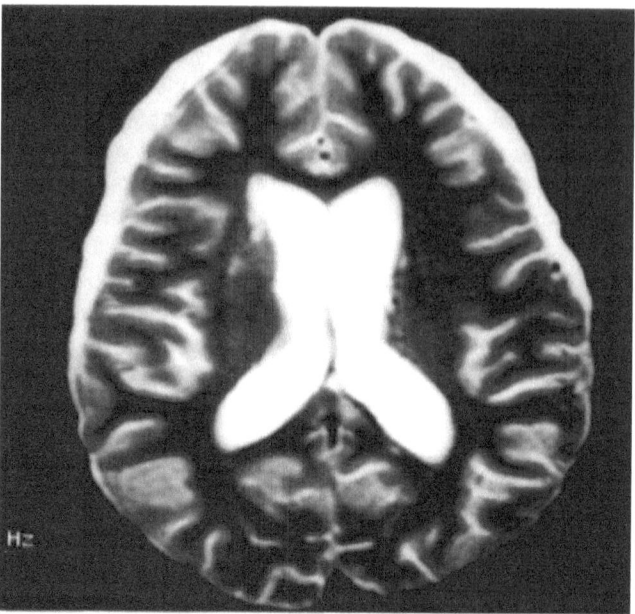

(b)

Figure 9.2 (a-b) Magnetic resonance scan of a patient in a persistent vegetative state more than one year following a severe head injury. It shows cerebral atrophy with secondary ventricular enlargement and multiple white matter and basal ganglia lesions (black spots), which represent sites of old haemorrhage and neuronal disruption.

BRAIN STEM DEATH

Brain death is defined as the irreversible loss of brain stem function. The need to diagnose brain stem death only arises when mechanical ventilators are in use. Because the vasomotor centre is low in the brain stem it is possible for the circulation (heartbeat, pulse and blood pressure) to be maintained when there is no chance of recovery of spontaneous breathing or regaining consciousness. The final event is usually severe brain swelling or raised intracranial pressure which obstructs blood flow into the head so the brain stem loses its blood supply and infarcts. Strict criteria for diagnosis must be adhered to because no one should discontinue ventilation when there is still hope of survival. Patients who are brain stem dead and have no possibility of recovery should be certified dead as soon as possible and ventilation discontinued. To continue ventilating a patient with no hope of recovery wastes valuable resources and may cause another death due to lack of an intensive care bed or ventilator.

Legal criteria for the diagnosis of brain death in your country should be followed. Some countries insist on an electroencephalogram (EEG) being done but this is subject to error and is not the practice in most developing countries. Nuclear (radio-isotope) brain scans and cerebral angiograms are also used in some centres for confirmatory evidence. If there is a transplantation programme it is worth contacting the appropriate team, providing the patient is not dying of a contagious disease or neoplasm and that cardiac function is intact. The following is a guide if there are no established criteria in your hospital. Brain stem death should be established by two senior doctors on two separate occasions. It is not important to have a long-time interval between the two occasions; an hour should be sufficient.

Practice point

The diagnosis of brain death is clinical and relies on simple testing of brain stem reflexes. However, the reversible factors must be corrected before brain stem death can be legitimately diagnosed.

Preconditions

1. GCS is 3.
2. Patient is on a ventilator with no spontaneous breathing.
3. Pupils are fixed and dilated.
4. Suffering from a condition known to cause irrecoverable brain damage.
5. The core body temperature (rectal) >35.5°C.
6. Serum potassium >3.5 mmol/1 and no other major electrolyte disturbances.
7. Muscle relaxants and sedatives should have worn off. Their action may be prolonged in renal failure.

Brain stem reflexes

1. **Apnoea**. If blood gases are available the PaCO2 should be allowed to rise above 55 mmHg (7.5 kPa) to stimulate the respiratory centre while avoiding hypoxia. To do this, the ventilator is disconnected and an oxygen catheter is passed down the endotracheal tube with a flow rate of 12 litres/min. The arterial blood gases (if available) are checked after 5 minutes, to ensure the PaCO 2 has reached a satisfactory level. If the brain stem is dead there should be no spontaneous breathing.
2. **Pupils**. The pupils are fixed and dilated in response to light.
3. **Corneal reflex**. There is no corneal reflex to touching the cornea with cotton wool.
4. **Gag reflex**. There is no gag or cough response with stimulation of the oropharynx and carina using an endotracheal plastic suction catheter.
5. **Oculocephalic reflex** (doll's eye reflex). The head is turned from side to side and flexed and extended with the eyes pointing in the direction the head is turned, rather than straight ahead which occurs when the brain stem reflex is intact.
6. **Oculovestibular reflex**. 20 ml of iced water is syringed into the external auditory canal on each side separately. There must be no wax in the external ear canals. There should be no eye movements or nystagmus. An assistant will need to hold the eyelids open.
7. **Pain reflex for cranial nerves**. Pressure at the supraorbital margin, where the supraorbital nerves are located will produce no facial grimace or other movement.

If the patient has a positive response to any of the above tests then brain stem death cannot be diagnosed.

LOCOMOTOR OR GAIT PROBLEMS

There are many causes of gait disorder that require a detailed history and examination to diagnose. Neurological, musculoskeletal and vascular disease may cause locomotor or gait problems. Neurological causes may be due to motor, sensory or coordination deficits. Musculoskeletal causes may be due to disease affecting the bones, muscles or joints. Vascular problems present with claudication, rest pain, ulceration or gangrene and may be due to any vascular disease such as atherosclerosis, thromboangiitis obliterans (medial sclerosis), vasculitis or trauma. The gait examination is an essential part of any neurological assessment and can give the keen observer a lot of information about the possible site of a lesion. When assessing gait, it is important to distinguish between upper motor neuron weakness with spasticity and hyperreflexia and no muscle wasting until late, from lower motor neuron weakness with flaccidity, hyporeflexia or areflexia and muscle wasting. In the former case, the lesion is placed in the brain or spinal cord level down to but not including the anterior horn motor neuron, whereas in the latter, the lesion is at the motor neuron level from the anterior horn cell distally to the level of the motor end plate on the muscle cells.

The main causes of gait disorder are:

1. **Pain**
   The patient limps to avoid the pain (antalgic gait):
   - nerve compression: sciatica,
   - vascular ischaemia: claudication,
   - joint disease,
   - bone disease,
   - myositis and muscle injury,
   - soft tissue inflammation and infection.
2. **Balance disorder**
   - cerebellar ataxia - wide-based unsteady gait
   - loss of dorsal column function - impaired proprioception
   - drug induced, e.g. alcohol, phenytoin
3. **Extrapyramidal disorder**
   In Parkinson's disease the gait is small stepping, often slow to initiate, festinating (hurrying), with a flexed posture and no arm swing. In dystonia there is a sustained simultaneous contraction of agonist and antagonist muscles, which produces bizarre postural deformities of the limbs and sometimes the trunk. Dystonia therefore disturbs the pattern and equilibrium of the gait.
4. **Hemiparesis**
   There is unilateral spasticity and stiffness, rigidity and hyperreflexia following a stroke.
5. **Nerve injury**
   For example, foot drop or common peroneal nerve injury with wasting of the anterior compartment of the leg.
6. **Spastic paraparesis**
   The lower limbs are weak, spastic, stiff, slow and small stepping. The patient may have difficulty carrying their own weight. There will also be sensory and possibly sphincter disturbance. The arms may also be involved if the pathology is cervical (spastic quadriparesis).

7. **Mechanical causes**
   - leg length discrepancy
   - restricted joint movements, e.g. chronic arthritis
8. **Cerebral palsy**
   Cerebral palsy is a group of disorders resulting from brain injury that occurs in the antenatal or perinatal period. There are many causes with the commonest being **prematurity** with intraventricular and subependymal haemorrhage and resultant deep white matter loss called **periventricular leukomalacia**. The haemorrhage is often secondary to an ischaemic insult. Other causes of the brain injury are anoxia, mechanical injury, kernicterus, infection in utero, e.g. toxoplasmosis, rubella, cytomegalovirus and genetic abnormalities. The brain damage is static although the clinical manifestations may change as the child grows and matures. There is retardation of motor development and primitive reflexes are retained leading to the development of abnormal posture, coordination and movement. The incidence is 2.0 to 2.5 per 1000 school-age children.

   The four basic **types of cerebral palsy** are:
1. spastic,
2. dyskinetic:
   - choreoathetosis- continuous involuntary jumping, jerking and writhing movements
   - dystonia- sustained involuntary contraction of muscle causing disturbed and contorted postures,
3. ataxic,
4. mixed.
   There are six types of spastic form (75 percent of cases) are:
   1. spastic hemiplegia,
   2. spastic quadriplegia (double hemiplegia),
   3. spastic diplegia- leg involvement out of proportion to the arms,
   4. tetraparesis involvement of three limbs,
   5. spastic monoplegia,
   6. spastic paraplegia (lower limbs only involved) (rare).

   The affected children often exhibit choreoathetosis, dysarthria with slurred speech and varying degrees of intellectual disability. However, it should be appreciated that even the most severely affected individuals may have a normal intellect. The child with spastic diplegia has a characteristic gait with toe walking (equinus deformity of the feet due to Achilles tendon shortening), flexed knees and hips, and often a compensatory lumbar lordosis. The upper limbs are also commonly affected but to a much milder degree. There may be spontaneous improvement in many of the milder cases, but for the more severely affected, walking becomes increasingly difficult and they may require a wheelchair. In the developing world simple physical therapies are all that can usually be provided. A simple release and lengthening of the Achilles tendons or hamstrings can be performed by an orthopaedic surgeon with experience in cerebral palsy cases. Careful judgement is required before embarking on surgery.

The lower limb function can be improved with combinations of physiotherapy, botulinum toxin injections in spastic muscles and orthopaedic surgery to lengthen tendons (Achilles and hamstrings), and alter hip joint function (e.g. osteotomies of the upper femurs). Selective dorsal rhizotomy is a complex neurosurgical procedure where in selected cases, an extensive lumbar laminectomy is performed and the dorsal rootlets from L1 to S1 are individually electrically tested via a lumbar laminectomy to determine which are responsible for the maintenance of the spasticity and these are sectioned. These procedures can only be provided in a specialised paediatric multidisciplinary setting where advanced orthopaedic, neurosurgical, physiotherapy and rehabilitation facilities are available.

EPILEPSY AND STATUS EPILEPTICUS

Convulsion, seizure or fit are three terms that all mean the same. They may arise as a result of many illnesses (Table 9.2, page 444) and, when the illness is cured, there will be no recurrent fits; or they may be due to epilepsy. Epilepsy means that fits are recurrent and that there is an underlying focus in the brain (however small and undetectable) responsible for inducing recurrent fits. Fits need to be differentiated from tetany, rigors, spasms of tetanus (associated with muscle rigidity and sweating) and faints.

The different types of fit are classified below. In the tropics many epileptics suffer severe burns from falling into an open fire during a seizure. In the management of epilepsy traditional remedies are common, and are interwoven with witchcraft, magic and taboo. Epileptics may sometimes be perceived as demon-possessed.

We strongly advise that in every case physical causes are sought. Even then there will be many cases where the cause is not found and it may be important for a doctor to intervene to prevent an epileptic being ostracised or regarded as being 'possessed' by a religious community. A diagnosis of epilepsy also carries implications for driving and employment (see below).

Case report

A 25-year-old nurse presented to the emergency department having collapsed. She was said to have fitted. Careful questioning found no evidence of frothing of the mouth, biting of the tongue or incontinence.

Bystanders did not notice any spasms. The emergency doctor diagnosed a faint and sent her home. Unfortunately, he failed to consider why she had fainted. She was readmitted a few hours later in hypovolaemic shock from a ruptured ectopic pregnancy.

Case report

A 22-year-old woman was referred for repeated spasms thought to be epilepsy. These were not associated with incontinence or biting the tongue. When her blood pressure was checked she developed carpopedal spasm (Trousseau's sign) and she had a positive Chvostek's sign on tapping the facial nerve. Her serum calcium was 1.56 mmol/l despite a normal serum albumin. She was discovered to have a thyroid nodule which proved to be a medullary carcinoma of the thyroid.

***Lesson**: this woman had tetany from an excess of calcitonin secreted by the tumour. She was treated by total thyroidectomy.*

Seizure classification

Generalised

Generalised seizures are bilaterally symmetrical, have no local onset, consciousness is lost from the onset.
1. **Generalised tonic-clonic (GTC)** (grand-mal seizure). This does not include partial seizures that generalise secondarily.

2. **Absence** (petit-mal seizure). Impaired consciousness with mild or no motor involvement - these automatisms[54] occur more commonly with bursts lasting more than 7 seconds and are usually simple, e.g. lip smacking or chewing. There is no post-ictal confusion, and an aura is rare. May be induced by hyperventilation for 2-3 minutes. EEG shows spike and wave pattern at three per second.
3. **Bilateral myoclonus** (a sudden involuntary jerking of a muscle or group of muscles).

Infants and children:
- infantile spasms: head thrown back, arms up, waist flexed
- atonic seizures (**'drop attacks'**)
- tonic seizures (the body, arms or lower limbs become suddenly very stiff or tense)

Partial (begin locally; focal seizure)

A new onset of focal seizure represents a structural lesion until proven otherwise.

1. **Simple** (usually no loss of consciousness)
   - with motor symptoms (including Jacksonian)
   - sensory (special sensory or somatosensory)
   - with autonomic symptoms
   - affective
2. **Complex**: there is often an aura - e.g. auditory, olfactory, then there is an alteration of consciousness, with an initial motionless stare followed by automatisms. The seizures are followed by a period of confusion (not usually present in absence seizures). They may have a temporal lobe or extratemporal origin.
3. **Partial with secondary generalisation**
   - simple partial evolving to generalised
   - complex partial evolving to generalised
   - simple partial evolving to complex partial evolving to generalised

Unclassified epileptic seizures

---

[54]*Automatisms: complex stereotyped behavioural acts occurring during seizures, e.g. lip smacking, chewing, fumbling of the hands, picking at clothes, scratching, dressing, undressing, rearranging objects, shuffling the feet. The person has no recollection of these movements following the seizure.*

It is important to distinguish generalised tonic-clonic seizures (primary generalised) from partial with secondary generalisation (often, a focal onset may not be observed). A new onset of seizure without an obvious cause should prompt a search for an underlying pathology, which will involve a careful clinical assessment and investigation for a space occupying lesion, or general brain disorder, as described.

Status epilepticus

Clinical recognition

Status epilepticus is defined as generalised tonic-clonic seizures which continue for more than 5 minutes, or as two or more generalised tonic-clonic seizures without a return to consciousness between seizures. When the fitting has been prolonged, the clinical appearance may become subtle and recognition requires careful observation. Note that continuous seizures in comatose patients may manifest as continuous twitching of the eyelids, fingers or toes, or nystagmoid jerking of the eyes. One out of six patients presenting with their first seizure will be in status epilepticus.

Pathophysiology

A failure of the mechanisms that normally abort an isolated seizure is the basic problem and can arise as a result of abnormally persistent, excessive excitation or ineffective inhibition. The actual site and pathways are unknown and the mechanisms poorly understood. Status epilepticus lasting 30 minutes may cause cerebral injury, particularly in the limbic structures such as the hippocampus. There may also be severe stresses on metabolism with adverse effects on the heart, kidneys and lungs.

Treatment

1. Ensuring an adequate airway is present - turn the patient on their side, administer oxygen, suck out secretions. Most patients breathe adequately providing their airway is clear.
2. Supporting the circulation.
3. Making sure hypoglycaemia is not the cause.

4. Administering intravenous diazepam 2-4 mg per minute until the seizure stops, or until a total of 30 mg has been administered (adults).
5. A slow intravenous infusion of phenytoin (less than 50 mg/minute) in 0.9 percent saline, to a total of 20 mg/kg of body weight).
6. Clonazepam, if available, can be used as an alternative to diazepam. The dose is 0.25 mg to 0.5 mg with repeated injections up to a dose of 1 mg slowly IV.
7. Midazolam is another alternative to diazepam. Dose: 0.05 mg/kg IV at <0.01 mg/min, or 0.3 mg/kg up to 10 mg buccal administration.
8. Some countries have paraldehyde which is an alternative to midazolam or clonazepam if these drugs are not available. Paraldehyde is administered in a glass syringe (not plastic) by intramuscular injection or 10ml of paraldehyde mixed in 100ml of 0.9 percent saline and infused intravenously over 10-15 minutes.
9. If all of this fails to control the seizures the patient will require intubation, ventilation and barbiturate infusion such as thiopentone. Note that the patient may develop respiratory depression from repeated doses of diazepam and may require intubation on this basis.
10. Hyperthermia occurs frequently and should be treated by passive cooling (e.g. sponging, fanning and paracetamol).

Table 9.2 The causes of convulsions.

Infection

    Meningitis, encephalitis, HIV, malaria, abscess, parasites

Pyrexia

    Febrile fit

Metabolic

    Hypoglycaemia,

    Hypocalcaemia (tetany), hypomagnesaemia

    Electrolyte abnormalities, renal failure

    In-born errors of metabolism

Toxins

    Lead, drugs including overdose of lignocaine

Trauma

    Cerebral contusion

Figure 9.2 *(Continued)*

Intracranial haematoma

Chronic subdural

Post-traumatic epilepsy

Vascular

Hypertensive encephalopathy

Arteriovenous malformation

Cavernous malformation

Venous sinus thrombosis

Mass lesion

Neoplasm, chronic subdural haematoma or abscess

Congenital

Tuberous sclerosis (tuber)

Sturge-Weber syndrome

Cortical dysplasia

Cerebral palsy, mental retardation

Post-traumatic seizures

Post-traumatic seizures are divided into **early** (less than 7 days) and **late** (greater than 7 days) after head trauma. A third group of 'immediate' posttraumatic seizures occur very shortly after the impact injury, but carry a good prognosis, usually do not recur, and do not require any ongoing prophylaxis. Early posttraumatic seizures have a higher incidence in children than adults, but late seizures are much less frequent in children. Most children will develop posttraumatic seizures within 24 hours of the injury. There is an incidence of 10-13 percent of late onset post-traumatic seizures within 2 years after a serious head injury for all age groups. Late seizures are focal or tonic-clonic in type.

Patients at high risk for developing post-traumatic seizures are those with a GCS <10 on admission, intracranial haemorrhage, compound depressed skull fractures with brain injury, cortical (haemorrhagic) contusion on CT, early seizure within the first 24 hours after injury, penetrating brain injury, or history of significant alcohol abuse. There is increasing doubt about the efficacy of prophylactic anticonvulsant therapy following head injury.

Prophylactic anticonvulsants reduce the risk of early seizures but after one week, there is no benefit in continuing the drugs.

However, the three factors that increase the risk of late epilepsy significantly are an acute intracranial haematoma evacuated within 2 weeks of injury, an early fit, or a compound depressed fracture of the vault. When any of these three factors exist, or following the development of a late posttraumatic seizure, or where there is a prior seizure history, the maintenance of anticonvulsant therapy is indicated for 6-12 months. In all the other patients with significant head injury, it is recommended that antiepileptic drugs (phenytoin or carbamazepine) are tapered after one week of therapy. Levetiracetam or phenytoin are commonly used as prophylactic antiepileptic drugs.

Carbamazepine or sodium valproate are alternatives. Any further seizures while the patient is off the drugs, will require two years of prophylactic therapy, and if fit free during this time, the anticonvulsants can be ceased. It may be difficult to acquire and maintain these drugs for prolonged periods in the developing world. If available, an EEG is often performed before discontinuing antiepileptic drugs. Stopping anti-convulsive therapy has medico-legal implications, but EEG does not have a good predictive value in this situation, and will not be readily available in the developing world.

The side effects of phenytoin are: gum hypertrophy, anaemia, skin rashes, drowsiness, lethargy, ataxia, mental confusion, gastrointestinal upset, lymphadenopathy, hyperglycaemia, hepatic dysfunction, hirsutism, acne, and teratogenic effects in pregnancy. If any rash occurs, the drug should be ceased immediately and the patient changed to levetiracetam or carbamazepine, otherwise the rash may progress severely and involve the mouth and throat. The side effects of levetiracetam are drowsiness, weakness, anorexia, tiredness and dizziness. Side effects of carbamazepine are drowsiness, gastrointestinal upset, hepatic disturbance, haematological changes including aplastic anaemia (rare), agranulocytosis, skin reactions, and teratogenic effects in pregnancy.

Postoperative epilepsy

Surgery for cerebral abscess, intracranial tumour including burr hole biopsy, and aneurysm, carry a significant risk of postoperative epilepsy. In these operations, prophylaxis is recommended with levetiracetam or phenytoin as the drugs of choice. The drug is commenced the night before surgery or during the surgery. In children, we taper the drug after a week, and would only restart if seizures develop. The risk of seizures is highest in the first week after surgery. In adults, phenytoin or levetiracetam is continued for 3-6 months and then tapered off. If seizures occur despite adequate phenytoin or levetiracetam (confirmed on plasma levels if available), then carbamazepine or sodium valproate should be added. Seizures do not occur after posterior fossa surgery so prophylaxis is not required.

Driving and epilepsy

Patients with recurrent seizures should not drive until they are seizure free for 6 months to a year but this time period may vary with local regulations. Supratentorial craniotomy or significant head injury preclude driving for three months. Patients with a malignant glioma should in general, not be driving, because of the ongoing risk of epilepsy, and the likely mental deterioration as the tumour progresses.

Surgery for epilepsy

Where comprehensive and well-resourced epilepsy programmes are in place, some patients with chronic and intractable epilepsy are considered for surgery. Thorough investigation is performed using MR and functional imaging, nuclear brain scans, video-EEG monitoring, neuropsychological testing, and sometimes direct cortical monitoring with implanted electrode grids.

Selective temporal lobectomy, which includes **amygdalo-hippocampectomy** is effective in patients with complex partial seizures due to mesial temporal sclerosis. Elimination of seizures is obtained in 70-80 per cent of cases. Drop attacks may be helped significantly by **corpus callosotomy.**

Hemispherectomy may be indicated for intractable seizures arising from a damaged or malformed hemisphere associated with hemiplegia.

Lesionectomy in focal and some generalised epilepsy cases may be indicated for tumour, developmental lesions such as cortical dysplasia or a tuber in tuberous sclerosis.

Unfortunately, the advanced diagnostic facilities and surgical skills are unlikely to be available in the developing world where there may be many patients who might benefit.

CONVULSIONS IN CHILDREN

John D. Vince

Convulsions in children present either in the form of an acute medical emergency or as a child with a history of fits. A logical approach to both situations is required. The following clinical approach has been written assuming that CT and MRI scans may not be available for those who must treat childhood convulsions in the tropics and low resource settings.

Classification

The typical grand mal convulsion, recognisable by medical and lay person alike is only one form of seizure. Other types are more difficult to recognise but are convulsions nevertheless. Seizures can be classified in a number of ways, each classification having its drawback. The common types of fit are described in Table 9.3, page 456 in a roughly chronological order of most frequent occurrence. Fits in children can be further classified depending on the presence or absence of fever at onset.

Fits with fever

Indicative of underlying brain pathology

In these instances, such as meningitis, cerebral malaria or encephalitis, the fit can be thought of as being the result of the inflammatory processes in the brain. Since these illnesses are both common and serious, they must be considered in all fitting children.

Caused by a fever in the absence of acute brain pathology - febrile convulsion of childhood

The term febrile convulsion of childhood is specific for a convulsion occurring in a child aged 4 months to 5 years, who has no history of afebrile fits, who has no history of previous CNS damage, and who has a fever > 38°C which is not associated with a specific central nervous system infection (meningitis, encephalitis, cerebral malaria). The most common cause of the fever is an upper respiratory infection. It should be remembered also that the fever of malaria may cause a febrile convulsion. The distinction between a febrile convulsion due to 'simple' malaria and a fit due to cerebral malaria is based on the presence of signs of neurological involvement · in particular persisting disturbance of consciousness and localising signs.

Three to four per cent of normal children will have a febrile fit · and a third of those who fit will have more than one. In the majority of cases the fit is classified as simple · short lasting (less than 15 minutes), generalised (no focal features) and with minimal postictal drowsiness or neurological disturbance.

Typically, by the time the child is brought to medical attention the fit has finished and the child is awake, hot and bothered. Such simple febrile convulsions are not associated with long-term CNS damage. In a proportion of children with febrile convulsion the fits are complex (i.e. they last longer than 15 minutes, have focal features, or are recurrent in the same febrile illness). Such complex febrile fits are associated with a high recurrence rate, a higher risk of subsequent epilepsy (afebrile seizures) · though the risk is still relatively small · and are more likely to be associated with previous CNS damage than are simple febrile fits.

Afebrile fits

A single afebrile fit may be an indicator of metabolic disturbance (such as hypoglycaemia) or of non-infective intracranial pathology such as a space occupying lesion. The term epilepsy is used to describe recurrent afebrile seizures of any type.

Management of the fitting child

Management is much easier for two people than for a single operator · call for help. Management can be divided into five aspects · but more than one aspect can and should be undertaken at the same time.

The management plan is shown in brief in Figure 9.3, page 452 and described in detail as follows:

Clear and maintain the airway

- Nurse the child on his/her side.
- Suck out secretions or vomitus.
- Use a plastic airway if available.
- Empty the stomach through a nasogastric tube.

Prevent CNS damage by correcting hypoxaemia and metabolic disorder

1. Give oxygen if available by nasal catheter, nasal prongs or mask.

2. If the child is not breathing, get air or (preferably) oxygen into the lungs with one of the following techniques:
   - bag and mask ventilation,
   - nasopharyngeal catheter and frog breathing (oxygen required at 2-4 litres/min),
   - endotracheal tube and ventilation,
   - mouth to mouth resuscitation.

3. Check for hypoglycaemia with Dextrostix

   If hypoglycaemia (blood glucose < 3 mmol/1, 55 mg/dl) give i.v. 5ml/kg of 10% dextrose over 5-10 minutes or, if not available give i.v.50 percent dextrose 1 ml/kg as a slow bolus (over 1-2 minutes) followed by dextrose saline drip to run at two-thirds maintenance requirements and continue regular Dextrostix checks.

Stop the fit

1. Use midazolam 0.05 mg/kg IV, at <0.01 mg/min or 0.3 mg/kg up to 10 mg by buccal administration.
2. Or diazepam 0.5 mg/kg p.r. or 0.25 mg/kg i.v. Repeat if no control after 5 minutes.
3. Or Paraldehyde 0.2ml/kg by deep intramuscular injection.
4. Change to alternative if no control after further 10 mins.
5. If still fitting, after 10 minutes give either:

- **Phenobarbital (Phenobarbitone)** 15-20 mg/kg i.v./i.m. over 5 min or,
- **Phenytoin** 15-20 mg/kg i.v. over 30 min,
- **Midazolam, propofol, or thiopentone infusions** are alternatives but intubation will be needed.

6. Phenobarbitone or Phenytoin are used for prophylaxis of further fits. Observe for potential adverse effects of therapy as diazepam may cause respiratory depression in neonates.
   - The combination of diazepam, phenobarbital (phenobarbitone) is a potent cause of respiratory depression in neonates, so prepare to ventilate for a short period. Rapid administration of phenytoin may cause cardiac arrhythmias.
   - Diazepam and phenytoin should never be given i.m. because it wastes time and drugs.

Treat the cause of the fit (Figure 9.3, page 452)

1. Do a careful physical examination. Don't forget the tympanic membranes and throat.

2. If the child is febrile investigate appropriately with:
   - lumbar puncture if there are signs of meningitis (unless there is papilloedema or the child is extremely ill)
   - dextrostix (and quantitative blood glucose if available) - good idea to do this in all cases
   - blood slide for malaria parasites in an endemic area.
   - blood culture
   - urine culture if no obvious cause of the fit
   - others if indicated and available

3. Treat as outlined below.

If there are signs of meningitis and the CSF is cloudy, blood stained or LP is unsuccessful, or if the child is too sick to do LP then treat for meningitis with Ceftriaxone or Ceftazidine if available- or chloramphenicol or high dose crystapen if not. Also check for malaria in endemic areas and treat for cerebral malaria using the available antimalarial drugs (usually Artemisinin combinations). Treat hyperthermia by cool (not cold) sponging (this is effective and involves the parents in the child's care) or with paracetamol. Treat with antibiotics if bacterial infection obvious or suspected (e.g. otitis media abscess).

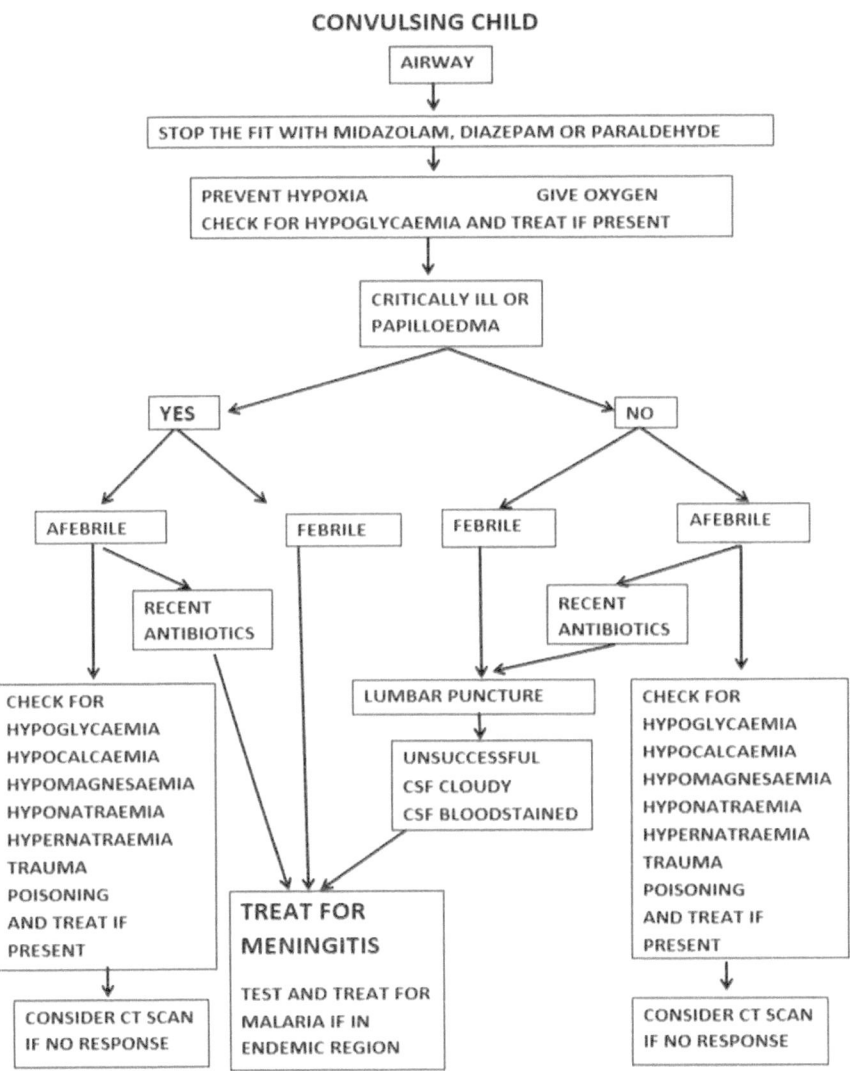

Figure 9.3 The management of a fitting child.

4. If the child is afebrile investigate appropriately:
   - Dextrostix (and qualitative blood sugar if available).

- Consider LP if the child is unwell or there are signs of meningitis,or the child has received antibiotics in the last few days (to exclude partially treated meningitis).
- Blood slide for malaria parasites. (to exclude partially treated malaria)
- Others if available:
  - serum calcium,
  - urea and creatinine and electrolytes,
  - liver function tests.

A CT scan may be indicated if available and no cause has been found using the simple investigations listed above. If the cause is suspected (e.g. hypocalcaemia) treat appropriately.

If the cause is not obvious and the fits are not controlled then treat empirically for metabolic causes:

- Calcium gluconate 10 percent 0.5 ml/kg i.v. slowly over 5 min
- Magnesium sulphate 50 per cent 0.2 ml/kg i.m.
- Pyridoxine 50 mg i.v. if available or 50-100 mg oral (or nasogastric tube)

If fit is completely 'unexplained' remember the possibility of head injury (search for bruises and localising signs) and poisoning (search for clues in the history and examination).

Prevent further fits

Unless the child has a simple febrile fit, give a loading dose of either phenobarbital (phenobarbitone) 15-20 mg/kg i.v. or i.m. over 5 min or phenytoin 15-20 mg/kg i.v. over 30 min if one of these has not been given already. Continue maintenance anticonvulsants for the duration of the illness, or for several months if the fits have been very difficult to control.

Practice point

The longer the fit lasts, the more likely there is to be permanent brain damage resulting from the fit itself. Never walk away from a fitting child until the convulsion has been controlled. Don't leave it to someone else!

The child with a febrile fit

As indicated above, by the time the child with a simple febrile fit is seen by medical personnel, the fit is usually over and the child is hot and bothered. If there are no signs of meningitis and the child is feeding well, it is not necessary to do a lumbar puncture, but the child should be observed carefully for several hours to make sure there is no change in his/her condition.

1. If it is the child's first or second fit and you are not sure if the child has signs of meningitis: do a lumbar puncture to exclude meningitis.
2. If the child has recurrent febrile fits (two or more):
   - If there is an obvious cause for the fever, and there are no other signs of meningitis - Treat the cause of the fever and observe the child.
   - If there is no obvious cause for the fever or
   - If the child looks sicker than you would expect or
   - If there is any suspicion of meningitis such as stiff neck – Do a lumbar puncture to exclude meningitis providing there is no papilloedema.

Practice point

Don't feel bad about obtaining clear CSF. That's a positive finding, in the interests of the child.

Management of the child with recurrent seizures

Recurrent febrile seizures

This is a debatable topic. There is no evidence that simple febrile seizures are harmful in themselves, though complex seizures may be. On the other hand seizures are disconcerting for the child and parents alike. Only phenobarbital (phenobarbitone) and valproate have been shown to be effective prophylactics, and both drugs may have side effects. Our policy is to use phenobarbital (phenobarbitone) if a child has three or more febrile seizures and to continue its use, in the absence of side effects, until the child has been seizure free for a year, after which it is slowly withdrawn over one week. This is combined with advice to parents of all children with a febrile fit to reduce the child's fever with sponging and paracetamol, and to nurse the child on his/her side should there be further episodes. In some countries, parents of children with recurrent seizures are advised to give rectal diazepam if the child fits - or develops a high fever. This is not the author's routine practice. A strong argument can be made for prescribing prophylactic phenobarbital (phenobarbitone) after a single, and certainly after two, complex febrile fits.

Recurrent afebrile seizures - epilepsy

The availability of anticonvulsant drugs in the tropics may be limited. Nevertheless, with appropriate use, reasonable control can be achieved in most cases.

In selecting drug therapy, the following rules should apply:
1. Aim to use a single drug if possible.
2. Use a drug that is readily available for the patient (this will vary depending on access to Health Centre or Hospital}.
3. Give the correct dose of the drug.
4. Change to another drug only after a fair trial of the one initially selected. (Remember that it takes about 5 days to achieve adequate therapeutic levels for most anticonvulsants if no loading dose is given.)
5. Use more than one anticonvulsant only if satisfactory control with one drug is not achieved.
6. Try and review the patient frequently when starting treatment, to ensure adequate compliance and control.

The available anticonvulsants, indications for their use, and side effects are shown in Table 9.4, page 458 and Table 9.5, page 459. Phenobarbital (phenobarbitone) and phenytoin are readily available, have the advantage of a single daily dosage regime, but have side effects. They are the drugs of choice in neonates. Carbamazepine, while less familiar to many medical and nursing staff, is extremely useful, covering all the types of seizure covered by phenobarbital and phenytoin, and being the drug of choice for benign focal epilepsies of childhood, temporal lobe epilepsy and, initially for myoclonic jerks, drop attacks and infantile spasms.

A twice daily - rather than the usually recommended three times daily - regimen is practicable in most cases. There are newer anticonvulsants such as vigabatrin, lamotrigine and gabapentin which are used for poorly controlled epilepsy in well-resourced settings, but these are usually not available in the less well-off regions of the tropics. Infantile spasms, myoclonic jerks and akinetic seizures may be very difficult to control. Should carbamazepine not be successful, nitrazepam should be tried initially with the carbamazepine and then on its own. Patients may develop apparent 'resistance' to nitrazepam - but its effectiveness may be restored by a drug 'holiday' of 2-3 weeks. In severe cases the 'holiday' can be covered by an alternative anticonvulsant (valproate or steroids). Should nitrazepam fail, or be impractical because of side effects (excessive salivation and bronchial secretion being the most troublesome), it will be necessary to use prednisolone. For the management of children with petit mal, ethosuximide and sodium valproate are both effective. It is important to remember that there are some conditions that may mimic seizures. These are syncope, breath holding attacks, tics and hysteria. Prolonged breath holding attacks may sometimes end in a fit. A careful history will almost always distinguish these conditions from genuine seizures.

The management of children with epilepsy consists not only of rational drug prescribing, but also of trying to ensure that they achieve a normal life style appropriate for their age and background if this is at all possible. This may involve writing letters to teachers and headmasters to support applications for school entry, and encouraging participation in sports. Clearly activities such as climbing coconut or betel nut trees should be discouraged - but providing the epilepsy is under good control, swimming should be allowed in the presence of other competent swimmers.

Table 9.3 Classification of fits in children.

---

1. Neonatal fits

Changes in normal activity

Deviation / flickering of eyes

Changes in breathing pattern

Apnoea

Unusual cry

Lip smacking

Repetitive protrusion of tongue

'Cycling' movements of limbs

Tonic-clonic seizures - focal or generalised

Tonic seizures - opisthotonic, decerebrate posture

Table 9.3 *(Continued)*

Myoclonic jerks - repetitive jerking of part of face, or of one or more part of one or more limbs

2. Infantile spasms (salaam spasm)

Sudden tonic spasms, often of trunk, may involve the neck only

Begin usually at 3-9 months

80% associated with severe CNS damage either before or after. Usually cease by 2-4 years but may be replaced by other seizure types

3. Myoclonic jerks

Sudden jerking movements of neck or one or more limbs

May occur with akinetic seizures

4. Akinetic seizures

Sudden loss of tone causing falling to ground drop attacks

Myoclonic and akinetic seizures begin usually in preschool child

May also be associated with tonic clonic seizures

High incidence of CNS damage particularly in the severe form Lennox-Gastaut syndrome

5. Tonic-clonic fits

Typical grand mal 'seizure'

May be aura, tonic then clonic phase, often incontinence and often postictal drowsiness

6. Petit mal (absence attacks)

Onset usually 5-10 years

Sudden cessation of activity - staring into space

May be blinking or upward deviation of eyes

Mouthing movements

Fine movements of the hands

Usually last 5-10 seconds but may be repetitive

A majority of patients conditions resolve by late adolescence.

7. Benign focal seizures of childhood

Usually focal motor seizures often of face

May be sensory features

Often just before or just after sleep or on waking

Onset usually 5-10 years

Excellent prognosis

Common clinical problems

Table 9.3 *(Continued)*

---

8. Psychomotor (temporal lobe) seizures
Complex psychological and perceptual disturbances (e.g. taste, smell or visual aura)

Purposeless motor activity (e.g. lip smacking)

May be autonomic disturbances

Usually starts after the age of 5 years

Prognosis is relatively poor. However, the newer antiepileptic drugs are improving control. If there is a structural lesion, such as mesial temporal sclerosis (which is the most common cause), or a temporal lobe tumour, or developmental lesion, resective surgery may be indicated (see section on epilepsy surgery page 314).

Table 9.4 Drugs used in the treatment of recurrent seizures.

Drug	Dose		Indications	Main side effects
	Loading	Maintenance		
Phenobarbital *phenobarbitone*	15 mg/ kg orally	5 mg/ kg daily	Grand mal Benign focal Temporal lobe	Behaviour disorder
Phenytoin	15 mg/ kg orally	5 mg/ kg daily	Grand mal Benign focal Temporal lobe	Gum hypertrophy Ataxia Rash Hirsutism Acne Blood dyscrasia
Carbamazepine		5-15 mg/ kg b.d.	Grand mal Benign focal* Temporal lobe* Infantile spasms Akinetic seizures Myoclonic jerks	Rashes Liver dysfunction Leucopenia Nausea and vomiting
Nitrazepam		0.25-0.5 mg/ kg b.d.	Infantile spasms Myoclonic jerks Akinetic seizures	Initial drowsiness Hypersalivation Increased bronchial secretion 'Resistance'
Sodium valproate		5-15 mg/ kg b.d	Grand mal Petit mal Benign focal Temporal lobe Infantile spasms, Akinetic seizures, Myoclonic jerks	Weight gain Gastrointestinal upset Liver toxicity Sedation Alopecia Thrombocytopenia

Table 9.4 *(Continued)*

Drug	Dose		Indications	Main side effects
	Loading	**Maintenance**		
Ethosuximide		2.5-12.5 mg/ kg t.d.s.	Petit mal	Gastrointestinal upset Thrombocytopenia
Prednisolone		1-2 mg/ kg/ day	Infantile spasms	Cushing's syndrome Growth retardation

Table 9.5 Drugs suitable for use in specific types of epilepsy.

Neonatal seizures	Phenobarbital, phenytoin
Grand mal	Phenobarbital, phenytoin, carbamazepine
Petit mal	Ethosuximide*, sodium valproate
Benign focal	Carbamazepine*
Psychomotor (temporal lobe)	Carbamazepine*
Infantile spasms	Carbamazepine, nitrazepam, prednisolone
Myoclonic jerks	Carbamazepine, nitrazepam, prednisolone
Akinetic seizures	Carbamazepine, nitrazepam, prednisolone

* Drug of choice

Unfortunately, a sizeable proportion of the children with the most severe epilepsy will have underlying brain damage and developmental delay, and some may be hyperactive. Physiotherapy is likely to be important, and parents can be shown how to prevent contractures in children with cerebral palsy. Advice can be given on simple 'helps', such as sitting supports and eating and drinking utensils to make life easier for the children's parents, and to give the child more independence. Most parents appreciate regular contact with the health professional, even if there doesn't appear to be much progress. The management of a child with epilepsy is not always straightforward. However, simple drugs will do the job in most cases and most epileptic children can be well controlled. Even in the most severe cases, improvement can be achieved.

ACUTE VISUAL LOSS (FIGURE 2.9, PAGE 26)

The causes of sudden visual failure are best classified according to anatomical location.

Eye

- Retinal artery or vein occlusion
- Vitreous haemorrhage
- Retinal detachment
- Acute glaucoma
- Uveitis

- **Acute optic neuritis**
  This is caused by inflammation of the retrobulbar optic nerve, i.e. the optic nerve behind the globe of the eye, so that there is no papilloedema present. Only a small proportion will have papillitis (inflammation of the optic nerve head on fundal examination). There may be tenderness over the globe of the eye and pain on eye movement. It is usually unilateral and multiple sclerosis is the usual cause. It may occur in repeated attacks. The patients are usually young (18-50 years).
- **Ischaemic papillitis**
  The optic nerve become ischaemic due to arteritis or vascular occlusion. The optic disc appears swollen and pale. These conditions require urgent referral to an ophthalmologist.
- **Amaurosis fugax**
  Episodes of monocular visual loss, lasting one to two minutes; like a shutter or curtain coming down over the eye. Retinal artery emboli may be seen on fundoscopy and it is usually due to carotid stenosis in the neck (see Chapter 8, page 399).

Compression of the optic nerve

This usually results in a painless loss of vision. The many types of mass lesions in the orbit that compress or involve the optic nerve are described in Chapter 6.

Compression of the optic chiasm

This is usually due to an enlarging pituitary tumour from below. Meningiomas are less common. With a pituitary tumour, the visual loss is bitemporal in approximately 60 per cent, unilateral blindness with a contralateral temporal field cut is present in approximately 15 per cent, homonymous hemianopia occurs in 10 per cent and temporal scotomatous defects and temporal loss occur in 10 per cent of cases.

Retrochiasmal visual pathway lesion

This includes damage to the optic tract and radiation, which will produce a homonymous hemianopia or quadrantanopia. These patients may not be aware of their visual defect and have normal pupillary reactions. Some have a sector of preserved vision in their fields which they use. It is easy to label these patients as being 'functional'. The causes are stroke and cerebral tumour. Cortical blindness results from bilateral occipital- cortical damage, usually from bilateral posterior cerebral artery lesions.

HEADACHE

The history should include length of history of headache, frequency of attacks and their duration, the site and quality of the pain, the mode of onset, any associated features and precipitating, aggravating or relieving factors.

Serious causes of headache

Subarachnoid haemorrhage

This will cause a sudden explosive headache, which may radiate down the neck and is associated with photophobia and meningism (neck stiffness and positive Kernig's sign - restricted straight leg raising). The patient may appear ill, febrile, and be drowsy, confused, irritable and resist examination. They may have nausea, vomiting, or focal neurological signs (see Chapter 8, page 402).

The headache of raised intracranial pressure

This headache may build up over several days to weeks, is often episodic and may be localised or generalised. It is classically worse on waking, and may be precipitated or aggravated by exercise or any activity causing a further pressure rise, e.g. cough, straining or sexual intercourse. There is often associated nausea and vomiting, and papilloedema. There may be some neck stiffness associated with tonsillar herniation. As the pressure increases further, there may be short periods of loss of consciousness (cerebellar fits). This is due to acute rises of intracranial pressure associated with obstructive hydrocephalus. Focal neurological signs may be present.

Giant cell arteritis (temporal arteritis)

There is patchy inflammation of external carotid branches, but also sometimes intracranial arteries and the retinal vessels. This may eventually lead to a thrombotic occlusion of the retinal arteries and blindness. It usually affects patients over 60 years of age, and is associated with general malaise, joint pains, night sweats, weight loss and anorexia. The headache is continuous and throbbing in nature with localised tenderness over the affected scalp vessels: most often the superficial temporal artery, which may feel swollen and thickened. The patient may have increased pain on chewing. The ESR will be elevated (greater than 60 mm/hour). The treatment is prednisolone 60-80 mg per day. The diagnosis can be confirmed with a biopsy of the segment of superficial temporal artery, which can be done under local anaesthetic.

Causes of recurrent or chronic headache

Migraine

Migraine is an episodic lateralised headache which is associated with prostration and vomiting. It is usually idiopathic and there is often a family history. The intensity duration and frequency vary considerably. It affects 10-20 percent of the population to some degree, e.g. many only have one to two attacks a year. There may be warning transient ischaemic symptoms often with visual patterns or flashing lights, scotomata, field loss or blurred vision. Giddiness occurs in about 25 per cent, but other neurological problems such as hemiparesis, hemisensory disturbance, speech disturbance or diplopia are uncommon. These last about 10 minutes followed by the build-up of an intense throbbing headache which probably represents a vasodilatation phase. During the attack there may be photophobia, scalp tenderness and dilated scalp vessels. Many triggers to migraine are recognised including certain foods (chocolate, spices, cheese, citrus fruit etc.), trauma, the contraceptive pill, exertion, red wine, and stress. The treatment is outside the scope of this book.

Cluster headache

Cluster headache is less common than migraine, more common in men than women and starts in early middle age. The pain is intense and occurs around the eye and is associated with conjunctival injection, eye watering and rhinorrhoea. Clusters of attacks may be separated by weeks or months and each attack lasts 10 minutes to 2 hours. The migraine drugs are used to treat it.

Tension headache

Tension headache is a chronic and persistent headache, often present all day, may last days to months and does not interfere with sleep. It may not respond to simple analgesics. It may be related to muscle contraction, nervous anxiety and/or depression. It may be described as a tight band on the head, a weight, heaviness, crushing pain or pressure around or over the head and is often associated with other pains. About 75 per cent of the patients are women. There should be a normal physical examination. A change in the pattern of the headache may indicate a serious underlying cause.

Cervical spondylosis

Degenerative arthritis in the neck may cause pains radiating up into the occiput and occipital region, in the distribution of the second and third cervical roots. It is often associated with muscle spasm and there may be radicular symptoms and signs in the upper limbs.

Post-traumatic headache

Headache is common after head injury and even minor head injuries may result in persistent severe headache. Compensation may affect the course of posttraumatic headache adversely. Post-concussional syndrome includes headache, dizziness, light-headedness, blurred vision, impaired concentration, irritability and depression. The pain is very variable in quality and often aggravated by exertion and mental effort and relieved by rest. Post traumatic amnesia testing for patients with concussion is discussed in Chapter 3, page 91. A chronic subdural haematoma needs to be excluded.

Chronic subdural haematoma

After a trivial head injury, elderly patients often present with dull generalised headache, present for several weeks, associated with impaired alertness, memory and general apathy. The symptoms and signs often fluctuate. The patient may present with a confusional state or dementia. One-third will have papilloedema. Most appear drowsy, vague or confused. There may be focal limb signs. About 20 percent will have bilateral subdural haematomas.

Benign intracranial hypertension (BIH) (pseudotumour cerebri or idiopathic intracranial hypertension (IIP))

The patient presents with chronic headaches with bilateral papilloedema but no space occupying lesion on imaging. The ICP may reach extremely high levels (30-40 cmH$_2$O) with the patient alert, because there is no differential in pressure or brain shift throughout the intradural space. The CSF is normal. BIH may occur in children, but is more common in overweight young adult women. There may be an enlarged sella turcica on plain skull X-ray which may be mistaken for a pituitary tumour. This appearance is due to an 'empty sella', which is an open sella filled with CSF with the pituitary gland squashed against the back wall of the pituitary fossa. CT scan shows a normal brain, with small ventricles.

BIH is usually idiopathic but in some cases, there is an occlusion of a venous sinus, particularly the transverse sinus. Where there is limited access to medical care or non-compliance, septic thrombosis following chronic ear infection is an important cause of this problem, but otherwise most venous sinus obstruction is due to a haematological cause. Other associations are the oral contraceptive, excess vitamin A, tetracyclines, iron deficiency anaemia, chronic renal failure and some endocrine disorders. The main differential diagnosis of benign intracranial hypertension in the tropics is chronic meningitis, or cryptococcal meningitis, but other causes such as malignancy affecting the CSF (carcinomatous meningitis), cerebral vasculitis, lead poisoning and gliomatosis cerebri (diffuse infiltrating glioma causing brain swelling), should also be considered.

These patients need to be monitored closely, particularly in relation to visual fields and acuity because if the papilloedema progresses, the patient may suffer permanent impairment of vision or even go blind. A lumbar puncture revealing high pressure is diagnostic and also therapeutic following drainage of CSF. Lumbar punctures with CSF drainage to lower the CSF pressures to normal every 2 or 3 days for 1-2 weeks, may allow the condition to subside and many cases are self-limiting. The condition may also improve spontaneously if affected obese women lose weight. The addition of diuretics such as acetazolamide may also help. If the condition progresses, or fails to improve with the conservative management a lumboperitoneal shunt, placed from the lumbar intraspinal subarachnoid space and the tubing passed subcutaneously to enter the peritoneal cavity anterolaterally via a separate incision. This is an effective means of permanently lowering the ICP.

Other causes of headache

1. Chronic sinus infection, including the sphenoid sinus.
2. Ocular pain, e.g. acute glaucoma or inflammation of the eye.
3. Chronic focusing problems, e.g. astigmatism.
4. Dental pain, e.g. dental abscess or temporomandibular joint dysfunction.
5. Chronic ear infection.
6. Systemic disorders such as hypertension or fever.

FACIAL PAIN

Acute pain

1. **Sinus infection**. This causes a throbbing facial pain overlying the involved sinus. There may be accompanying nasal obstruction and purulent discharge although an occluded ostium will prevent any discharge. There may be local tenderness over the sinus and plain X-rays help confirm the diagnosis.
2. **Dental disease**. There is a throbbing severe pain associated with local tenderness and soft tissue swelling, and perhaps a purulent discharge from the gum. The affected tooth may be loose and affected by obvious decay.
3. **Ocular inflammation**. The acute red eye may cause local pain and requires referral to an ophthalmologist.
4. **Herpes zoster ophthalmicus**. This presents with acute pain in the forehead and eye and within 3-4 days an herpetic skin eruption appears. The eyelids may swell severely and the eye becomes more painful and inflamed. Ophthalmological referral is necessary.
5. **Giant cell arteritis** (see headache section above). This may involve the facial artery with pain aggravated by chewing.
6. **Acute trauma**.

Recurrent facial pain

1. **Migraine** (see headache section).
2. **Cluster headache** (migrainous neuralgia) (see headache section).

Trigeminal neuralgia (tic douloureux)

The pain is described as severe and stabbing, like electric shocks lasting usually seconds only and affecting one side of the face. It is often triggered by touch, movement, washing, shaving, eating or temperature. The patient becomes fearful of the activities that produce the pain. There may be long periods of freedom from pain in between the episodes. Importantly, there are no abnormal neurological signs particularly in relation to the trigeminal nerve.

There is no sensory loss or disturbance of the corneal reflex. It is usually due to an artery pulsating against the trigeminal nerve as it enters the brain stem. This is usually the superior cerebellar artery.

Bilateral trigeminal neuralgia is very uncommon and is seen in patients with multiple sclerosis affecting the brain stem. Trigeminal neuralgia usually responds to carbamazepine, valproate, clonazepam, phenytoin or baclofen. Two-thirds of patients with trigeminal neuralgia will respond to carbamazepine. The surgery is described in Chapter 10 on page 491.

Glossopharyngeal neuralgia

This pain is similar to that of trigeminal neuralgia but affects one side of the throat or the ear, and may be triggered by swallowing. The medical treatment is the same as for trigeminal neuralgia. For intractable cases, intracranial section of the glossopharyngeal nerve and the upper rootlets of the vagus usually stops the pain.

Chronic facial pain

It is important to examine the cranial nerves closely. Ocular symptoms and signs may suggest an orbital tumour. Sensory loss on the face or nasal symptoms and signs may suggest a nasopharyngeal carcinoma or lymphoma. Lower cranial nerve involvement may suggest a tumour eroding the skull base.

Post-herpetic neuralgia

After an attack of herpes zoster ophthalmicus (shingles) about 15 percent of patients will develop chronic severe pain in the site of the previous infection. Antidepressants such as amitriptyline may be helpful.

Temporomandibular joint dysfunction

This is a much over-diagnosed problem and may be associated with an audible clicking of the jaw joint, with pain in front of the ear. There may be malocclusion of the bite and sometimes locking of the jaw. Referral to a dentist, or a maxillofacial surgeon will be necessary.

Atypical facial pain

This is often a continuous and variable pain, often in middle-aged women and is little affected by simple analgesics. Many of the patients are depressed. All investigations are negative. It is a diagnosis of exclusion.

FACIAL PALSY

The deficits produced by facial nerve lesions may include reduced taste (chorda tympani nerve), hyperacusis (louder sounds due to loss of the stapedius reflex), and reduced lacrimation and salivation.

The upper half of the face has bilateral supranuclear involvement, so that a unilateral upper motor neuron facial palsy will cause only weakness of the contralateral lower half of the face, whereas a lesion affecting the facial nerve nucleus or the facial nerve will cause weakness of the entire ipsilateral side of the face.

It is best to think anatomically to work out the cause of a facial palsy (Table 9.6, below).

Table 9.6 The causes of facial palsy.

Unilateral upper motor facial neuron palsy
1.   Vascular - haemorrhage or infarction
2.   Tumour
3.   Demyelination
4.   Abscess
Unilateral lower motor neuron palsy
1.   Brain stem. There may be an associated sixth nerve palsy
Vascular
Tumour
Demyelination
Encephalitis

Table 9.6 *(Continued)*

---

2. Cerebellopontine angle

   Acoustic neuroma

   Meningioma

   Epidermoid

3. Facial canal in the petrous temporal bone

   Fracture of the skull base

   Middle ear sepsis

   Bell's palsy (see separate section)

   Herpes zoster of the facial nerve ganglion (geniculate ganglion)

   Tumour invasion of the skull base

4. Peripheral nerve lesion

   Parotid tumour

   Parotid surgery

   Facial trauma

Bilateral complete facial palsy

1. Bilateral nuclear

   Vascular-infarction, haemorrhage

   Demyelination

   Tumour

   Infection

   Syrinx

   Congenital (Mobius' syndrome) – rare

2. Bilateral infranuclear

   Guillain-Barre syndrome (acute post-infectious polyneuropathy)

   Bell's palsy - rarely bilateral

3. Muscle disease

   Myasthenia gravis

   Myotonic dystrophy

   Facio-scapula-humeral dystrophy

Bell's palsy

Bell's palsy is a spontaneous onset of lower motor neuron facial paralysis which develops over 24-48 hours and may be partial or complete. There is a danger of corneal exposure injury, i.e. corneal ulceration, if the eyelids cannot be closed. There may be some pain or discomfort behind the ear at the onset. If the facial nerve proximal to the chorda tympani nerve is involved, then taste on the anterior two-thirds of the tongue is also affected. The cause of Bell's palsy is obscure but may represent a viral infection of the nerve, with acute swelling. This may result in demyelination and then slow regeneration must occur if recovery is to take place.

There is an increased incidence in patients with hypertension, diabetes and multiple sclerosis. Prednisolone 40-60 mg per day, given for 5 days, may be used in the early stages to try and reduce the swelling of the nerve and any permanent damage. Recovery may be incomplete in severe cases. If herpes zoster is responsible (geniculate zoster), there may be pain in the ear and vesicles in the external auditory meatus, acute deafness and vertigo as well as the facial palsy.

TORTICOLLIS

Birth torticollis

Congenital wry neck or torticollis begins during the first month of life, and is due to a shortening of the sternomastoid, which develops a firm spindle shaped mass in the midportion of sternomastoid which is an inflammatory pseudotumour. This mass settles after 2-3 months and the muscle becomes fibrotic and shortened. Histologically, there is acellular connective tissue and an ischaemic mechanism seems the most likely cause, perhaps triggered by birth injury. The head of the normal newborn can be turned 90°, but in the affected infants the head is turned to one side, with the occiput pointing towards the side of the sternomastoid problem and there is restricted motion to the opposite side. In long-standing cases there may be an associated secondary plagiocephaly with facial asymmetry.

Management

Turn the infant's head opposite way when asleep. The sternomastoid is stretched up to 10 times, twice a day by extending the neck and turning it in the opposite direction. If the torticollis is not settling with expectant management, and plagiocephaly is developing there is a place for partial section of the affected sternomastoid muscle.

Torticollis in older children and adults

The causes of torticollis in older children and adults are listed in Table 9.7, next page.

The management of torticollis

The primary cause is treated and acute torticollis may be eased with halter cervical traction, which consists of a chin-occiput strap and gentle traction for 2 weeks, then a soft collar.

Spasmodic torticollis

Spasmodic torticollis is defined as involuntary turning of the head on the trunk, sometimes with additional forward flexion (anterocollis), backwards extension (retrocollis) or lateral flexion (laterocollis). When it affects the thoracolumbar spine it is called torsional dystonia. The cause is unknown but recent psychophysical studies have shown abnormalities in the way patients with torticollis judge the position of their bodies and how they recognise 'straight ahead'. The sternomastoid and adjacent muscles are contracting continuously often with intermittent spasms causing the torticollis and often marked hypertrophy of the affected muscles. The treatment of chronic spasmodic torticollis is problematic. Mild cases can be treated with partial section of the sternomastoid, although this is unlikely to solve the problem because other cervical muscle groups are usually involved. Botulinum toxin has also been used in mild cases, but only has a temporary effect, is expensive, and not readily available in low resource settings. More invasive surgery for severe cases involves upper cervical laminectomy, sectioning of the C1 to 3 motor rootlets intradurally, and bilateral accessory nerve section at the C1 level. This operation carries a significant risk of destabilising the neck, causing swallowing problems and shoulder paresis. It is only undertaken by a specialist neurosurgeon.Stereotactic pallidotomy or thalamotomy or deep brain stimulation are also used in some severe cases of dystonia with spasmodic torticollis.

Table 9.7 The causes of torticollis.

Acute

1. A neck injury
2. Cervical disc prolapse
3. Infection
   - cervical abscess
   - retropharyngeal abscess
   - cervical TB
4. Wry neck
   - self-limiting spasm of sternomastoid ? post trauma, ?myositis

Chronic

1. Chronic osteomyelitis or TB
2. Posterior fossa tumour with tonsillar herniation
3. Fourth nerve palsy with secondary torticollis to reduce the diplopia
4. Tumour of spinal cord or spinal column
5. Cervical cord syrinx
6. Chronic subluxation of cervical spine especially locked facet(s)
7. Spasmodic torticollis (see below)
8. Congenital disorders of the cervical spine, e.g. hemivertebra (rare)

Torticollis due to syringomyelia

MR is used to diagnose syringomyelia and this may be associated with cerebellar tonsil herniation. CT may show tonsillar herniation crowding the foramen magnum. CT myelography may be an alternative to MR in LMIC. The management is initially posterior fossa decompression of the tonsils and if this fails to relieve the syrinx, a secondary direct drainage of the syrinx either into the subarachnoid space or into the pleural or peritoneal cavity via a shunt tube is indicated to prevent progression of the neurological deficit.

Pain and peripheral nerve disorders

PERIPHERAL NERVE INJURY

The **Seddon Classification** of peripheral nerve injury:

Class 1 Neurapraxia. The mildest type of peripheral nerve injury. This is caused by blunt injury or prolonged pressure on the nerve. There is a short segment of demyelination but the axons remain intact. There is no Wallerian degeneration. There is initially a block of nerve transmission. The nerve function recovers fully in a few days to weeks.

Class 2 Axonotmesis. This nerve injury is due to crush or traction. The axon and myelin covering is damaged but the nerve sheath ie epineurium and perineurium, which is connective tissue, is intact. There is a block to transmission. There is Wallerian degeneration distal to the injury. Recovery may occur slowly without surgery but sometimes surgery is required to remove scar or perform a neurolysis.

Class 3 Neurotmesis. The most serious nerve injury. The axons and nerve sheaths are severed. Wallerian degeneration occurs distal to the lesion. There is a block of transmission. Motor, sensory and autonomic function are severely affected. A clean cut through the nerve has scope for immediate repair and more rapid recovery than a ragged laceration.

A peripheral axon will grow at a rate of approximately 1 mm per day with a greater speed proximally, and a slower speed distally. Reinnervation of intrinsic hand muscles is very unlikely to occur from an ulnar lesion at the brachial plexus level or foot reinnervation from a lumbar plexus injury. The difficult decision in peripheral nerve injury is when to explore; the history of mechanism of injury and the clinical examination are vitally important. If there is clearly a wound when the nerve could have been injured, this should be explored acutely and the peripheral nerves in the vicinity identified. Whether the nerve is a digital nerve or the sciatic nerve, the best results will be obtained if the nerve is repaired in the acute phase. A direct blow to a peripheral nerve may cause a neuropraxia or axonotmesis and most will improve. If there is no improvement in 3 months they should be explored. A neurolysis is performed - the nerve is freed from external scar (entrapment) and any discontinuity is repaired. This may permit partial recovery. Internal neurolysis, where individual fasciculi are freed requires microsurgery and results are often disappointing. Tinel's sign is a tingling felt distal to a nerve injury, elicited by tapping with the examiner's fingers at the point of denervation - this point will move progressively distally as the nerve regenerates. The limb distal to the injury should be kept moving through its full range with active physiotherapy, that the patient can learn to perform and repeat. After 3 months the motor end plates degenerate on the target muscles rendering reinnervation and therefore recovery incomplete, no matter how good is the surgical repair. Nerve conduction studies can be helpful in determining how much regeneration has occurred, but this test will not be readily available.

Nerve repair (Figure 10.1, page 476 and Figure 10.2, page 478)

The principles of repair are to obtain evenly incised ends using a scalpel blade before the anastomosis, but beware of excising too much from each end lest the ends become difficult to appose. Use a microscope if possible to appose the epineurium of the major fasciculi with 8/0-10/0 nylon (this is the type of suture that is available for ophthalmology) and then suture the perineurium with interrupted sutures with 6/0-8/0 nylon - as few sutures as are necessary to appose the ends. There should be minimal if any diathermy for haemostasis, as minimal dissection as is necessary to mobilise the nerve ends so that vascularity is not compromised and there is no tension on the ends. If there is ongoing tension there will be a poor functional result and the anastomosis may completely dehisce. The adjacent joint can be flexed to relieve tension and a plaster of Paris back slab placed across the joint for immobilisation at the end of the procedure. If this is not sufficient then a single or multiple cable nerve graft will be required. The sural nerve is an ideal source.

Brachial plexus injury

There is an increasing trend to explore brachial plexus injuries acutely, particularly if they are partial. However, this remains controversial and is unlikely to be practical in many parts of the developing world. If there is evidence of nerve root avulsion on myelography - the presence of pseudomeningoceles is a guide - these nerve roots should not be explored. The presence of a triple response (wheal, flare) to scratching the skin in the presence of a complete root injury in that dermatome implies complete root avulsion (proximal to the dorsal root ganglion, which is where the synapse occurs for the reflex).

The presence of a Horner's syndrome with a brachial plexus palsy presents with a constricted pupil (meiosis), ptosis, lack of ipsilateral sweating on the face, and indicates a disruption of the sympathetic outflow from the spinal cord at Tl due to avulsion of the Tl root from the spinal cord. It is a bad prognostic sign. A stab wound or open laceration to the brachial plexus should be explored and major nerve roots repaired. Repair may involve primary anastomosis or bridge nerve grafts from e.g. sural, or transposition of intercostal nerves, depending on the pattern of injury. The surgeon and anaesthetist should be prepared for repair of major vessel injury such as the subclavian artery as well as brachial plexus repair. Brachial plexus injuries that occur at birth from forced extraction of a foetus with excessive traction and angulation of the shoulder and neck can produce permanent deformity. There is an increasing trend to explore and repair these plexuses with microsurgery, and will not usually be applicable in a developing country.

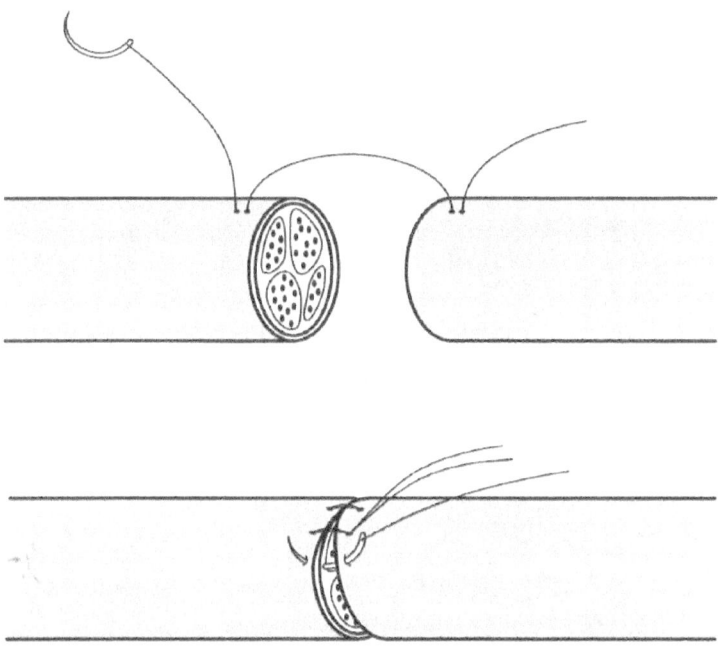

End to end anastomosis of epineurium

Figure 10.1 (a) End-to-end anastomosis of epineurium.

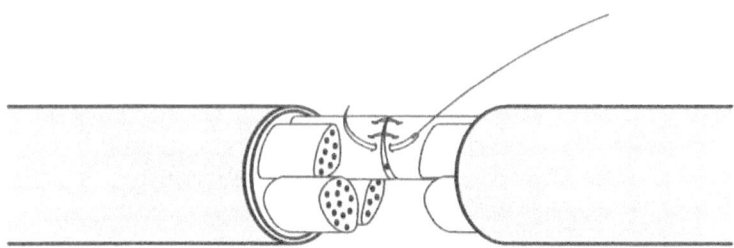

End to end anastomosis of nerve fascicles

(b) End-to-end anastomosis of nerve fascicles.

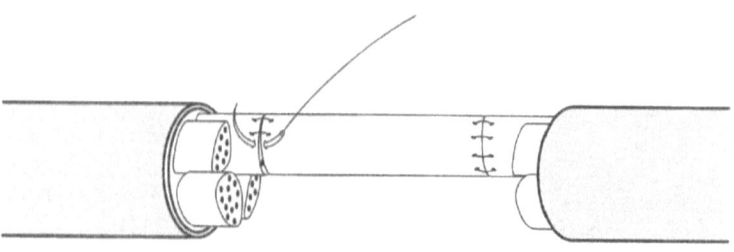

Placement of interfascicular sural nerve grafts

(c) Placement of interfascicular sural nerve grafts.

Figure 10.1 (a-c) Techniques of peripheral nerve repair.

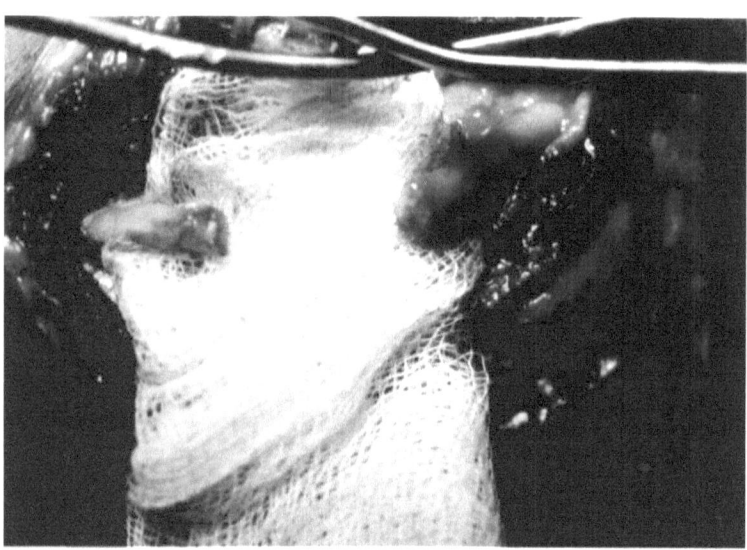

(a) Ends displayed and prepared for repair.

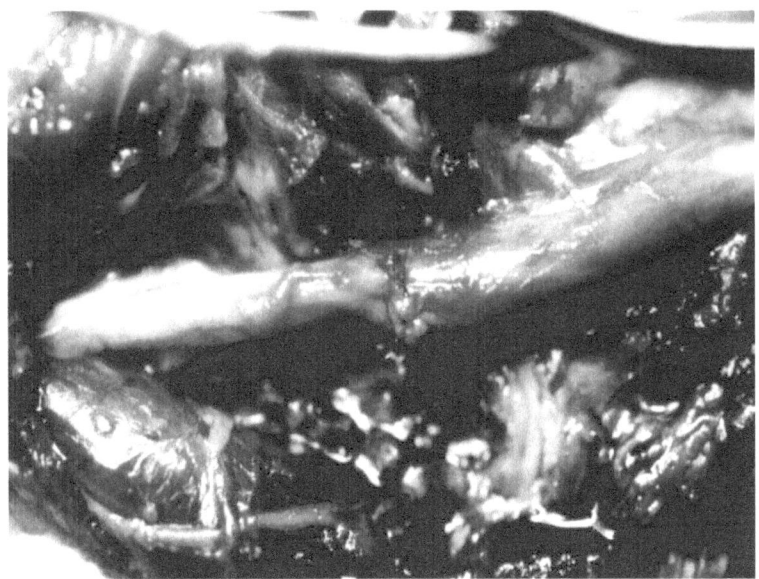

(b) Epineurial repair complete.

Figure 10.2 (a-b) Traumatic transection of ulnar nerve.

Radial nerve

The radial nerve palsy which accompanies a fractured radius shaft is best managed conservatively, and most will recover. There is a trend towards exploration at the time of internal fixation but as this will be unlikely to be employed in the developing world and is not recommended.

PERIPHERAL NEUROPATHY

Neuropathies can be caused by direct injury, pressure or entrapment, or develop secondarily to other diseases. Neuropathy may also arise as a side effect of some drugs. The medical causes of neuropathy are many and their treatment is beyond the scope of this book. Table 10.1, page 480 lists some common causes.

Mononeuropathies may well be mechanical or due to trauma. Polyneuropathies are likely to be due to some systemic disorder. Some cases prove to be idiopathic despite the number of causes listed in the table. Generalised peripheral neuropathy presents as paraesthesiae affecting feet, legs and sometimes the hands in a stocking and glove distribution. There may be a mixed motor and sensory element with muscle weakness and wasting.

Entrapment neuropathies (Table 10.2, next page)

Carpal tunnel syndrome

This is an uncommon disorder in the tropics. It presents with paraesthesiae in the thumb, index, middle and sometimes ring, fingers of the hand, which is often worse at night and wakes the patient so they have to get up and shake the arm, in order to relieve the symptoms. There is often pain in the palm and/or fingers. It may follow a previous fracture or trauma to the wrist, and is more common in young females. The condition may be helped by nocturnal splinting and diuretics; but if it does not settle, surgical decompression of the median nerve by division of the flexor retinaculum is indicated. This can be done with local anaesthetic infiltration, but alternatively with an intravenous (Bier's) arm block or general anaesthetic.

A pneumatic tourniquet on the upper arm is helpful but not essential. A vertical incision is made in the mid-palm, deepened through the palmar aponeurosis; and then the flexor retinaculum which is a strong, taught ligament, is divided using a small scalpel blade (size 15) until the median nerve or long flexor tendons with their overlying synovial sheath are encountered. The retinaculum may spring open as it is progressively divided. Care should be taken not to damage the branches of the median nerve distally, particularly the recurrent motor branch to the short thenar muscles. A probe should be passed over the median nerve proximally and distally to make sure there are no residual compressive fibrous bands.

The division can be extended either way to decompress the nerve fully. The wound is closed with a few sutures in the subcutaneous fat and then a separate skin layer. A compression bandage is applied and the arm elevated. There is usually an immediate relief of symptoms after surgery.

Table 10.1 Common causes of peripheral neuropathy in the tropics.

Infection	Mechanical	Miscellaneous	Drugs	Toxins	Endocrine
Leprosy HIV	Trauma	Vitamin B deficiencies	Vincristine	Lead	Diabetes
Tetanus	Entrapment	Alcoholism	Phenytoin	Mercury	Hypothyroidism
Poliomyelitis	Avulsion	Porphyria	Nitrofurantoin	Trichloroethylene	
Botulism	Stretching	Carcinomatosis	Isoniazid	Industrial poisons	
Diphtheria		Amyloidosis	Metronidazole		
Brucellosis		Sarcoidosis			
		Guillain-Barre syndrome			

Table 10.2 Peripheral entrapment neuropathies.

Nerve and site of injury	Common or colloquial name
Median nerve at wrist	Carpal tunnel syndrome
Ulnar nerve at the elbow	Tardy ulnar nerve palsy
Radial nerve in axilla	Crutch palsy
Radial nerve at back of humerus	Saturday night palsy
Common peroneal nerve at fibular head	Tailor's palsy

Tardy ulnar nerve palsy

This is also an uncommon condition in the tropics. The ulnar nerve may be traumatised or entrapped against the posterior aspect of the medial epicondyle of the humerus. It is held in the osseous grove by a fascial covering. The palsy presents with progressive paraesthesiae in the ring and little fingers, and weakness and wasting of the intrinsic muscles of the hand. Eventually clawing of the fingers develops. The patient may complain of pain along the medial side of the forearm. Sensory loss does not occur above the wrist. There may be a previous history of trauma to the elbow. The shorter the history before exploration, the more complete the recovery is likely to be. The operation can be carried out under local anaesthesia, but preferably an intravenous (Bier's) arm block or general anaesthetic are used. A tourniquet is not essential. A gently curved incision is made just anterior to the medial epicondyle, extending about 5 cm above and below the elbow joint. Flaps of skin are raised and the medial epicondyle region exposed. The ulnar nerve is identified immediately posterior to the epicondyle. A neurolysis is performed by dividing adhesions around the nerve, dividing the adjacent medial intermuscular septum of the arm, and the two heads of flexor carpi ulnaris so that the nerve is freed above and below the epicondyle.

Do not divide the medial and internal areolar mesentery of the nerve which contains the blood vessels that supply the nerve. If the nerve is still stretched significantly when the elbow is flexed, the epicondyle can be excised to further release the tension on the nerve. This is done by preserving the periosteum and flexor muscle origin over it by doing a subperiosteal dissection using diathermy, removing the prominence using rongeurs until it is a smooth surface, applying bone wax, then closing the periosteum over the bare bone with absorbable suture.

The wound is then closed in two layers. The improvement after surgery is slow and the intrinsic muscle wasting in the hand may never reverse fully. Transposition of the ulnar nerve anteriorly, although it takes the tension off the nerve, tends to devascularise the nerve and is not to be recommended. Ulnar nerve entrapment may also occur at the wrist where the deep palmar branch of the nerve enters Guyon's canal between the pisiform and hook of the hamate, and the transverse carpal and volar carpal ligaments. There will be progressive paralysis of the intrinsic muscles of the hand but sensation should be spared.

Radial nerve palsy (Saturday night & crutch palsy)

Compression of the radial nerve occurs as the radial nerve leaves the axilla as a result of the crutch pressure. Another common site for a radial palsy is where the radial nerve passes around the back of the humerus, where it can be compressed by pressure from the arm on a hard surface such as the floor, during an alcoholic stupor. Previous weight loss reduces the cushioning effect of soft tissues which protect the nerve. It presents as wrist drop. Thumb extension is lost but usually the only area of numbness is in the anatomical snuff box. Where there is a history of external compression no exploration is indicated as the patient will recover. Treatment should focus on splintage and physiotherapy to avoid contractures and joint stiffness.

Common peroneal nerve at the fibular head

The common peroneal nerve passes from the popliteal fossa to the lateral aspect of the fibular neck. At this point the fibrous band of the peroneus longus arches over the nerve. Forced inversion of the foot will tighten this arch against the nerve, thus the neuropathy may be initiated by an inversion and plantar flexion injury of the foot caused by a slip and fall on wet grass or during sport.

Once the pain in the ankle has subsided it is found there is still pain on the lateral aspect of the lower leg and a foot drop. Prolonged inversion of the foot or sitting cross-legged (yoga or tailoring), may result in a palsy occurring in the uppermost leg. Direct trauma may also occur due to a blow or due to pressure from Lloyd-Davies or other stirrups during anaesthesia.

Treatment is expectant with splintage and physiotherapy to avoid contractures and joint stiffness. The prognosis for recovery is good. If there is no improvement over 4-6 weeks a decompressive neurolysis may hasten recovery (Figure 10.3, next page).

Meralgia paraesthetica

Compression of the lateral cutaneous nerve as it passes through or beneath the inguinal ligament to reach the anterolateral thigh may cause chronic numbness and burning pain in the anterolateral thigh, which can easily be mistaken for an upper lumbar root disorder. There is decreased sensation in the distribution of the nerve as the only objective finding. It is often associated with obesity and usually improves markedly when the nerve is sectioned, just proximal to the inguinal ligament. Freeing the nerve, particularly if it passes through the ligament, is less reliable than section of the nerve.

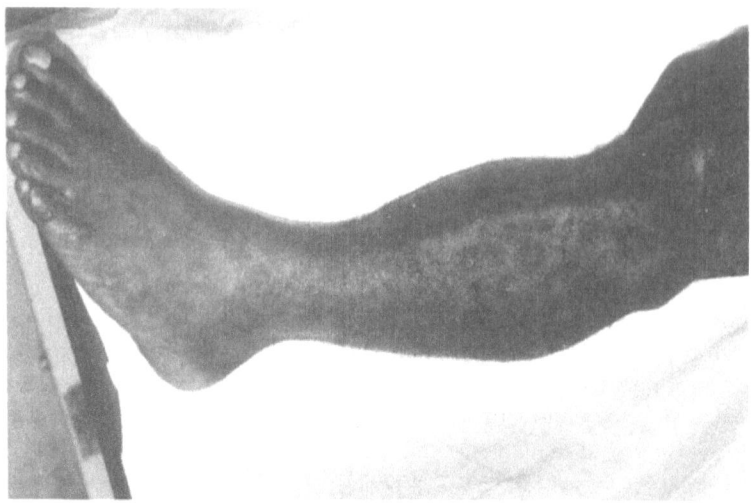

Figure 10.3 Chronic wasting of anterior compartment muscles of left leg with foot drop. Common peroneal nerve injury at the posterolateral side of the knee due to a knife wound.

CHRONIC PAIN AND NEURALGIA

Definitions

Pain is an unpleasant sensory and emotional experience associated with actual or potential tissue damage. Nociception is the process whereby signals in the CNS evoked by activation of sensory receptors result in a response to a noxious stimulus.

The pain pathway (Figure 10.4, page 485)

Somatic pain is experienced by impulses passing from sensory receptors in either fast or slow fibres. A-delta, large, myelinated fibres transmit impulses rapidly, whilst C fibres are smaller, unmyelinated and slow. Pain and temperature fibres pass to the dorsal root ganglion and terminate in layers 3- 6 of the dorsal horn of the spinal cord. The pathway crosses to other side with in one or two segments of the cord and passes up in the lateral spinothalamic tract to the ventral posterolateral nucleus of the thalamus. From there the next relay is to the sensory cortex (postcentral gyrus of parietal lobe). Chemical mediators are important in the local appreciation of pain: injury or tissue damage releases bradykinin and prostaglandins, which activate and sensitise nociceptors. Activation of nociceptors results in substance P and other peptides being released, which in turn act on mast cells to release histamine which directly stimulates the nociceptors.

Visceral or autonomic pain tends to be diffuse and involves sympathetic nerves. It may be stimulated by ischaemia, spasm, distension or inflammation. Pain may be referred to distant sites innervated by the same nerve root (e.g. shoulder tip pain in peritonitis - C3, 4, 5).

There are many neurotransmitters and additions to the list are constantly being made.

- The main somatic neurotransmitter is acetylcholine.

- The preganglionic autonomic neurotransmitter is acetylcholine.

- The postganglionic sympathetic neurotransmitter is norepinephrine (noradrenaline) (exceptions being sweat glands and muscle vasodilator endings which use acetylcholine), and postganglionic neurotransmitter for parasympathetic is acetylcholine.

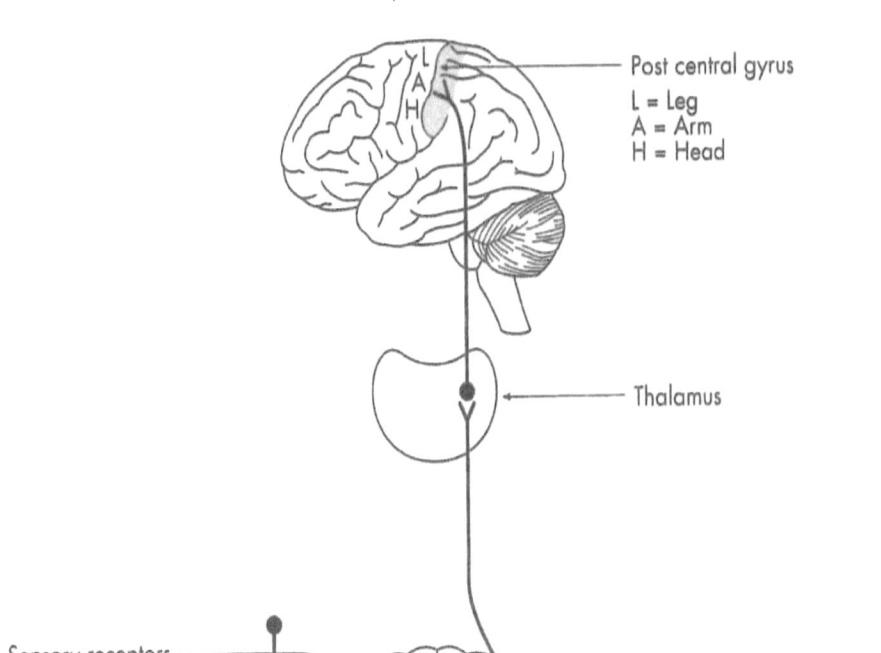

L = Leg
A = Arm
H = Head

Post central gyrus

Thalamus

Sensory receptors

Lateral spinothalamic tract

Spinal cord

Figure 10.4 Anatomy of the pain pathway.

Classification of pain

It is important to differentiate between acute and chronic pain, as acute pain should be easily relieved by an increasing hierarchy of analgesics, and an attack on the cause of the pain, whereas chronic pain may be much more difficult to subdue. It is helpful to divide chronic pain into benign causes and malignant causes.

The major types of pain are:

1. **Nociceptive**
   - Somatic, which is well localised, sharp, stabbing, aching or cramping and results from tissue inflammation or injury, or from nerve or plexus compression or tumour infiltration. It responds to treating the underlying pathology or by interrupting the nociceptive pathway by neurectomy.
   - Visceral, which is poorly localised, and responds poorly to primary pain medication. Local wall blockade using phenol, e.g. coeliac block for pancreatic cancer pain may be effective.

2. **Deafferentation pain.** This is a form of central pain and is due to aberrant pain circuits developing in the central nervous system, either in the spinal cord and/or the brain itself. It is described as crushing, tearing, tingling, or numbness and may be associated with burning dysaesthesia, or lancinating pain and hyperpathia (pain on touching the skin). This pain does not respond to section of nerves and responds poorly to ablative procedures in the central nervous system.

3. **Sympathetically maintained pain** such as reflex sympathetic dystrophy and causalgia. Sympathetic stimulation maintains the pain due to fusion of sympathetic nerves with somatic sensory nerves.

Management of chronic pain

The pathophysiology of pain is extremely complex. Cultural and emotional responses also play an important part but these modifications are unpredictable and ill-understood.

The clinical approach to a patient with chronic pain includes:

1. **Take a pain history**, which should include questions about the site, severity, onset, character, duration and frequency of the pain, aggravating and relieving factors. Helpful questions to assess the impact of pain upon a person's life include 'can you sleep at night and what does the pain stop you doing? Then the effect of analgesics or other pain treatments should be assessed.

2. **Examine** the patient, try to provoke and relieve the pain

3. **Special tests:** a self-portrait can be drawn to show the site and nature of the pain or the patient can be asked to score his/her pain on an analogue scale.

4. Determine what proportion of the pain may be due to **emotional factors** such as depression or anxiety.

5. **Relieve pain** with analgesics, blocks, antidepressants or sympathetic blockade (see Table 10.3, page 489). Pains in numb areas are unlikely to respond to opiates. Opiate addiction is unlikely to occur with pain due to malignancy. Analgesia should be given in adequate doses to break the pain cycle, and make the patient forget the pain. This may mean giving the drug in high enough doses and more frequently. It should not be necessary for patients with malignancy to die in pain. The combination of non-opiate and opiate produces additional analgesia with fewer side effects. For pains that do not respond to normal conventional analgesics there are several options. Gabapentin (Neurontin) and pregabalin (Lyrica) are used for neuropathic pain; tramadol - dependence may develop with long term use; antidepressants such as amitriptyline (25-75 mg nocte) for dysaesthetic or resistant chronic pains.

Anticonvulsants may also be effective for neuropathic pain (eg. sodium valproate (Epilim) 200 mg b.d. or 500 mg nocte or carbamazepine (Tegretol) slowly increase up to 1000mg per day). The use of spinal opiates via an implanted infusion pump, or a passive plastic reservoir implanted beneath the skin of the abdominal wall with a connecting catheter placed intradurally into the lumbar theca and passed up to the thoracic subarachnoid space, has also been a major advance in the control of severe malignant pain, which eventually requires very high oral doses of opiates to control and is associated with all the unwanted side effects of the oral route. The spinal route allows for a much lower dose (several milligrams per day of morphine) with an insignificant level of clouding of consciousness and disturbance of the respiratory centre. However, these prosthetic devices are expensive and may not be available in many developing countries.

Chronic benign pain can be very disabling for the patient and is difficult to treat. Opiate analgesics are usually ineffective and it is advisable not to gradually increase these drugs, as addiction will result and there will be very poor relief of pain. There are often significant psychological or psychiatric issues involved, and compensation claims may also be contributing to the maintenance of the pain. There may also be secondary psychological gain from the pain and some individuals would fear they would fail to cope if their pain were taken away. Such issues need to be dealt with if pain is to be relieved. It is important to treat any correctable causes for the pain, such as a recurrent ruptured disc or spinal instability etc., before concentrating only on the pain. Once a correctable organic cause is excluded, the treatment in Western countries involves the inevitable multidisciplinary pain management team with physician, psychiatrist, and perhaps anaesthesiology and physiotherapy input. In the developing world setting, such multidisciplinary services are not readily available, and the individual practitioner will usually have to handle the problem alone.

6. **Surgery:** Sympathectomy may be indicated for some patients with rest pain due to arterial insufficiency, or reflex sympathetic dystrophy. Excision of an amputation stump neuroma may also relieve stump pain in a patient with a well healed amputation stump. Cordotomy and stereotactic surgery to interrupt the pain pathway are rarely beneficial because of the incidence of side effects such as incontinence and other unwanted cord damage, and their effect is usually short lived (months). They are unlikely to be available in the developing world and, in any case, we believe the simpler options for treatment are usually better.

One procedure, which is becoming more popular for the treatment of chronic benign pain, is spinal cord stimulation. This involves placing a thin grid or column of electrodes into the epidural space, either via a percutaneous route or via a small open laminectomy and the electrodes are placed in the mid-thoracic or cervical region, depending on the level of the pain. It is connected via a subcutaneous lead to an implantable battery-operated pulse generator and produces high frequency electrical stimulation directly to the dorsal aspect of the spinal cord, and reduces chronic pain. It is particularly useful for chronic back and lower limb pain, following failed spinal surgery, phantom limb pain, amputation stump pain and other forms of central deafferentation pain. It has also been used successfully to treat the rest pain due to ischaemia of the lower limbs. It is expensive technology, and again is not readily available in the developing world. It reduces pain significantly in about 50 percent of selected patients.

Specific pain syndromes

Postherpetic neuralgia

This is a pain in the distribution of a nerve affected by an acute herpes zoster attack (shingles), the pain being due to destruction of cells in the posterior nerve root. The condition is most common in the elderly and also in immunocompromised patients with HIV. Idoxuridine (topical) or aciclovir (800 mg 4-hourly) reduces the severity of an acute attack. Analgesics do not normally relieve postherpetic neuralgia. Gabapentin, pregabalin, anticonvulsant or anti-depressant may be helpful.

Table 10.3 Treatment options for chronic pain.

Analgesics
Non-opiates
Aspirin
Paracetamol
Non-steroidal anti-inflammatory
Nefopam
Opiates
Codeine
Morphine and others
Buprenorphine
Other agents
Gabapentin (Neurontin)
Pregabalin (Lyrica)
Tramadol
Anticonvulsants such as carbamazepine, valproate, phenytoin
Antidepressants (amitriptyline)

Nerve blocks
Somatic pain
Intercostal
Trigeminal
Focal point such as facet joint
Extradural
Lntrathecal
Autonomic pain
Stellate ganglion sympathectomy
Lumbar sympathectomy
Intravenous guanethidine
Coeliac plexus block

Trigeminal neuralgia

This is a unilateral, sharp, paroxysmal usually brief, electric shock like severe pain which occurs most often in the middle-aged, and affects females twice as often as in males. It usually affects the mandibular and/or maxillary divisions of the nerve, and less commonly the ophthalmic. There may be mild sensory loss on the affected side of the face in a minority of patients. The diagnosis is based on the history. Carbamazepine (up to 1500 mg daily in divided doses) or phenytoin (100 mg 8-hourly), or sodium valproate should be given. Patients in whom these drugs are unsuccessful may have a percutaneous rhizotomy for longer term relief (see below). A nerve block with local anaesthesia will be ineffective. Alcohol injection or cryoanalgesia of an affected nerve in the face (e.g. infraorbital) may relieve the pain to some degree but produces complete focal sensory loss. The cause is usually an artery which compresses the proximal trigeminal nerve (nerve root entry zone) in the posterior fossa. The most effective and long-lasting operation for trigeminal neuralgia is the microvascular decompression where a posterior fossa craniotomy is performed and, under the microscope, the offending blood vessel (usually the superior cerebellar artery) is dissected away from the nerve and an interposition pledget of Teflon used to prevent the continuous pulsation against the nerve root entry zone. An alternative to this technique, which is usually used in the elderly patients or those not fit for craniotomy is the percutaneous rhizotomy technique, as it is simple to perform. It can also be repeated. The downside is that there is varying degrees of facial numbness following the procedure and the pain relief does not last as long as the MVD. Under local anaesthesia, a needle is passed lateral to the mouth (see below), and guided up through the foramen ovale (the bony foramen in the skull base for the mandibular division of the trigeminal nerve) and into the cave of Meckel.

The trigeminal ganglion and its rootlets are situated in this dural 'pocket' bathed in CSF. Radiofrequency lesions at 70°C or glycerol injection (0.25-0.4ml) into the retrogasserian rootlets of the trigeminal nerve, i.e. the rootlets just proximal to the trigeminal ganglion in the cave of Meckel, is the preferred target, but the lesions may be made in the ganglion itself. First division lesions may result in some corneal sensory loss and may require a tarsorrhaphy if corneal exposure keratitis develops. Inflating the 0.75cc balloon of a 4 French Fogarty embolectomy catheter passed via a needle in the same way as the other percutaneous procedures into the Cave of Meckel is an alternative technique which may also be effective. In the developing world where these various techniques are unavailable, water at 70°C injected into the trigeminal ganglion can act as an alternative for the second and third divisions (not the first because of the risk of intracranial spill). This will cause a destructive heat lesion in the nerve albeit in a less controlled fashion than the radiofrequency lesion technique.

Technique: This could be performed in the X-ray department because lateral X-rays of the skull are required to confirm the position. Use local anaesthesia with infiltration of the cheek and subjacent tissue. The patient may also require some sedation when the lesion is made. There is normally some pain when the needle enters the appropriate division of the trigeminal nerve. The entry point is made 2.5 cm lateral to the angle of the mouth, and is aimed at a point in space level with a transverse line drawn from 3 cm in front of the middle of the tragus to meet a vertical line in the mid-pupillary axis. This is the approximate marking of the foramen ovale, through which the mandibular division of the trigeminal nerve exits the skull. A long lumbar puncture needle is bounced on the floor of the skull until it enters the cave of Meckel along this trajectory. This is checked with a lateral X-ray. When the needle is passed posterior to the clival edge, it is entering the first division. At the level of the clivus and within 3 mm of the clivus, the needle is in the second division. The third division is 3-5 mm below this point. A volume of 1 ml of water at 70°C is injected into the appropriate division, with the patient sedated, once the position is achieved. The differential diagnosis of facial pain has many causes apart from trigeminal neuralgia and includes atypical facial pain, postherpetic neuralgia, posttraumatic neuralgia, temporomandibular joint incongruence or arthritis, sinusitis, dental problems and malignancy (see Chapter 9, page 475).

Amputation stump pains and phantom limb pains

If the stump is well healed and delayed pain develops, the origin of the pain is most likely to be a neuroma, which could be treated by local anaesthetic injection, cryoanalgesia or excision. It is therefore sometimes worth exploring the stump in the hope of finding a neuroma. Phantom limb pains are difficult to treat and there are many methods in use, none of which are particularly effective, although spinal cord stimulation has been successful in some cases. Anticonvulsant drugs may be tried, the most effective being clonazepam (0.5 mg nocte up to 1.5-2 mg t.d.s.). Other drugs described above for chronic c pain may also be helpful.

Brachialgia

Severe intractable pain may develop in a limb following brachial plexus avulsion from the spinal cord. It is a central deafferentation pain and usually involves feelings of crushing, twisting or distraction of parts of the limb, as if fingers are being ripped away from the hand. It does not respond to opioid analgesics. Amputation of the useless limb will not control the pain, and the patient will then likely develop disabling phantom pain. Lumbar plexus avulsion is much less common but the same principles apply. The neurosurgical procedure, which has been of benefit in many of these patients, is dorsal root entry zone lesioning (DREZ) of the spinal cord, or radiofrequency heat lesions where small multiple lesions are made in the substantia gelatinosa of the dorsal horn, over the affected segments where the rootlets were avulsed. A higher success rate, up to about 70 per cent, is achieved if the radiofrequency lesions are extended above and below the affected roots. There is a risk of causing motor weakness on the side of the lesions as well as sphincter disturbance.

Ischaemic rest pain

This is due to severe peripheral vascular disease. Sympathectomy may be indicated together with investigation for and treatment of correctable peripheral vascular problems in the hope of salvaging the limb in the long term. Diabetics with rest pain may not benefit from sympathectomy because their diabetes may already have induced a neuropathy. Treat as for other types of neuropathic pain.

Back pain

This is discussed in Chapter 5 on page 203.

Complex regional pain syndrome, reflex sympathetic dystrophy, sympathetically maintained pain and Sudeck's atrophy

This is a condition that is part of the complex regional pain syndrome. The pain is sympathetically maintained and can be blocked by sympathetic blockade. It is hypothesised that there is, after injury, an abnormal communication at the microscopic level between sympathetic nerves that normally supply blood vessels and sweat glands, and sensory nerves mediating pain, resulting in the following clinical features:

1. Pain which is out of proportion to the injury.

2. Changes in the colour and temperature of the affected part.

3. Disuse atrophy or osteoporosis in the long term (Sudeck's atrophy).

Sympathetic blockade may be achieved by:
1. Phentolamine infusion which blocks alpha receptors ⁻ activated by norepinephrine (noradrenaline) release.
2. Alpha blockade with phenoxybenzamine orally (higher incidence of side effects).
3. Guanethidine block (inject using Bier block with a tight tourniquet proximally): blocks norepinephrine (noradrenaline) release.
4. Lumbar sympathetic block (using local anaesthetic) for the lower limb.
5. Cervical sympathectomy for the upper limb.

Patients who have a combination of autonomic disturbance and pain, but who fail to respond to sympathetic blockade are classified as having sympathetically independent pain, the autonomic disturbance being a secondary response to the pain, rather than a primary sympathetic involvement in the pain pathways. It is postulated that these patients who suffer chronic pain have sensitisation of pain receptors in the affected area and the pain pathway. Oral steroids may also help by reducing inflammation, thought to be part of the pathogenesis of reflex sympathetic pain. Causalgia is a burning pain in the distal limb following nerve trunk injury. It is also sympathetically maintained and may be relieved by sympathetic blockade.

LEPROSY

J.K.A. Clezy

Leprosy is caused by *Mycobacterium leprae*, a bacterium unique in human disease in that it has a striking affinity for Schwann cells, where it interferes with myelin production. Demyelination occurs, accompanied by varying degrees of inflammation depending on the extent of the host's specific T cell-mediated immune defect to this organism. Most people are completely immune. A mild defect allows a brisk inflammatory response which kills most of the bacilli, and produces disease at the tuberculoid end of the spectrum. At the lepromatous pole bacteria multiply freely, slowly destroying nerves, often without much in the way of inflammation for months or years.

The most obvious effects are on the skin and the peripheral nerves. A description of the various forms of leprosy, from the **tuberculoid** end of the spectrum to the **lepromatous** end, the latter being the most aggressive, are beyond the scope of this book. This section concentrates on the peripheral nerve pathology and its management. The public health priority is to recognise and treat leprosy early and effectively before there is major peripheral nerve damage, which if not treated promptly is irreversible. The numbers of cases are falling due to the success in many countries of BCG vaccination, which was more effective in preventing leprosy than tuberculosis, and improved leprosy control. The recommended medical treatment for leprosy using the WHO multiple-drug therapy regimen is shown in Table 10.4, next page. The multi-drug regimen was introduced because of the development of dapsone resistance since the 1960s. The next priority is to prevent further tissue damage in patients with paralysis and sensory loss. The number of leprosy cases requiring surgery has fallen in the past two decades. The bacillus prefers cool sites, which helps explain the curious distribution of nerve involvement. Amongst nerves that may become palpable are the greater auricular, the superficial radial at the wrist, the ulnar at the elbow, the median at the wrist, the common peroneal at the knee and the tibial at the ankle.

The only commonly involved nerve that is almost never palpable, is the facial, presumably because its branches are too fine. In Papua New Guinea, and in East Asia and the Pacific generally, the radial nerve is commonly thickened (and paralysed) in the spiral groove, but

494

curiously this nerve is rarely affected in India, where most of the textbooks were written, or in Africa. The median nerve is only rarely involved at the elbow, presumably because it is right alongside the brachial artery which keeps it warm. Similarly, the tibial nerve in the popliteal fossa is safe. Other mixed nerves are rarely involved, and only when a prominent skin lesion in their sensory territory allows bacteria to track proximally to reach the motor component of the nerve.

Table 10.4 WHO multiple drug treatment for leprosy.

Leprosy type*	Rifampicin 600 mg once monthly	Dapsone 100 mg daily	Clofazimine 300 mg once monthly (supervised) or 50 mg daily (unsupervised)	Duration months§
Multibacillary	Yes	Yes	Yes	>24
Paucibacillary	Yes	Yes	No	6

*Any patient whose skin smear is positive for acid-fast bacilli should be treated as multibacillary.
§Treatment should continue till skin smears are negative.

The mixed nerve most commonly affected in the arm is the ulnar, with sensory fibres almost always affected before motor fibres. Depending on the population, a varying percentage of ulnar lesions have an associated median lesion. Isolated median paralysis is rare. In the leg the common peroneal is often paralysed with little in the way of damage to other nerves. Acute episodes, called reactions long before their mechanism was understood, occur spontaneously, but more often in response to treatment.

Type I reaction occurs anywhere except in pure lepromatous disease, and results in acute swelling of skin lesions and any involved nerves. Skin lesions may ulcerate, and affected nerves may rapidly lose function, which may usually be reversed by steroid treatment. Fever and general malaise may occur, but are not prominent features.

Type II reaction occurs at the lepromatous end of the spectrum, and is a much more generalised response. The key sign is erythema nodosum, appearing as crops of tender nodules on the extensor surfaces, particularly on the legs. Fever is common, as are arthritis, orchitis, lymphadenitis, iritis and diffuse nerve pains. Nerve damage is usually slow. All features of type II reaction respond quickly to thalidomide, but in the interests of preserving nerve function steroids should also be given, and always are when thalidomide is not available.

Practice point

Do not prescribe thalidomide to women of reproductive age because of the teratogenic effects preventing limb development in the foetus.

Sensory loss occurs in skin patches, in the territories of one or more of the above-mentioned nerves, or in the extremities of lepromatous patients due to involvement of terminal nerve filaments in the skin, whether or not any patch is present. Ulceration of extremities is due to unnoticed trauma to anaesthetic areas. Just as in any other case of sensory loss, prevention is much better than cure. Care, and self-care, of leprosy patients therefore includes identification and protection of anaesthetic areas. For the hand this means protection from heat and rough tools, in particular, and in the foot, it means use of well-fitting footwear that spreads the weight effectively. Ordinary shoes may do more harm than good. Established ulceration requires rest and elevation. Splintage is usually necessary.

Sepsis is not often a major problem, and antibiotics are too frequently used when rest is what is required. Osteomyelitis is secondary and late, and rarely requires treatment, although prominent metacarpal heads often need removal in order to deal with persistent areas of high pressure on the sole. A well-moulded plaster cast will allow a plantar ulcer to heal even though the patient continues to take weight on it, but casts should only be applied when heat and swelling have gone. When the ulcer is healed, the patient must wear protective shoes of some sort. Deformities produced by paralysis of various muscle groups are progressive, and are best treated early, once it is obvious that paralysis is permanent and the disease itself is under control. Standard techniques of tendon transfer to correct claw hands and dropped feet were developed by Paul Brand and others in the 1950s, but require considerable experience.

No tendon surgery will be successful without the help of a physiotherapist skilled in the care of leprosy patients. The management of a neuropathic limb is described below.

THE NEUROPATHIC LIMB

The two commonest reasons for the development of a neuropathic limb in the tropics are leprosy and diabetes mellitus. While the number of cases of leprosy is declining, diabetes is on the increase in many developing countries exposed to Western diets and lifestyles. In the South Pacific and many parts of sub-Saharan Africa maturity onset diabetes is a major epidemic and surgical wards are full of patients with infected feet.

Pathology

Motor neuropathy results in muscle paralysis and muscle imbalance. In the feet this results in clawing of the toes and may also result in foot drop. Increased weight bearing then occurs on the areas of the foot in contact with the ground, normally the metatarsal heads, which predisposes these points to ulceration. Sensory loss makes the patient unaware of small fissures and wounds, so that walking causes further damage. The injured limb is not rested as it should be. Autonomic loss means the skin is dry, more prone to fissures and that the normal vascular response to injury is impaired. Trophic ulcers, soft tissue infections and, ultimately osteomyelitis and gangrene are the outcome. In diabetes soft tissue infection is more aggressive due, perhaps, to an impaired inflammatory response as well as small and/or large vessel vasculopathy. Infection spreads through the foot and limb, often necessitating major amputations. Loss of vision may make it difficult for the patient appreciate small skin abrasions and fissures on his foot.

Management

Treat acute problems

Treat soft tissue infection by drainage of abscesses, excision of necrotic tissue (which often means amputation of a digit or forefoot in the diabetic), intravenous antibiotics and bedrest with elevation. Radical debridement of dead tissue early gives the best chance of healing and preventing further tissue destruction by micro-organisms. Any skin or wound problem is potentially serious and must be treated by protecting the area and avoiding further damage.

The walk to and from the clinic may destroy the anaesthetic foot. Protect and rest ulcers and wounds.

Prevent disability

1. **Prevent contractures**: this often means splinting and physiotherapy. As well as splinting a foot or wrist drop, splinting may be indicated for wounds crossing joints or palmar creases so that the wound heals without a contracture. Splinting may also be indicated for infective tenosynovitis.

2. **Protect the hands and feet** from further damage: provide footwear or other walking aids. Protecting the neuropathic hand involves teaching the patient to avoid actions (e.g. touching a hot cooking pot) in his workplace or home, which may damage fingers.

3. **Instruct the patient to inspect their feet**, to care for their feet and to rest their often painless, injured feet when there is an ulcer or fissure.

4. The patient must accept **responsibility for their neuropathic limbs**. They should be set realistic objectives in the care of their feet. These should be measurable and recordable to help motivate him.

5. Develop a **team approach** to the problem involving the patient, the shoemaker, the physiotherapist and the nurse or other health worker. The doctor or surgeon is in the best position to lead the team.

6. In a few selected cases **surgery** may assist in preventing or minimising disability.
   a. Tendon transfers are indicated where the patient will regain a particular movement or function, he has lost, there is a functioning tendon available, and the transfer will not compromise some other important function of the limb. There should be adequate after-care and physiotherapy backup. Tendon transfers are contraindicated if there is a soft tissue or joint contracture which would limit the movement to be regained by the transfer or if the patient is poorly motivated and unlikely to co-operate with a care programme designed to prevent further tissue loss. Joints must be fully mobile before transfer. It is therefore important to prevent contractures by passive movement and splinting right from the start.

b. Release of contractures.
c. Amputation or arthrodesis of badly contracted digits may be indicated.
d. Tarsorrhaphy may be indicated for the anaesthetic eye.

Numerous other procedures are described for neuropathic hands and feet, particularly in patients suffering from leprosy. Unfortunately, in diabetes, the vasculopathy is often so severe that no matter what is done the patient ends up with more and more extensive amputation.

Chapter Eleven

Common operations

The procedures described in this chapter are those which a general surgeon may have to undertake in a remote setting with limited resources, or in a country with limited or no neurosurgical services. The procedures chosen are generally within the technical capability of the general surgeon, but some prior exposure to neurosurgery is recommended. The procedures chosen are either urgent and potentially life-saving, such as evacuation of an acute extradural haematoma; are urgent and may correct or prevent serious neurological impairments, such as spinal cord decompression; or are purely elective but may transform the life of the sufferer, such as repair of a frontal encephalocele.

GENERAL PRINCIPLES OF OPERATIVE NEUROSURGERY

The basic equipment required is listed in Chapter 11, page 614. The principles are outlined in Table 11.1, page 510.

Principles

Anaesthetic: For cranial and spinal surgery, the patient should be intubated, muscle relaxed (paralysed) on controlled ventilation. An end tidal CO_2 monitor will help guide the level of ventilation.

Position: The patient's head should be positioned so that the approach to the target area is optimised and can be acquired by the shortest, direct route. The operating field should be uppermost so that the brain tends to fall away from, rather than into, the exposed site. It will be helpful to place the head of the table up to 10-20° to increase venous return and thereby reduce brain swelling. Avoid excessive twisting of the neck. Place a sandbag or pillow under the shoulder opposite to the side the head is turned to lessen the torsion on the neck. A urinary catheter is inserted for craniotomies. The patient's pressure points around the elbows knees and ankles are well padded to avoid pressure injuries to the skin. For the prone position pads or pillows are placed under the pelvis and the chest will lessen direct pressure on the abdomen. This will help to avoid compression of the vena cava which impedes venous return. **Retraction**: Neural tissue is unforgiving. Excessive deformation or retraction can irreversibly affect the function of the structure. Any retraction should be slow, progressive and gentle. Retractors on the brain should be released every few minutes if possible, to allow the microcirculation to recover. The degree of retraction should be as small as possible to perform the chosen manoeuvre. Place cottonoids beneath the retractors to prevent laceration of the cortex by the sharp edge of the metal retractors or other instruments (Figure 11.1 (a), page 503). **Eloquent cortex**: Avoid manipulating or incising the brain in the so-called eloquent areas. These are the speech, motor, sensory and visual areas.

Haemostasis

The techniques for securing haemostasis are as follows:

1. Apply special or ordinary curved artery forceps to the scalp, to evert the galea. If you have Raney clips, these are what is usually used on the scalp edge in HIC.

2. Scalp edge - diathermy major galeal bleeders when curved artery forceps are removed.

3. Ligate the superficial temporal artery if severed when the scalp is incised.

4. Apply bone wax to the bleeding bone edge.

5. Diathermy the middle meningeal artery - if no diathermy is available or it cannot be controlled with diathermy, underrun the vessel with silk or a similar non-absorbable suture.

6. Diathermy major bleeding vessels on the dura or occlude with silver clips. Bipolar coagulation is much preferred to monopolar.

7. Apply Surgicel to the oozing brain surface.

8. Bipolar diathermy to discrete haemorrhage from intracerebral vessels or vessels on the surface of the brain.

9. Irrigate the brain and dural surface with Ringer's solution or normal (0.9%) saline.

10. Dural hitching stitches are useful to prevent postoperative epidural haematoma. The dura is hitched to the pericranium or to the bone edge, through multiple drill holes.

If general oozing is a problem:

1. Be patient - pack, tamponade, apply gentle direct digital pressure and wait 5-10 minutes - most of the bleeding will probably stop (Figure 11.1 (b), page 504).

2. Try topical thrombin in Gelfoam soaked pledgets.

3. Elevate the head of the table 10°-20°.

4. Lower the blood pressure (if it is not critical to do so) to 90-100 mmHg systolic.

5. Apply hydrogen peroxide.

6. Apply crushed muscle and gentle digital pressure.

7. Leave a suction drain in the epidural or subgaleal plane with the dura closed watertight.

Venous sinus bleeding can be torrential and is best controlled with suturing of a fascial or crushed muscle patch over the rent. If the blood loss is too great, place a crushed muscle plug over the area, covered with Surgicel and cottonoid and wet gauze, tamponade the leak with your fingers or those of your assistant and wait at least 5 minutes (Figure 11.1 (b), page 504). The bleeding will stop. Beware of air embolism through the open venous sinus - especially if the head of the patient is elevated. Air embolism will cause sudden cardiovascular collapse. Postoperative haematoma can be life threatening and is not easy to diagnose early without CT scan, particularly if the anaesthetic drugs are slow to reverse. Reoperation for haematoma may become necessary - but permanent morbidity may still result. Meticulous attention to haemostasis will minimise this complication.

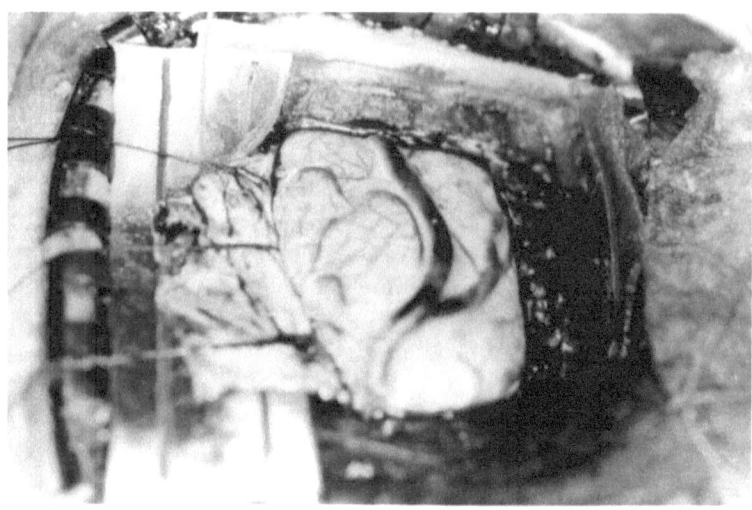

(a) i Shows the brain in contact with the falx before retraction. The dural flap is reflected medially.

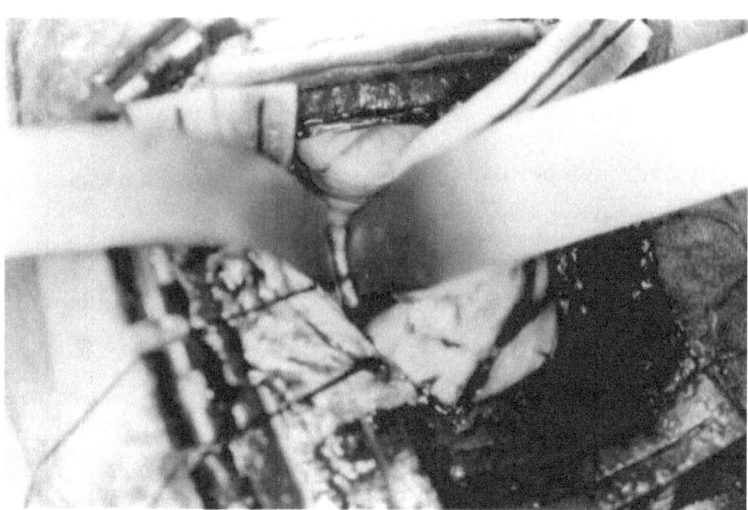

(a) ii Shows the retractors in position. The left retractor is on the edge of the falx and sagittal sinus, the right retractor is on the posterior frontal lobe. The cottonoids (linteen strips) are seen beneath the retractors protecting the brain.

Figure 11.1 (a) Placement of the retractors to gain exposure to the interhemispheric fissure. This is the approach to a falcine meningioma.

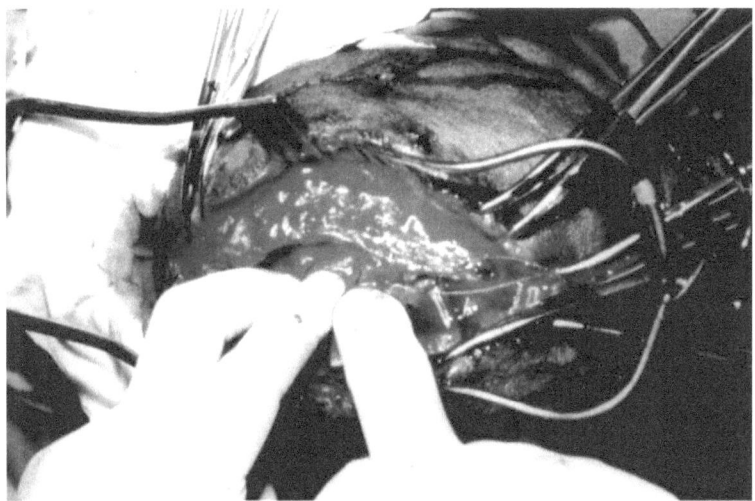

(b) Operative photograph showing digital pressure over the sagittal sinus to control haemorrhage. Crushed muscle, Surgicel, linteen strips and gauze underlie the fingers.

Figure 11.1 (a-b) Operative techniques.

Air embolism

An air embolus may occur if a large vein or venous sinus is open, and the head is higher than the heart. The cardiac output suddenly drops, with a precipitous fall in blood pressure, and there may be a 'machinery' murmur over the heart on auscultation. The treatment is to lower the head, flood the field with saline or Ringer's solution, wax the bone edge, occlude the open sinus with a muscle plug or Gelfoam and cottonoids. The anaesthetist will administer 100 percent oxygen, and try to aspirate the air from a central line in the right atrium, which is placed on induction if air embolism is considered to be a risk.

Air sinus exposure

If the frontal sinus is widely opened during a frontal craniotomy the sinus is best exenterated to prevent delayed mucocele. The mucosa is stripped, the back wall of the sinus is partly removed with rongeurs. The sinus is packed with Gelfoam soaked in antibiotic solution, the pericranium is stripped from the scalp and folded over the open sinus and sutured to the dura (Figure 11.2, next page). If there is only a small opening in the sinus, pack it with Gelfoam, then cover the opening with a pericranial patch. If the mastoid air cells are opened during a temporal or occipital craniotomy, they should be occluded with bone wax, and a watertight dural closure obtained. If there are large openings, then a pericranial or muscle patch should be sutured over them. CSF rhinorrhea and meningitis may result if the sinuses are not closed. This occurs via the Eustachian tube when the leak goes through the mastoid air cells.

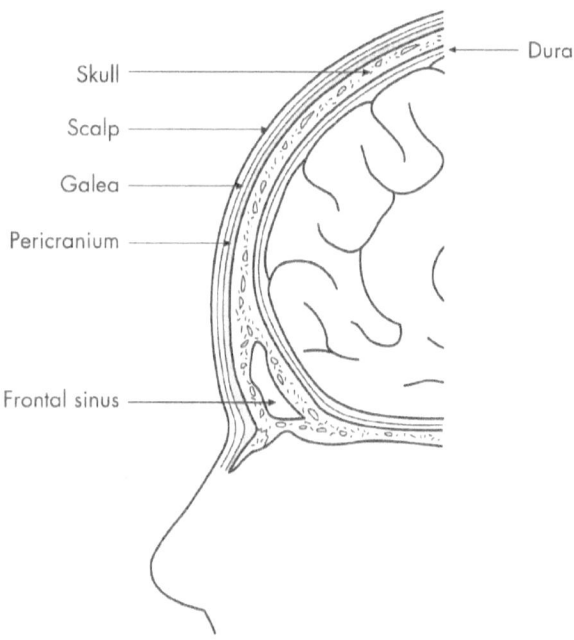

Figure 11.2 (a) Normal anatomy.

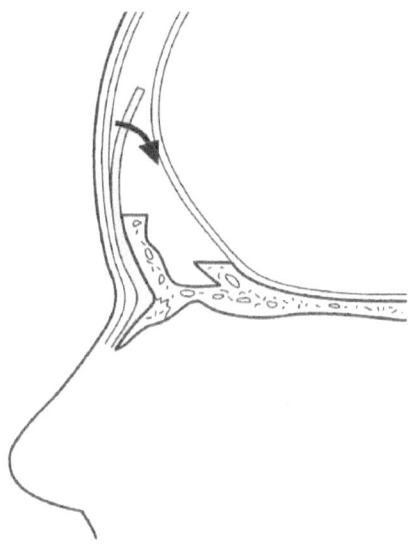

(b) Craniotomy has been performed. Posterior wall of the frontal sinus largely removed, and mucosa of frontal sinus stripped and curetted out. Pericranial layer separated from outer table of skull ready to rotate posteriorly over the exposed sinus.

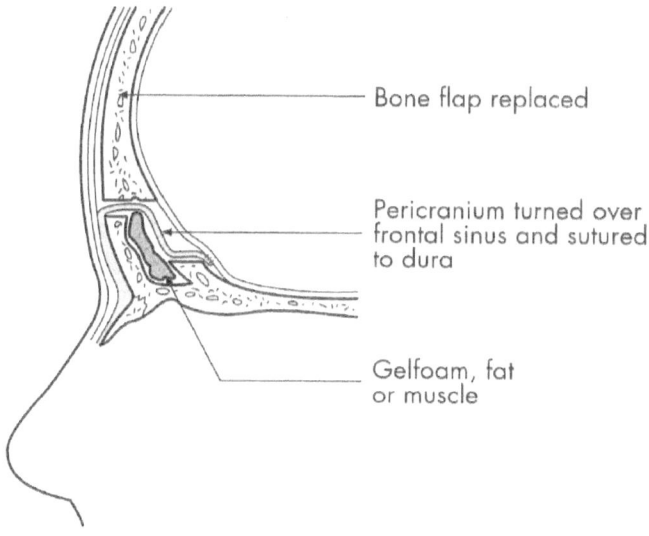

Bone flap replaced

Pericranium turned over frontal sinus and sutured to dura

Gelfoam, fat or muscle

(c) Pericranial flap sutured in position to dura posterior to the frontal sinus. Frontal sinus packed with Gelfoam, fat or muscle. Watertight seal. Bone flap replaced.

Figure 11.2 (a-c) Repair of frontal sinus to prevent postoperative CSF leak.

Antibiotics and the prevention of infection

Great care should be taken to maintain sterility throughout the case. Neurosurgical infection is always serious and easily becomes life-threatening. There is evidence that prophylactic antibiotics prevent postoperative infection in neurosurgery. These can be given at the time of anaesthetic induction and theoretically this one dose is enough. Continuance after the operation is unnecessary unless the wound is contaminated or infected. The combinations of penicillin and chloramphenicol, flucloxacillin or cloxacillin and ampicillin, or a single cephalosporin like cefalotin (alternate name is cephalothin) or ceftriaxone are suitable alternatives.

Anticonvulsants

There is evidence that post-craniotomy epilepsy is prevented by anticonvulsant. This is started the day before surgery or, if the case is an emergency a loading dose is given intraoperatively. Phenytoin is the drug of choice because it can be given parenterally. It is usually continued for one week postoperatively as a prophylactic. If the patient has had previous seizures it is continued longer. They should not drive for 3 months, because the major risk of seizures is during this period. Levetiracetam is an alternative to phenytoin, if available. A depressed fractured skull with cortical laceration, an intracerebral haematoma, acute subdural haematoma, cerebral tumour or cerebral abscess all place the patient at higher risk of ongoing epilepsy and are all indications for keeping the anticonvulsant duration longer - up to 1 year if seizure free, or indefinitely while having seizures. They should remain on anticonvulsant for 2 years from the time of the last seizure. All anticonvulsants are withdrawn slowly over several days, to prevent rebound epilepsy.

PHENOBARBITAL (PHENOBARBITONE)

i.v., i.m.-prep-admin

• i.v. Admin: Dilute at least 1:1, give at 1 mg/kg/min or slower. Monitor vital functions

• i.m. Admin: Use 200 mg/ml undiluted.

Dosage

Neonates

Seizures i.v.: Loading dose 20 mg/kg given in 2 doses, 3-4 hours apart then, i.v., oral: Maintenance: 3-4 mg/kg/day in 1-2 doses

Infants and children

Seizures i.v., i.m.: Loading dose: 20-30 mg/kg stat i.v., i.m.,
oral: 3-6 mg/kg/day in 1-2 doses

Febrile convulsion prophylaxis: Oral: 3-4 mg/kg at night

Adults (usual dose)

i.v., i.m.: Up to 600 mg/day Oral: 100-300 mg/day

DIAZEPAM

Dosage

Children

i.v.: 0.1-0.3 mg/kg/dose (max 10 mg). Repeat every 1-4 hours as needed (max 30 mg in 8 hours)

Oral: 0.1-0.3 mg/kg/dose 8-12 hourly starting at lower dose and increase to desired effect.

Rectal: 0.3-0.5 mg/kg/dose

Adults

Oral: 5-40 mg/day in divided doses.

PHENYTOIN

i.v.-prep-admin

• Admin: 6 mg/ml or more dilute

• Loading dose: Over 60 min

• Usual: Over 15-30 min

• Do not mix with glucose. Can be mixed with saline if used within 1 hour.

• AVOID EXTRAVASATION.

• i.v. boluses may cause severe myocardial depression.

Dosage

Loading dose in an emergency i.v.: 15-20 mg/kg

Neonates

i.v., oral: Week 1 of life: 4 mg/kg/dose 12 hourly

Week 2-12 months: 4 mg/kg/dose 6 hourly

Infants and children

i.v., oral: 4-8 mg/kg/day in 2-3 doses

Adults (usual dose)

i.v., oral: 7 mg/kg/day in 2-3 doses.

The burr hole

A burr hole is a basic component of all cranial neurosurgery which can stand alone, or form part of a craniotomy. The scalp is prepared and infiltrated with 0.5 percent Marcaine with 1:200 000 adrenaline (bupivacaine hydrochloride with epinephrine) (alternative plain 0.5 percent Marcaine, or Xylocaine (lignocaine) 1 percent or 2 percent, plain or with adrenaline (epinephrine). As a general principle, be aware of the maximum dose of local anaesthetic allowed for the age of the patient, to avoid hypertension or cardiac arrhythmia from overdose, and avoid injection directly into blood vessels for the same reason, i.e. aspirate before injecting and move the needle through the tissues as you inject. Try and infiltrate the scalp rather than the subgaleal tissues for best effect. The local anaesthetic will reduce scalp edge bleeding and also provide some post-operative analgesia.

Make sure the instruments are sharp. A linear 3 cm incision is made, the periosteum is split off the skull with a sharp periosteal elevator subjacent to the wound, and a small self-retaining retractor inserted. In the absence of a high-speed drill, the skull perforator attached to the Hudson brace is used to create a conical opening in the skull, which will create a small hole through the inner table to reveal the blue or white dura beneath. Keep probing with a forcep until you feel the bone give way in the base. If you are not sure when the perforator is through the skull, you will feel it pass through into the cancellous bone and then it becomes more difficult to cut the bone as it passes through the firm inner table. Avoid undue pressure as you pass through the inner table for fear of cracking the skull and plunging. Use the conical or cylindrical burr to create a cylindrical opening in place of the conical opening. When the burr becomes difficult to turn it is usually through the full thickness of the skull.

In the adult skull, some pressure must be exerted particularly when the outer table of the skull is perforated. You should then ease up on the pressure. The squamous temporal and the child's skull are relatively thin. Do not press too hard on the brace in these situations or it may plunge through the skull and brain. If there are no brace, perforator or burrs available, a bone gouge and large mallet, a trephine or even a carpenter's brace and bit are worthwhile alternatives in a desperate situation. Lift out the small bone remnants at the base of the opening with an artery forcep or smooth periosteal elevator. Do not leave fragments indented beneath the edge of the bone, as this may promote epidural haematoma formation and perpetuate bleeding into the burr hole. On completing the burr hole, inturned bone chips are removed from the underside of the bone edge using a blunt hook or a smooth periosteal elevator. Diathermy the central dura with bipolar coagulation and then lift with a sharp hook and incise it with a scalpel (15 or 11 blade) and diathermy the edges thus created. Control of bleeding from beneath the edge of the bone can usually be achieved with small pieces of Surgicel impacted beneath the bone edge. If this fails, use a curved dissector such as a Watson-Cheyne, and pass it beneath the bone and diathermy under the bone against the dura. Bone wax may also be necessary along the bone edge. If this fails, place Surgicel along the edge preferably before opening the dura, place a pattie over the Surgicel or wet gauze to tamponade the hole and leave it for 5 minutes. Usually on removing the pattie the burr hole is dry.

Routine scalp closure

The scalp is best closed in two layers with an inverted galeal stitch or absorbable suture such as Vicryl or Dexon and a continuous or interrupted non-absorbable skin suture such as 3/0 nylon. It is important that the wound is closed watertight to prevent CSF leak, which could lead to meningitis and infection. Accurate skin apposition should be the goal in order to increase complete wound healing rates and thus reduce infection.

TRAUMA

The pathology and clinical management of trauma to the head is discussed in Chapter 3, page 76.

Table 11.1 Principles of neurosurgical operating.

- Have a good knowledge of the anatomy
- Have a well-planned approach and strategy
- Have an accurate picture of the neurological state before operation so it can be compared after operation.
- **Check the side of the pathology or the level in the spine before making incision**
- Shave the skin in the operating room just before surgery. This will reduce the risk of postoperative wound infection by avoiding contamination of small skin wounds created by the razor blade

Table 11.1 *(Continued)*

- Position the patient's head to optimise exposure
- Draw incision line before draping (scratch skin with needle if no indelible marker is available)
- Catheterise the bladder of all patients having craniotomies and major spinal surgery, particularly if neurological compromise is already present
- Meticulous sterile technique:
    - -scalp preparation and draping
    - -infection in neurosurgery is a disaster and may cause death or serious morbidity
- Obtain continued accurate haemostasis throughout the procedure
- Ensure delicacy of touch, and accuracy of attack
- Minimal brain retraction
- Protection of brain surface with cottonoids
- Adequate anaesthesia with control of ICP and brain turgor
- Avoid eloquent brain areas
- Avoid entering the venous sinuses
- Do not obliterate major cerebral veins
- Adequate lighting - headlight can be helpful
- Close and obliterate air sinuses if opened - to prevent CSF leak and infection
- Irrigate the subdural structures with Ringer's solution or saline before final dural closure to reduce the amount of residual air and blood in the head
- Prophylactic antibiotics
- Prophylactic anticonvulsants - duration post-operation - at least 1 week, usually 3 months.
- Means of controlling brain swelling intraoperatively
    - -well chosen patient position
    - -adequate ventilation, patent airway
    - -patent neck veins - untwist neck
    - -elevate head of operating table
    - -aspirate CSF - intraventricular and cisternal
    - -hyperventilation to $PaCO_2$ 25-30
    - -mannitol - 0.5 g/kg over 10-15 min i.v.
    - -check for remote subdural, extradural,
    - e.g. pin site, or contrecoup injury with increasing swelling
    - -check for intracerebral haematoma
    - -barbiturate – thiopentone
    - -isoflurane
- Close the dura watertight, if possible; a fascial or muscle patch can be used to accomplish this manoeuvre. Temporalis fascia or pericranium is very useful

---

Exploratory burr holes

Indications

Suspected intracranial haematoma (acute or chronic) or abscess where and there is no CT scan available.

Strategy

The burr hole is made overlying the suspected pathology, however in the case of a suspected acute epidural haematoma, three burr holes are made on each side of the head until the collection is located (Figure 11.3, next page). Shave and prepare the whole head for a craniotomy, unless the side is obvious. The first burr hole is made over the suspected site of the collection, which for most epidural haematomas is in the temporal region on the side of the scalp contusion and swelling, and the side of the pupillary dilatation and sluggishness.

The temporal burr hole is placed approximately at the mid-zygomatic point, approximately 3-4 cm above the zygoma. If this site proves negative, frontal and then parietal burr holes are performed. The frontal burr hole is made just behind the hairline in the mid-pupillary line, and the parietal burr hole is made over the parietal eminence (the most prominent part of the parietal bone). The three burr holes are then repeated on the other side. If an epidural haematoma is present, the dark semi-solid blood will be obvious when the skull is breached. The epidural haematoma operation is then carried out (see below). The presence of an acute subdural haematoma will give the dura a bluish hue, and will make it tense. If a subdural collection is a possibility, the dura should be opened, and if present, a craniotomy will be necessary. If there is no collection and the patient has a primary brain injury with cerebral swelling, the dura will be tense and usually pale. When the dura is opened to exclude a collection, swollen and sometimes necrotic brain will swell or exude out of the burr hole. Posterior fossa burr holes may be performed if there is a suspected posterior fossa collection with a fracture in this region and overlying scalp and soft tissue swelling, neck stiffness and headache. The diagnosis· of a posterior fossa collection is often a diagnosis of exclusion unless seen on a CT scan.

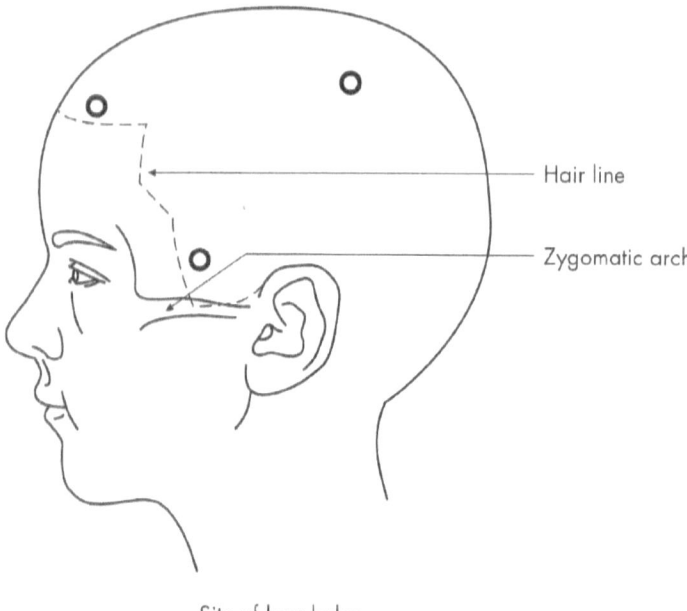

Site of burr holes

Figure 11.3 The siting of exploratory burr holes following head injury. Temporal, frontal and parietal positions.

Method

Described in the general principle section

Evacuation of an extradural haematoma (Figure 11.4, page 515)

Indications

1. Deteriorating conscious state post head injury. Exploratory burr hole performed and epidural haematoma identified.
2. Poor conscious state since head injury with focal signs suggestive of intracranial collection. Exploratory burr holes performed and epidural haematoma identified.

Strategy

The single burr hole overlying the collection is enlarged by either craniectomy or craniotomy. For the inexperienced surgeon a craniectomy is preferable because it is more rapid. If a temporal craniotomy is performed a craniectomy is extended inferiorly if necessary to follow the haematoma onto the floor of the middle cranial fossa beneath the temporal lobe dura.

The clot is usually semi-solid and cannot be removed through a single burr hole. The enlarged opening is necessary. The clot is completely evacuated. A headlight is helpful to check the areas beyond the bone edge, particularly inferiorly under the temporal lobe. The bleeding is often coming from a single meningeal artery on the dura and it is important to locate this bleeding point, and either under-run it with silk or seal it by diathermy.

General dural ooze is often a problem following the removal of a large haematoma, particularly one that has been present for several hours, and this bleeding is controlled with a combination of Surgicel, diathermy, Gelfoam and the essential dural hitching sutures around the edge. It is often necessary to place a drain in the epidural space if there is ongoing ooze. This should be a closed drainage system and a suction drain is satisfactory, such as a redivac drain or Jackson Pratt drain with plastic bulb attached which can be repeatedly suctioned and emptied post-operatively. If no closed drainage system is available, and the wound is very oozy, then an open drain will be an adequate substitute.

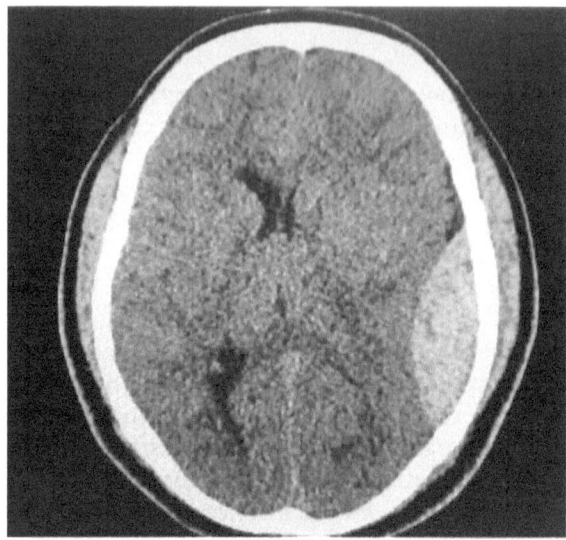

Figure 11.4 (a) CT scan showing an acute left temporo-parietal extradural haematoma.

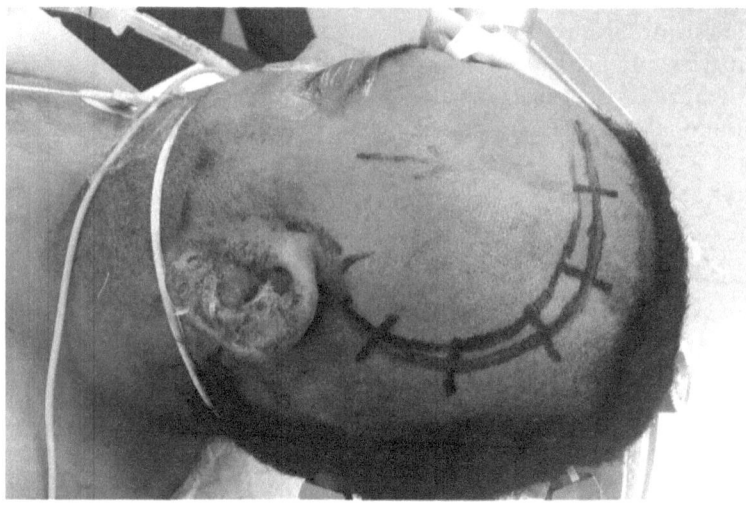

(b) Patient anaesthetised, scalp shaved and incision line marked. This is a large fronto-temporo-parietal flap. In this case the head is fixed in a 3-pin headrest. Paraffin wax is placed in the left external auditory canal to prevent alcoholic or iodinated solution entering the ear canal and causing injury.

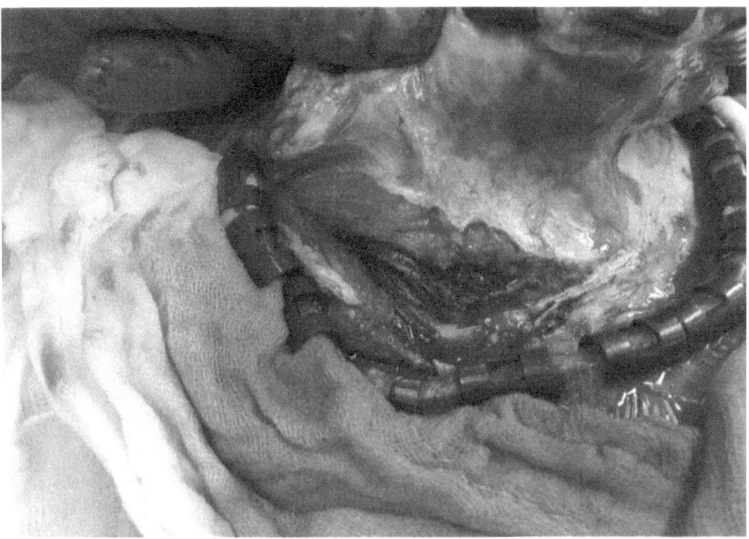

(c) The scalp incision is made, Raney clips are placed on the scalp. Temporalis fascia and temporalis muscle are divided.

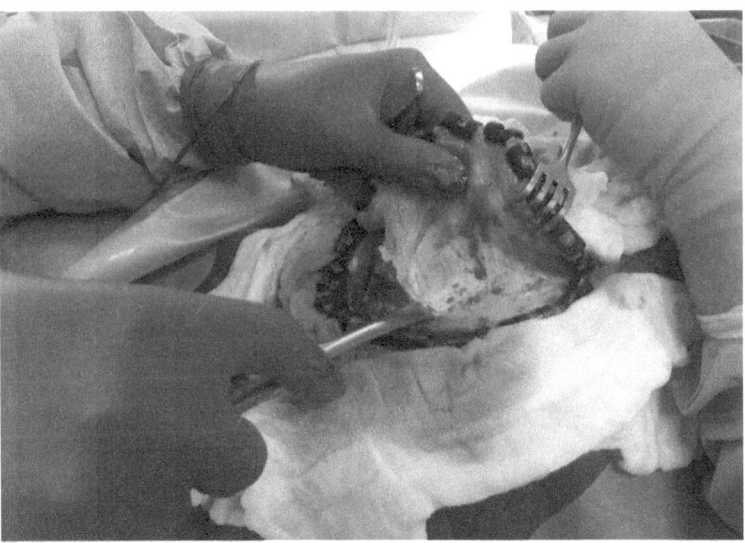

(d) Temporalis muscle with temporalis fascia being raised and turned forwards using a broad sharp periosteal elevator.

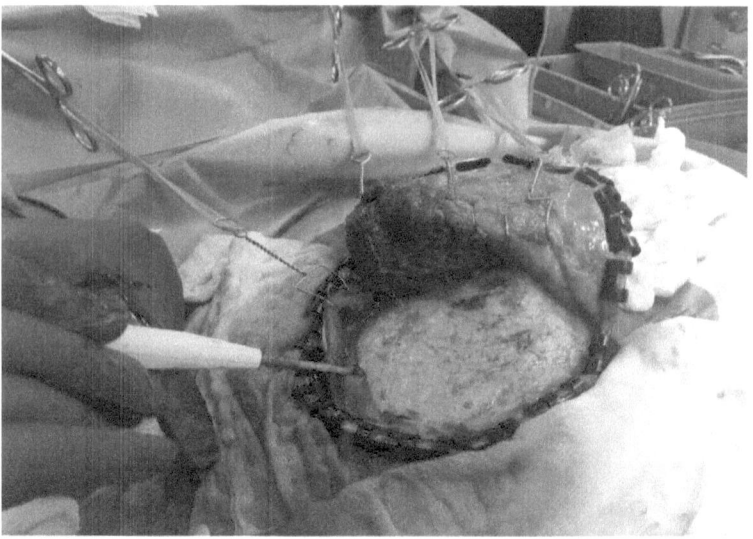

(e) The scalp and temporalis muscle are retracted forwards using double hooks and rubber bands. The skull is exposed ready for the craniotomy. Note the vertical fracture line in the posterior temporal bone being pointed out by the diathermy tip.

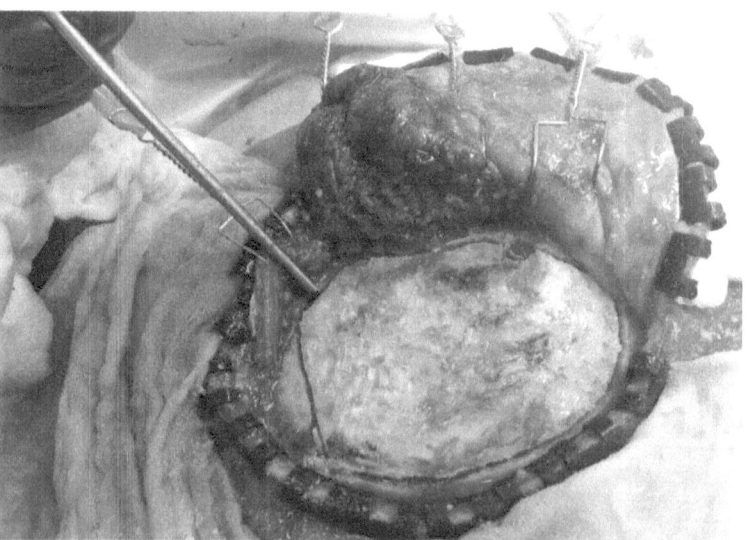

(f) The bone flap has been cut using the craniotome and is ready to elevate.

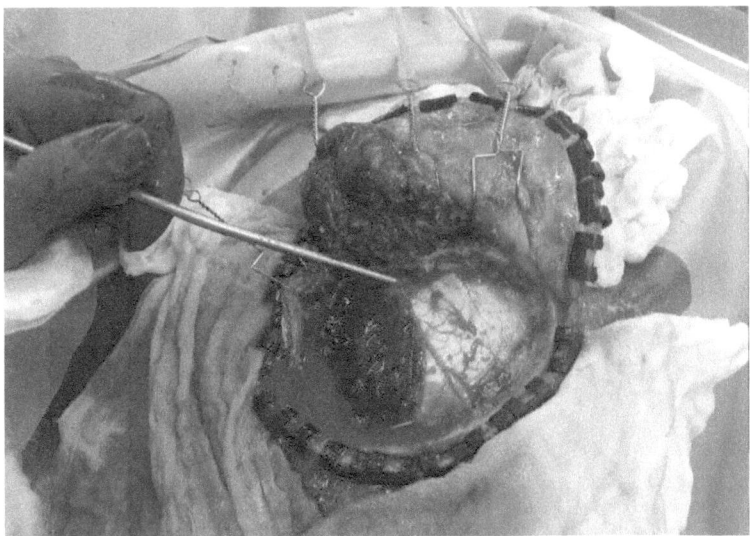

(g) The epidural haematoma is exposed. Note there is evidence of fresh bleeding and solid clot.

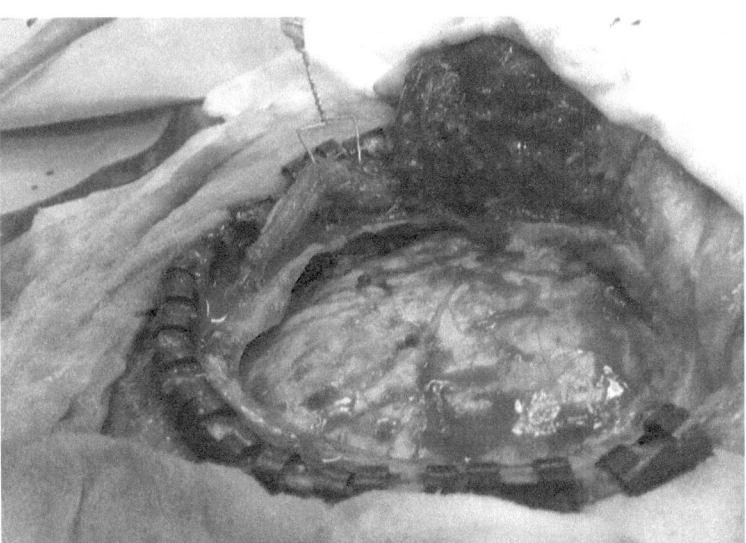

(h) The haematoma has been evacuated and the middle meningeal artery (MMA) has been coagulated proximally. The MMA can be seen traversing the dura. Note the space between the dura and the temporal bone overlying the middle cranial fossa where the haematoma was evacuated. This requires some tamponade with gelfoam, surgicel and dural hitching sutures.

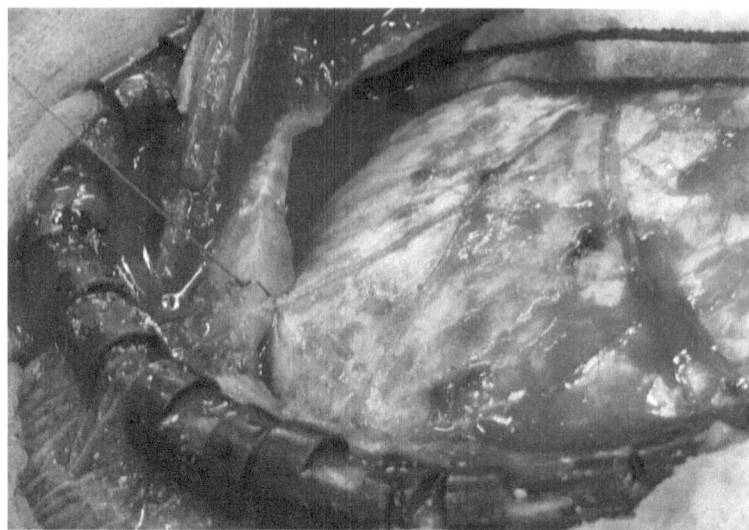

(i) Dural hitching suture of 3/0 prolene being applied to prevent recurrent extradural formation. Dural hitching suture in position. Multiple of these sutures were applied to hold all of this dura up to the bone edge. In this case small drill holes were made in the bone but if no drill is available, the sutures can attach to temporalis or pericranium (periosteum of the skull).

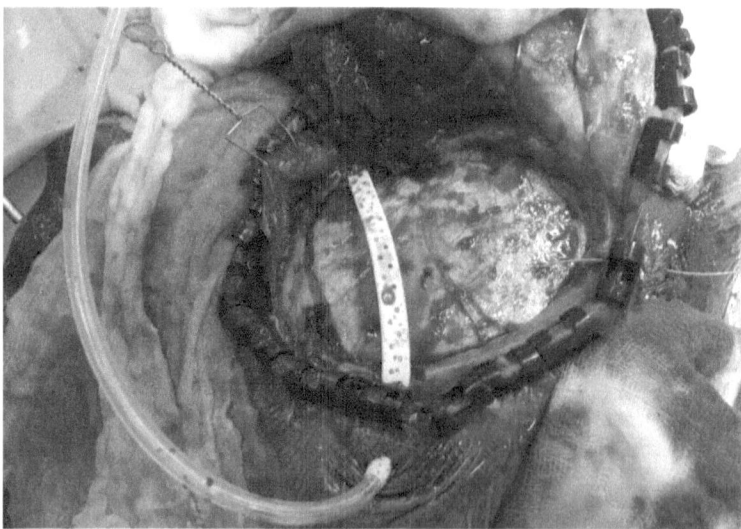

(j) Drain tube in position with the tip placed down in the middle cranial fossa. The other end is brought out a separate stab incision in the scalp. This is a Jackson-Pratt suction drain but other suction drains or even a rubber or Penrose drain could be used. A parenchymal ICP monitor is used in this case (the thin wire coming out of the dura) and is brought out separate incision scalp.

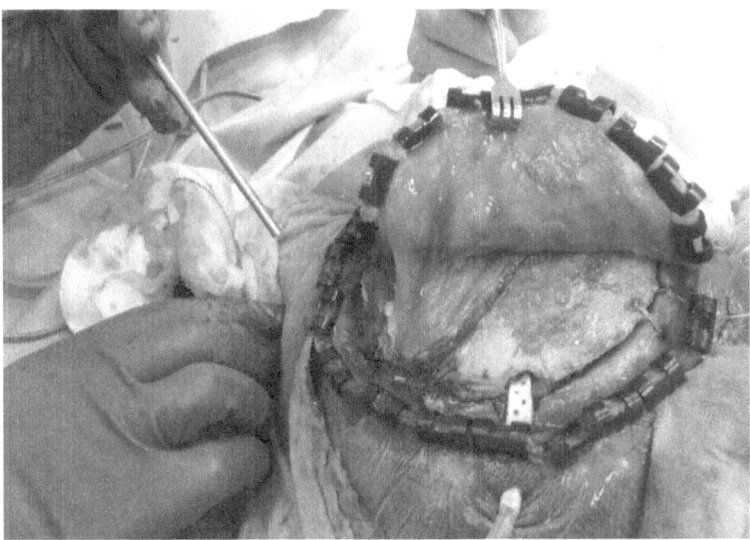

(k) Bone flap re-anchored with miniplates and screws. Sutures with heavy silk or nylon can be used if plates are not available. The temporalis is re-apposed with 1/vicryl.

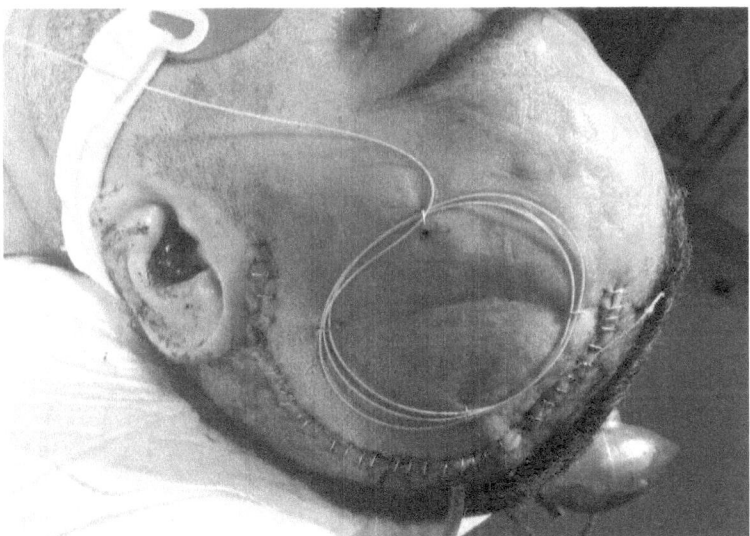

(l) The scalp is closed and the drain tube secured with a suture. The parenchymal ICP monitor is the thin wire coiled on the scalp.

Figure 11.4 (a-l) The sequence of operative steps in the evacuation of an acute extradural haematoma.

Avoidance of complications

Beware that the drains may not take away a postoperative collection, and if the patient is not improving or deteriorates, there may be a re-collection; and re-exploration may be indicated. The mortality rate from acute extradural haematoma should be around 4 per cent or less, but if patients are delayed in presentation, with a poor conscious state, and bilateral neurological signs, particularly extension to pain or no response to pain, or fixed, dilated pupils; they are likely to do badly. Time is critical in extraction of an epidural haematoma. Mannitol can be used to gain an extra half hour to an hour or so, by reducing intracranial pressure. Beyond this time, the haematoma may expand to fill the space left by the shrinkage of the brain following osmotic diuretic administration.

Subdural haematoma

Acute subdural haematoma

Indication

Deteriorating conscious state following high velocity trauma, or comatose since time of injury, focal neurological signs suggesting mass lesion, usually skull fracture, dilated pupil on ipsilateral side or bilaterally dilated pupils, scalp contusion± laceration.

Strategy

Perform a rapid craniotomy and/or craniectomy, depending on the urgency and the exposure required. Evacuate any extradural haematoma, open the dura widely and rapidly to allow the brain to swell uniformly. Evacuate haematoma, secure haemostasis, remove non-viable brain, secure haemostasis. Consider placement of ICP monitor and removal of bone flap.

Method

Create a generous scalp flap overlying the maximal point of trauma, lift temporalis with the scalp flap, raise a free bone flap and/or craniectomy, open the dura widely, secure meningeal bleeders, and evacuate subdural haematoma including beyond edges of craniotomy. Headlight and malleable brain retractor are essential for this gentle retraction of the brain away from the dura on all sides of the craniotomy. Active bleeding from the sagittal sinus region is difficult to control but the best way is to use crushed muscle, e.g. temporalis and/or large pledgets of Surgicel impacted over the sagittal sinus and bridging vein to tamponade the haemorrhage. Do not attempt to extend the craniotomy up to the sagittal sinus, because the bleeding will likely become uncontrollable. Cortical bleeders are controlled with diathermy or Weck clips and non-viable macerated brain is removed, e.g. temporal lobectomy. The underside of the frontal lobe and temporal pole, and perisylvian region are the most common areas contused and damaged in an acute subdural haematoma because of the impact of this part of the brain against the sharp edge of the sphenoid wing and the adjacent bone, i.e. bursting injury of the brain. If the bone flap is removed and stored in the abdominal subcutaneous fat, it can be replaced when the brain is sunken and soft and this can be assessed by the position of the scalp flap. This may occur usually several weeks of even months following the injury.

Progressive brain swelling is a frightening situation for the surgeon. Ask the anaesthetist to give another dose of mannitol or hypertonic saline. Check that CO_2 levels are adequately reduced, that the patient is being ventilated satisfactorily, elevate the head end of the table, consider looking around the edges again to exclude a distant subdural haematoma, particularly under the temporal lobe, and consider needling the brain with a brain needle and aspirating to make sure there is no large expanding intracerebral haematoma. If the brain remains swollen and turgor is tense, consider placing a ventricular catheter, either on the side of the subdural or on the opposite ventricle via a separate burr hole. One danger of evacuating CSF from the opposite ventricle is that shift may increase and worsen the patient's clinical state therefore, beware of this alternative. Another possibility is bleeding on the other side of the head so the surgeon may wish to perform burr holes on the other side to check for this correctable situation. If all of these are negative, and the brain continues to swell, the outlook is very poor, and usually the patient will not survive.

Control of massive brain swelling is difficult. This 'malignant' brain swelling continues unabated despite measures to correct it. The best way to handle this is to lay the dura over the brain without closing it. (Dural closure is impossible in this situation.) Replace the temporalis muscle and place a few holding sutures on the edge of this muscle and then close the scalp rapidly. Debridement of necrotic brain can sometimes help this situation.

Chronic subdural haematoma

This is usually drained via a frontal and parietal burr hole, and for a large collection a temporal burr hole may also be inserted. The chronic subdural is usually yellow to dark brown coloured fluid or dark blood which exits under high pressure when the dura is opened. The brain is often depressed 1·3 cm from the dura. There may be a thick outer membrane to penetrate using diathermy and there may be one or two middle membranes, which also require penetration. This is best done with bipolar coagulation. A CT scan will give guidance as to whether these are present or not. Once the fluid collection is drained, the subdural space is irrigated with warm (body temperature 37°C) Ringer's or saline solution. An infant feeding tube can be passed well beyond the margins of the burr hole to irrigate the far extremes of the subdural collection and try and remove as much of the old blood as possible. Be very careful passing this tube to make sure it does not enter the brain itself. Passing the tube over a smooth periosteal elevator placed beneath the edge of the burr hole is a good way to do this.

Once all the washout is relatively clear, the infant feeding tube is left in the subdural space as a drain for 24·48 hours until any residual bloodstained fluid is drained and the effluent is a clear yellow colour or CSF-like fluid, or until drainage stops. This indicates that the brain has fully expanded. The tube is best passed posteriorly and brought out through the posterior burr hole and then through a separate stab incision in the scalp and tied in position. This will reduce the risk of infection. If it is brought out through the same incision line there is a slightly increased risk of infection. The drain is placed dependently well below the head level and attached to the end of the bed. It should be a closed drainage system and the drainage of the fluid into a blood collection bag is a satisfactory, cheap method. The patient should be placed mildly head down (5·10°) with one pillow for 24 hours then lie flat with one pillow. If they are unable to tolerate the head down position due to mental confusion, lack of co·operation or cardiovascular problems, then they should lie flat with one pillow.

They are best kept in bed flat for 5-7 days to minimise the 10 per cent risk of recurrent subdural haematoma. Rescanning is not necessary in the first few weeks, because there is often some residual fluid. The clinical state of the patient gives the best guide to whether recurrence has occurred. The patient will develop recurrent headaches, focal neurological signs, epilepsy, drowsiness and re-investigation will then be necessary.

Decompressive craniectomy (Figure 11.5, page 526)

Decompressive craniectomy (DC) has become a common operation to reduce intracranial pressure due to brain oedema (in either one or both hemispheres) and/or intracranial haemorrhage. Decompressive craniectomy is a major operation and will require some prior neurosurgical experience and familiarity with performing a major craniotomy. The main indications are traumatic brain injury or cerebral ischaemia due to cerebral artery thrombotic occlusion. DC involves removing a large segment of skull either unilaterally or bilaterally and not replacing it at the end of the procedure. An alternative is the hinged craniotomy which does replace the bone but allows it to float up under the scalp flap whilst the brain is swollen but gradually sink into the final position when the swelling subsides.[55,56] This procedure avoids the need for a second operation to replace the bone flap (cranioplasty) and is thus very suitable for LMICs.

Where surgical instruments are limited, the surgeon may remove the skull piecemeal using bone rongeurs but this will not result in a large DC and will leave a skull defect that may be difficult to repair by cranioplasty in the setting of LMIC. The operative surgery technique is described in the section below on blast injury (page 530). The surgeon requires specific training to embark on a DC. To perform the operation competently is technically quite challenging and is not the equivalent of performing a small localized craniectomy. The latter procedure is more frequently being performed by general surgeons in LMICs. In LMICs, DC is often undertaken as an emergency procedure when the patient has severe traumatic brain injury with an acute subdural haematoma. The thought process is

[55]Gutman, M. J., E. How and T. Withers. The floating anchored craniotomy. Surg Neurol Int 2017; 8: 130.
[56]Schmidt JH, 3rd, Reyes BJ, Fischer R, Flaherty SK. Use of hinge craniotomy for cerebral decompression. Technical note. J Neurosurg. 2007;107(3):678-82.

that having the DC would obviate the need for the ICP monitor because the ICP is lowered satisfactorily by the DC. See the section on ICP monitoring in Chapter 3 on page 131. This is not universally the case but may be the only alternative in LMIC.[57] Where the DC is performed by inexperienced surgeons, the decompression is often partial or smaller than would be achieved by a neurosurgeon with experience in doing the procedure. A smaller craniectomy may be adequate to evacuate an acute or subacute subdural haematoma but it may not be adequate to reduce the ICP due to brain swelling. The swollen brain may herniate and be further injured where there is a small craniectomy.

It should be noted that extradural haematomas can be usually be evacuated via a craniotomy (rather than craniectomy) and the bone is then replaced. DC is also used as a late salvage operation in advanced centres when continuous ICP monitoring is being used and the intracranial hypertension becomes intractable despite maximal medical therapy. Delayed DC may also be indicated in patients with severe cerebral contusions where the contusions increase in severity over days and there is increasing surrounding oedema. For those patients with diffuse axonal injury who survive following the DC, there will be a significant number who are severely disabled or in a persistent vegetative state.[58,59] However, the mortality will increase if surgery is not performed.

The decision to embark on early DC is relatively straightforward if the patient has an acute subdural haematoma or a blast/penetrating injury but prognostic factors such as age, GCS, pupil reactions, motor response and imaging findings should all be considered in making the final decision. The declared wishes of the patient pre-injury and the families wishes should also be considered. The decision to perform an early DC for diffuse swelling is challenging because medical management can also be used to control ICP. However, if no ICP monitoring available a decision for medical monitoring is less feasible.

There are usually no rehabilitation services available for the severely disabled patients or for patients in a persistent vegetative state are unlikely to survive long in LMIC. In many LMIC, the

[57]Rubiano AM, Maldonado M, Montenegro J, et al. The evolving concept of damage control in neurotrauma: application of military protocols in civilian settings with limited resources. World Neurosurgery. 2019. doi: 10.1016/j.wneu.2019.01.005. [Epub ahead of print]
[58]Cooper DJ, Rosenfeld JV, Murray L, Arabi YM, Davies AR, D'Urso P, et al. Decompressive craniectomy in diffuse traumatic brain injury. New England Journal of Medicine. 2011;364(16):1493-502.
[59]Hutchinson PJ, Kolias AG, Timofeev IS, Corteen EA, Czosnyka M, Timothy J, et al. Trial of Decompressive Craniectomy for Traumatic Intracranial Hypertension. New England Journal of Medicine. 2016;375(12):1119-30.

families will be expecting an operation for their family member with a severe traumatic brain injury but they should be fully informed of potential outcomes by the surgeon if DC is or is not performed. Unfortunately, prediction of outcome is uncertain in the first few days after a severe TBI so that many neurosurgeons would advise proceeding with DC to try and save the life of the patient. An International Consensus meeting on DC for severe TBI has provided guidance for neurosurgeons in various settings.[60]

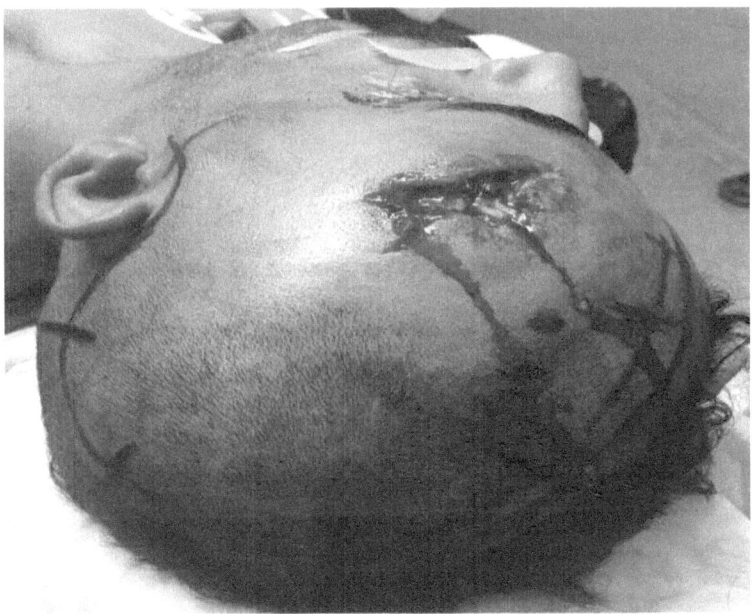

Figure 11.5 (a) Gunshot wound to the left forehead. Patient under general anaesthesia in the operating room. Head turned to the right side. Black incision line drawn on the scalp for left fronto-temporo-parietal decompressive craniectomy. Note the separate line for the midline adjacent to the incision line. This will prevent the craniotomy coming too close to the sagittal sinus.

[60]Hutchinson PJ, Kolias AG, Tajsic C, et al. Consensus statement from the International Consensus Meeting on the role of decompressive craniectomy in the management of severe traumatic brain injury: consensus statement. Acta Neurochir (Wien). 2019 May 28. doi: 10.1007/s00701-019-03936-y. [Epub ahead of print].

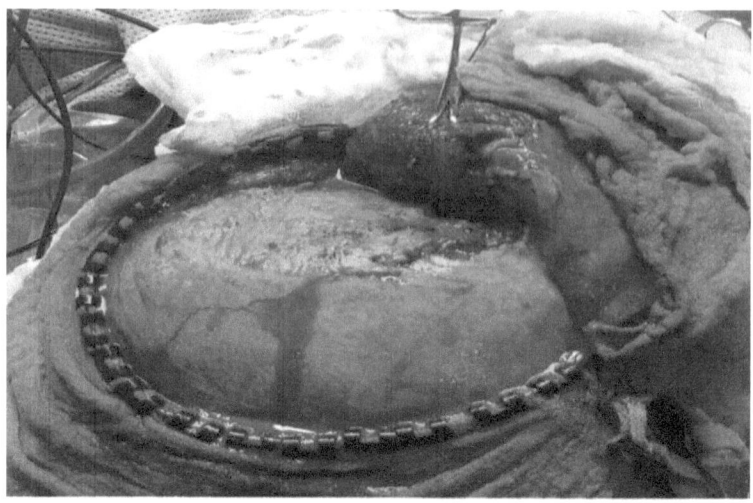

(b) Decompressive craniectomy left side. The scalp flap and temporalis muscle have been elevated to expose the left side of the skull.

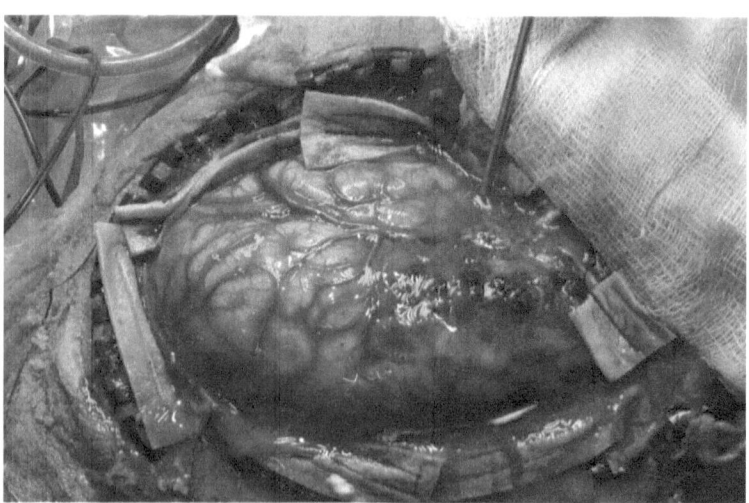

(c) Decompressive craniectomy left side. The bone flap has been removed using a craniotome and the dura is opened thus exposing the injured left hemisphere. The brain is swollen, haemorrhagic and congested, and there is contusion surrounding the penetrating injury to the left frontal lobe.

Figure 11.5 (a-c) Decompressive Craniectomy.

Chapter Eleven

Depressed fracture of the skull

Simple depressed fracture

Indication for elevation

If the skull has been depressed greater than the full thickness of the skull, it should be elevated.

Contraindication

If the depression is directly over the sagittal or transverse sinus, the non-neurosurgeon should avoid operating on this region because of the risk of major uncontrollable haemorrhage and air embolism.

Procedure

A scalp flap is raised around the fracture area. The periosteum is stripped away with a sharp periosteal elevator. A burr hole is placed in the surrounding non-depressed skull up to the edge of the fracture line and the fragments elevated with a smooth periosteal elevator. If the fracture is minor, this will suffice. However, if there are plates of bone acutely angled with the possibility of a dural tear, all of the fragments should be removed. Grasping the edge of the bone with a bone forceps (Horsley's, Wilms, or Pennybacker) may be needed to lever the fragments out, being careful not to lever the fragments into the brain. It is better to remove the fragments and repair a dural laceration and sometimes a cortical laceration, than to just elevate the fragments blindly. Having obtained haemostasis from any lacerated brain using bipolar coagulation and Surgicel, the dura is repaired watertight, and the bone fragments are replaced in approximately the same position as they were previously. They may require trimming and do not usually need anchorage with sutures or metal plates. The wound is then closed in layers. A layer of Surgicel over the bone fragments is helpful to hold them in position. Sometimes a small craniectomy is required extending the burr hole to gain adequate access to the underside of the fracture fragments. Beware of a split outer and inner table such that the outer table comes up but the inner table is left depressed when the fragments are removed. This situation should be corrected.

Compound (open) depressed fracture

The wound edges may require debridement. The bone fragments are removed and all foreign material removed and washed out. The wound can be irrigated with Betadine (povidone iodine). Beware of using alcoholic antiseptic preparations on the scalp in this situation, as they may enter the wound and damage the exposed brain beneath. It is preferable to use aqueous chlorhexidine and/or Betadine. The contaminated brain on the surface is debrided, the deeper hidden fragments of bone or foreign material are not usually retrieved particularly if the operator is experienced. The dura is repaired watertight, and often requires a pericranial patch. Monofilament suture such as polypropylene (Prolene) is satisfactory for this repair. If the bone fragments are heavily contaminated, or the wound has been open for more than 4 hours, the bone fragments should not be replaced; and the wound can usually be closed in layers. However, if there is a sizeable soft tissue defect, or gross contamination and the question of viability of tissue remains following debridement, then the wound should be packed and left open; but the dura does need to be closed watertight in this situation to prevent meningitis developing. A secondary closure may require a rotation or advancement flap to close the wound.

Infant depressed fracture

These fractures are usually a deformation of the bone (greenstick fracture), and can be easily elevated by drilling a small hole at the periphery of the fracture and passing a dissector or periosteal elevator beneath the fracture and lifting it very easily to the original contour. A small incision is made at the periphery of the fracture where the small burr hole is to be made. The infant skull is very thin and soft, and only a few turns of the perforator are necessary to breach the skull. This small opening can be enlarged by the removal of small fragments of bone at the edge of the burr hole with scissors or avulsion using an artery forceps.

Gunshot wound to the brain

If the patient is considered to be suitable for surgery (see Chapter 3), the head is shaved to examine the entire scalp for entry and exit wounds. These wounds are debrided so that primary closure will still be feasible, unless the defect is so large or so contaminated that delayed primary closure will be indicated. The skin incision is extended either with the gunshot wound in the middle of the flap, or included in the middle of a sigmoid incision. A bone flap or decompressive craniectomy is performed to gain adequate exposure of the injured brain. High velocity gunshot wounds result in significant brain swelling and this will require a wide decompressive craniectomy to adequately decompress the brain (see Figure 11.5, page 5.26). More localized lower energy injuries will be best managed with a more localised craniotomy. The superficial loose bone fragments are removed along with debris and hair and the bullet track is followed into the brain substance using irrigation and forceps to remove further debris. Haematoma in the trajectory of the bullet is evacuated and any sizeable vessel bleeding is easily controlled with silver clips and/or bipolar coagulation. The brain is irrigated with hydrogen peroxide solution and can be irrigated with Betadine as well, including the cerebral wound. The exit wound is then treated in a similar way. An ICP monitor is preferably inserted to aid postoperative management. The preoperative skull X-ray will give an indication as to how much metal is intracranial. These fragments should not be followed deep into the brain unless there is significant necrotic tissue and further debris along the track. If in doubt about what is viable and what is non-viable, it is better to leave the tissue rather than take it. A superficial cerebral debridement will usually suffice. The dura should be closed watertight even if a pericranial patch is necessary. Then the wound is closed if possible. Brain swelling is managed in a similar way to other head injury and a craniectomy, or leaving a craniotomy flap out, may be necessary to allow for the swelling to occur, to minimise a rise in intracranial pressure.

Stab wound to the head

Ideally, an angiogram (CTA) should be performed before surgery to define any vascular injury, though the facilities may not be available. If the patient is clinically well, the wound is debrided and closed. If the weapon is still in situ, then it should be removed under general anaesthesia and the track debrided in a similar way to the gunshot wound to the head, by raising a small bone flap, and by following the track of the stab wound if possible. If it looks like a clean stab, then it would be better to perform a very superficial inspection and not follow the wound deeply into the brain. Only a heavily contaminated wound should be followed. Any obvious haematoma is extracted. The dura is then closed watertight. If the patient has a fixed neurological deficit, this is unlikely to be altered by the surgery. If the patient is clinically deteriorating before reaching the operating room, this would imply a progressively enlarging haematoma; or if the deterioration is more sudden, a thromboembolic episode due to vessel injury is likely. Nothing can be done about this in the developing world setting, but an enlarging haematoma with progressive deterioration can be dealt with by evacuation of the haematoma. If on removing the weapon, the patient subsequently deteriorates, this would imply that a vessel or vessels have been pierced and, on removing the foreign body, haemorrhage is occurring. It could prove very difficult to deal with this problem without adequate investigation and instrumentation, and it may lead to the death of the patient. However, there is no alternative but to remove the foreign body under controlled conditions. The patient's family should be warned that the patient may die following removal of the foreign body.

Bomb blast injury

The principles of surgery for bomb blast injury are minimal debridement (to avoid causing more injury to the brain than what is already present) and maximal bone removal in order to widely decompress the swollen brain.[61] The key objective with any decompressive craniectomy for trauma, and especially blast injury, is to make it as large as possible. If the craniectomy is too small, the swollen brain herniates over the bone at the edges and lacerates or strangulates becoming ischemic or infracted. The surgical technique for unilateral and bilateral decompressive craniectomy has been well described.[62]

Practice point

Decompressive craniectomy is a major operation and will require some prior neurosurgical experience and familiarity with performing a major craniotomy.

---

[61]Ragel BT, Klimo P Jr, Martin JE, Teff RJ, Bakken HE, Armonda RA. Wartime decompressive craniectomy: technique and lessons learned. Neurosurgical Focus 2010;28(5):E2.
[62]Quinn TM, Taylor JJ, Magarik JA, Vought E, Kindy MS, Ellegala DB. Decompressive craniectomy: technical note. Acta neurologica Scandinavica. 2011;123(4):239-244.

It is vitally important for the surgeon to know the landmarks of the major venous sinuses so they are not injured during the craniotomy. Venous haemorrhage can be torrential and is made even more challenging and life threatening if the bone flap has not been lifted. An electric or compressed air driven craniotome will be required to perform a craniectomy because trying to do it with a Hudson brace and Gigli saw is neither practicable nor time efficient.

The scalp

The scalp should be completely shaved. The 3-pin head clamp is applied if available, otherwise the head is placed on the horseshoe rest. Care is used to place the pins away from where the scalp incision will be made. The ipsilateral shoulder is raised if the head is in a lateral position. Three types of scalp incision can be used when performing DC for military trauma:

1. A midline sagittal incision with a 'T-bar' extension which was described by Ludwig G. Kempe for his hemispherectomy operation.[63] The midline incision extends from the hairline to the inion (the occipital bony protuberance). The 'T-Bar' incision starts 1-2 cm anterior to the tragus at the root of the zygoma, extends superiorly to meet the midline incision just behind the coronal suture. This incision preserves the superficial temporal artery and occipital artery angiosomes.

2. The large reverse question mark incision which starts at the root of the zygoma, 2-3cm anterior to the tragus, extends back towards the asterion and then curves around the parietal eminence to the midline and forwards to the hairline. The scalp is reflected as a myocutaneous flap with the temporalis muscle.

3. Bicoronal incision for the bifrontal craniectomy. This extends from the root of the zygoma, 1-2cm anterior to the tragus extending up to the midline just behind the coronal suture and across to the other side.

Late breakdown of posterior wound margins was encountered with the reverse question mark incision particularly related to the patient lying on this region and where there were complex scalp

---

[63]Kempe L. Hemispherectomy, in Operative Neurosurgery. New York, Springer-Verlag. 1968.

lacerations incorporated in the scalp flap. For this reason, there has been a tendency amongst military neurosurgeons to favour the 'T' shaped scalp incision particularly when complex scalp lacerations were present.

The skull

Unilateral frontotemporoparietal DC.

The 4[th]Edition of the Brain Trauma Foundation guidelines recommend a frontotemporoparietal decompressive craniectomy in the civilian context be not less than 12cm by 15cm diameter.[64] Bell et al from their military experience recommend a hemi-craniectomy for frontotemporoparietal decompression at a minimum 14 cm anteroposterior by 12 cm supero-inferior dimensions.[65]

The surgeon should mark the midline and the line of the transverse sinus carefully so that the bone cuts avoid the venous sinuses. The posterior bone cut should be at least 2cm above the lambdoid suture. The craniotome is taken as low as it will go in the middle fossa, but it is important for the surgeon to remove the remaining squamous temporal bone and greater wing of the sphenoid down to the floor of the middle fossa using rongeurs. This will decompress the temporal lobe and upper brain stem. Air cells in the sphenoid or mastoid bone must be plugged with wax to avoid CSF leaks.

Bifrontal decompressive craniotomy

Burrholes are placed either side of the sagittal sinus as well as at the pterion and at the root of the zygoma just below the superior temporal line. The posterior edge of the bone cut can extend just behind the coronal suture and extend vertically downwards to decompress part the frontal and temporal lobes. The temporal bone is removed with rongeurs below the inferior cut as described above. A strip of bone can be left over the sagittal sinus to protect it. To avoid

---

[64]Carney N, Totten AM, O'Reilly C, Ullman JS, Hawryluk GW, Bell MJ, Bratton SL, Chesnut R, Harris OA, Kissoon N, Rubiano AM, Shutter L, Tasker RC, Vavilala MS, Wilberger J, Wright DW, Ghajar J. Guidelines for the Management of Severe Traumatic Brain Injury, Fourth Edition. Neurosurgery. 2016.
[65]Bell RS, Mossop CM, Dirks MS, Stephens FL, Mulligan L, Ecker R, Neal CJ, Kumar A, Tigno T, Armonda RA. Early decompressive craniectomy for severe penetrating and closed head injury during wartime. Neurosurgical Focus. 2010;28(5):E1.

entering the frontal sinus which creates further potential morbidity with CSF leaks and infection the lower bone cut can pass just above these air sinuses. This can be judged on the scout view of the CT scan or a plain radiograph if no CT is available. Cranialization of the frontal sinus will be required if the sinus is entered (see section on air sinus exposure on page 504).

Dura

The dura should be widely opened to optimize relief of intracranial hypertension and to allow for exposure and treatment of the hematomas/ penetrating injury. Be careful your scissors do not lacerate the swollen brain during this manoeuvre. **Unilateral Decompressive Craniectomy**. The dura is opened in a 'C' shape with multiple relieving spoke-wheel cuts. The dura is cut no closer than 2 cm from the superior sagittal sinus to avoid trauma to the sinus and bridging veins. Dural tack-up (hitching) sutures are used to avoid postoperative hematomas beneath the bone edge. **Bifrontal craniectomy.** The dura can be opened with cuts parallel to the sagittal sinus and the posterior bone margin or with a stellate opening. Some neurosurgeons have also divided the sagittal sinus inferiorly and released the falx. The basal dura needs to be repaired if it is lacerated. The use of a vascularized pericranial flap is preferred. This is also used to cover the cranialized frontal sinus. Tensor fascia lata can also be used. These grafts should be tacked down and can also be secured with tissue glue if available. Onlay graft material such as DuraGen may not be sufficient for the skull base repair.

Duroplasty with patches sewn in to create a water-tight closure and dural expansion would be ideal. However, in an emergency situation and to conform to the principles of damage control surgery, it is preferable that a dural substitute such as DuraGen[66] is laid over the dural openings. This does not require suturing. If this is not available sterile plastic sheeting can be laid over the dura and exposed brain and the scalp then closed in two layers so that it is watertight. This will allow the scalp to be lifted without the presence of adhesions to the cortex when it comes time for the cranioplasty.

---

[66]*Integra Life Sciences Corporation, Plainsboro, New Jersey, USA.*

Bone flap management

There are 3 options:

1. The bone is cleaned and washed as above and placed in a subcutaneous pocket in the left lower quadrant so the scar is not confused with an appendicectomy scar in the future.

2. The bone can be cleaned, then washed with bacitracin or gentamicin solution, placed in a sterile plastic bag and cryopreserved at -70 degrees C. This unlikely to be available in the developing countries.

3. In Afghanistan and Iraq because of the high levels of contamination of the bone encountered in the complex penetrating trauma and the high risk of sepsis if the bone was replaced at a later date, the practice has developed to discard the bone and repair the skull with CT-derived 3D printed prosthetic materials such a methyl methacrylate. Bell et al found just over half the military patients with severe CNS injury had concomitant systemic infections. The fluid collection around the abdominal bone implant could not be excluded as the source. The bone was discarded in almost all these cases.[67] The problem in the developing countries is that these printed prosthetic implants are not available. Hand-shaped titanium mesh or acrylic molds may be alternatives.

Principles of surgery for the blast injury

The surgery should be rapid but maintaining control. Large haematomas are evacuated. Devitalised tissue is then debrided. Superficial debridement and irrigation of brain wounds is carried out without overly aggressive searching for deep fragments of metal or bone. Hemostasis is completed. A parenchymal ICP monitor is placed and preferably a ventriculostomy so that CSF can be vented to help control ICP. The repair of facial injuries should follow abbreviated damage control principles with packing of facial wounds and limited fixation of facial fractures in the first operation.

---

[67]Bell RS, Vo AH, Neal CJ, Tigno J, Roberts R, Mossop C, Dunne JR, Armonda RA. Military traumatic brain and spinal column injury: a 5-year study of the impact blast and other military grade weaponry on the central nervous system. The Journal of Trauma. 2009;66(4):S104-111.

This can be pursued further during second and third stage surgery. ENT, ophthalmology and maxillofacial surgeons if available may also be required to manage these complex craniofacial injuries.

Intensive care management

The patient remains intubated and sedated in the ICU until the ICPs are normal and the brain swelling is subsiding. This may take 7 to 10 days. The head of the bed is elevated to help control ICP. The aim is for normal physiology to be restored as quickly as possible. Rewarming continues to normothermia. Abnormal acid/base, coagulation, electrolytes, hemoglobin are corrected. Early enteral feeding is commenced.

Early Complications

Rebleeding is not uncommon and is due to ongoing coagulopathy or failure to secure hemostasis at the first operation. This may be due to epidural, subdural or intracerebral hematoma. A rescan the day following surgery or earlier if there is clinical deterioration will pick this up. Wound ischemia breakdown may require wound revision and avoidance of pressure on this area of scalp. CSF leak from calvarial wounds should be prevented with dural patching and water-tight scalp closure in two layers. CSF leak is not uncommon with complex skull base fractures and dural tears. CSF leak increases the risk of early and late meningitis. Craniotomy revision may be required to repair the leak. Lumbar drainage may be required when brain swelling subsides to stop the CSF leak while the tissues are healing. Infection as a delayed complication and may require reoperation to drain subdural empyema or brain abscess. Hydrocephalus and syndrome of the trephine are delayed complications. Syndrome of the trephined or 'sinking skin flap syndrome' is a neurological deterioration due to atmospheric pressure affecting the brain which is not covered by the skull and is sunken in appearance. The best treatment is to replace the cranial bone flap and perform a cranioplasty.[68]

---

[68]Ashayeri K, Huang MJEJ, Brem, RGC. Syndrome of the Trephined: A Systematic Review.Neurosurgery. 2016;79(4):525-534.

Dural repair of the anterior cranial fossa

Indication

Persistent CSF leak from nose. The leak should persist for at least 2-3 weeks.

Procedure

The right thigh is prepared for the harvesting of fascia lata. The head is placed in a neutral position, resting on the horseshoe headrest. A bicoronal scalp incision is made just behind the hairline and the forehead scalp folded forwards. A bifrontal craniotomy is performed. The safest way for the inexperienced surgeon to do this is to raise a separate flap on each side with a strip of bone and the sagittal sinus and falx in the midline left intact. The inferior margin of the bone flap is close to the supraorbital margin. The dura is opened on each side and the frontal lobe elevated gently away from the floor of the anterior fossa. Inspect the floor of the anterior fossa medially and identify the olfactory bulb, sitting on the cribriform plate on each side just beside the crista galli.

On the traumatised side, a fracture will be noted on the floor of the anterior fossa extending often into the cribriform plate region and the olfactory bulb is atrophic, disrupted or avulsed. A small piece of temporalis muscle is crushed and placed in the cribriform plate region, covered with Surgicel, and then covered with the fascia lata graft. The falx attachment to the crista galli can be divided so that the graft can be placed across each side, if the fracture extends to the other side. It is best to try and preserve the olfactory bulb on the other side if it remains intact. Gelfoam is placed over the dural graft. If the frontal sinus is opened from the craniotomy then the pericranium should be folded down over it and sewn to the dural margin. The dura is closed watertight, the bone flaps replaced and the wound closed. So that there is less chance of the graft moving, do not use diuretics to shrink the brain. The patient should be kept lying in bed for 2 or 3 days, so that the graft has less chance of displacement.

Intracranial pressure monitoring

Indication

1. This will usually be done for severe head injury patients who cannot be monitored clinically or who will be ventilated, paralysed and sedated, especially if multiple injuries are present and a prolonged period of ventilation is to be anticipated.

2. Post-craniotomy for evacuation of acute extra-axial collection.

Strategy

Intracranial pressure cannot be monitored without breaching the skull. The simplest method of measuring the pressure is to place an infant into the subdural space or preferably a ventricular catheter into the frontal horn, then brought out through a separate stab incision and connected it to a pressure transducer, similar to that used to measure blood pressure, by filling the infant feeding tube or ventricular catheter with fluid.

The advantage of this technique is that CSF can be vented to help reduce the intracranial pressure. The disadvantage is the increased infection rate if the tube is left in for more than 48 hours. There is no clear evidence that prophylactic antibiotics would reduce the risk of this infection. The CSF should be cultured regularly to make sure no infection is developing when this technique is used. (It is difficult to pass an infant feeding tube into the ventricle without some rigidity to it).

Alternative methods of measuring ICP are:

1. Place a catheter in the subdural space; but the disadvantage of this is that when the brain is very swollen and tight the catheter readily becomes occluded.

2. Epidural transducers, which are prone to inaccuracy due to damping.

3. The Richmond bolt method, where a hollow metal bolt is screwed into the burr hole to allow fluid communication between the

subdural space and the pressure transducer via a tube, is also prone to inaccuracy due to damping and is not recommended.

4. Small pressure transducer on the end of a thin flexible wire placed 2-3 cm into the brain parenchyma (Codman). A lesser used alternative is the fibre-optic pressure transducer which is a more rigid catheter which is also placed directly in the brain parenchyma (Camino catheter). These newer devices are significantly more expensive and are usually not available in the developing world. The simpler fluid-filled systems are quite satisfactory.

Interpreting the result

The normal intracranial pressure is 0-10 mmHg. It is abnormal over 15 mmHg. Once the brain becomes tense and turgid, brain compliance is reduced and pressure waves may appear. Plateau waves are the most dangerous (ICP elevations 50 mmHg for 5-20 minutes) and urgent treatment is required. There is usually a simultaneous rise in mean arterial pressure. B waves have amplitudes of 20-30 mm and occur rhythmically every 30 sec to 2 min. These require treatment and will progress to plateau waves if untreated. C waves are low amplitude 4-8 Hz of little clinical significance. A sustained pressure above 22 mmHg for more than 2 min warrants urgent treatment (see Chapter 3, page 132).

Technique

1. **Subdural catheter**. The infant feeding tube can be placed in the subdural space following evacuation of a collection and this is then brought out through a separate stab incision in the scalp. If there has been no craniotomy, a burr hole is placed usually in the right frontal region above the hairline several centimetres away from the midline. The dura is opened with a cruciate incision. The catheter is passed through a stab incision beside the incision then gently over the cortical surface, filled with Ringer's or saline solution.

2. **Ventricular catheter**. A burr hole is placed in the line of the pupil just behind the hairline usually on the right side. The dura is opened with a cruciate incision. The catheter with stillette is aimed perpendicularly in the direction of the inner canthus of the eye on the same side. You will often feel a release in resistance

when the catheter passes through the ependyma into the CSF at about 5·6 cm from the cortical surface. The stillette is then removed and CSF will escape.

- Confirm that CSF is escaping adequately and then tunnel the catheter and bring it out through a separate stab incision. Anchor it to the scalp and close the scalp in two layers.
- Commercially available ventricular catheters are used in advanced centres. These are supplied with a metal stilette. These catheters are often unavailable in the developing countries because of cost.

Troubleshooting

1. If the catheter becomes blocked with a small amount of debris or clot, it can be syringed with 1·2 ml of saline, which should then be gently extracted until resistance occurs.
2. If ventriculitis develops (increasing white cell counts in the CSF) and the ICP monitor can be removed, place 5 mg gentamicin into the CSF and remove the catheter. The patient will need systemic antibiotics for 7 days, including initially Gram positive and negative cover until sensitivities are back, e.g. gentamicin and flucloxacillin or vancomycin, if staphylococcal resistance is a problem. If the catheter needs to remain in situ, treat the CSF with daily gentamicin and systemic antibiotics. If the ventriculitis starts to clear in 48 hours remove the catheter and re·site a new catheter on the opposite side.

Closure of scalp defects

Scalp defects that overlie chronic trauma are best closed with a rotation flap. Waiting for the wound to granulate usually fails, especially if there is bard bone without pericranium. Even if pericranium is intact the wound may never heal properly by second intention, i.e. granulation. The wound is extended in a generous curve, bearing in mind the blood supply of the flap. This new large flap is lifted from the pericranium and rotated forwards to fill the defect. The posterior defect resulting is covered with split skin at the time, and a firm dressing applied. The wound is debrided anteriorly and the flap moved into position to close the defect and the edge closed primarily, in two layers (Figure 11.6, next page).

Common operations

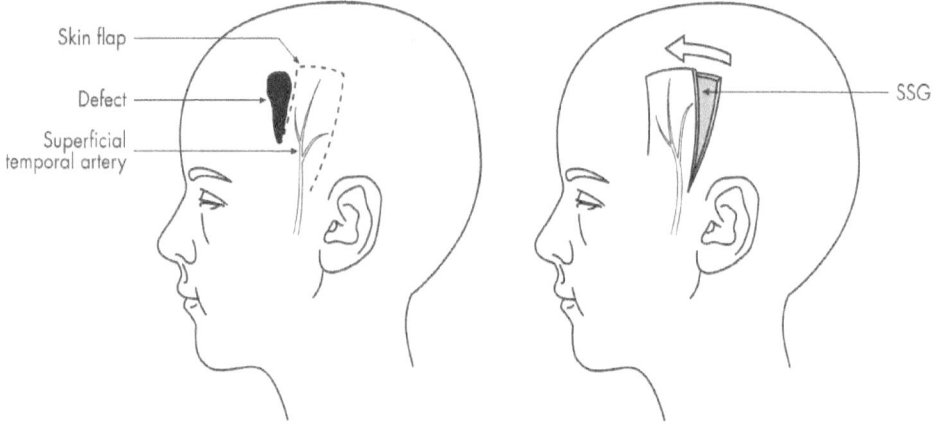

Closure of scalp defects using scalp flaps

Figure 11.6 (a) Temporal defect.

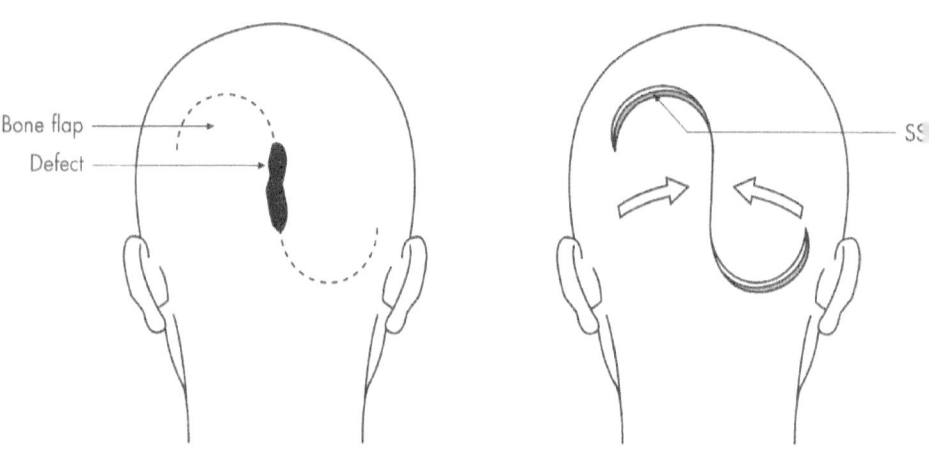

(b) Occipital defect.

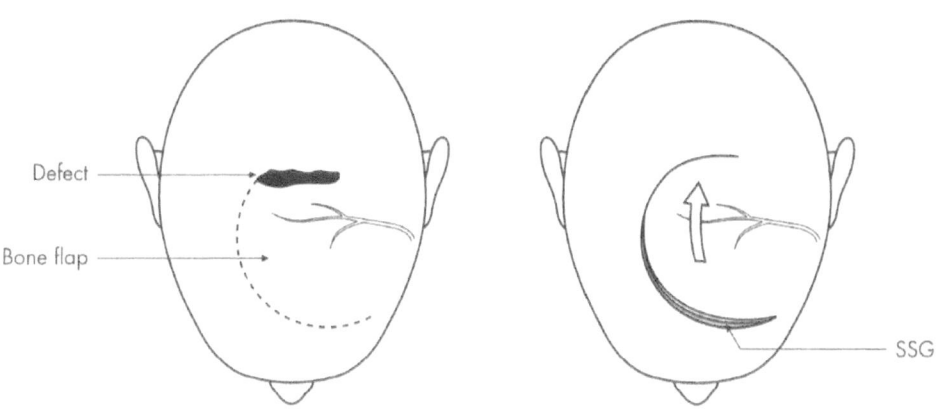

(c) Vertex defect.

Figure 11.6 (a-c) Closure of scalp defects using scalp flaps. The flaps are based on major scalp arteries. The scalp defects created by the movement of the flaps are closed with split skin grafts.

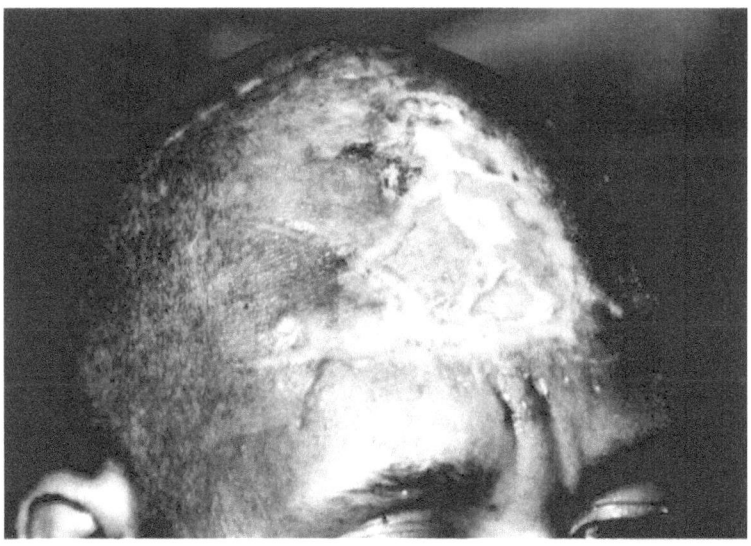

(d) i The defect.

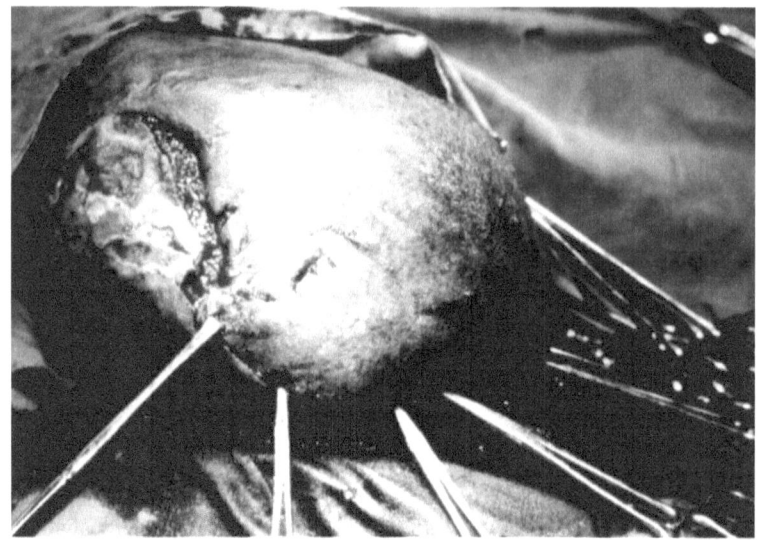

(d) ii Debridement of the defect, and fashioning a large scalp flap.

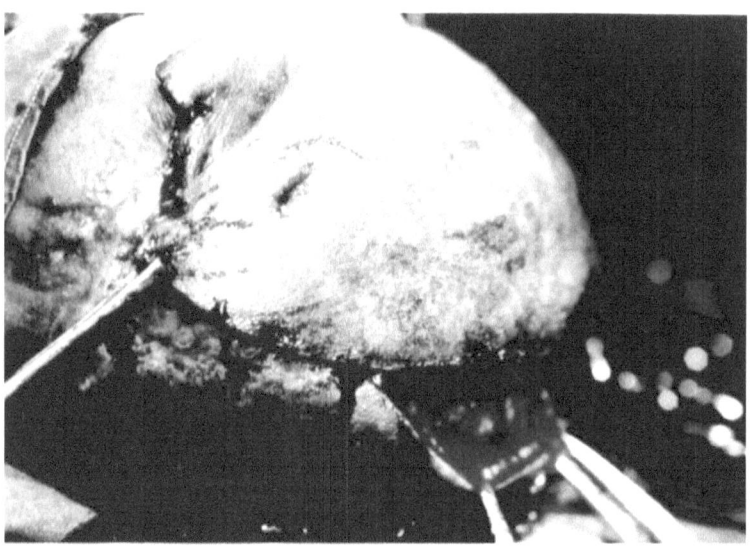

(d) iii Rotation of the flap to cover the defect.

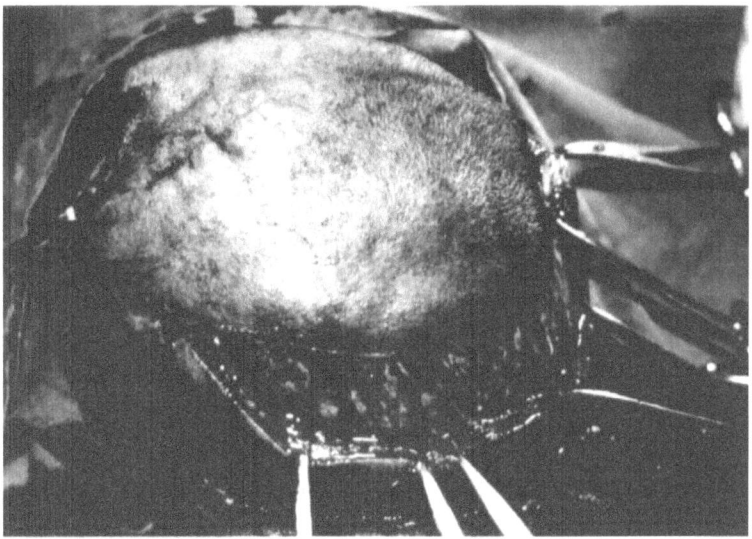

(d) iv The new posterior defect created by the rotation.

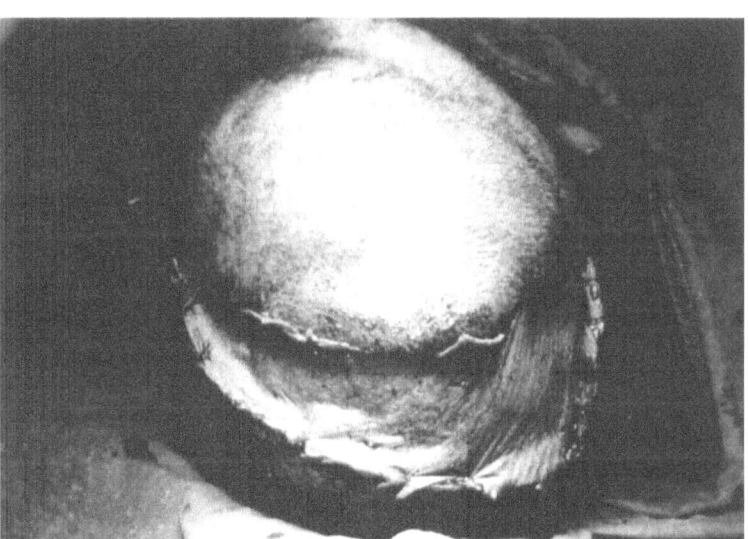

(d) v Closure of the posterior defect using a split skin graft.

Figure 11.6 (a-d) Closure of scalp defects using scalp flaps. The flaps are based on major scalp arteries. The scalp defects created by the movement of the flaps are closed with split skin grafts.

The technique of drilling holes in the outer table to expose cancellous bone and allow granulations to grow up through the holes and cover the bone surface, is limited. It takes a considerable time to form granulations and then would require skin grafting after this, leaving a poor cosmetic result in an exposed area albeit protecting the cranium (see Figure 11.7, below).

A more serious complication is the development of chronic infection in the bone before the granulations have grown over it with the possibility of intracranial extension. However, where the skill to rotate a scalp flap over the defect, or to excise a dead outer table of the skull is not available, and where blood transfusion is in short supply this is at least a temporising option to save the bone and get the wound to heal.

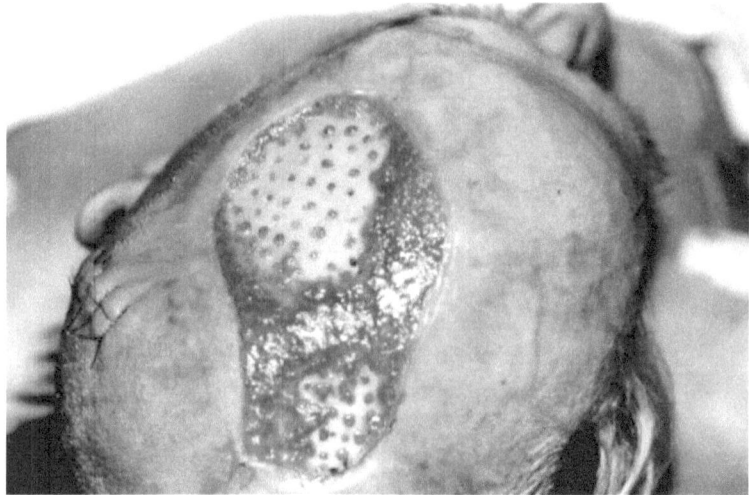

Figure 11.7 Multiple drill holes placed in outer table to create granulation tissue and allow closure of scalp defect. This operation produced epidural abscess and meningitis and did not lead to the closure of the defect. A rotation flap was still required once the infection had been treated.

Repair of cranial defects - cranioplasty

Where there has been a loss of skull bone either through infection, trauma or neoplasm, elective restoration of the defect may be indicated. Young children (less than 2 years of age) have a propensity to form new bone in from the edges of skull defects and from the osteoblastic potential of the dura. Sizeable defects may heal spontaneously. However, adults have a low propensity to heal discrete defects. The best material to use is the patient's own autologous bone, either from a rib which can be split in half and into narrow strips which can be wired or sutured in position, through small drill holes at either end. Alternatively, adjacent skull bone can be used. This is cut to the shape of the defect and transversely split into two, and each half is laid into each defect and fixed in position. This is called a **split skull cranioplasty.**

An alternative to using bone is acrylic (methyl methacrylate) which is mixed from a powder and liquid into a soft paste, which hardens over approximately 10 minutes. It is moulded into the shape of the defect on a base of plastic sheeting when semi-solid. The solidification is exothermic and generates a lot of heat, so it is advisable to remove it when semi-solid and getting hot, to avoid heat damage to the underlying tissues. When solidified, it can then be pared down to size and anchored into position with multiple sutures or fine stainless-steel wire. In better resourced settings, mini-plates and screws will be available to anchor the bone or acrylic in position. When performing the operation, the bone edge of the defect should be defined by stripping away the muscle and pericranium from the edge and dissecting the dura away from the inner table, so that sutures can be placed through drill holes to hold the graft. Any dural tear should be repaired at the time.

CONGENITAL MALFORMATIONS

The pathology and clinical management of hydrocephalus, encephaloceles and myelomeningoceles are discussed in Chapter 4.

Ventriculoperitoneal shunt (Figure 11.8, page 548)

The indication for insertion of a ventriculoperitoneal shunt is symptomatic or progressive hydrocephalus.

Strategy

The aim should be to place the tip of the ventricular catheter within the frontal horn anterior to the foramen of Munro so that the perforations avoid the choroid plexus. The catheter must be passed along the long axis of the lateral ventricle. A low-pressure valve is used in infants. For patients with very large ventricles, e.g. aqueduct stenosis, a high-pressure valve is used to prevent collapse of the brain mantle and chronic subdural collections, and for all other cases a medium-pressure valve is used. Great care should be taken to reduce the risk of infection.

The basic principle is that a low-pressure valve results in higher flow and high-pressure valve results in lower flow. Try and touch the shunt as little as possible (use instruments to hold it), try and open the packaging just before it is needed, give a dose of perioperative antibiotic, minimise operative time, try and do the case first in the morning before the theatre becomes contaminated, minimise the number of personnel in the operating room and try not to let the device touch the skin, i.e. cover the skin with gauze.

Position

The position of the patient is very important to ensure ease of insertion of the device. The head is turned into a lateral position resting on a horseshoe headrest or a sponge or doughnut ring at the end of the table. A towel is placed beneath the shoulders so that the neck is extended. The head of the table is elevated 10°. There should be a smooth line between the head, along the neck to the anterior chest wall so that the tunneller is not passing towards the underside of the clavicle. The approximate length of catheter required to reach just in front of the coronal suture line is measured on the head. It usually measures approximately 8 cm in an infant, and 10-12 cm for an adult. This should place the tip in the frontal horn of the lateral ventricle on the side of the burr hole.

Scalp incision

Figure 11.8 (a) Scalp incision.

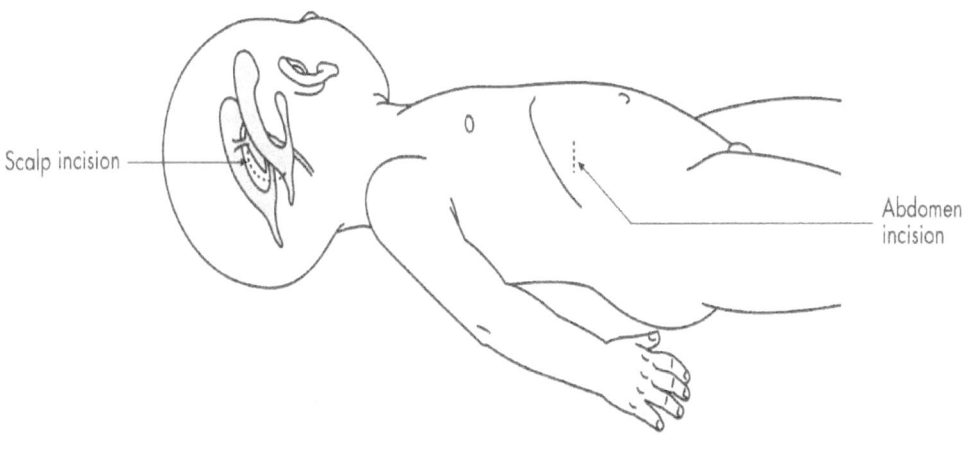

Scalp incision

Abdomen
incision

(b) Operative position showing orientation of ventricles to scalp incision and the
site of a right upper quadrant abdominal incision.

Common operations

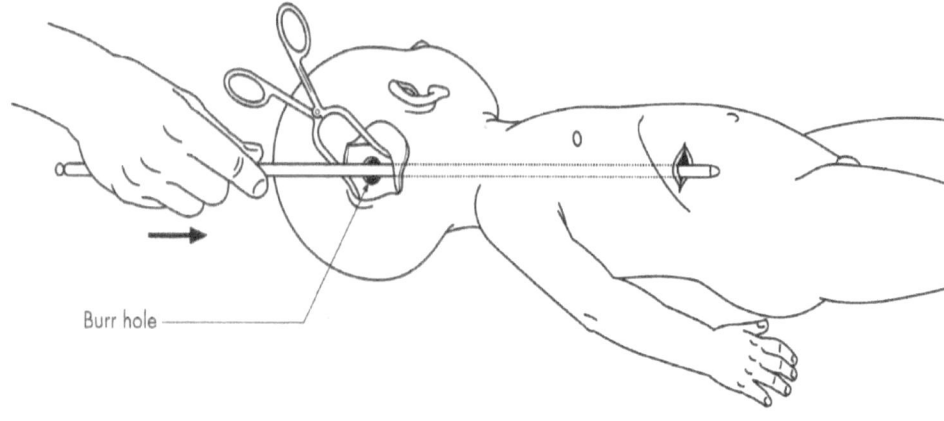

Burr hole

(c) Passing of the tunneller from the cranial to the abdominal wound.

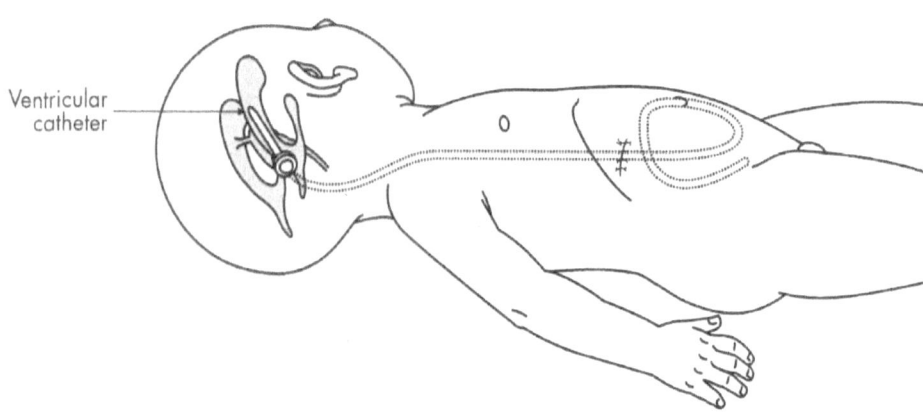

Ventricular catheter

(d) Final placement of shunt components.

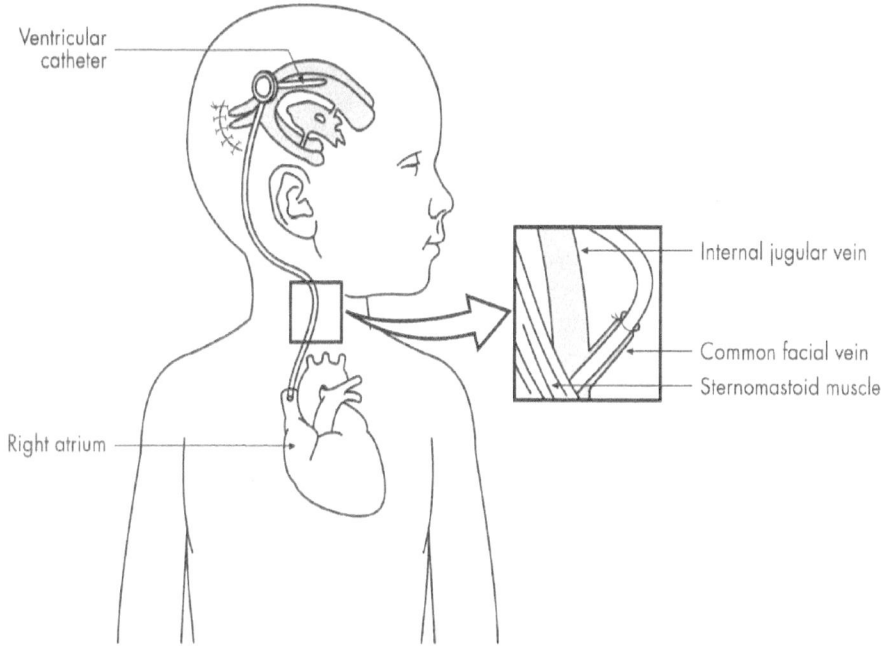

(e) Placement of a ventriculoatrial shunt with the atrial catheter entering the venous system via the common facial vein in the neck.

Figure 11.8 (a-e) Placement of ventriculoperitoneal shunt.

Procedure

The skin incision for an **infant** should be a semicircular generous scalp flap several times bigger than the valve, so that the scalp is not stretched unduly, and the edge of the valve is not placed directly beneath the skin incision. A similar incision, but smaller, with an arm extending inferiorly and posteriorly, i.e. reverse hockey stick incision, is appropriate for an **older child or adult**. A common mistake is to make the incision too low, close to the transverse sinus.

It should be made approximately 3 cm above the centre of the pinna and 4 cm behind the top edge of the pinna in the parieto-occipital region, usually on the right side. In the infant head, it can be placed even more posteriorly, so that a more direct line with the ventricle is achieved. A burr hole is inserted and at this point, before opening the dura, the abdominal incision is made. In infants, this is best made as an upper epigastric small midline incision directly through the linea alba, but in adults this is more difficult particularly if there is a lot of fat in the falciform ligament. It may be preferable in this case, to make a right upper quadrant incision splitting the rectus abdominis vertically. A tunneller is then passed between the two wounds. Disposable tunnellers usually come with the shunt set, and the peritoneal catheter is passed between the two wounds, and the tunneller removed. Make sure that the abdominal incision has actually entered the peritoneal cavity particularly from a midline approach. It is easy to mistake the extra-peritoneal fatty tissue for the peritoneal cavity. The slit valve at the end of the peritoneal catheter is opened and Ringer's fluid syringed through the peritoneal catheter to prove its patency.

Wrap up the lower end in an abdominal pack until the upper end is inserted and the shunt is tested. It is easier for the valve to be connected to the peritoneal catheter before connecting it to the ventricular catheter. The dura is opened with a small central cruciate incision just enough to place the catheter through. If it is a large incision, then CSF leak around the valve can be a problem, producing a scalp collection of CSF The ventricular catheter is passed with the stillette, initially slightly forwards of the perpendicular to enter the trigone (central) region of the lateral ventricle.

It is aimed towards the inner canthus of the opposite eye. A button stuck to the forehead can be felt through the drapes, and will indicate to the surgeon where the midline is located. Once the catheter has entered the ventricle, it should be angled more forwards and the stillette removed so that it passes along the axis of the ventricle and enters the frontal horn. 0bserve the flow of CSF. There should be a substantial flow of clear CSF. If it only drips out, it is not properly sited. Once the catheter is well placed in the ventricle, withdraw it 2 cm, then shorten the catheter to be 1 cm less than the length required to achieve the optimal position in the ventricle to allow for the valve length, then attach the ventricular catheter to the valve, secure the with a ligature of non-absorbable suture such as Prolene or silk. The valve is anchored to the pericranium, either over the burr hole if it is a Pudenz type flushing valve, or on the adjacent pericranium away from the burr hole if it is a Hakim type valve.

Test the valve patency and the flow of CSF by pumping the valve and observing the spontaneous flow from the lower end and the flow augmented with pumping. The catheter distal to the valve can be compressed and having emptied the valve, the valve should then refill if it is sited correctly. The peritoneal catheter is then placed in the peritoneal cavity passing down towards the pelvis.

It is anchored loosely to the peritoneum with a purse string absorbable suture, such as Vicryl or Dexon and then the rectus is closed in layers in the usual way, being careful not to tighten the suture around the catheter and kink it or block it. The upper end is closed in the usual layers and the patient should awaken readily.

Third ventriculostomy (Figure 11.9, next page)

The indications for this procedure are discussed in Chapter 4. The endoscope should be no greater than 4·6 mm in external diameter including working and irrigation channels. The irrigation fluid entering the ventricular system should be drained out the endoscope so that intracranial pressure does not rise. The availability of a camera and video system for the endoscope is essential. The procedure is performed under general anaesthesia. A burr hole is placed 4 cm lateral to the midline just anterior to the coronal suture and the dura opened with a cruciate incision.

The dural edges are diathermied and an incision made in the pia. The endoscope outer sheath with a smooth ended trochar is passed in a perpendicular direction into the lateral ventricle and the trochar removed. The CSF will often gush out. This trajectory will align the endoscope with the foramen of Munro and the third ventricular floor. The endoscope is then inserted through the outer sheath and the endoscope passed through the foramen of Munro into the third ventricle.

The two safest methods of perforation of the floor of the third ventricle are:

1. Placing a small pilot opening in the floor, using the grasping forceps, then enlarging the opening using a size 3 Fogarty balloon catheter (we prefer this method).

2. Passing the blunt tip of the endoscope directly through the floor with the angled edge of the endoscope placed anteriorly.

Bipolar diathermy, if available, can also be helpful with the opening. The opening is made in the midline where the floor of the ventricle is usually translucent between the mammillary bodies posteriorly, and the infundibular recess anteriorly. The basilar artery and its branches usually lie just in front of the mammillary bodies and can be seen through the floor.

Common operations

The opening in the floor must be made anterior to these blood vessels. Any bleeding is best handled by continuous irrigation of Ringer's solution or saline until it stops. Stenosis may develop if the opening is smaller than 4 mm. Beware of angling the endoscope too far in the sagittal plane as this may damage the structures at the foramen of Munro.

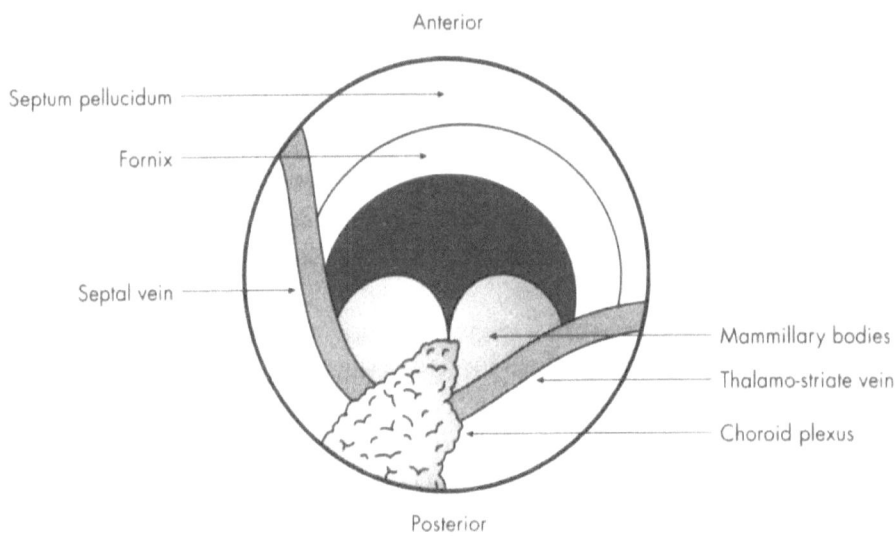

Figure 11.9 (a) Endoscopic view of the right foramen of Monro.

Anterior

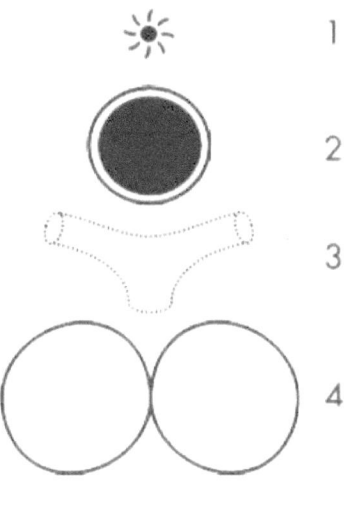

1

2

3

4

Posterior

Floor of 3rd ventricle

(b) Endoscopic view of the floor of the third ventricle.

Legend
1. Infundibular recess (the pituitary stalk lies below this point)
2. Completed opening in the floor of the third ventricle
3. Outline of subjacent basilar and posterior cerebral arteries
4. Mammillary bodies

Figure 11.9 (a-b) Placement of third ventriculostomy.

Encephalocele repair

Frontal encephalocele

Frontoethmoidal encephalocele

These can be repaired via a direct approach and the procedure is somewhat akin to an inguinal hernia repair in that the sac is isolated, plicated, and the roof over the hernia, in this case the nasal bridge is repaired with a bone or cartilage graft to close the bony defect.

A transverse incision is made, and the sac is defined from the surrounding tissue using sharp dissection. The sac is opened and the contents reduced. The sac is then plicated so that the hernia is eliminated. Usually the neck is too wide to close it with a ligature and plication is preferable. Nonabsorbable suture such as Prolene should be used for this.

Any non-viable tissue can be excised, although this is not usually present in a frontal encephalocele. To reconstruct the nasal bridge a piece of cartilage can be taken from a rib and fashioned to the shape of the nasal bridge and anchored into position with small wire sutures passed through fine drill holes in the bone. The wound is then closed in layers. This method has a higher recurrence rate than the transcranial repair which is described in the next section.

Frontonasal encephalocele

These are best repaired with a craniotomy because of the long neck which cannot be easily approached through the transfacial route. A bicoronal craniofacial approach is used by rotating the entire forehead scalp forwards, a bifrontal craniotomy is performed, raising a central flap which is taken low down on the forehead to just above the supraorbital ridge on each side, thus giving a good exposure to the floor of the anterior fossa. In these patients, there is a steep funnel-shaped floor through which the hernia passes at the apex of the cone. The dura is separated from the bone around the edge of the neck, and finally the neck is opened and the contents reduced. Usually, the contents will require excision as they are non-functional or non-viable and cannot be reduced intact. It may be preferable to transect the neck here and leave the solid tissue inferiorly to prevent any CSF leak. The dura is closed if possible, with non-absorbable suture, although it may be difficult to get a watertight closure particularly as the dura may still be stuck posteriorly to the bone edge. This is all the more reason to leave some hernial tissue below the transection. A bony disc is raised from the posterior cranial edge and impacted into the bony defect to prevent any recurrence. The craniotomy is then closed in the usual way. An extradural drain may be necessary if there is a large dead space.

Occipital encephalocele

The occipital encephalocele may be large and contain both CSF and cerebral hernia. It is important to try and reduce as much of the brain as possible, preferably all of it. Any non-viable tissue is resected. An elliptical incision is made over the hernial sac. The sac is opened and any meningocele thus emptied. The sac is separated from the surrounding tissues with sharp dissection and the neck defined. The hernia is reduced. This may require some bony removal on each side. The neck is then ligated or plicated in a similar way to the frontal encephalocele and usually the bony defect is too large to close at this stage. The scalp is then closed in layers. A secondary cranioplasty may be required at a later date. This can be achieved using rib graft or acrylic, if available.

Repair of myelomeningocele (Figure 11.10, next page)

Indication

In the developing world where severe physical disability is very difficult to manage, if not impossible, it is reasonable to take a conservative approach to the high open myelomeningocele lesions in the thoracic or cervical region. These are all associated with total paraplegia and double incontinence. The upper lumbar spine open myelomeningocele may also have a similar effect, but the low to middle lumbar lesions are associated with a better prognosis, in terms of ambulation and other complications.

A selective policy of repair was described by Lorber in Sheffield in the 1960s but would now be controversial in many countries, particularly those providing more support for the disabled. Some authorities recommend repair of all lesions and then face the consequent management of the disabled child. Other congenital anomalies need to be considered.

Common operations

The conservative approach involves shared decision making with the family, maintaining hydration, using sedation (e.g. barbiturate) to treat any distress, and letting nature take its course.

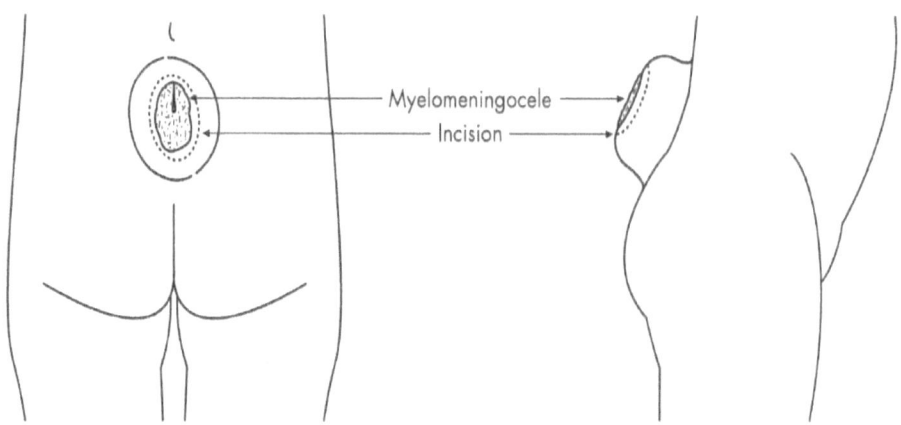

Figure 11.10 (a) i Line of the skin incision at the edge of the placode.

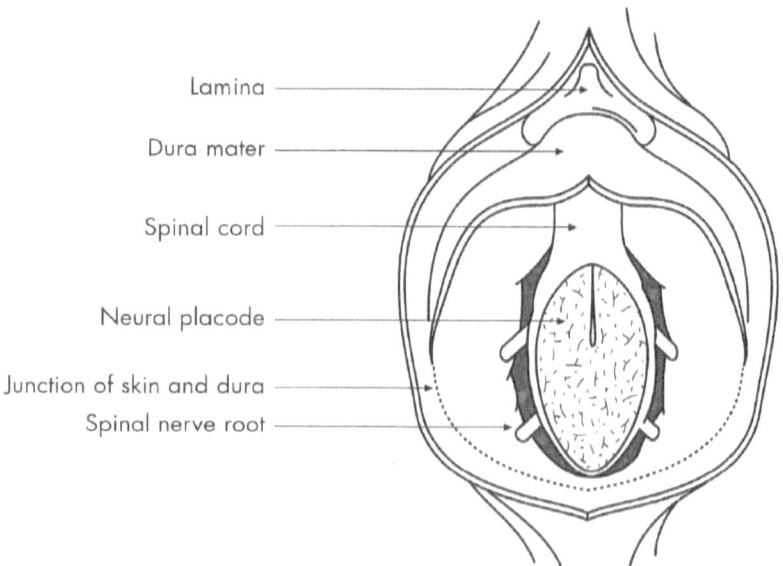

Lamina

Dura mater

Spinal cord

Neural placode

Junction of skin and dura

Spinal nerve root

(a) ii Dissection of the dura.

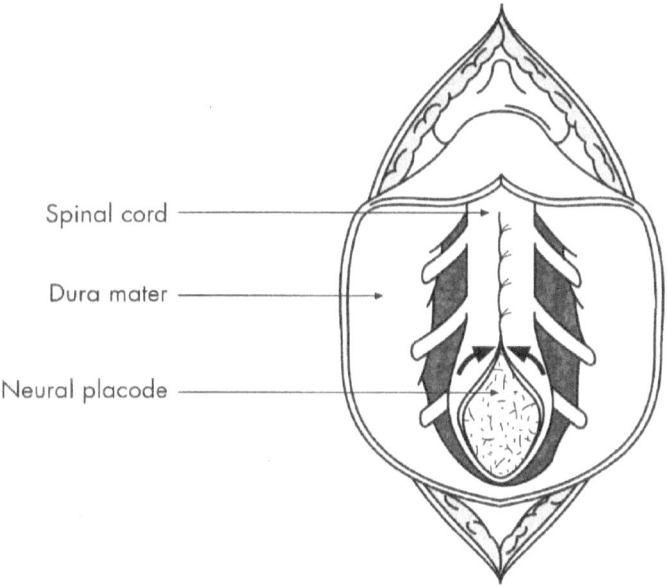

Spinal cord

Dura mater

Neural placode

(a) iii Closure of the placode to create a 'neural tube'.

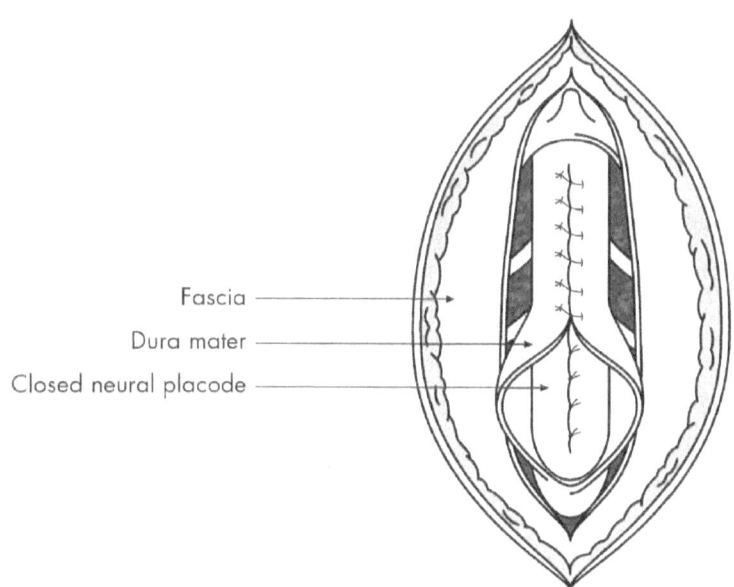

Fascia

Dura mater

Closed neural placode

(a) iv Closure of the dura.

Common operations

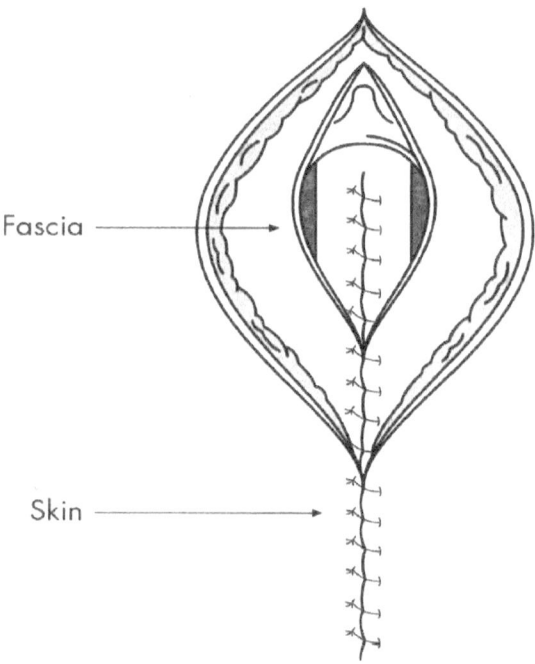

Fascia

Skin

(a) v Closure of the deep fascia and skin.

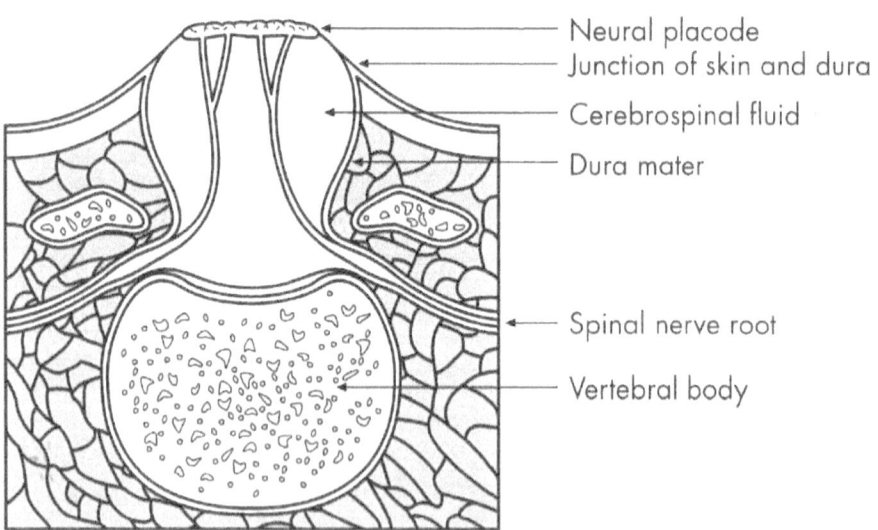

Neural placode
Junction of skin and dura
Cerebrospinal fluid
Dura mater

Spinal nerve root

Vertebral body

(b) i Pre-repair.

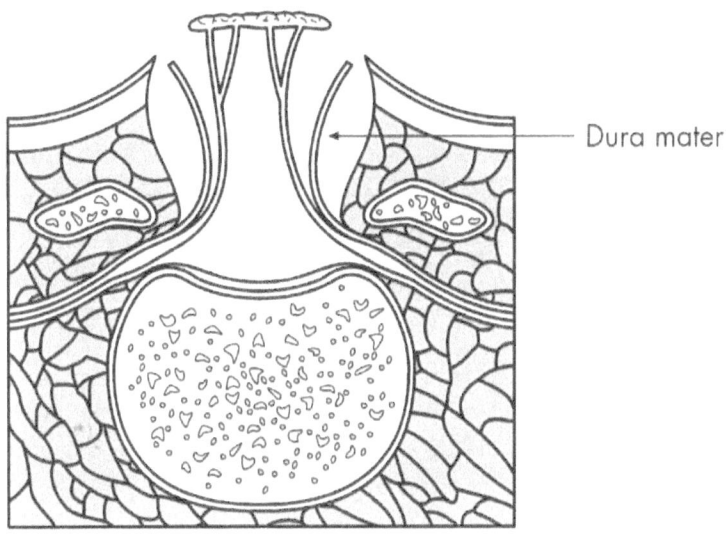

(b) ii Separation of the placode and dissection of the dura.

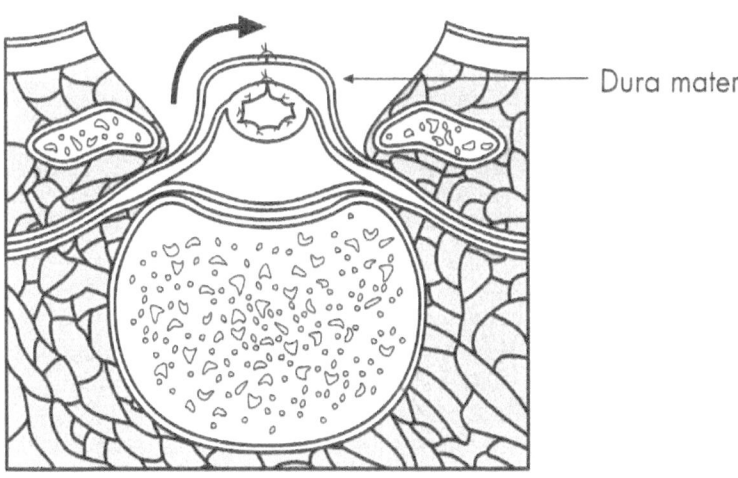

(b) iii Closure of the placode, closure of the dura.

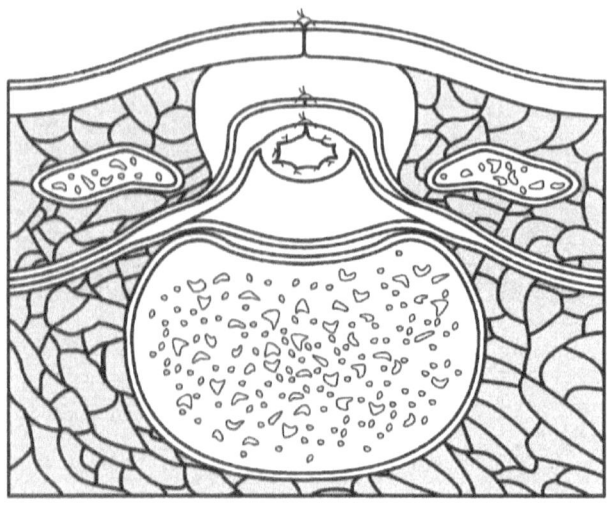

(b) iv Closure of the deep fascia and skin.

(b) i-iv Coronal view of the stages of myelomeningocele repair.

Figure 11.10 (a-b) Myelomeningocele repair.

For those lesions selected for repair, the recommendation is that the open myelomeningocele be repaired in the first 24 hours of life. It is important to examine the child, particularly in relation to the function of the lower limbs and determine what the motor and sensory levels are. A gentle prick of the skin with a blunted needle will allow determination of the sensory level (starting distally and moving proximally) by noting the movement of the limbs and the facial expression. Spinal reflexes involving withdrawal leg movements may be obtained with skin stimulation below the lesion level, but skin stimulation above the level of the lesion, if it is complete, will not produce any lower limb movement.

A lesion with a motor level clinically above L3·4 should be considered a high lesion. The motor level can be checked by looking at which muscle groups are wasted and watching the movements of the legs spontaneously and on pain stimulation with a gentle prick.

The assessment of the sphincter function is difficult in a neonate, but the continuous dribbling of urine indicates a neurogenic bladder and a patulous incontinent anus usually indicates sacral root involvement. The child may already have an enlarged head indicating hydrocephalus, and a careful search for other congenital abnormalities should be made, especially the heart and kidneys. An ultrasound will determine whether the kidneys are present. Other serious congenital anomalies will further strengthen the argument for conservative management in a neonate with a high lesion.

A neonate with L5-S1 involvement may just require supportive orthotic braces to walk satisfactorily. However, once the extensors of the knees are affected (L3-4) then ambulation may become more difficult as the child gets older and heavier, and eventually the adolescent may end up requiring a wheelchair.

A closed myelomeningocele does not need to be repaired urgently. The technique of closure is the same as for the open lesion, but the spinal cord is usually structurally intact in these cases. The recommended management for the hydrocephalus is to insert the shunt 2-3 days following the closure of the myelomeningocele. This allows time for enough wound healing to reduce the risk of shunt infection. Insertion of the shunt at the same time as the repair, increases the risk of shunt infection.

Operative strategy

The aim is to close the open neural tube, create a new watertight dural envelope for the spinal cord and nerve roots, and then to mobilise skin and subcutaneous fat to close over the dural defect. The nerve roots passing ventrally from the placode (the exposed flattened plate-shaped neural tissue of the spinal cord) should all be preserved. Any aberrant nerve roots passing dorsally to the edge of the defect can be sacrificed if necessary, to enable closure.

Operative method

The baby is placed under general anaesthesia and intubated, prone on the operating table, with the chest and pelvis elevated on sponge supports and the other pressure points attended to. This leaves the abdomen relatively free in order to reduce venous bleeding. The head is turned to the side and rested on a sponge support. Care is taken to prevent heat loss by providing an overhead strip heater if possible. If this is not available, the baby should not be exposed for prolonged periods.

The placode is circumnavigated with the scalpel, just inside the cutaneous margin so that no skin remains on the placode when it is buried. This will prevent any late epidermoid formation. Bipolar coagulation should be used to achieve haemostasis in this region, particularly on the placode. The placode can be turned in on itself to recreate the neural tube, and fixed in place with fine Prolene sutures through the outer pial layer. The dural sac is then refashioned by making a lateral incision on each side of the placode through the dura, which is then rotated over the placode. This incision will need to be taken superiorly above the placode to enable the placode to be buried entirely within the dural tube. This is sealed with fine Prolene. Any aberrant dorsal rootlets are divided. The ventral rootlets are spared. A partial single level laminectomy may permit more access to the upper end of the dura. The skin and soft tissues are then closed in two layers with Vicryl and nylon, aiming for a watertight closure. The skin flaps can be undermined at a subfascial level to lessen the tension. In rare cases, where the defect is large, bilateral skin flaps must be raised to close the defect. However, in the developing world setting this will not be necessary because a very large defect is usually a high lesion and in most cases the child will be managed conservatively.

It does not matter whether the wound is closed transversely or vertically; it depends on the shape of the ovoid wound and whichever closure creates the least tension. The wound should be kept covered and a plastic sheet placed over the dressing with an adhesive edge or taped on the inferior aspect to prevent faeces and meconium from getting onto the wound. The baby is nursed prone for several days after the operation, until the wound looks healthy and dry.

Avoidance of complications

1. Only excise as much skin as necessary to debride very thin or necrotic tissue otherwise it may be much more difficult to close the wound. This also applies to the closed myelomeningocele where excess skin can be excised at the time of wound closure, to create a wound without tension.
2. Be careful about achieving watertight wound closure to avoid CSF fistulas.

Repair of lipomyelomeningocele (Figure 11.11, next page)

Indication

These lesions present as a fatty subcutaneous lump in the lumbar or lumbosacral region. Their outer appearance belies the seriousness of their deep extent, as they may penetrate the dura and be intimately attached to the spinal cord, thus tethering it.

This may lead to delayed neurological deficit if the spinal cord and its nerves are anatomically intact. The delayed deficit may manifest as back pain, lower limb pain, limping, and gradual leg weakness which may manifest as unilateral or bilateral regression in walking ability and tolerance, and finally urinary and bowel sphincter disturbance. On examination, there may be walking on the toes, prominent pes cavus, spasticity, muscle wasting, weakness or sensory deficit. If the spinal cord and/or spinal nerves are malformed *in utero*, the child will be born with muscle wasting and abnormal posturing of the leg(s).

There is controversy in the neurosurgical literature about whether these lesions should be repaired prophylactically, as the neurological state, particularly sphincter function, may be worsened following the surgery. There is a greater likelihood of worsening if the lipoma is attached to the central or ventral aspect of the spinal cord through which the nerve roots pass. Preoperative investigation with MRI is advisable in the ideal circumstance. Preferably, the child should be reviewed by a neurosurgeon, because the repair of these lesions is technically challenging and difficult. However, if no neurosurgeon is available and neurological deterioration is occurring, then it may be appropriate for an experienced general surgeon to at least detether the cord.

Common operations

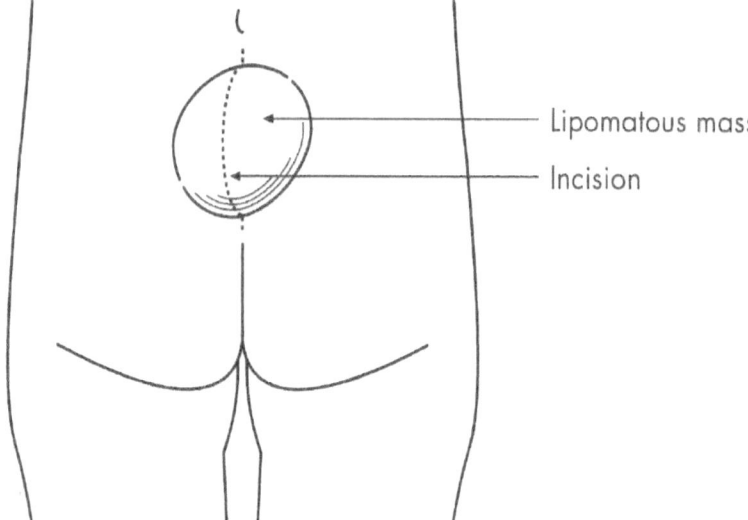

- Lipomatous mass
- Incision

Figure 11.11 (a) Incision line.

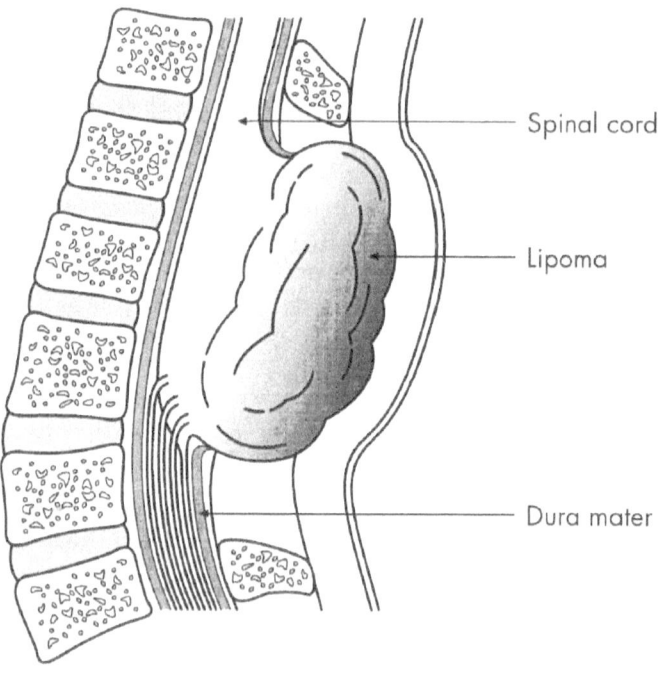

- Spinal cord
- Lipoma
- Dura mater

(b) Sagittal view of the lipomyelomeningocele attached to lower spinal cord, with dura fused to the lesion.

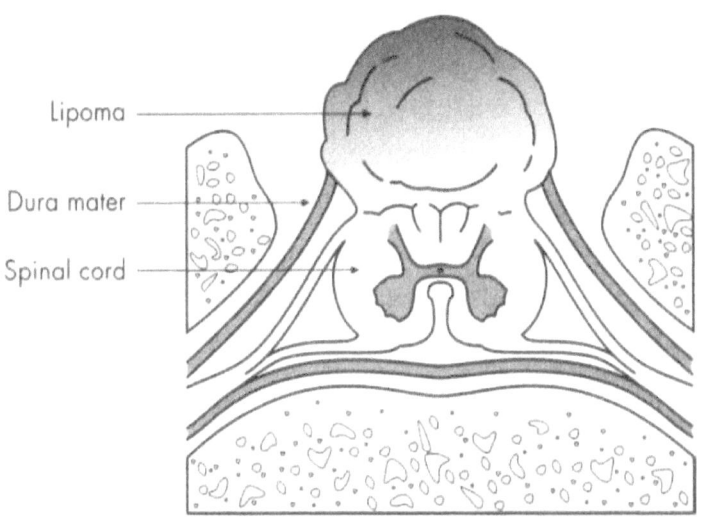

Lipoma

Dura mater

Spinal cord

(c) Coronal view of the lipomyelomeningocele before excision.

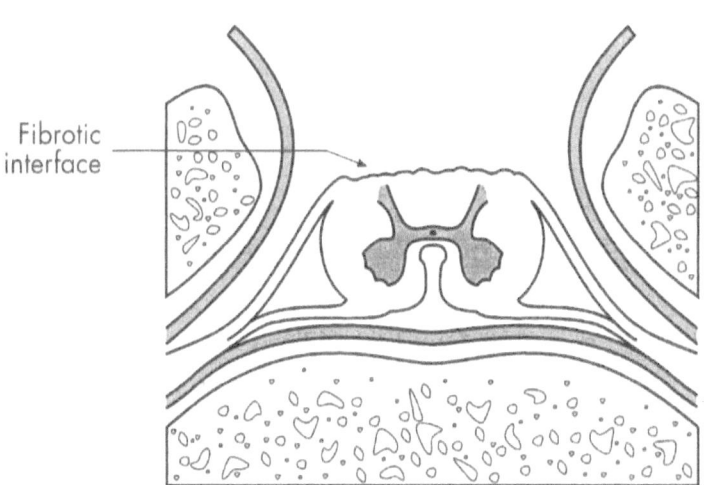

Fibrotic
interface

(d) Coronal view showing excision of the lesion with dorsal aspect of the spinal cord exposed. The dura is ready to close.

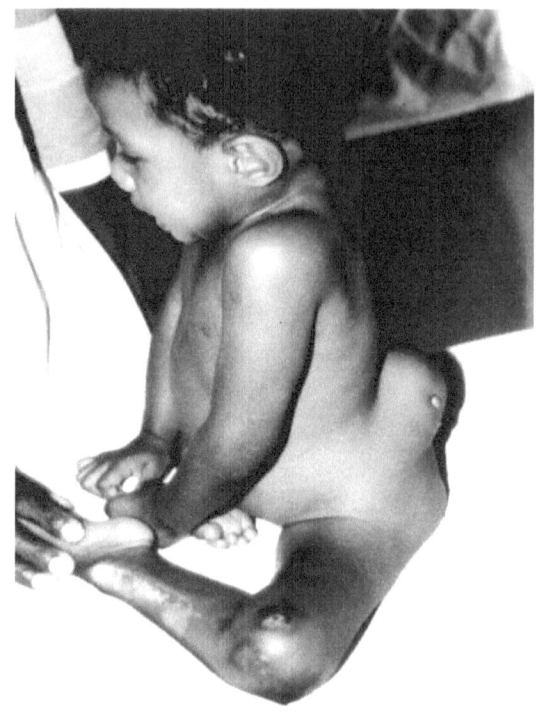

(e) i

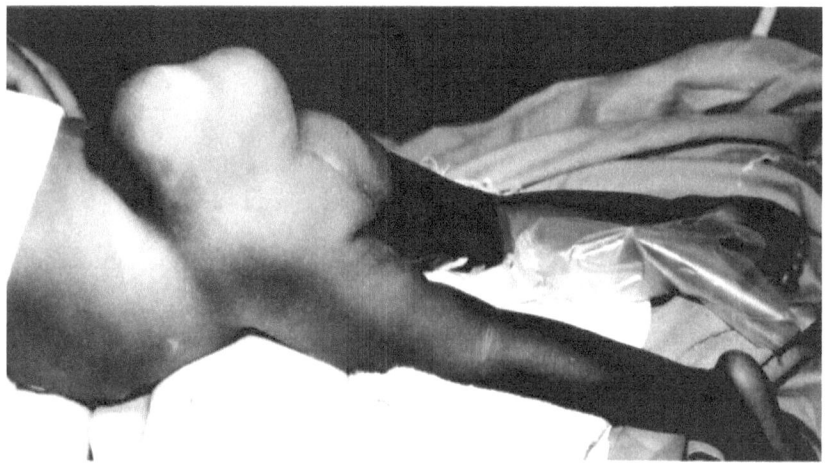

(e) ii

(e) i-ii Two children with untreated lipomyelomeningoceles. Both have severe neurological deficit in the lower limbs.

Figure 11.11 (a-e) Lipomyelomeningocele.

Strategy of repair

The surgeon should excise the subcutaneous component of the lipoma, enter the spinal canal through the normal spine above the lipoma. This would involve a laminectomy and durotomy, and exposure of the spinal cord within the dural sac down to the level of the lipoma. The nerve roots must be preserved and the lipoma should be ideally resected from the spinal cord. However, if it is a complex lesion, the inexperienced surgeon may wish to leave the lipoma attached to the conus of the cord and its nerve roots, but separate it from the overlying extra spinal lipoma. This at least would take the tension off the spinal cord, and hopefully relieve the presenting problem. It is not advisable for an inexperienced surgeon to perform the operation as a prophylactic measure.

Operative method

The patient is placed under general anaesthesia, prone on the operating table with the pelvis and chest supported and the pressure taken off the abdomen. A midline incision is made, extending through and above the lipoma. The normal spine above the lipoma is exposed and a one- or two-level laminectomy and durotomy performed. The spinal cord is traced down to the level of the lipoma. The lipoma is transected, and the subcutaneous component excised. The Cavitron ultrasonic aspirator is an ideal instrument to shave the fat off the spinal cord in layers, but this instrument may not be available. As an alternative, sharp dissection and bipolar coagulation, are used. It is preferable to leave a remnant of fat on the spinal cord, rather than injure the underlying neural tissue or spinal nerves. Thus if there is any doubt about what level the surgeon is resecting, this tissue should be left behind. The spinal cord will ultimately retether in its new location, but the detethering at this stage may be enough to reverse any neurological deterioration.

The dural sac is closed and a fascial patch placed in the dural opening may be required to give the spinal cord enough room, and to create a watertight closure, as there will be a sizeable dural defect created when the fat is excised. The dura is closed watertight with non-absorbable suture (e.g. prolene) and the wound is closed in layers. The patient can be nursed prone for several days to try and reduce the re-tethering problem and to allow the wound to heal without any direct pressure on it. A urinary catheter is required until the child is mobile.

Avoidance of complications

1. Do not follow the fat around the cord ventrally, when removing it, as this will interfere with the spinal nerve roots.
2. Do not cut spinal nerve roots unless in an unusual dorsal location and clearly aberrant.
3. Aim for a watertight closure and be careful to close the wound in layers with at least two layers to the paraspinal muscles to prevent CSF leaks. Do not use a spinal suction drain because this may precipitate development of a CSF fistula.
4. Obtain good haemostasis before closure to avoid wound haematoma.

Craniosynostosis

The most straightforward craniosynostosis operation is linear craniectomy. This can be applied to the lambdoid suture in plagiocephaly, the sagittal suture in scaphocephaly, and if no specialist craniofacial unit is available, to the coronal suture for coronal synostosis. Removal of the sagittal suture carries risk of sagittal sinus injury and if the surgeon is inexperienced, a bilateral strip craniectomy can be performed either side of the sagittal suture, and preserving a midline strip of bone. The sagittal craniectomy is performed from the anterior fontanelle to the junction of the lambdoid sutures posteriorly (the lambda).

The lambdoid craniectomy is performed from, and including the junction of the lambdoid sutures, down to the junction with the temporal bone at the asterion. The coronal craniectomy is carried from the lateral edge of the anterior fontanelle down to the skull base. Small burr holes are placed at the extremes of the craniectomy and the bone removed preferably with a power tool, but a Gigli saw is an alternative. An approximately 3 cm width craniectomy is performed at each of these sites. New bone will form in the gap.

THE SPINE

Application of skull traction

Indication

Fracture, dislocation of the cervical spine.

Skull tongs: Gardner-Wells or Crutchfield (Figure 11.12, next page)

Technique: This can be done under local anaesthesia in the ward. The temporal scalp is shaved and prepared with skin antiseptic and infiltrated with local anaesthetic (preferably 0.5 percent Marcaine and 1:200 000 adrenaline (bupivacaine and epinephrine)). A small incision is made on each side and the sharp pointed screws inserted through the outer table of the skull. Care must be taken not to place them through the squamous temporal bone.

They are placed in line with the external auditory meatus and approximately 2-3 cm above the top edge of the pinna. For mild extension of the neck they are placed 1-2 cm in front of this point, and for mild flexion of the neck they are placed 1-2 cm behind this point depending on the direction of reduction required. The patient's head is supported on a pillow. A pulley is attached to the end of the bed, and weights applied as described in Chapter 5.

Check X-rays will be required daily until the fracture is aligned. This can be the definitive treatment of a fracture dislocation but traction will be required for 6-8 weeks and then the patient placed in a hard collar. The deficiency of this treatment is the long period of bed rest required and the accompanying risk of bed sores, deep vein thrombosis, urinary infection, and other complications and the prospect of malunion or ongoing instability. If the skills and equipment for internal fixation are available, this will be a preferable method after initial stabilisation in skull traction. If the patient is to be under traction for 6-8 weeks, they will require regular rotation and adequate pressure care.

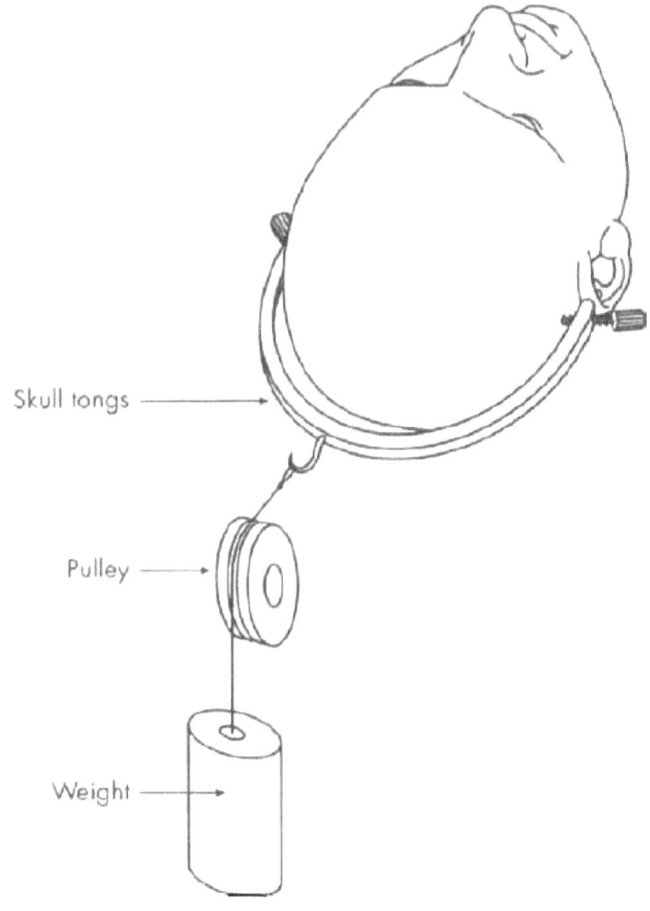

Skull tongs

Pulley

Weight

Gardner-Wells skull tongs

Figure 11.12 Application of Gardner-Wells skull tongs. Skeletal traction applied for fracture dislocation of the cervical spine.

Hoens's traction (Figure 11.13, next page)

This is an alternative method of skeletal traction when there are no tongs. Under local anaesthesia, four burr holes are inserted 3 cm from the midline, 3 cm apart centred on the line joining the mastoid process. Two heavy braided wires are passed between the holes on each side using the Gigli saw guide. These wires are joined to a rope which is set up as for the skull tongs.

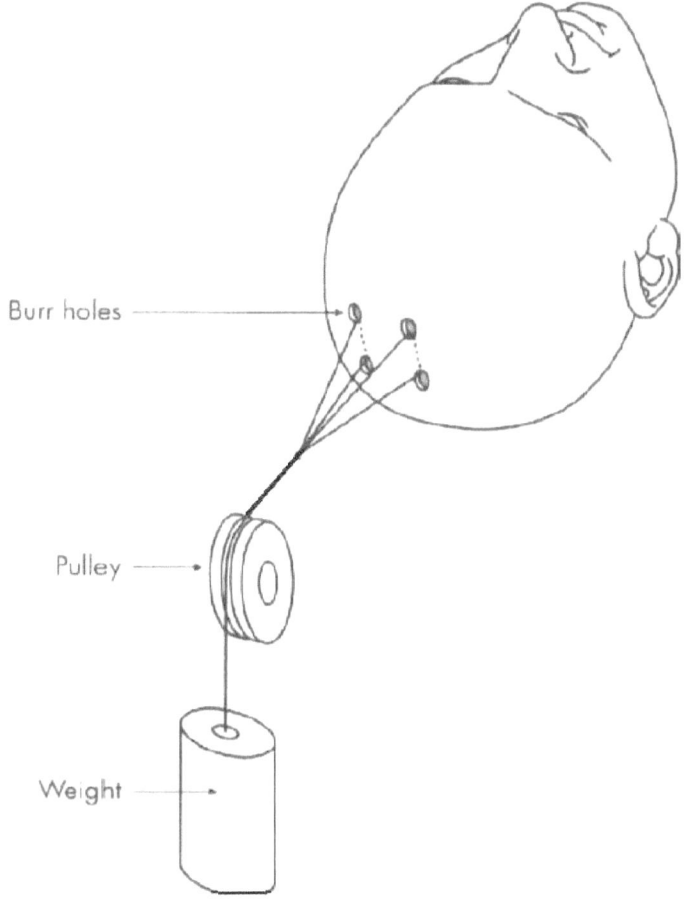

Hoen's skull traction

Figure 11.13 Application of Hoen's traction.

Principles of spinal surgery

The principles are the same as for the cranial surgery if the patient is prone - make sure there is no direct pressure on the abdomen - place pillows under the chest and pelvis to remove pressure from the inferior vena cava and thus reduce bleeding from the venous plexus in and around the spine. Try and bend the table into a jack-knife position to open up the spinous processes. The lateral position is an alternative for spinal surgery, although it is more awkward for the surgeon.

Initial incision: stay in the midline raphé down to the spinous processes. This is a relatively bloodless plane. Strip the paraspinal muscles in a subperiosteal plane using a diathermy stick on coagulation or blend mode while retracting them with a heavy toothed forcep or osteotome (eg. Cobbs elevator). The muscles are stripped off the spinous processes and laminae (see Figure 11.16, page 585).

Practice point

Make sure that when you operate on the spine that you have identified the correct side and the correct spinal level. Intra-operative X-rays are used to check the level.

Lumbar laminectomy and discectomy

Indication

Persistent sciatica with signs of nerve root compression due to disc prolapse with confirmation by radiological investigation.

Strategy

A posterolateral disc protrusion can be removed with an interlaminar approach on one side which includes a resection of the medial portion of the intervertebral facet joint (laminotomy). However, a larger disc prolapse with a central component will require a complete laminectomy at the appropriate level. The commonest discs to rupture are L4-5 and L5-S1. L3-4 is much less common. The disc space should be cleared of soft central disc fragments, otherwise the risk of recurrence is high. It is advisable for the surgeon performing this operation, to have previous spinal surgery experience. Spinal fusion is not usually required following a routine discectomy.

573

Technique

Prophylactic intravenous antibiotics are administered at induction (usually a cephalosporin or penicillin - depending on local antibiotic policy and microbial resistance patterns). A headlight and perhaps a set of loupes will be helpful to provide a brighter operative field allowing better identification of structures. The patient is placed under general anaesthesia, intubated, prone on the operating table, with the head turned to one side, resting on a soft support, such as a sponge ring. The standard position as described in the principles section is attained. The back is shaved, prepared, draped, and a midline incision made centred over the proposed interspace. Remember that the L4-5 level is usually level with the iliac crests and there should only be one main interspace below this level, although in thin people, the S1-2 interspace can be mistaken for the L5-S1 interspace on palpation of the back.

The incision is deepened in the midline and the paraspinal muscles reflected off one or both sides using the diathermy in a subperiosteal plane, depending on the size and site of the disc prolapse as discussed above. If the specific unilateral muscle retractor is not available, the muscle should be taken down on the opposite side as well to allow a bilateral retractor to be inserted. The level is checked by the relative movement of the vertebral elements. A finger is placed on the interlaminar spaces and the spinous process is grasped with a bone forceps, such as the Horsley and pulled away from the adjacent one. If the interspace opens up this excludes the S1-2 level. The sacrum also has a hollow note when tapped in comparison with the bony elements of the lumbar spine, which have a duller note. The sacrum tends to curve upwards inferiorly with the deepest point of the curve being the L5-S1 interspace. Having confirmed the level, the bone is removed using a power drill with a 'matchstick' head burr. The ligamentum flavum (thick yellow ligament) lies immediately beneath the laminae. A segment of this ligament can be incised with a size 15 blade, being careful not to penetrate the dura beneath, although there will likely be some epidural fat between the ligament and the dura. An angled punch is placed beneath this ligament and is used to remove the ligament, adjacent lamina, and also the adjacent facet joint of the vertebrae above and below. When sufficient bone is removed, the edge of the dural sac and the axilla of the nerve root will be seen.

Using a blunt forceps or probe, the surgeon should palpate the region and identify the disc prolapse, which will be lying directly beneath and lateral to the nerve root, which will be stretched tightly over the surface of the disc and usually deflected medially. The nerve root must be separated from the disc and identified definitively as the nerve root. This dissection must be done with the minimum of trauma to the nerve root and the blunt ended nerve root retractor (Krayenbühl) is useful for this purpose. The plain dissecting forceps are also helpful. It is wise not to use sharp dissection because of the risk of incising the nerve root. A dose of intravenous dexamethasone is helpful at this stage, to try and minimise the neurological deficit following nerve root retraction. The nerve root is retracted medially and the disc exposed. The epidural veins, which are often quite prominent, should be diathermied preferably with bipolar coagulation and are then cut with fine scissors, or a scalpel blade, so that the disc alone is exposed when it is incised. Persistent epidural bleeding is controlled with Surgicel packing.

The disc is incised using a scalpel blade, while the assistant holds the nerve root medially. There may be free fragments of disc which are 'delivered' on retracting the root and these are removed individually with the rongeurs. The disc space is then entered with straight and angled rongeurs or alligator forceps to remove the multiple disc fragments remaining. A sharp curette is helpful to loosen the fragments attached to the vertebral endplate cartilage. A central disc prolapse will require medial retraction of the nerve root and the dura. Great care must be taken not to pass the instruments too deeply, otherwise the anterior annulus may be perforated and the major vascular structures anterior to the spine damaged. The disc space is irrigated with saline solution to wash out any free fragments. The lumbar nerve root should also be well decompressed inferolaterally, by removing enough bone from the inferior lamina and adjacent articular process of the facet joint. A few pieces of Surgicel are laid in the region of the nerve root and disc space for continued haemostasis.

Any large pieces of Surgicel impacted against the nerve root should be removed at this stage. The wound is then closed in layers, with a heavy absorbable suture for the muscle; the deep fascia is closed separately, and then the skin in two layers. Any dural tear should be repaired using fine Prolene. When the dura is torn, CSF escapes, the dura collapses and epidural bleeding tends to increase. Hence there is a need to close the dural leak quickly, so that this does not happen. A suction drain tube is placed into the epidural space if there is copious epidural bleeding, which has not been fully controlled with the Surgicel. It is brought out through a separate stab incision. It is not advisable to place a drain if there is an active CSF leak, because there is a high risk of CSF fistula developing.

Cervical disc prolapse

In the developing world setting, decompression is best done by a foraminotomy, which involves a hemilaminectomy approach at the appropriate level. The patient is best placed in a prone position with the head fixed in the threepin headrest. If this is unavailable the patient can be placed in a lateral position, with the head resting on a horseshoe ring, at the appropriate level. The head of the table is elevated to reduce venous pressure and bleeding. The correct spinal segment is identified at operation by placing a needle at the relevant interspinous level and performing a lateral X-ray on the table or using the image intensifier, if available. A more reliable method is to count down with the finger from the spinous process of C2, downwards. C2 spinous process can readily be distinguished from the arch of the atlas (without a spinous process) above it. This requires a more extended incision to be able to pass the finger down from above. The paraspinal muscles are reflected in a subperiosteal plane off the affected side only.

The operation is very similar to the lumbar discectomy exposure, except that it is in the neck. The hemilaminectomy (interlaminar approach) at the relevant level is extended out laterally to include the facet joint and the exposed ligamentum flavum is excised. The power tool with a cutting 'match-head' burr, and the angled bone punches of varying sizes are recommended. The lateral edge of the dura and the axilla of the relevant cervical root are exposed. The root is decompressed laterally. There are often large epidural veins around the nerve root which will require coagulation and Surgicel. It is often impossible to retrieve the disc from in front of the nerve root without retraction and damage to the nerve root. If there are sequestrated fragments it may be possible to lift them out gently from beneath the nerve root, using a blunt dissector such as a Watson-Cheyne, however, most cases will improve with the dorsal decompression alone. If there is a large soft disc component, this may be better decompressed via an anterior approach with an anterior cervical discectomy and fusion. However, this requires neurosurgical or orthopaedic expertise and is not recommended for the beginner. The results of decompressing a nerve root following cervical disc rupture are excellent for pain relief and improvement of neurological signs, provided the operation is done soon enough, before irreversible nerve root or spinal cord damage has developed.

Costotransversectomy (Figure 11.14, below)

Indication

Costotransversectomy is used for decompression of the spinal cord when there is compression anteriorly and is also used for access to the vertebral bodies from a posterior approach, without compromise (i.e. retraction) of the spinal cord. It is particularly suited to the general surgeon, who has not had experience with anterior approaches to the spine and is reluctant to pursue thoracotomy with the resources available. The most common indication is tuberculosis, secondly pyogenic osteomyelitis with anterior cord compression, and thirdly, anterior tumours particularly metastatic disease with anterior compression and collapse of the adjacent vertebrae with gibbus deformity.

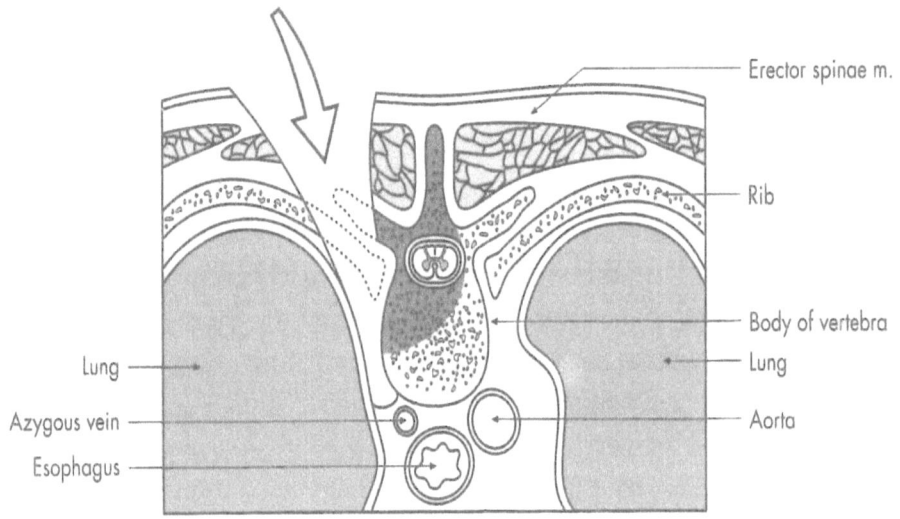

Figure 11.14 Costotransversectomy: the dorsolateral approach to the spine with resection of the transverse process, neck and head of the adjacent rib, and partial corpectomy, laminectomy, and excision of the spinous process. The paraspinal muscles may be reflected off the vertebrae for added exposure.

Operative strategy

The aim is to approach the anterior spinal column from the dorsolateral approach, thus avoiding any need for retraction on the spinal cord (Figure 11.14, previous page). The lamina is partly removed on the side of the approach, and the head and neck of the rib, the transverse process, the facet joint and pedicle on the side of the lesion are excised. The intercostal nerve is skeletonised at its junction with the dura. The pathological process is biopsied and excised, and then a reconstruction of the spine may be attempted, although this is difficult from the costotransversectomy approach. The side of attack will depend on the side of the maximal pathology, but the inexperienced operator will find a left-sided exposure easier because it avoids the azygous veins and the inferior vena cava.

Operative method

The patient is placed prone on the operating table, with support under the chest and pelvis, so that the abdomen is sitting relatively free of pressure to avoid obstruction of venous return, which would increase spinal bleeding from the epidural venous plexus considerably. A skin marker is put on the appropriate skin level, by doing an A-P and lateral X-ray before the operation with a metal marker on the skin. This is most easily done using fluoroscopy but if this is not available, plain films will suffice. A 'T' incision is used, or a gently curved incision away from the midline. The paraspinal muscles are reflected off the spinous processes and laminae, but also are split transversely, and dissected off the underlying ribs. The appropriate neck and head of rib are removed, along with the transverse process and laminae at the level of pathology. The pleura should be dissected off the rib and away from the exposure. Any rents in the pleura should be repaired and rendered airtight. There may be some tumour in the soft tissues and erosion of the bone, to confirm the level even before any bone is removed. A high-speed drill with a round cutting burr is very useful for removing the bone, and is much easier than using rongeurs and a bone punch, which are the alternatives.

The facet joint is then removed and the pedicle. This does not create significant instability in the thoracic region because of the buttressing of ligaments, facet joints and ribs surrounding the operation and on the opposite side. The lateral dura is identified and protected along with the intercostal nerve. The tumour or infection can now be biopsied and cultured, necrotic bone fragments are removed and the paraspinal and epidural abscess drained. An infant feeding tube can be passed up and down the spinal canal to confirm patency. The dura should be pulsating at the end of the decompression. The reconstruction could possibly be performed by impacting fresh rib fragments into the defect to prevent further collapse. A drain in the epidural space is necessary. If there has been a dural tear, this should be closed watertight, and if possible, a drain avoided, because of the risk of causing a CSF fistula, particularly if there is suction on the drain. The wound is then closed in the usual layers.

Anterior decompression of the spinal cord via thoracotomy, thoracolaparotomy or transcervical approaches

Introduction

This is a difficult operation and should not be attempted unless the surgeon and anaesthetist are familiar with thoracotomy.

Costotrans-versectomy is often a satisfactory alternative. There may be considerable bleeding and a blood transfusion is often required.

Indications:
1. Spinal cord compression due to tuberculosis with progressive paraplegia and sphincter involvement despite anti- tuberculous therapy and steroid.
2. Malignant cord compression (primary and secondary) with predominant anterior compression and destruction of vertebral bodies.

Strategy

A posterolateral thoracotomy is performed to gain access to the anterior thoracic spine. A right-sided thoracotomy is preferable to a left-sided approach because the aorta is an obstacle on the left, and the artery of Adamkiewicz may be vulnerable. This is the main radicular artery supplying the thoracolumbar spinal cord and usually is a branch of the left T11 intercostal artery, but may arise from T8 to T12. Interruption of this vessel will carry a high risk of paraplegia. A thoracolaparotomy with splitting of the diaphragm is used for the low thoracic upper lumbar region; and for the mid to lower lumbar region an extraperitoneal approach is used. The anterior cervical region can be exposed via an incision, usually on the right side of the neck for a right-handed operator, either obliquely in front of sternomastoid or transversely in the skin crease lines and then deepened in the bloodless plane between the carotid sheath structures posteriorly and the pharyngolaryngeal structures medially, with the dissection proceeding to the prevertebral fascia and the longus colli. Bone for reconstruction of the spine can be harvested from the iliac crest on the same side as the exposure.

Operative procedure

For a thoracotomy, the patient is placed in a lateral position, with the arm turned forwards. A posterolateral thoracotomy approach is used with retraction of the scapula upwards. The intercostal space chosen for the entry should be two levels above the level of the vertebral body involvement. This allows the surgeon to work from above down, which is the preferred angle. Removal of the posterior 5-10 cm of a rib may permit a wider thoracotomy exposure and a segment of rib can be used for the bony reconstruction. The lung is retracted and preferably collapsed unilaterally, if a double lumen endotracheal tube is available. The lung can be gently retracted even if a single lumen endotracheal tube is all that is available and adequate access can be gained to the thoracic spine. The parietal pleura is opened over the area of abnormality and often the abscess or tumour will be apparent when the lung is retracted. Azygous veins and intercostal arteries may require ligation to gain access to the spine. Long thoracic instruments will be required to handle these blood vessels, which will usually require ligation, although the smaller veins can be diathermied (Figure 11.15 (a), next page). The paraspinal abscess and necrotic bone fragments or tumour are excised. The dura is exposed and the spinal cord decompressed.

The inexperienced surgeon may find radical debridement and exposure of the dura quite difficult, particularly if the instruments are deficient, and only a partial decompression may be possible. If the dura can be exposed it should be pulsating well at the completion of the decompression and an infant feeding tube catheter can be passed up and down the canal to make sure that the obstruction has been relieved. The spine is then reconstructed by impacting the rib or iliac crest grafts into position into the healthy bone above and below the decompression. Two or three bony blocks are sufficient (Figure 11.15 (b), page 582 and Figure 11.15 (c), page 583). It is not usually possible to close the parietal pleura. The thoracotomy is closed in the usual way. An intercostal drain tube connected to an underwater sealed drainage system is placed before closure.

The drain can usually be removed after 24-48 hours after clipping of the drain, and a chest X-ray up to 6 hours later, to make sure that pneumothorax has not occurred. The lung should be reasonably well inflated before the intercostal tube is removed. Comment: In HIC, adjustable vertebral cages are used to replace vertebral bodies and various techniques of multilevel fusion of the spine performed to avoid further angulation and instability.

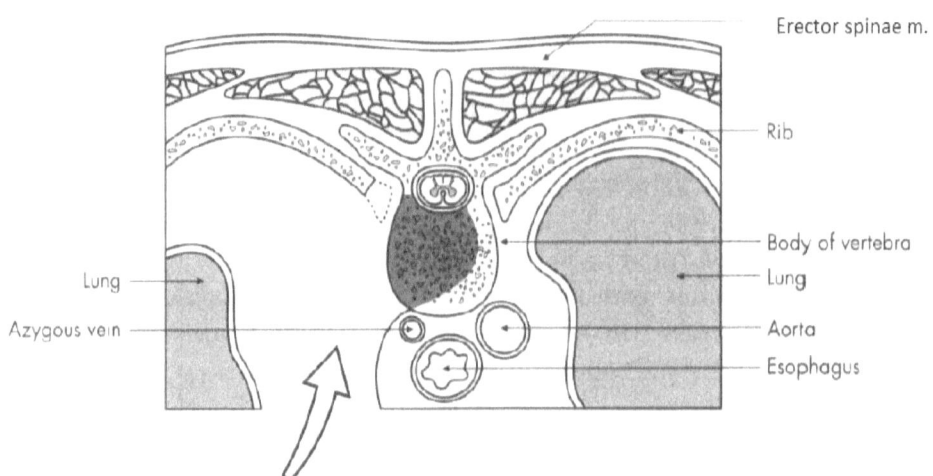

Figure 11.15 (a) Horizontal section showing transthoracic approach.

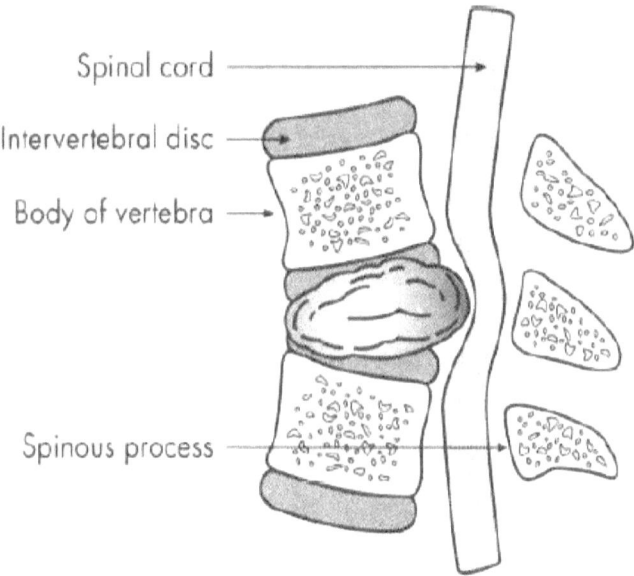

Spinal cord

Intervertebral disc

Body of vertebra

Spinous process

(b) i Vertebral body and adjacent discs replaced by neoplasm or infection with angular kyphosis and compression of the spinal cord.

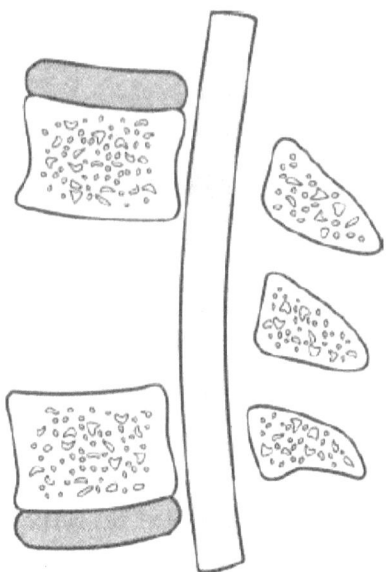

(b) ii Vertebrectomy including adjacent diseased discs. Decompression of spinal cord.

Common operations

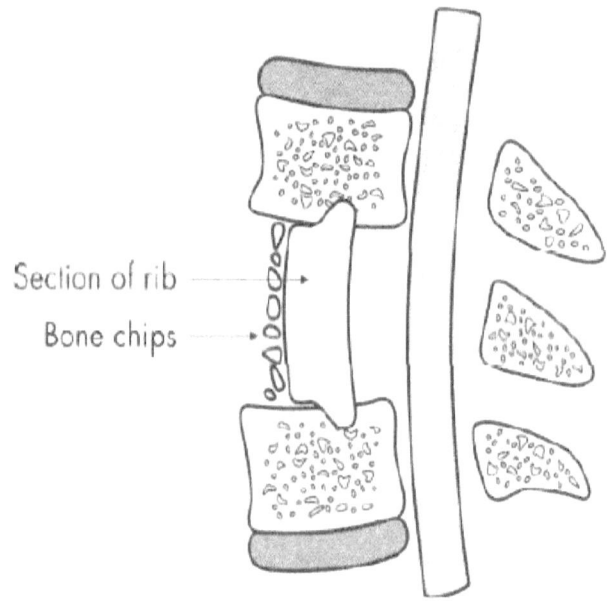

(b) iii Reconstruction of the spine using rib graft and bone chips.

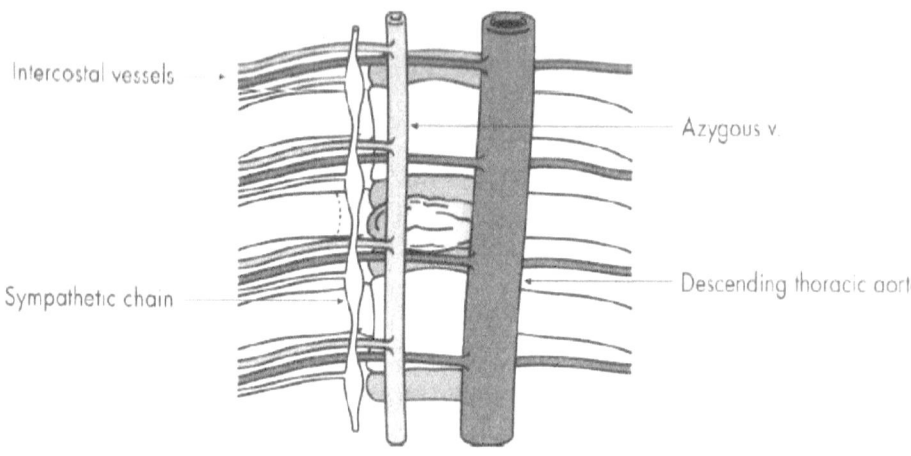

(c) i Exposure of anterior spine showing adjacent vascular and neural structure.

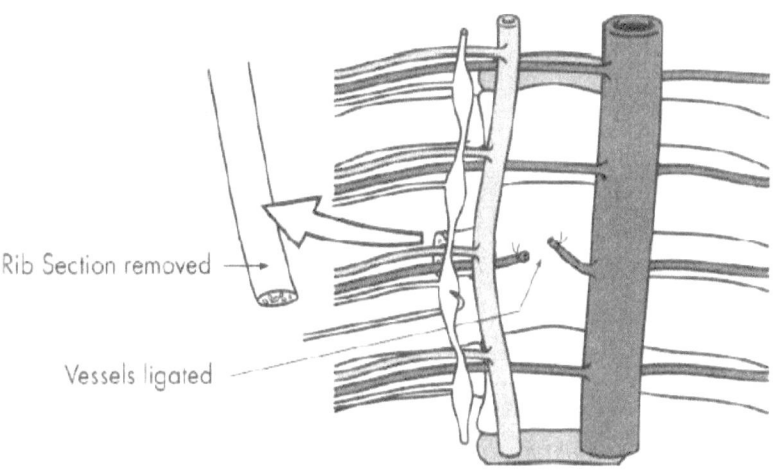

Rib Section removed

Vessels ligated

(c) ii Resection of rib for a reconstruction. Ligation of adjacent intercostal artery. Lateral displacement of sympathetic chain with blunt nerve hook.

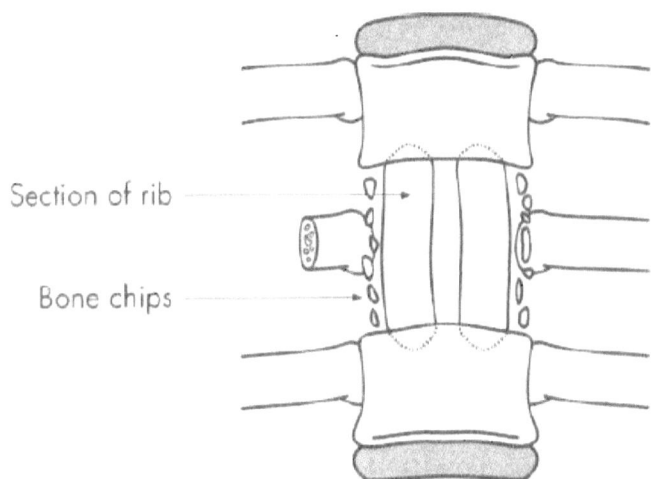

Section of rib

Bone chips

(c) iii Anterior view of the reconstructed spine with two sections of rib graft and bone chips.

Figure 11.15 (a-c) Anterior approach to the thoracic spine via thoracotomy.

Lumbar canal stenosis (Figure 11.16)

Indications

Indications are neurogenic claudication or persistent sciatica with exclusion of vascular causes of claudication, and imaging showing typical lumbar canal stenosis. This disease usually affects the lower lumbar spine, but may affect all levels of the lumbar spine and there may be a congenital element to the degree of stenosis of the canal. CT scan is the best diagnostic test.

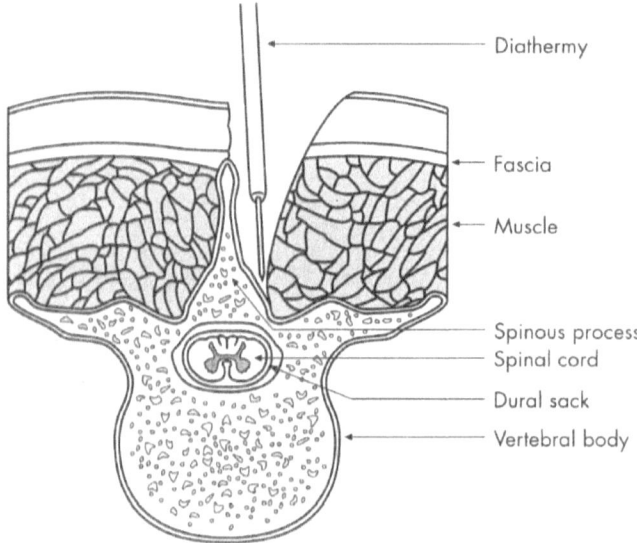

Figure 11.16 (a) Subperiosteal diathermied dissection of muscle off the spinous process and laminae.

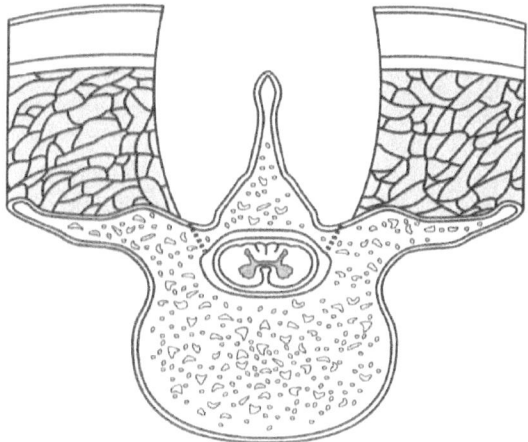

(b) Exposure of spinous process and laminae.

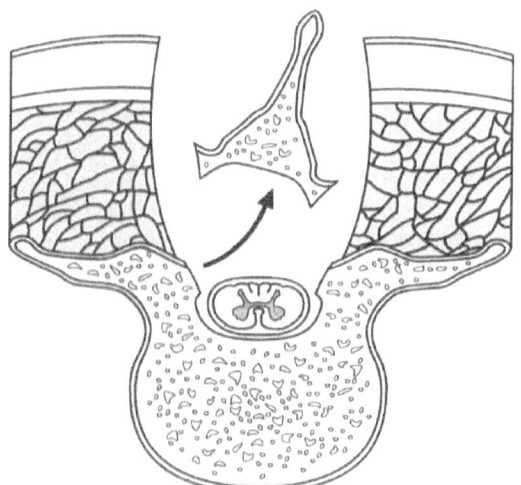

(c) Laminectomy.

Figure 11.16 (a-c) Exposure of the spine and laminectomy.

Strategy

A complete laminectomy is performed over the affected levels, being careful not to neglect the L1-2 level if this is also affected. Specific nerve root involvement clinically will require decompression at the laminectomy. An important part of the operation is to de-roof the lateral recess of the spinal canal, in which the lumbar roots lie before they exit the spine, so that the dural sac and nerve roots on each side are well decompressed and visible by the end of the procedure. About half the facet joint is removed on each side to enable this exposure. There is a small risk of instability developing, although most of the patients having this operation already have advanced arthritis and varying degrees of ankylosis of the facet joints. Greater caution is required if spondylolisthesis is present, because there will be a higher risk of slip. It is advisable for the surgeon performing this operation, to have had previous spinal surgery experience.

Operative procedure

The patient is placed in the same position as described for lumbar discectomy. The spinous processes and laminae are exposed in the same way as described for lumbar discectomy and the level checked as described above. The spinous processes and laminae are excised using rongeurs and the angled Cloward or Kerrison punch is the best instrument to clear the lateral recess of excess osteophyte and ligamentous overgrowth. The epidural fat is usually atrophic and deficient at each laminar level of 'hourglass' deformity, so great care must be taken in removing this bone, not to tear the dura underneath. Discectomies are not usually required during this operation. A suction drain (redivac) tube is usually placed in the epidural plane and brought out through a separate stab incision. The wound is then closed in layers as described for the discectomy operation.

Spinal subdural empyema

Subdural empyema may also occur in the spine secondary to osteomyelitis and epidural infection; or secondary to penetrating injuries or postoperative septic complications. The principles of treatment are the same as for the cranial condition, where the primary pathology must be dealt with, i.e. the spinal and epidural abscess must be drained adequately and the spine reconstructed (see spine fixation descriptions in this chapter); but then the spinal dura must be opened, the purulent material in the subdural space evacuated and the space irrigated with warm (37°C) Ringer's solution or saline. Passing an infant feeding tube can assist with the irrigation above and below the laminectomy

Gunshot wound to the spine

These wounds should be explored in a similar way to the gunshot wounds of the head. A laparotomy or thoracotomy may also be required to cope with the further damage from the bullet track. The track should be followed down into the spine, using a standard midline approach with reflection of the paraspinal muscles and a laminectomy. Bone fragments and debris are removed from the epidural plane along with haematoma. The dura is then opened in the midline and the spinal cord inspected. Any haemorrhage is controlled with bipolar coagulation or titanium clips. Haematoma is extracted from around the spinal cord and in the spinal cord, and any bullet or bone fragments which are palpated or seen in the bullet track are extracted, and a thorough debridement performed. The spinal cord should be treated very gently and no spinal cord tissue should be removed because of the increased neurological deficit that will result. The dura should be closed primarily and if need be, a patch of deep fascia from the back is sewn into position. This will prevent CSF fistula. The wound is then closed primarily in the usual layers.

Stab wound to the spine

This is handled in a similar way to gunshot wound to the spine. The foreign body is removed under controlled conditions with the patient prone on the operating table. The entry wound is extended, preferably into the midline, the paraspinal muscles are reflected, the foreign body traced down to the spine and removed. A laminectomy is performed, the dura inspected, any opening in the dura is extended and intradural haemostasis obtained, clot removed. The dura is then closed watertight and the wound closed in layers in the usual way. Any fixed deficit is likely to remain although some improvement may occur as oedema settles.

SPACE OCCUPYING LESIONS AND TUMOURS

Glioma

No CT availability

When a space occupying lesion in the cerebral hemispheres has not responded to conservative treatment, and the patient is deteriorating, the surgeon should perform a ventriculogram then a burr hole and aspiration at a site based on the clinical localisation to detect and treat a possible abscess. This is described in Chapter (2). If the aspiration is negative the surgeon with some experience in neurosurgery should perform a generous exploratory craniotomy over the presumed site of the lesion. Craniotomy is also indicated if yellow straw-coloured glioma cyst fluid or necrotic/ haemorrhagic cerebral tumour mush is obtained. Sometimes it is difficult to distinguish abscess content from necrotic tumour. Mannitol 0.5 g/kg i.v. is administered on opening the scalp. This will help reduce the turgor of the brain, and make the operation somewhat easier and safer. The dura is opened widely to expose the cortex. A typical glioma will result in a swollen tense brain, with widened pale gyri.

There may be hypervascularity and evidence of necrotic, discoloured, grey/blue tissue on the surface if it is a malignant glioma. If the surface is normal, a brain needle is passed at various angles into the deep white matter, and aspirated as it is withdrawn. The actively growing wall of the glioma has a tougher consistency with some resistance to penetration compared with the surrounding white matter. The cortex is opened with a 2-3 cm linear incision overlying the site of the identified or presumed pathology, and the assistant should retract the edges of the cortex gently with malleable spatulas. A wide-bore sucker can then be passed into the tumour itself and the central necrotic contents aspirated. Haemostasis of the edge of the cavity can be controlled with bipolar coagulation and Surgicel. Cotton wool or gauze can be laid in over cottonoids to tamponade the resection cavity until it is dry, which may take 5-10 min, and then these materials are removed. If a solid fleshy tumour is encountered when the deep white matter is opened, multiple biopsies are taken. Some of the mass may be resected with suction and coagulation. If a smooth-walled glioma cyst is encountered, this is left to drain through the cortical incision and the walls of the cyst left undisturbed. A description of lobectomy is beyond the scope of this text.

CT scan available

CT will help the surgeon to decide what the likely pathology is and where it is located, before the operation is undertaken. It may eliminate the need for operation, or on the other hand, may guide the surgeon more accurately to the site of the pathology. It is even possible to put a scalp marker on, overlying the lesion, just using the CT scanner alone with multiple parallel needles stuck to the scalp, so that the needle overlying the lesion can be counted on the CT scan and the scalp marked at this point. Once the tumour is encountered the procedure is the same as described above. Comment: Neurosurgeons in HIC have the advantage of frameless strereotaxy which enables precise navigation to the lesion and helps define its boundaries at least initially.

Closure

The dura should be closed watertight, and the bone flap firmly re-anchored with heavy sutures, e.g. silk or nylon. If the bone flap is loose, the tumour will tend to fungate through the dura and underneath the scalp creating an ugly swelling, and prolong the life of a disabled individual by lowering the intracranial pressure.

Posterior fossa exploration for tumour (Figure 11.17, next page)

It is well worth exploring a posterior fossa mass in children because a significant number may be benign and curable by surgery, and good palliation can be provided if there is a malignant cerebellar tumour. A urinary catheter is inserted. You will need a headlight for the intracranial component. The patient is placed prone on the operating table with padding beneath the upper chest and the pelvis. The head is rested on a padded ring, paying particular attention to eye protection. If a three-pin headrest is available this is preferable to resting the face on a ring. The head of the table is elevated and mannitol is administered. Initially, an occipital burr hole is placed 6 cm above the external occipital protuberance and 2 to 3 cm from the midline. A ventricular drain is placed into the occipital horn (an infant feeding tube can be used for this purpose). No CSF is drained at this stage. Next, a midline incision is made extending from just above the external occipital protuberance to about C3 level. This is deepened in the midline where there is a relatively avascular plane. The suboccipital muscles are split in a subperiosteal plane off the occipital bone and also off the posterior arch of C1.

Be aware of the vertebral arteries on each side laterally at this level (piercing the atlanto-occipital membrane). Four burr holes are inserted, the upper two just below the superior nuchal line and the lower two just above the foramen magnum.

If no craniotome is available to create a craniotomy, a craniectomy can be performed using the bone rongeurs, joining all of the burr holes. The dura is then opened with a Y-shaped incision, carrying the vertical limb of the Y just one side of the occipital dural sinus in the midline. Where the tumour extends into the upper cervical canal, the arch of the atlas will need to be excised and the dural incision extended inferiorly.

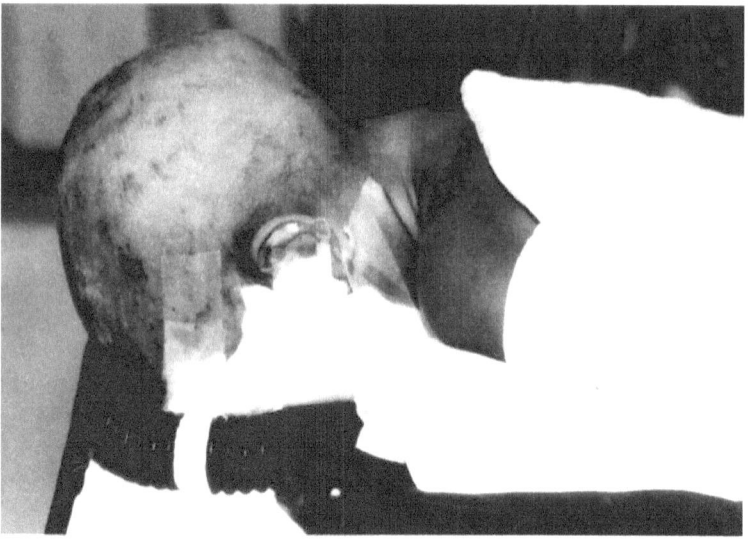

Figure 11.17 (a) The patient placed prone with the face resting on a padded ring. Note that the neck is flexed and the eyes are well padded.

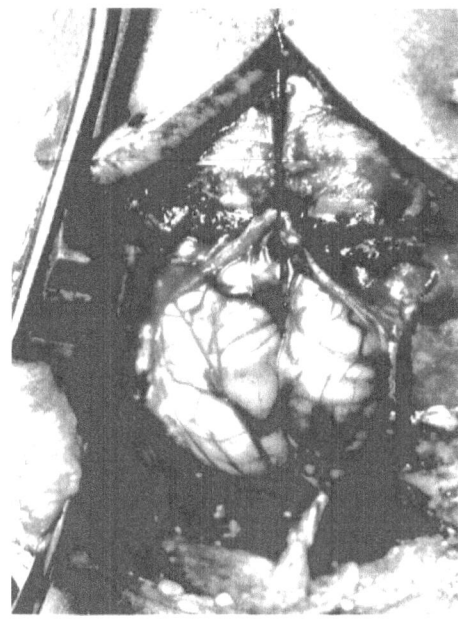

(b) Operative photographs of posterior fossa exploration, showing an exposed cerebellum with tumour coming to the surface and widening the cerebellar folia.

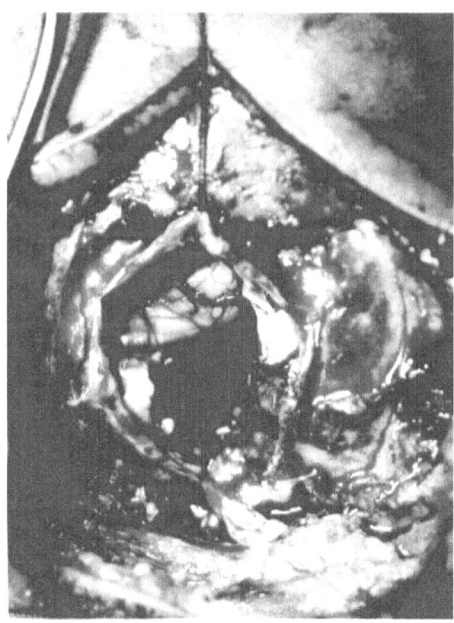

(c) The appearance of the posterior fossa following excision of the tumour.

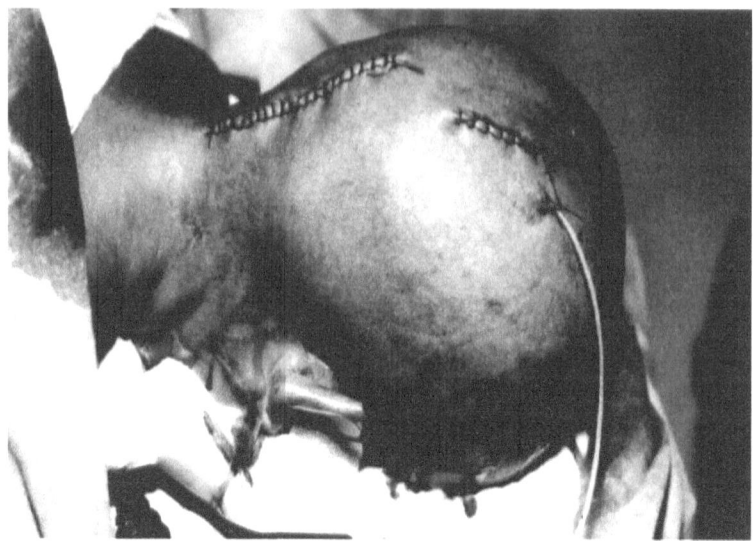

(d) The incision lines extending from above the external occipital protuberance to the mid-cervical region in the midline and a separate occipital incision for occipital burr hole and placement of ventricular drain.

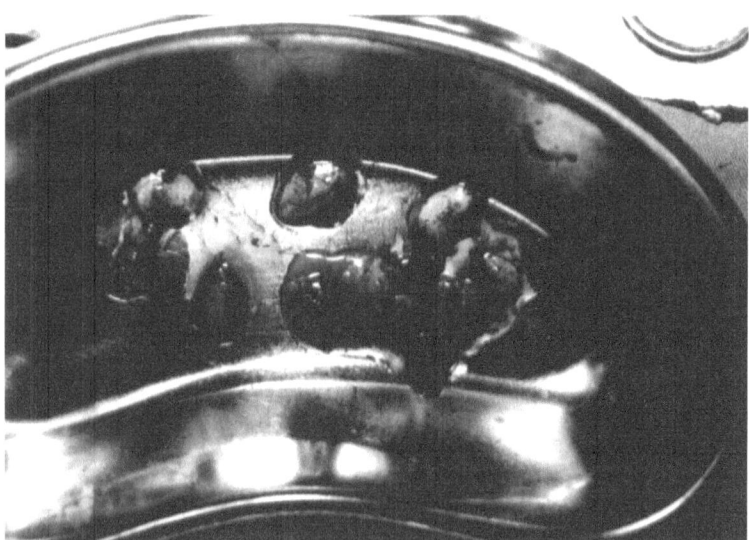

(e) Fragments of tumour in kidney dish, to be sent for pathology.

Figure 11.17 (a-e) Posterior fossa exploration for tumour.

The cerebellum may bulge forth when the dura is opened. The inferior aspect of one of the cerebellar hemispheres is gently elevated medially using a retractor blade; the cisterna magna will be seen as a glistening translucent membrane. This can be pierced with a sharp hook and CSF will gush forwards to lessen the pressure on the posterior fossa. Also, at this stage, some CSF can be let off through the ventricular drain to even the pressures above and below the tentorium. A brain needle is passed into the cerebellar hemisphere with the suspected tumour, and an attempt made to aspirate fluid from any cystic component. Often, midline cerebellar tumours will present in the vermis region and fill the foramen of Magendie. If the tumour is located in the hemisphere, a transverse incision is made over the widened folia (The thin gyral formation of the cerebellum) and deepened into the tumour, which is then evacuated using suction and diathermy. It may be possible to enter a cyst and remove a mural nodule in the wall which would be the most straightforward procedure. The wall of the cyst is left behind.

If there is a midline cerebellar tumour, the medulloblastomas are usually soft and easily suckable, and can be quite bloody. The tumour is resected and the roof of the fourth ventricle opened up so that by the end of the resection, the floor of the fourth ventricle can be seen. For the inexperienced surgeon, take it step by step and do not plunge the sucker too deeply, as it may enter the brain stem. The ependymomas are tougher tumours and without a microscope and Cavitron ultrasonic aspirator might be quite difficult to remove macroscopically.

The astrocytoma will be usually removable by suction and diathermy and will probably have cystic elements in it. Care is taken at the end of the procedure to secure haemostasis and achieve an accurate watertight closure of the dura. Use a muscle or fascial patch to complete this closure. The muscle and deep fascia are closed with heavy absorbable suture (e.g. Vicryl), subcutaneous fascia then closed and lastly the skin. The ventricular drain is left in after the operation and is usually clipped off. However, if the patient deteriorates it can be opened to control hydrocephalus. It is usually removed at 24-48 hours. If a ventriculoperitoneal shunt is required at a later date, it is performed as a separate procedure.

Case report

A 3-year-old girl presented with chronic headache, neck pain, back pain, weak legs, inability to walk, incontinent of urine, with papilloedema, stiff neck and general irritability. Skull X-ray was normal. A ventriculogram was planned but for logistic reasons could not be performed. Therefore, the child was taken to theatre with a suspected diagnosis of cerebellar tumour. At posterior fossa exploration a solid cerebellar tumour was identified (see Figure 11.15, page 581). The tumour was debulked using suction and diathermy and the pressure relieved in the posterior fossa and the ventricular system by placing a ventricular drain. After surgery she improved rapidly, made a good recovery and was discharged back to her village.

The long-term outcome is unknown. The tumour was an astrocytoma. The diagnosis of posterior fossa tumour in this case was purely clinical and was largely based on the fact that she had signs of raised intracranial pressure, but also had neck pain and neck stiffness, which pointed to a problem in the posterior fossa. Although we were not on very strong ground, we felt that this was the most likely diagnosis and that exploration was warranted. Ideally, a CT or ventriculogram would have helped confirm the clinical diagnosis.

Meningioma

Cerebral convexity

Only small convexity (surface) meningiomas should be explored by the surgeon with little neurosurgical experience. The small meningiomas will not usually be diagnosed without CT, although a calcified lesion (which is unusual in the small tumours), may be seen on skull X-ray. The larger lesions and those near the sagittal sinus are difficult to remove and will require neurosurgical expertise. The strategy of removal is to perform a craniotomy overlying the lesion, to cut the dural edge just peripheral to the lesion and to develop a plane between the cortex and the tumour using cottonoids. This plane is usually well defined. When the dura is first exposed, there may be large dural vessels passing towards the tumour, and these should be coagulated or clipped to reduce the tumour blood supply. The tumour is debulked centrally, trying to minimise retraction on the brain, but rather retracting on the tumour to deliver it from the niche it has created in the brain. Meningiomas are usually fleshy with fibrous septa passing through them, and cannot be sucked away with the standard sucker, unless the centre has become softened and partly necrotic. Debulking is best performed using cutting diathermy and pituitary rongeurs. The tumour can then be imploded and further separated from the cortex, and is then lifted out with its overlying dura. Removing the bone flap can be very bloody, when there is a large meningioma beneath, and this should be done quickly with the facility for blood transfusion if necessary. When the meningioma is attached to the sagittal sinus it is best to shave it off the sinus, leaving a wall of tumour adherent to the lateral wall of the sinus and fulgurate it with diathermy coagulation, rather than risk massive haemorrhage from the sagittal sinus.

Skull base

Meningiomas that arise from the skull base and indent the underside of the brain and envelop or stretch the cranial nerves are technically challenging and also require an experienced neurosurgeon. Beware of tackling tumours close to the optic nerves, carotid artery, cavernous sinus or the cranial nerves of the posterior fossa, as these lesions are difficult to remove and are best tackled by an experienced neurosurgeon who has access to microsurgical instruments. It is possible for the experienced neurosurgeon to remove these lesions without using a microscope and this was the way it was done before the 1960s, but better results are now obtained with magnification.

Pituitary tumour (Figure 11.18, page 598)

Indications

The indications are discussed in the section on pituitary tumour which is presented in Chapter 6.

Strategy

A right frontal craniotomy is performed with elevation of the right frontal lobe, exposure of the right optic nerve and the tumour will be debulked and haemostasis achieved.

Operative method

Extra illumination with a headlight is required. Mild dehydration of the brain with mannitol (0.5g/kg) gains further exposure with less retraction. Elevation of the head of the table 10-15° is important for reducing brain swelling and the head can be placed in a neutral position resting on a doughnut ring, or with some support either side of the head to stop it rotating during the case. A urinary catheter is inserted. Steroid (6mg dexamethasone), and prophylactic antibiotics, are administered intravenously. A curved incision is made, extending from the midline to the right temple just in front of the ear. A five-hole free flap craniotomy is raised. The temporalis is divided vertically and reflected off the temporal bone. The craniotomy is raised and the dura opened with a flap. The craniotomy lower edge should be taken down close to the supraorbital ridge and should avoid the frontal sinus medially and the sagittal sinus.

The frontal lobe is elevated and the olfactory tract is noted on the underside of the frontal lobe where it crosses the lesser sphenoid wing, as the elevation proceeds posteriorly. An assistant will be required to hold a retractor on the underside of the brain but the retraction should remain gentle and the operator will need to keep an eye on the degree of retraction so that trauma is not occurring to the brain. You will note the optic nerve entering the optic canal at this point. Further retraction will reveal the pituitary tumour sitting medial to the optic nerve and stretching the optic chiasm upwards and backwards.

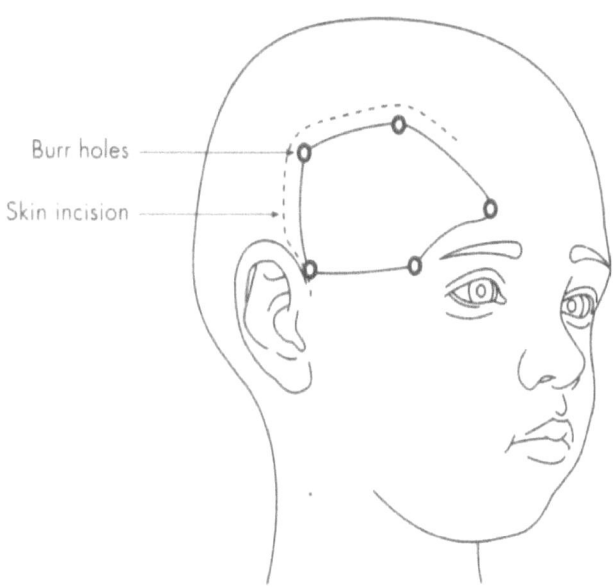

Burr holes

Skin incision

Figure 11.18 (a) Position of scalp incision and frontotemporal craniotomy.

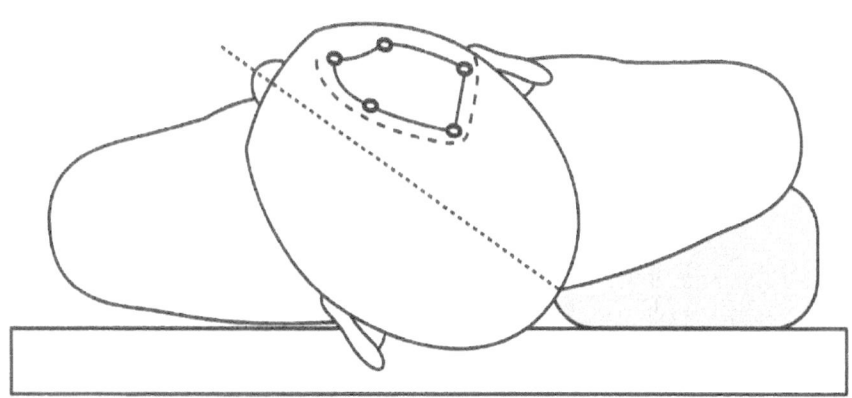

(b) Position of head and trunk on operating table.

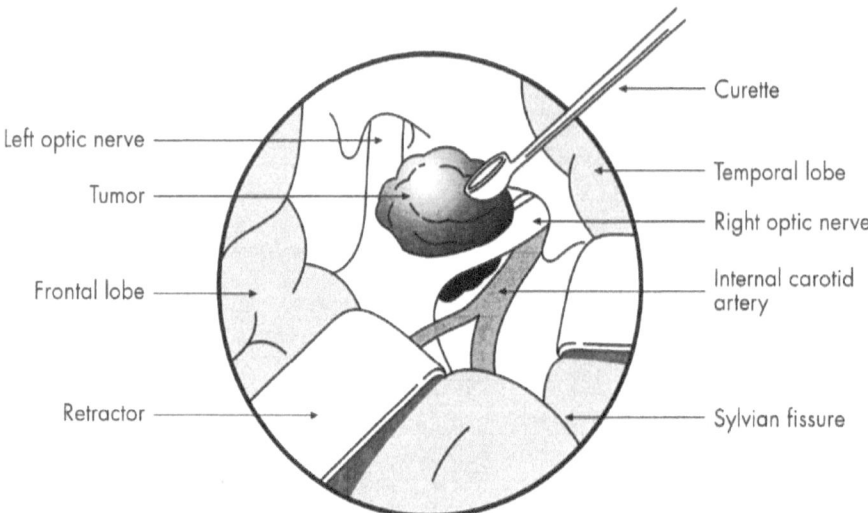

Left optic nerve

Tumor

Frontal lobe

Retractor

Curette

Temporal lobe

Right optic nerve

Internal carotid artery

Sylvian fissure

(c) Trans-sylvian exposure of the optic chiasm, the right internal carotid artery and pituitary tumour, which is seen between optic nerves and lateral to the right optic nerve.

Figure 11.18 (a-c) Craniotomy for excision of pituitary tumour.

Several biopsies of the tumour are taken, using rongeurs or peeling some away with forceps if no rongeurs are available. The tumour is then sucked away and the optic nerve and chiasm decompressed. You will then most likely see the left optic nerve come into view and more of the chiasm. Be careful not to injure the pituitary stalk which may be seen more posteriorly beneath the chiasm once the tumour has been decompressed. Haemostasis is completed with Surgicel and some moist sterile cotton wool can be placed in the pituitary fossa for 5-10 min while venous bleeding is settling. If the bleeding does not stop, some crushed temporalis muscle placed in the pituitary fossa and then impacted with some Surgicel and moist cotton wool can be used. Every attempt should be made to protect the optic chiasm and optic nerves from trauma with the sucker or other instruments. Once you are satisfied that haemostasis is complete, the wound is closed in layers, fixing the bone flap in position with multiple sutures through drill holes.

The patient is kept on dexamethasone for at least a week to 10 days on a tapering dose and will then be placed on maintenance cortisone acetate (37.5 mg per day), until it can be established that the residual pituitary is functioning. Diabetes insipidus may occur in the first day or two after the operation, and is usually transient.

If there is no vasopressin or desmopressin available, you will need to keep up with the fluid loss by increasing the intravenous fluids (5 per cent dextrose) to match the urine output and keep a close watch on the serum sodium which may rise precipitously if the patient's hydration is not maintained.

INFECTION

The pathology and clinical presentation of infections affecting the central nervous system are discussed in Chapter 7. Selected procedures are described below for the surgery of brain abscess, subdural empyema, mastoiditis and osteomyelitis of the skull.

Brain abscess (Figure 11.19, next page)

Aspiration

If the location of the abscess is uncertain, a ventriculogram may be helpful to show the displacement caused by the abscess. A burr hole is placed over the suspected abscess site. The pia is opened and a brain needle passed directly perpendicular and aspirated. If this fails, the needle is angled at approximately 45° to locate the abscess. A depth of up to 5 to 7 cms should be enough to locate it, if it is present. The angle could be increased to approximately 60° if the 45° angle fails.

The walls of loculi should be gently penetrated with the brain needle. The pus is evacuated as completely as possible with a slow gentle withdrawal and sent for culture. The cavity is irrigated with Ringer's solution or saline with aspiration of this fluid. A catheter may be left in the cavity for re-aspiration and the installation of daily antibiotic, e.g. gentamicin 4-8 mg.

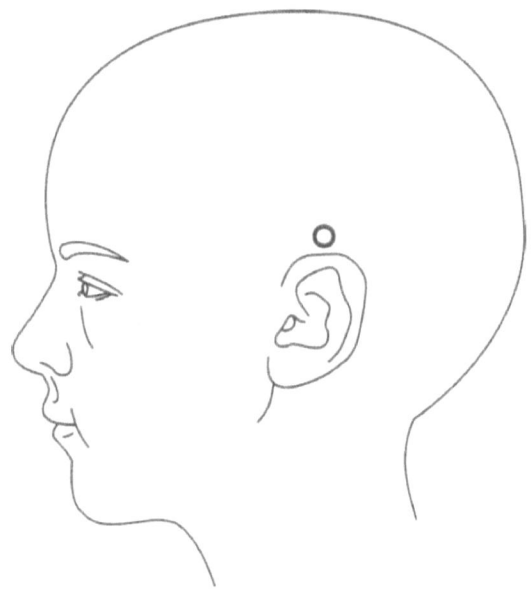

(a) i Site of burr hole.

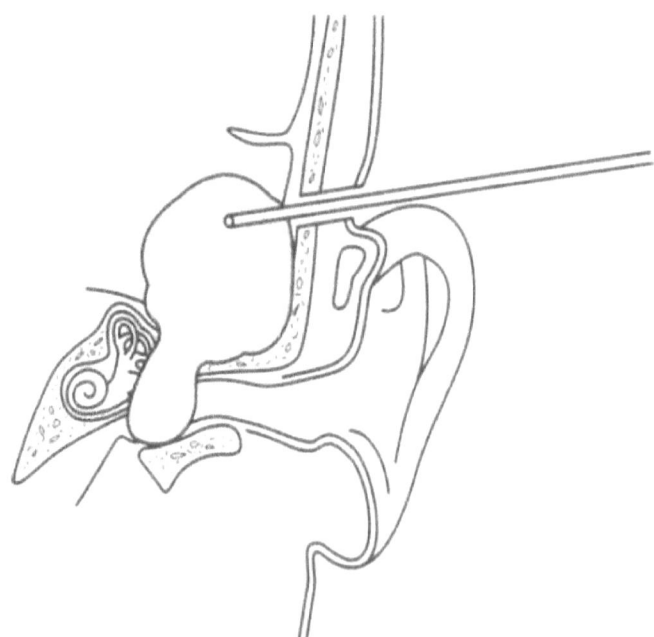

(a) ii Needle passing through temporal bone into abscess cavity.

Figure 11.19 (a) Temporal lobe abscess.

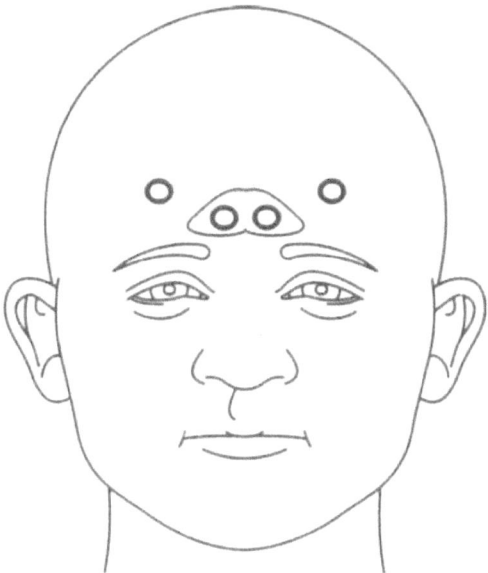

(b) i Site of burr holes overlying frontal sinus and overlying frontal lobe on each side.

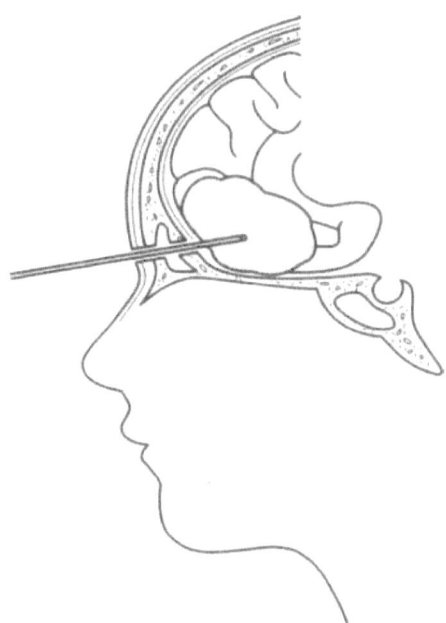

(b) ii Needle aspiration of frontal lobe abscess through frontal sinus.

Figure 11.19 (b) Frontal lobe abscess.

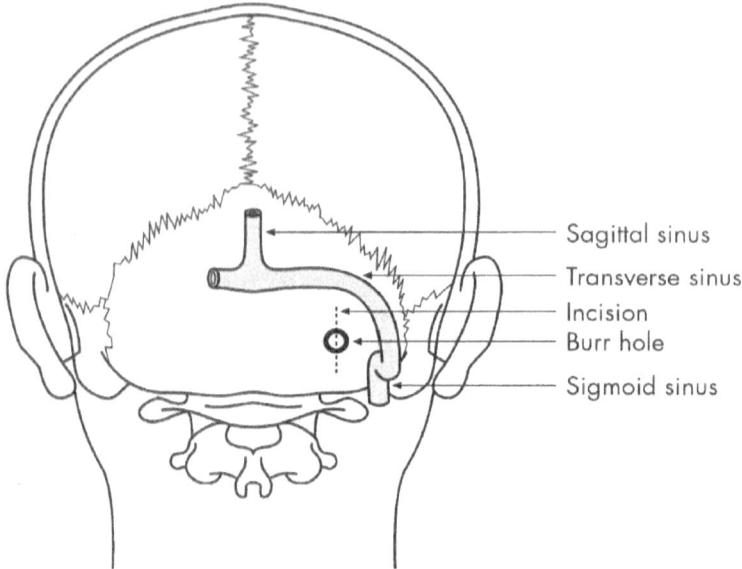

(c) Posterior fossa abscess - site of incision and burr hole.

Figure 11.19 (a-c) Aspiration of brain abscess.

An injection of 5-10ml iopamidol (lsovue) may be made through the catheter to outline the size of the cavity on plain X-ray and lasts about 6-8 hours. This can be repeated every few days to demonstrate shrinkage of the abscess and confirm resolution. The abscess may take several weeks to resolve. Systemic antibiotics with broad aerobic and anaerobic cover are required for all abscess cases. The antibiotics of choice are usually ampicillin, gentamicin and metronidazole, or ceftriaxone and metronidazole. The pus should be cultured if possible and the antibiotics changed according to sensitivities. Anaerobic cover with metronidazole should be continued if anaerobic cultures are not possible, because a high proportion of these lesions have anaerobes.

Drainage of a temporal lobe abscess (Figure 11.19 (a), page 601)

Place the patient supine with the head turned to the side. A burr hole is made just above the centre of the upper edge of the pinna. A brain needle is passed perpendicular to a depth of 5 cm, then in all four directions to 45° at 5 cm depth. Chronic mastoiditis will require a mastoidectomy in addition. Beware of opening the dura deep to the mastoid bone because the sigmoid sinus will likely be encountered.

Drainage of a frontal lobe abscess (Figure 11.19 (b), page 602)

A burr hole is made in the mid-forehead on the presumed side of infection via a transverse skin crease incision. The dura is opened with a cruciate incision and the edge diathermied. A brain needle is passed perpendicular to a depth of 6 to 7 cm and then in all four directions to 45°, at 6 to 7 cm depth. If frontal sinusitis is suspected make the burr hole over the sinus - just to one side of the midline. Clear the sinus contents and strip the frontal mucosa. A second burr hole will be necessary for the back wall of the sinus. Epidural pus may be encountered. Open the dura and probe the brain at 90°, then to each side. Beware of the midline dural venous sinus. The brain will likely be adherent to the dura if an abscess is present. The frontal sinus should be exenterated of content and mucosa) lining, and, if available, packed with Gelfoam soaked in gentamicin. The skin is closed, and no drain in the sinus is necessary.

Drainage of a cerebellar abscess (Figure 11.19 (c), page 603)

The abscess may be subjacent to a chronic mastoiditis. Place the patient in a lateral position with the head flexed forwards. A vertical incision is made 3 cm medial to the posterior edge of the mastoid process. The suboccipital muscles are quite thick in this region and the skin incision will need to be about 4 cm length to enable adequate muscle retraction. A burr hole is performed and the dura opened.

A brain needle is passed forwards to a depth of 5 cm and in each direction at 45°, probing for the abscess. The remainder of the treatment is the same as for frontal abscess.

When an abscess wall is well developed, excision may be indicated. However, this technically challenging surgery is not recommended in the absence of CT scanning and greater neurosurgical experience.

Excision

If the patient's condition is not improving after aspiration of the abscess; either a repeat aspiration procedure may be helpful, or a craniotomy is performed overlying the abscess area and the abscess excised. A 2-3 cm cortical incision is made over the abscess and a corridor pathway made down to the abscess. The wall may be well developed and a plane is progressively developed around the periphery of the wall, and the abscess shelled out in its entirety, without any significant disruption to the surrounding white matter. If the abscess is large, the exposed wall may be opened and the abscess imploded as its contents are progressively evacuated. The wall is thus gradually delivered. Surgicel should be avoided if possible, because it is acting as a foreign body in this situation and may increase the risk of recurrent abscess formation. The cavity is irrigated. The dura is closed watertight and the craniotomy closed in the usual way. No drain tube is necessary in this situation. If the abscess is communicating with the adjacent frontal sinus or middle ear cavity, then a dural repair will be required to prevent further infection and CSF leak. Therefore, the craniotomy size should allow elevation of the frontal lobe or the temporal lobe from the anterior or middle fossa respectively and inspection of the dura adjacent to the affected brain. The pericranial or fascia lata patch graft is laid into position if there is a defect, and preferably anchored with prolene or silk sutures.

Subdural empyema

The presence and extent of subdural empyema is best diagnosed on a CT scan. It is commonly related to primary infection in the air sinuses or following penetrating trauma, or after surgery. The patient may show clinical signs of meningitis and become rapidly obtunded, develop toxaemia, with superadded epilepsy, when the subdural empyema develops.

If no CT scan is available, a clinical diagnosis will have to be made. Plain X-rays may show opacified air cells or sinuses.

Strategy

The primary pathology should be dealt with in addition to draining the subdural empyema, e.g. an opening is made over the frontal sinus through a small transverse forehead incision and once the sinus is drained, the back wall of the frontal sinus can be opened and the dura opened beneath it and the brain inspected. The dura should be closed watertight following inspection, so the bony opening will need to be large enough to do this. The subdural pus often spreads along the falx and over the convexity, therefore multiple burr holes are required to evacuate this spreading collection. Mastoidectomy may be required before evacuation of the intracranial pus if this is the primary focus.

Operative procedure

Frontal pathology

The primary frontal sinus pathology is dealt with as described above, then multiple burr holes are inserted from just behind the hairline in the parasagittal region, 2-3 cm from the midline and also a temporal burr hole is inserted.

Parieto-Occipital pathology

One burr hole is placed above the transverse sinus skin marking and one in the occipital bone beneath the transverse sinus if pus in the posterior fossa is suspected. The dura is opened at each of these sites, and this can be done with a cruciate incision with the edges being diathermied. At each of these burr holes, the cortex is depressed with a blunt dissector and the subdural space probed for a purulent collection with a blunt dissector such as a Macdonald's. Swabs are taken of the pus for microbiological culture and possibly antibiotic sensitivity assays. If there is pus present, the subdural space is irrigated with copious warm (37°C) Ringer's or saline solution, until the washout is clear. The passage of an infant feeding gavage tube (6 or 8 Fr) is very helpful in this regard, in irrigating more deeply in the interhemispheric fissure and over the convexity. The drain tube can be brought out through a separate stab incision for the installation of topical antibiotics, e.g. gentamicin (8 mg) or vancomycin (4 mg) but not penicillin, which is highly epileptogenic.

The patient should be placed on prophylactic anticonvulsants. The mortality of subdural empyema is high unless the condition is treated aggressively and promptly. Repeated CT scans will be necessary to assess resolution of the problem.

Cortical (simple) mastoidectomy (the Schwartze operation) (Figure 11.20, next page and Figure 11.21, page 611)

Indication

In the tropics, the indication for mastoidectomy is evidence of infection involving the mastoid air cells which has spread from the middle ear and is not responding to antibiotics. It can be a lifesaving operation which must be done by the generalist if there is no ENT surgeon. The patient has persistent pain, purulent discharge from the ear, and increasing deafness. The signs are fever, tachycardia, general malaise, tenderness over the mastoid, swelling over the mastoid process, and sagging of the meatal roof near the tympanic membrane.

There may be extension of pus beneath the sternomastoid sheath (**Bezold's abscess**), or beneath the periosteum of the mastoid, or into the zygoma. A sixth nerve palsy may result from extension of the infection to the petrous temporal bone (**petrositis - Gradenigo's syndrome**). Spread of the middle ear infection into the labyrinth will cause vertigo, nausea, vomiting and nystagmus. A facial palsy may develop with advanced middle ear epidural abscess, subdural abscess, brain abscess (temporal lobe, cerebellum), or lateral (transverse or sigmoid) sinus thrombosis. These septic complications may be masked to some degree by antibiotics. A skull X-ray with a basal or Towne's view shows opacification of the mastoid air cells. If available, CT is also helpful to show the extent of infection.

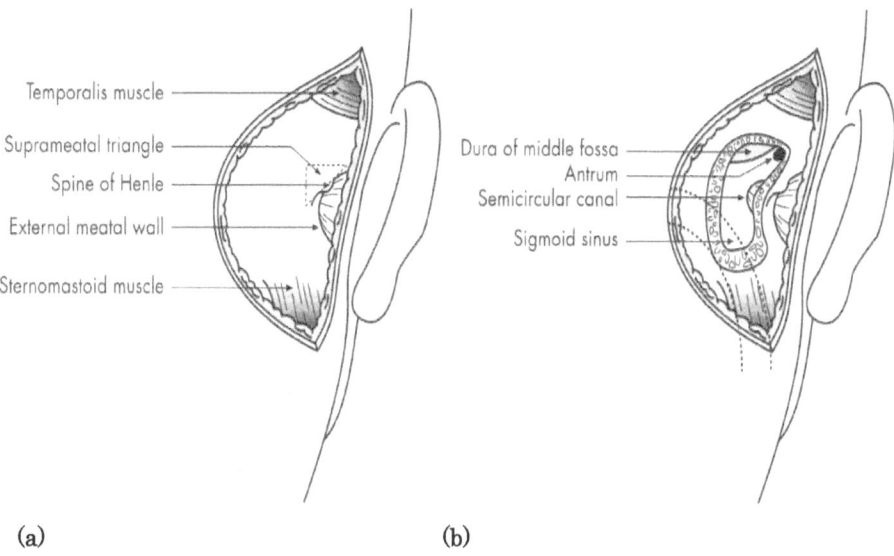

Temporalis muscle

Suprameatal triangle

Spine of Henle

External meatal wall

Sternomastoid muscle

Dura of middle fossa

Antrum

Semicircular canal

Sigmoid sinus

(a)

(b)

Figure 11.20 (a-b) Surgical anatomy of mastoidectomy.

Operative procedure

General anaesthesia is used. An operating microscope and power (ENT) drill should be used if available. The patient is supine with the head turned to the side. A small pillow under the shoulder may relax the neck position. The hair is shaved from the mastoid region. A curved incision is made 1 cm behind the retroauricular skin fold, commencing at the upper attachment of the pinna and extending to below the mastoid tip. Note that the facial nerve lies subcutaneously in the infant in this region. Incision is deepened to the periosteum and the periosteum is reflected posteriorly off the bone to expose the mastoid process and the superior and posterior borders of the bony meatus. The fibrocartilaginous meatus is not completely detached to avoid trauma and subsequent meatal stenosis. The temporalis muscle is reflected upwards and a mastoid retractor inserted.

The bony landmarks of the **suprameatal Macewen's triangle**, including the **spine of Henle** are identified and the direction of the bony meatus are used as guides to the exploration (see Figure 11.20, previous page).

The suprameatal triangle corresponds to the lateral wall of the mastoid antrum (which communicates with the middle ear cavity). Its wall is 2 mm thick at birth but gradually increases in thickness to reach 12-15 mm in the adult. The superior side of the triangle is formed by the supramastoid crest and is level with the floor of the middle cranial fossa. The anteroinferior side of the triangle is the posterosuperior margin of the orifice of the external acoustic meatus including the **spine of Henle**, and lies approximately along the course of the descending part of the canal for the facial nerve. The posterior side is formed by a vertical line that is a tangent to the posterior margin of the meatal orifice. The cortex of the mastoid is removed with the drill or a broad gouge and hammer, including the outer wall of the tympanic antrum. This is done by enlarging the opening in the mastoid immediately above and behind the meatus leaving the cortical wall of the bony meatus intact. The complete operation results in a triangular shape of bony removal with the transverse/sigmoid sinus exposed posteriorly and inferiorly, the dura of the middle fossa above and the bony meatus and the lateral semicircular canal anteriorly (see Figure 11.20, previous page).

The mastoid tip should be included in the de-roofing. Pus is sent for culture. Digital pressure at the upper and lower end of the exposed transverse sinus will help demonstrate its patency. All of this clearly requires experience and some knowledge of the temporal bone anatomy. The inexperienced surgeon may have to be satisfied with a partial mastoidectomy with decortication of the exposed mastoid and breakdown of mastoid air cells containing pus with particular attention being paid to the Macewen's triangle de-roofing and avoidance of the structures at the margins of the bony removal. This will prevent damage to surrounding structures but may not clear all infection.

The dura of the middle cranial fossa and the transverse/sigmoid venous sinus may be seen, and if a hole in the venous sinus is made it is controlled with a muscle patch or Surgicel, with overlying gauze and digital pressure until the bleeding stops. Do not pack the venous sinus tightly with bone wax or large quantities of muscle or Gelfoam as this may occlude the sinus and cause secondary cerebral swelling. The cavity is drained with a corrugated drain and the skin is closed. The external ear is then cleared of debris and pus.

Mastoiditis in a child is often simpler to deal with than in adults because the pus tends to come to the surface through thin bone or the petrosquamous suture. The operation can often be limited as a result.

Complications of surgery

Injury to the facial nerve, middle ear structures, labyrinth, and lateral venous sinus, CSF fistula, and meatal stenosis.

Case report

A 10-year-old boy presented with generalized seizures and was in a coma when he arrived in the emergency department of the Port Moresby General Hospital. He was febrile and had obvious pus exuding from his left external auditory canal. An urgent CT head scan was obtained and showed a large mass lesion centred in the left temporal region extending upwards. It had an enhancing wall and was clearly a large cerebral abscess. Intravenous anticonvulsants and antibiotics were administered.

The boy was taken urgently to the operating theatre where a temporal burr hole was performed and copious pus aspirated. A left mastoidectomy was then performed and the middle ear was cleared of pus. Postoperatively, he gradually improved. Note: Patients can deteriorate very rapidly with a brain abscess and therefore draining a cerebral abscess is a surgical emergency (Figure 11.21, next page).

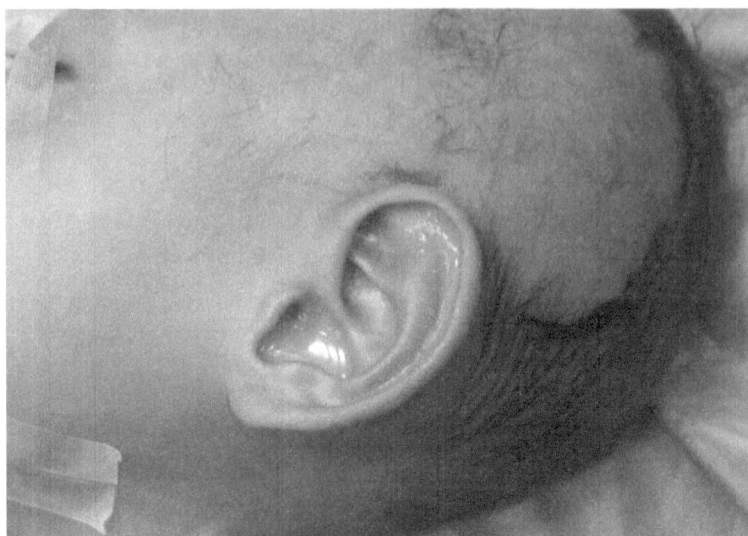

Figure 11.21 (a) The scalp is shaved ready for the temporal burr hole. Note the pus exuding from the left ear.

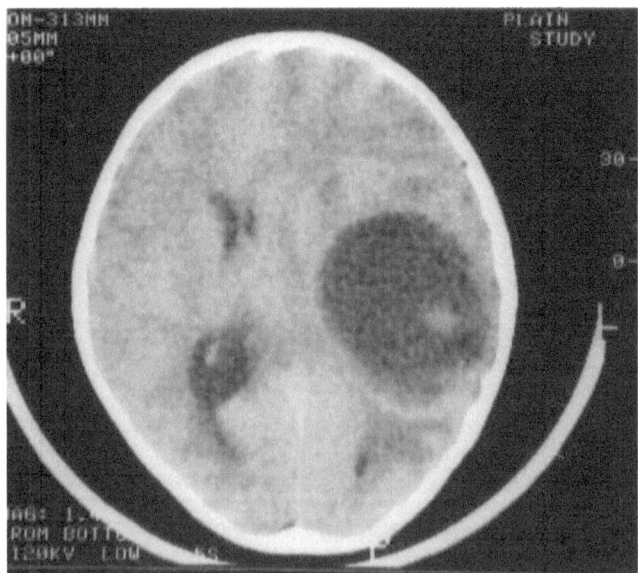

(b) CT scan without contrast showing a large mass lesion in the left temporal region.

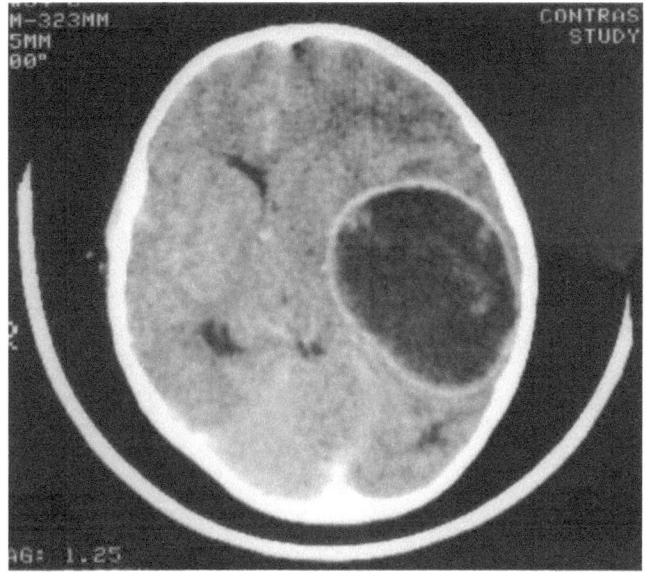

(c) CT scan with contrast showing enhancement in the wall of the abscess.

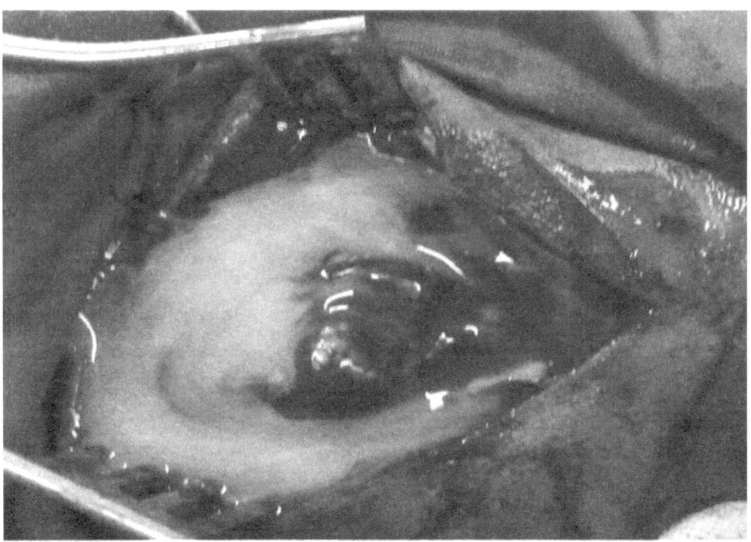

(d) The temporal burr hole has been performed and copious pus is spontaneously exuding from the small opening in the cortex which was used to aspirate the abscess.

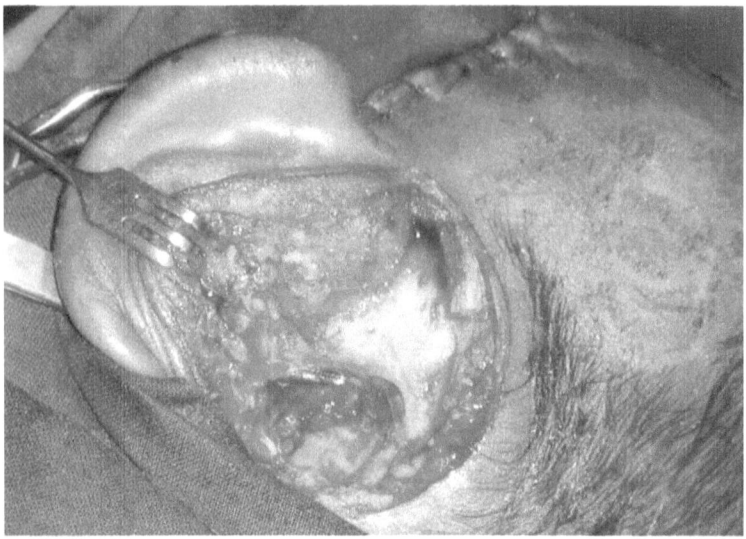

(e) Mastoidectomy. Note the exposure of the mastoid bone and the cavity created following mastoidectomy.

Figure 11.21 (a-e) Mastoidectomy and temporal lobe abscess drainage via burr hole.

Osteomyelitis of the skull

Osteomyelitis may develop from an open fracture, from sinusitis spreading into the adjacent bone, or from metastatic infection. There is usually a tender inflamed thickened oedematous scalp overlying the infection. The patient has toxaemia and is febrile. Skull X-ray shows a moth-eaten erosion of the bone, and perhaps evidence of adjacent sinus opacification. The operative treatment is urgent and involves exposing the infected bone, draining any subgaleal infection, removing any foreign material from a previously open fracture, removing dead and infected bone back to normal vascular bone using rongeurs.

This may mean removing large areas of bone. Any epidural abscess is drained and the scalp closed. Secondary repair of the bony defect will be required. Intravenous antibiotics are indicated, in the perioperative period and for up to 6 weeks after operation, depending on the nature of the organism cultured. Any sinusitis is treated on its merits and is treated at the same time as the skull debridement.

APPENDICES (FIGURE 11.22, PAGE 616 AND FIGURE 11.36, PAGE 626)

1. Operating room equipment requirements

In addition to a general set of instruments, certain special instruments will be required. Instruments marked with an asterisk are essential for cranial or spinal surgery.

- Sharp periosteal elevator - to strip periosteum on the outside of the skull
- Smooth periosteal elevator - to strip periosteum on the inside of the skull
- Adson toothed forceps - to hold dura
- Bayonet forceps - non-toothed forceps to diathermy bleeding points and manipulate tissue. The unipolar diathermy is touched against forceps while it grasps the bleeding vessel. The bayonet allows the line of sight along the instrument without the fingers getting in the way.
- Bailey (De Martel) Guide x 4 - to pass the Gigli saw under the bone
- Gigli saw blades x 10 (disposable) - to cut the bone flap
- Gigli saw handles - used to hold the Gigli saw at each end
- Bone rongeurs:
  single action - Adson, Beyer - used to remove bone
  double action - Echlin, Beyer - used to remove bone. Very helpful in spinal surgery such as laminectomy
- Gardner-Wells skull tongs - to attach to the skull for cervical traction and immobilisation of cervical spine fracture
- Dandy scissors - for cutting small deep structures. These are curved to preserve the line of sight.
- Rhoton suckers:
  8 cm 7 Fr, 8 cm 10 Fr
  10 cm 7 Fr, 10 cm 10 Fr] suckers with a gentle bulbous tip to use on and in the brain.
- Bipolar forceps 1-1.5 mm tip - bayonets the most useful.
- Bunnell hand drill or dental drill, including fine drills and burrs for drilling holes in the bone edge to fix the bone
- Hudson brace - to hold the perforator and the burr
- Hudson extension - for posterior fossa burr holes
- Triangular shaped perforator and conical burr. Large and small sizes are helpful depending on the age of the patient. Spherical shaped burrs can also be used. The perforator - cuts the conical

opening of the burr hole. The Conical burr converts the opening in to a cylindrical burr hole.

- Penfield dissector No. 3 - to lift dura away from inner table.
- Self-retaining retractors for cranial and spinal operations are required
- Needle holders
- Scalpel blades and holders
- Standard suckers
- Scalpel blades (23, 11, 15) and holders
- Self-retaining retractors for cranial and spinal surgery
- Needle holders: large and small
- Blunt hook - to dissect in and around small spaces: e.g. nerve root in canal
- Sharp hook - to tent up a membrane: e.g. dura or arachnoid or for fine sharp dissection.
- Malis bipolar machine
- Crile class haemostatic forceps x 20
- Dandy haemostatic forceps x 20 - to turn back galea and obtain scalp haemostasis
- Malleable brain retractor - to elevate or retract the bra in
- Nerve root retractor - Krayenbuhl - to retract spinal nerve roots
- Brain needle – to pass into the ventricle or other fluid-filled space in the brain.
- Punch - Kerrison rongeur – 2 mm, 3 mm, 4 mm – to remove small amounts of overhanging bone egde without damage to underlying structures.
- Fibreoptic headlight - very helpful for seeing into deep recesses
- Raney clip applicator and Raney clips (plastic disposable) - apply to scalp for haemostasis (Omni Medical Designs, Livonia, Michigan, USA).

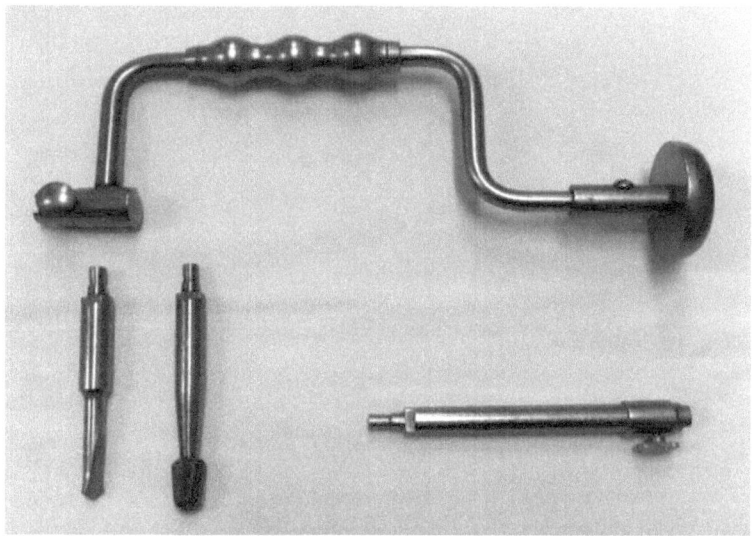

Figure 11.22 Hudson brace with small and large sized perforators and conical burrs. The extension for posterior fossa surgery is also shown.

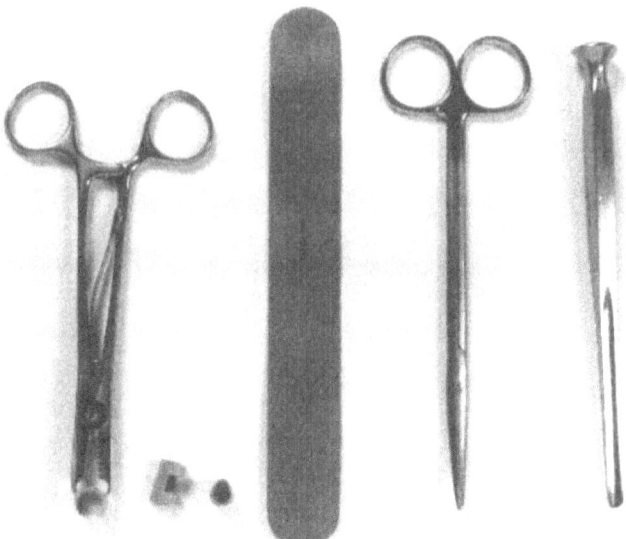

Figure 11.23 From left to right: Raney scalp clip applicator for haemostasis on edge of scalp. These Raney clips are plastic (Omni Medical Designs, Livonia, Michigan, USA). Malleable brain strip retractor. Metzenbaum dissecting scissors. Bone gouge (bone curettes are also useful but are not shown).

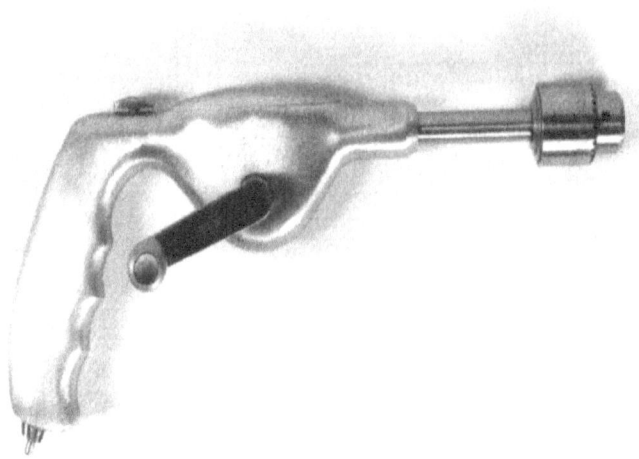

Figure 11.23 *(Continued)* Bunnell hand drill for drilling small holes in the bone, e.g. for anchoring craniotomy flap.

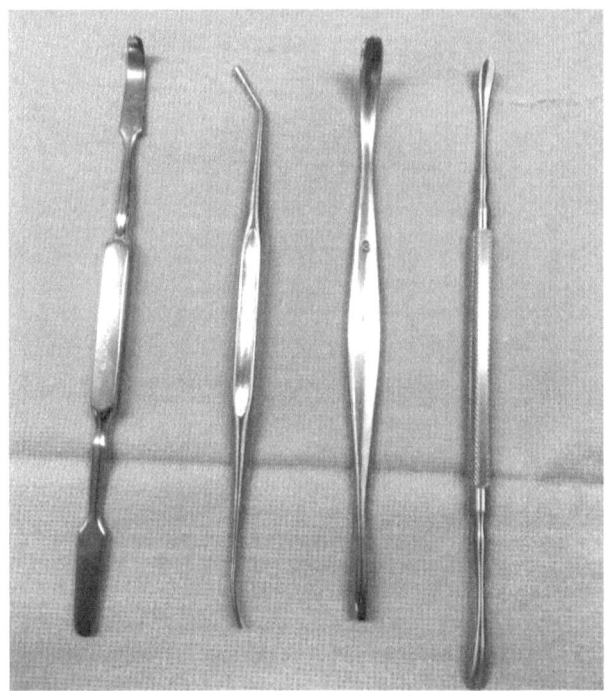

Figure 11.24 Various dissectors. From left to right: Macdonald's, Watson-Cheyne, Penfield number 3, Freer's.

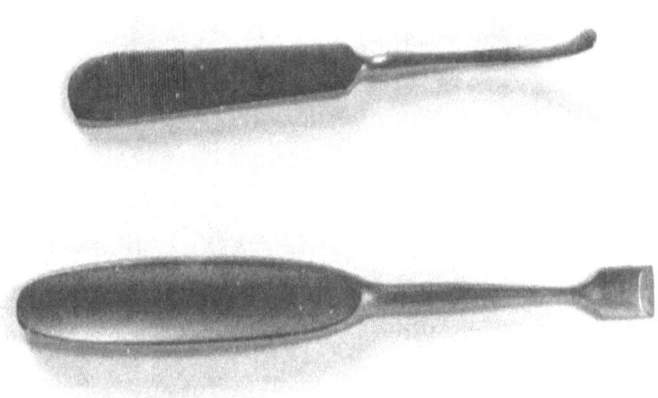

Figure 11.25 Smooth periosteal elevator (upper). Sharp periosteal elevator (McKissock spade) (lower).

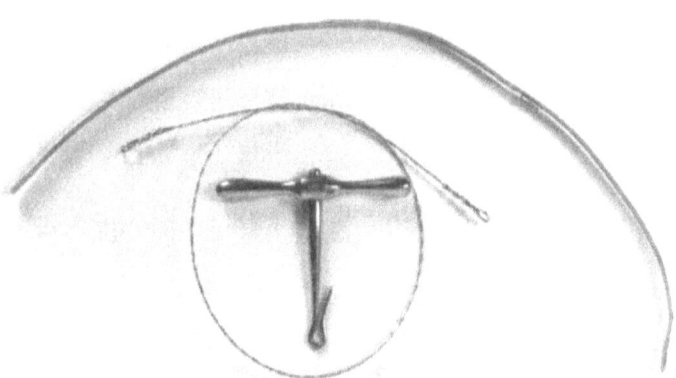

Figure 11.26 Gigli saw with saw blade and one hook shown. The set comes with two hooks which are attached to the loops at either end of the saw blade and the dural guide is used to draw the saw blade through between the burr holes. The loop at the end of the saw blade attaches to the small hook on the dural guide.

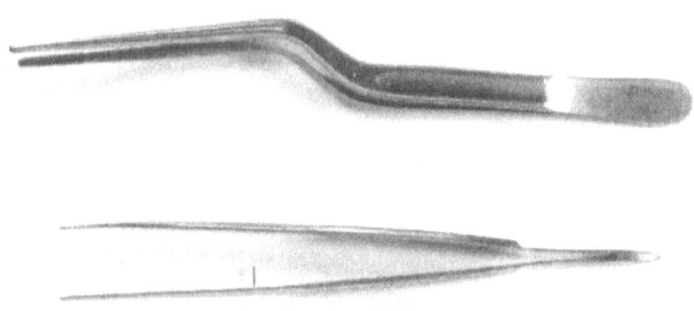

Figure 11.27 Bayonetted dissecting forceps (upper) and plain fine dissecting forceps (below). Toothed forceps (fine Adson or Gillies type and heavy toothed forceps are not shown).

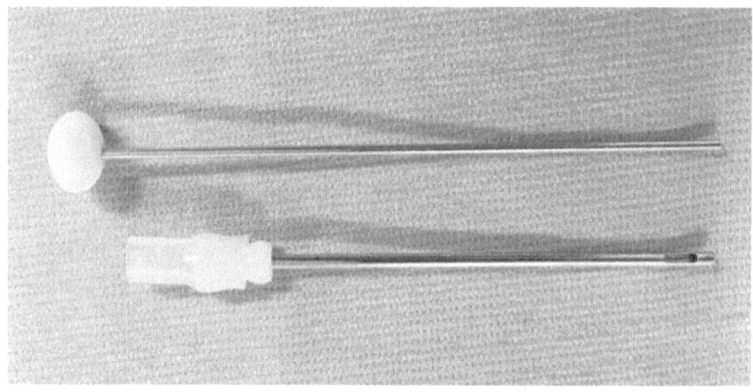

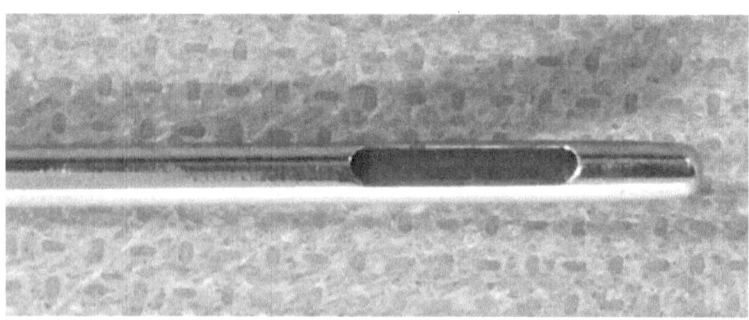

Figure 11.28 (a-b) Brain needle with stillette. Note the smooth curved tip and the side port for aspiration.

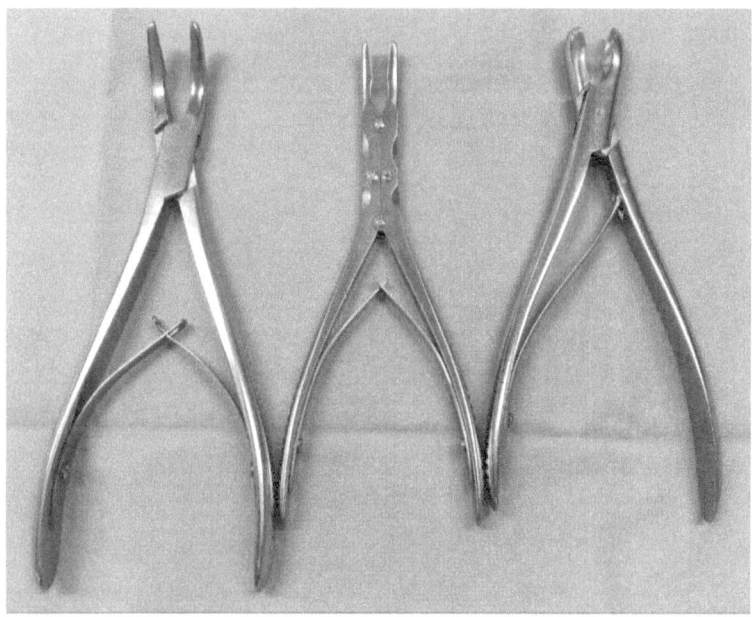

Figure 11.29 Bone rongeurs of various types (narrow and wide blades).

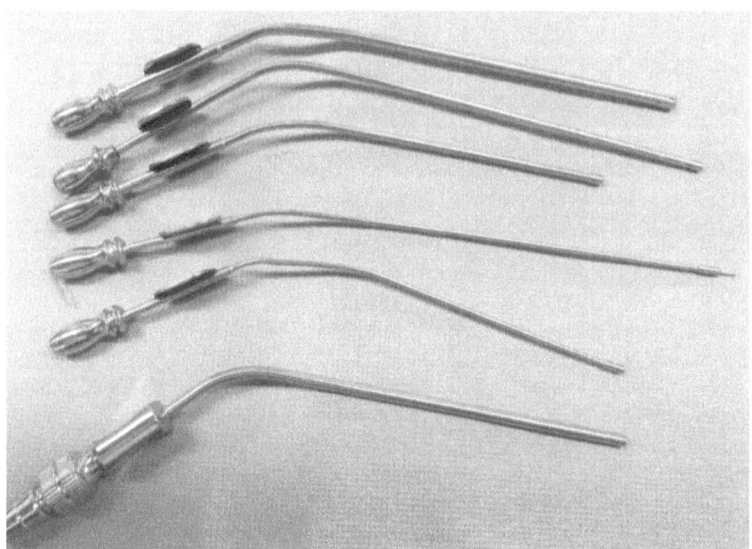

Figure 11.30 (a)

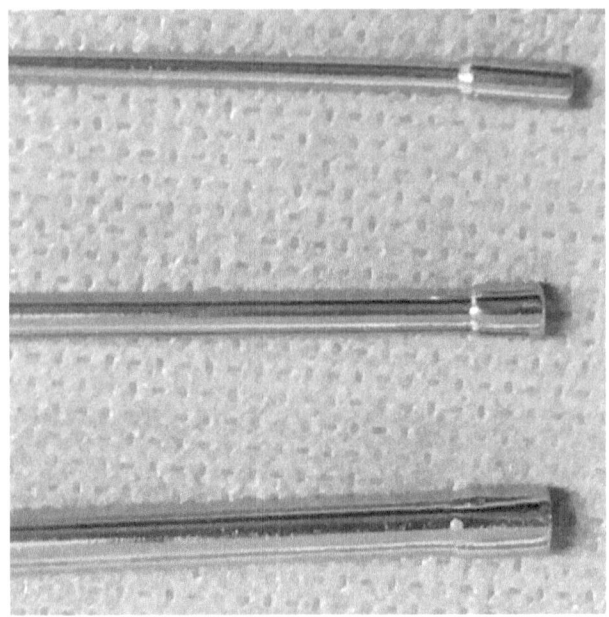

(b)

Figure 11.30 (a-b) *(Continued)* Suckers. a. Standard wide bore neurosurgical sucker lowest in the photograph. All the others are Rhoton micro-suckers with bulbous smooth tips. These come in varying sizes from 5 Fr to 10 Fr short and long length. b. Enlarged Rhoton sucker tips.

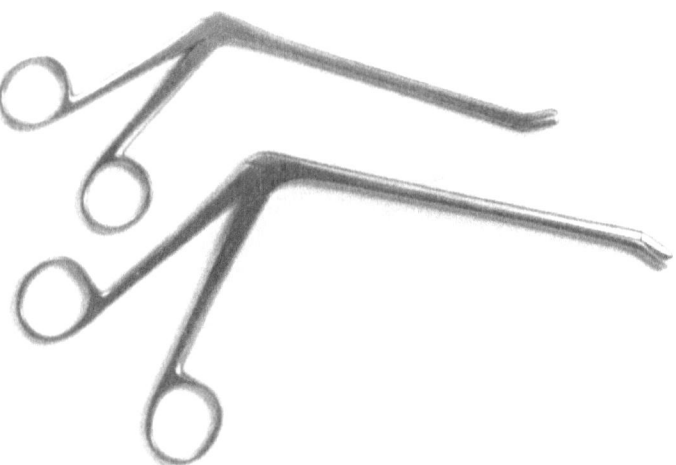

Figure 11.31 Tumour (pituitary) rongeurs of varying angle (straight not shown) for grasping and removing pieces of tissue, particularly disc material and to take biopsies of brain tumours at craniotomy.

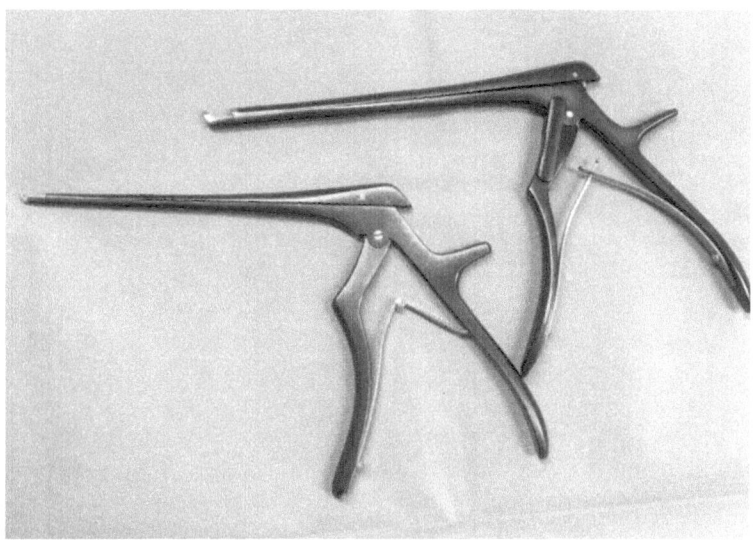

Figure 11.32 (a) Angled bone punches of varying size (2 mm, 4 mm), (Kerrison or Cloward). These are used to precisely remove small pieces of bone without injuring underlying structures such as a nerve root during spinal surgery.

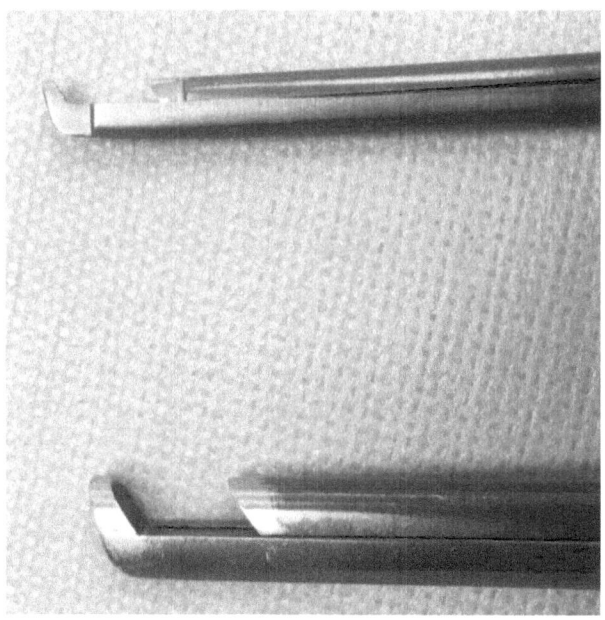

(b) Enlarged view of the instrument tips.

Figure 11.32 (a-b)

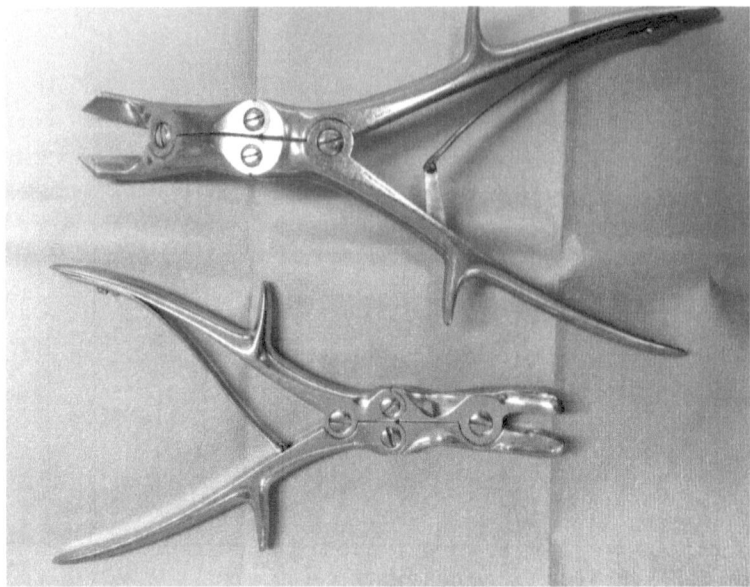

Figure 11.33 Double action bone shears (on the top) for removing spinous processes. Double action rongeurs (on the bottom) for removing bone in a laminectomy procedure.

2. Power tools

These will make neurosurgical exposure much easier but are not essential. Midas Rex craniotome (Medtronic) - uses electricity - used to cut bone flaps. The matchstick head burr is used for drilling burr holes and shaving bone. Spherical cutting burrs are also available in various sizes for this purpose.

The foot plate attachment with a cutting blade form the craniotome for cutting the bone flap. A space between the dura and the bone needs to be developed to insert the footplate so that the dura is not torn. Alternatives to the electric craniotome are the Codman craniotome - uses compressed air and the Osteon drill (Zimmer) - uses compressed air. These instruments are also used to cut, burr or drill bone.

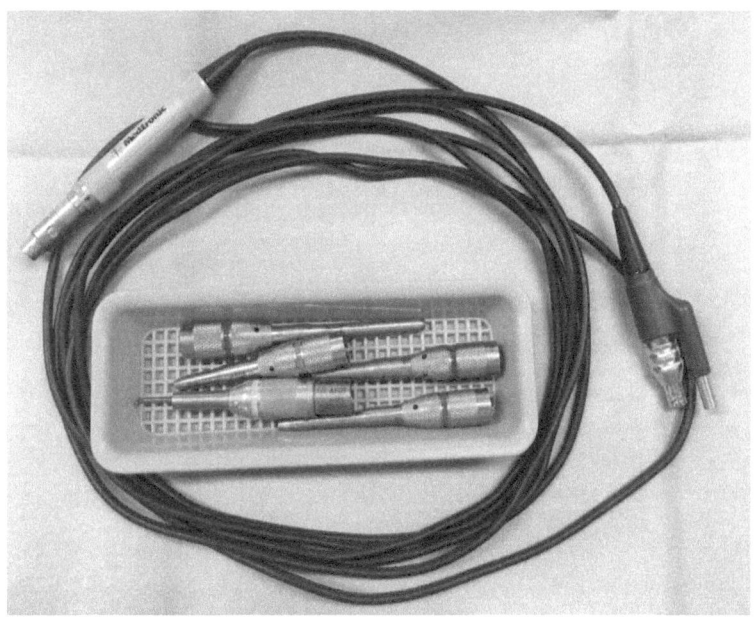

Figure 11.34 (a)

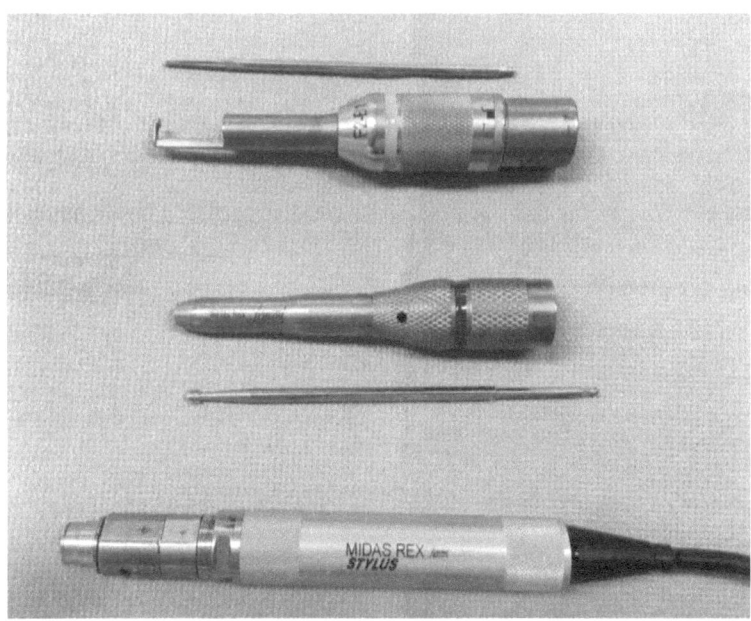

(b)

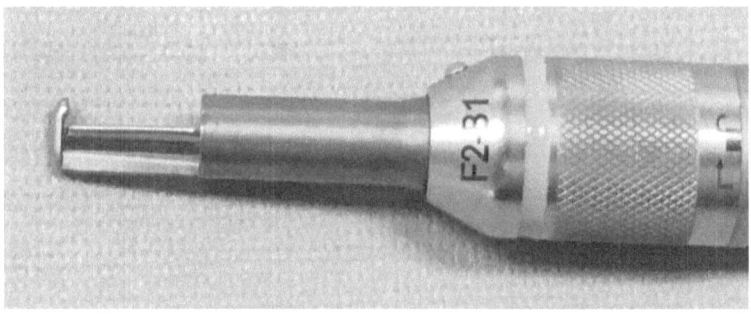

(c)

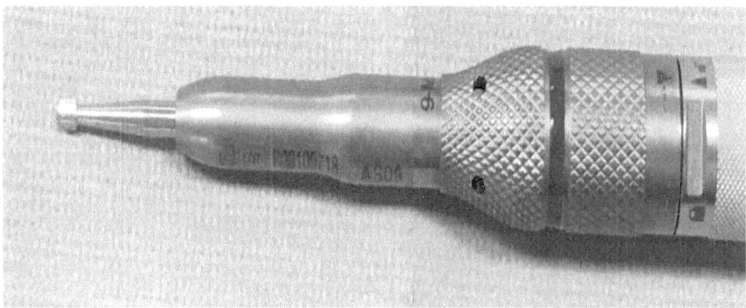

(d)

Figure 11.34 (a-d) Midas Rex craniotome (Medtronic) - electric - is used to cut bone flaps. Note the matchstick head burr for drilling burr holes and shaving bone. Spherical cutting burrs are also available in various sizes. Note also the foot plate attachment and the cutting blade which forms the craniotome for cutting the craniotomy flap. A space between the dura and the bone needs to be developed to insert the footplate so that the dura is not torn.

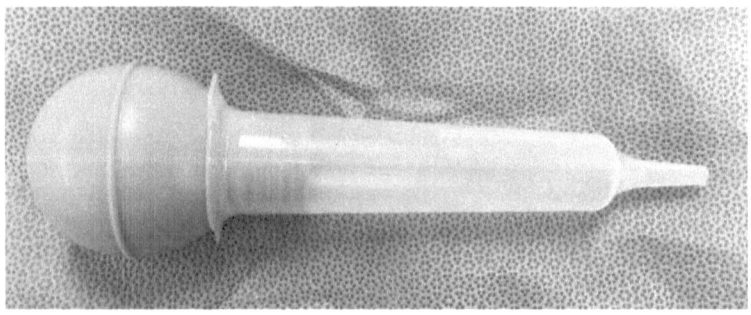

Figure 11.35 Dakin syringe (CR Bard Inc, Covington, GA, USA). Filled with warm saline or Ringer's solution to irrigate the operative field.

625

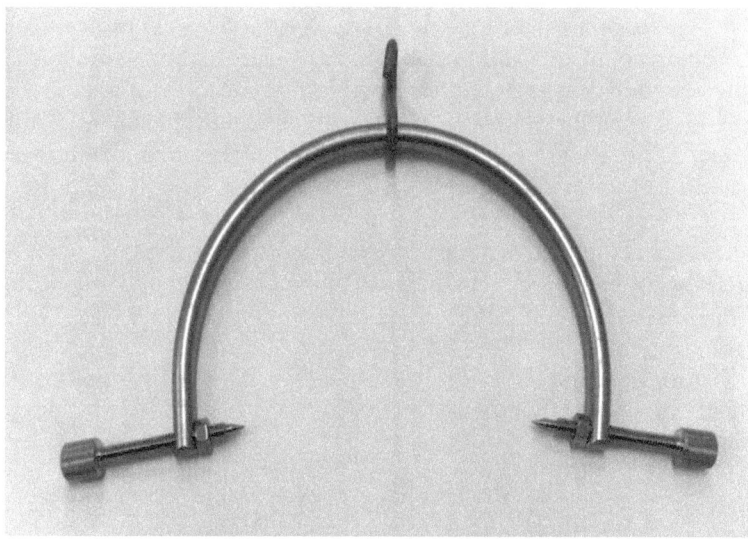

Figure 11.36 Gardner-Wells skull clamp for cervical spine skeletal traction.

3. Haemostatic agents

Very few bleeding points in neurosurgery can be ligated, so many alternative techniques and agents have been employed.

Diathermy It is possible to do many neurosurgical procedures with standard diathermy, but bipolar diathermy will be advantageous, particularly at stopping bleeding in the brain itself. The standard diathermy tends to char widely and stick on the brain, which does not quell the haemorrhage when the forceps is removed, and may make it worse.

Surgicel (Johnson & Johnson) is cellulose mesh and is very useful to stop haemorrhage on moist surfaces. It is left in situ.

Gelfoam (The Upjohn Company) is a gelatin sponge and is used to fill dead space and act as a buttress to quell haemorrhage: e.g. placed between the dura and the bone edge and held in place with sutures. It is not directly haemostatic.

Avitene sponge (Alcon (Puerto Rico) Inc) is a fibrillary material made of collagen and is very effective at stopping haemorrhagic ooze.

Topical thrombin (Parke Davis Pty Ltd) is thrombin in liquid form prepared just before use, from a powder in the ampoule · it is then injected or sprayed onto the oozing surface. Small pledgets of Gelfoam, approximately 4 x 4 x 1 mm, fully immersed in the thrombin can be placed in the bleeding space and held with a patty.

Cottonoids (patty's and Linteen strips) are flat squares and long rectangular strips of matted cotton to which strings are attached, so that they can easily be retrieved from deep spaces. These are placed on the brain to protect it against the trauma of instruments abrading its surface end passage, and are placed over bleeding points and compressed over the area with a Surgicel or thrombin soaked Gelfoam pledger. If these are not available, wet gauze can be placed over the brain and kept moist, as an alternative.

Bone wax (Ethicon Ltd). Invented by Sir Victor Horsley in 1890s. Valuable in stopping continued ooze from cancellous bone. It is impacted on the cut face of the bone using the surgeon's index finger interposed with gauze or a smooth periosteal elevator, or Watson-Cheyne dissector.

Titanium clips (Weck, Ligaclips) are useful to clip dural or cerebral vessels particularly if deeply placed or if diathermy is unavailable.

Irrigation fluid. Ringer's solution is preferable because it is most physiological, but saline can be used if Ringer's is unavailable. The brain or spinal cord and neural structures should be kept moist during operative procedure. The fluid is irrigated through a chip syringe or a Dakin syringe - plastic disposable Dakin syringes are available, (C. R. Bard Inc., Covington, Georgia 30014, USA). An ordinary plastic syringe will suffice, if the above are not available. Do not irrigate the brain directly with penicillin solution because it is highly epileptogenic.

4. Equipment supply

Shunt products are very expensive if purchased in the West. There are cheaper shunts available from India and Japan. The Chhabra shunt costs less than 5000 rupees which converts to under $75US depending on the exchange rate.[69] The Phycon shunt valve system from Fuji is an alternative.

---

[69]*http://www.surgiwear.co.in/neurosurgery/implants-1/hydrocephalus-shunt-systems/chhabra-slit-n-spring/chhabra-slit-n-spring-hydrocephalus-shunt-system-vp.html*

Neuro-rehabilitation and medicolegal issues

L.R. Atkinson & J.V. Rosenfeld

INTRODUCTION

The goal of this chapter is to present the scope of rehabilitation for patients with neurological damage, with an emphasis on the provision of rehabilitation within communities disadvantaged through geographical isolation or through a lack of facilities and resources.

The brain, the spinal cord and the peripheral nerves may be damaged by trauma, infection, vascular accidents and birth injuries. The tissue repair and the ultimate patient recovery is much slower than with other tissue injury such as skin and even bone. Recovery is related to the age of the patient; with increasing age the chance of a full recovery decreases. Previous injury, nutritional state, drug abuse, alcoholism also may modify recovery patterns. When the nervous tissue is damaged, repair and recovery pass through 90 per cent of the process in the first 6 months but recovery will continue on for up to 2 years.

Rehabilitation enables the patient with disabilities to reach their full potential, by minimising disability, and training them to master their disability. Good rehabilitation is also aimed at the early detection and treatment of delayed complications following the initial illness. Rehabilitation and spinal injury centres are usually non-existent in the developing world. The primary physician, in the broad sense, will be required to initiate a rehabilitation programme while the patient is still an inpatient, secure the necessary prostheses or aids to daily living, and instruct the patient and their relatives and family in their use. A physiotherapist, if available, will be of great value in developing and implementing the rehabilitation plan. Rehabilitation is a much-neglected facet of patient care in the developing world and with some thought and planning, can go a long way towards making the life of a crippled or otherwise disabled patient more tolerable and enjoyable. The goal of rehabilitation should be for the patient to regain as much independence as possible. The old adage 'use it or lose it' is a good philosophy to practise in order to maintain function in the disabled patient at any age.

The patient may need to relearn to do some daily tasks that were previously simple and automatic, e.g. transferring, washing, eating, toileting, walking and even the balance required for sitting. The patient's family must become an integral part of the rehabilitation treatment, and are usually very keen to do all they can to help their disabled kin. They should be trained to carry out basic physiotherapy procedures and help the patient in the mobilisation process and with activities of daily living. The family carers need much support to cope with their new role. Simple modifications to the home environment can have a significant impact on the patient's activity and ease of living and the family can assist in implementing these changes. Cultural beliefs and practices also need to be considered. The rehabilitation goals for a woman may be seen to be different from those of men and great sensitivity will be required to steer a diplomatic and fair course when these issues surface.

Table 12.1 Definitions.

Rehabilitation might be defined as the development of the person's fullest physical, psychological, social, vocational and educational potential consistent with his or her physiological and anatomical impairment and environment limitations

Impairment is the loss or an abnormality of psychological, physiological or anatomical structure or function (WHO 1980)

A disability is any restriction or lack (resulting from the impairment) of the ability to perform an activity in the manner or within the range consistent with the normal for a human being (WHO 1980)

A handicap is a disadvantage for an individual resulting from an impairment or the disability that limits the fulfilment of the role that is normal depending on the age, sex, social and cultural factors for that individual (WHO 1980). A handicap involves orientation, physical dependence, mobility, occupation, social integration and economic self-sufficiency.

THE REHABILITATION PROCESS

A detailed physical and mental assessment should be performed as a baseline and an individualised rehabilitation plan should be devised which includes a daily treatment schedule and realistic goals to be set. The physician and other therapists should have a regular weekly conference to discuss the progress to date and formulate an ongoing plan. The expected response to therapy and the predicted prognosis should be discussed with the family and preferably with the patient, if they can comprehend. Do not give a definite prognosis to the patient and family until there has been time to assess the recovery trend. This may take a week or two. Try and ascertain the patient's wishes for the extent of therapy to be administered. The initial assessment for the rehabilitation needs is presented in Table 12.2.

Table 12.2 The initial rehabilitation assessment.

- Premorbid level of function (information obtained from the relatives)
- Full general and neurological examination
- Determine the extent of physical disability and likely prognosis
- The motivation of the patient
- Level of function with the activities of daily living
- Examination for cognitive, behavioural, and affective (mood) problems
- Can the hospital meet the rehabilitation requirements?
- What support is available from the relatives?
- Community support available including education and retraining
- The home environment including the geographical layout and the social and cultural influences
- Current and future drug requirements

PREVENTION OF COMPLICATIONS

Prevention of complications commences as soon as the patient is admitted. The patient, if able, and their relatives need instructions in what to do. Attention to the following is recommended:

- General nutrition is provided with a full balanced diet or early nasogastric feeding of vitamised or crushed food if commercial preparations are unavailable.
- Early mobilisation as soon as practicable.
- Active daily exercise of a weak limb will help to maintain or build its strength and prevent joint stiffness and muscle wasting.
- Pressure care, with frequent and regular turning and early attention to pressure sores. The scalp in the occipital area is particularly susceptible to pressure necrosis in a comatose patient lying supine directly on the back of the head for many days.
- Chest physiotherapy with encouragement to deep breathing and coughing.
- Moving the paralysed limbs through the full range of motion to prevent or minimise contractures.
- Splinting of the floppy paralysed limb.
- Keeping urine and faeces away from the skin.
- The patient should be given the appropriate walking aids to prevent falls and instructed in their use.

NEUROTRAUMA REHABILITATION

The severity of this traumatic brain injury (TBI) is measured by the Glasgow Coma Scale, the period of posttraumatic amnesia and by the CT scan if available. The period of posttraumatic amnesia shows a consistent relationship with the degree of organic brain damage. Most recovery occurs in the first 6 months following a head injury.

The Glasgow Outcome Scale is a simple and standard measure of outcome. This has five levels:

1. Good outcome
2. Moderate disability with patient independence
3. Severe disability resulting in a loss of independent function
4. Vegetative
5. Dead.

The rehabilitation management of the patient with traumatic brain injury may be considered in four stages and commences from the day of admission.

Stage 1: The neurosurgical stage

Following injury, the patient needs retrieval and resuscitation. Improved outcomes have resulted from the Early Management of Severe Trauma (EMST) and the Advanced Trauma Life Support (ATLS) programmes that minimise the effects of hypotension, hypercapnia and poor oxygenation. This stage includes the management of coma in the intensive care unit. Improved long-term results have been obtained with intubation, ventilation and intracranial pressure monitoring in these patients. In this stage the care of the tracheostomy tube and splinting of limbs is an initial part of the rehabilitation. Effective long-term rehabilitation often depends on an early explanation, counselling and support for the patient's family. The Glasgow Outcome Scale and the Glasgow Coma Scale are useful indications of outcome, even at this stage.

Stage 2: The stage of clouded consciousness

The patient with a traumatic brain injury may take days or weeks to pass through this stage. The severe TBI patient may remain comatose and enter the persistent vegetative state (see Chapter 9). In Stage 2, the patient still has post-traumatic amnesia (PTA). A simple set of questions gives an indication of memory and orientation.

- What is your name?
- Which city is this?
- What is today's date?
- What month is it?
- What year is it?
- When is your birthday?
- How old are you?
- What is the name of an important person the patient would be familiar with, e.g. local politician, or media personality?

Further tests are the **Mental Status Quotient (MSQ)** or **Folstein Mini Mental Status Examination (MMSE)** (see Appendix 7, page 661) which has a scale of 0 to 30 and is of particular value in evaluating patients in this stage.

This is a very taxing stage for the nursing and allied health staff. It is stressful for the relatives. In this stage the patient may be drowsy, apathetic and relatively immobile; alternatively, the patient may be restless, noisy, agitated and incontinent. He or she may need restraint and this will need to be explained to the relatives to indicate that this is a positive sign of recovery. Towards the end of Stage 2 the rehabilitation process will require the removal of any tracheostomy. The patient is likely to have a slowness in swallowing. The oral diet at this stage needs to be thickened up and feeding may require careful supervision. The MSQ test and the MMSE are useful indicators of a return of continuous memory.

Stage 3: Once the posttraumatic amnesia settles, the tracheostomy tube is removed, and continence returns, the effect of rehabilitation will become more rewarding. The patient should now be back on a normal diet. In ideal circumstances - usually 3-6 weeks after a severe head injury - the patient is transferred to a rehabilitation facility supported by physiotherapy, occupational therapy, speech therapy and nursing staff. These facilities are not accessible in the developing world, so it is important that each hospital has a 'rehabilitation signpost' in which one healthcare individual is identified as the resource person for rehabilitation.

The patient will require a stepwise mobilisation, with initial lifting of the patient from the bed to a chair. This is followed with assisted transfers to the chair, assisted standing, walking with assistance and then independently. The patient is then directed towards a course of independent self-care. Emphasis is placed on establishing personal hygiene practices such as shaving, dressing and toileting.

The Rappaport Disability Rating Scale

See Appendix 8, page 662 for the full scale.

The Rappaport scale is an instrument for assessing quantitatively the disability of severe head injuries so that the patient's progress in rehabilitation can be followed through different levels of awareness and functioning to their return to the community.
1. The scale reflects changes in four categories:
2. Levels of arousal and awareness (as in The Glasgow Coma Scale).
3. The cognitive ability to deal with self-care.
4. The degree of physical dependence on others.
5. Psychological adaptability reflected in the ability to return to useful work, school or previous household functioning.

Scores are given for eight items that are within the above four categories. Rating of these items ranges from no ability to complete ability, with the lowest score indicating the highest level of ability (inverted scores).

Advantages of the Disability Rating Scale

The scale takes into account the reacquisition of cognitive function, the level of independence in activities of daily living, and social factors, i.e. employability. The scale therefore provides a sensitive index of a patient's physical, cognitive and social status.

- It can be used in the very early stages of head injury as well as long after discharge.
- It is sensitive to slight changes in the patient's condition over time, therefore
- is a good scale to use for long-term follow-up.
- It is easily learned and can be completed quickly.
- Reliability between users of the scale is high.
- Proven validity in reflecting the degree of clinical impairment in severely head-injured patient.
- Proven independent validity as it is significantly related to neurophysiological measures of brain dysfunction.

Once the patient has reached the independent self-care level, discharge to a day hospital service is a realistic option. The emphasis of therapy is on extended periods of daily living including the return for a patient to cooking, cleaning, domestic work, using public transport, money management and shopping.

Stage 4: The final stage is a return to employment or previous lifestyle. **Neuropsychological deficit** may improve over the first 2 years but usually remains unaltered after this. Most patients with moderate to severe head injury are young and therefore physical and psychological deficits may endure for many years. The adverse psychosocial sequelae of head injury are common and affect motivation, planning, foresight, judgement and impulse control. There may also be an alteration of mood with secondary depression. The cognitive deficits also need to be considered and include short- and long-term memory, language function, concentration, visual perception, visuomotor skills, planning and organisation of thoughts and comprehension. Any of these mental disturbances will interfere with the ability of the patient to cooperate with the rehabilitation programme. Be careful to differentiate dysphasia from a confusional state. The **Folstein Mini-Mental State examination** can be done in about 10 minutes (see Appendix 7, page 661). A score below 22 indicates a significant cognitive problem. Note that the patient needs to be literate to be able to complete the testing. **The Racho Los Amigos Cognitive Scale** is also a useful measure of cognitive impairment (see Appendix 9, page 663).

Physical deficits and the activities of daily living

The presence of a weak limb or hemiparesis may be compounded by a cerebellar ataxia interfering further with balance, visual field loss or neglect, dysphasia interfering with comprehension of instructions or self-expression, or parietal lobe dysfunction causing disorientation, sensory neglect, or dyspraxia in the affected limbs. The activities of daily living should be assessed in detail and include dressing, grooming, washing, eating, control over bladder and bowel function, getting on and off chairs or the toilet, and walking or using a wheelchair. Built up seats or toilet seats can be very helpful for the patient who does not have the strength or control to cope with standard seats.

Relatives

At all stages the relatives need to be given education, answers to questions, advice on future prognosis and discharge planning. Even in hospitals with limited facilities it is important to establish a health care professional who is responsible for rehabilitation. This person can then develop links with community facilities and community agencies and guide the TBI patient back to the family and to a degree of independent living.

Behavioural changes

Long-term behavioural changes are common in TBI patients, particularly those with a low Glasgow Coma Score on presentation. Minimal behavioural change is seen in the postconcussional syndrome where the patients complain of headaches, dizziness, fatigue, blurred vision and poor concentration. Most settle in 3 months but one percent remain symptomatic after a year. More severe behavioural complications include irritability, slowness of thought processes, excess fatiguability, perseveration (the repetition of meaningless words and phrases), sleep disorders, a reduced sex drive, and reactive anxiety/depression. Damage to the frontal lobes of the brain may result in a frontal lobe syndrome in which the executive functions of the brain are particularly affected. These include expressions of language, empathy for others, planning complex activities, a lack of problem solving, and an impairment of the ability to anticipate the consequences of actions. There may be a degree of denial and some patients are disinhibited. The patient may maintain a high intelligence but still be unemployable. On discharge they prove to be vulnerable, particularly as they seem to be physically normal. They are prone to antisocial behaviour. They may become socially rejected and isolated. They place large pressures on their families as a result of their domestic behaviour. Families and the patient need considerable support and explanation.

The cranial nerves

Injury of the cranial nerves may complicate recovery in the traumatic brain injured patient. The olfactory nerve is the most often injured. However, the loss of smell and the associated impairment of taste is slowly recognised and of minimal long-term impact. A direct injury to the optic nerve results in a permanent impairment. However, often the optic tracts are damaged by deep haemorrhages causing visual field impairments, which need to be defined with visual field assessments. This assessment may help during the patient's return to independent living.

Damage to the third, fourth and sixth cranial nerves can cause annoying diplopia. However, recovery usually occurs over 6 months, although the third nerve is less likely to recover. Ophthalmological intervention may modify the diplopia if it persists. When the fifth cranial nerve is damaged the most troublesome problem is numbness over the face and corneal sensory loss. This may recover slowly, but a temporary tarsorrhaphy may be indicated if keratitis or corneal ulceration is developing.

Deafness due to a sensory neural injury in association with a temporal bone fracture is unlikely to recover, although on occasions the patient has a conductive deafness resulting from a dislocation of the ossicles, and a surgical reconstruction is possible, with a return of hearing. Damage to the ninth to twelfth cranial nerves is uncommon.

Use of the Disability Rating Scale at Princess Alexandra Hospital, Brisbane, Australia

The Disability Rating Scale was introduced to the Princess Alexandra Hospital Head Injury Unit in Brisbane, Australia by the Occupational Therapists in June, 1986, in an attempt to monitor improvements in patients. It was seen as a highly sensitive scale for rating change in all aspects of recovery. It has since proved to be an extremely assistive device to Occupational Therapists, as it not only deals with a person's physical disabilities but also identifies residual deficits in cognitive status, levels of independence and employability.

These aspects often appear to be of major concern to a head injured person long after discharge. Each new patient admitted to the head injury unit is given an initial Disability Rating Scale Score. While an inpatient, progressive scores are kept on a 4-weekly basis. After discharge, patients are reviewed regularly through the Head Injury Follow-up Clinic, where scores continue to be updated. All scores have been recorded since the Disability Rating Scale was introduced and at present are being collated into a research study, dealing with the Disability Rating Scale as a predictive device.

The **Disability Rating Scale** has been accepted by the medical team at the Princess Alexandra Hospital Head injury unit. It is regarded as an excellent indicator of residual cognitive and social problems that most head injured patients experience, especially post-discharge, and also as a good indicator of improvement in the rehabilitation phase. Disability Rating Scale scores are now being reported to the team by the Occupational Therapists and are being recorded in the patient's hospital file.

Disability Rating Scale as a predictive measure

The outcome score is directly related to the patient's initial score on the Disability Rating Scale. Therefore, a patient with a high score when assessed initially, is less likely to achieve a greater level of recovery over time compared with a patient who has a lower score (ie. a less severe level of disability) initially. The features of the Disability Rating Scale are:

- It is useful in deciding when a patient has plateaued in rehabilitation, i.e. no change in score over a number of weeks.
- It is sensitive to change and improvement in the patient.
- It acknowledges the effect that cognitive and social deficits have on the overall level of disability of the patient.

REHABILITATION OF BRAIN HAEMORRHAGE OR STROKE PATIENTS

Patients who regain sitting control, continence of bowel and bladder and some return of muscle strength within the first week or two of the stroke, tend to have a better functional outcome. Visual field defects, visuospatial problems, prolonged coma, and altered mental state predict a worse functional outcome. A large haemorrhage involving the basal ganglia and ventricles causing midline shift has a worse prognosis than a more superficial bleed. Patients who are unable to sit on the edge of the bed with minimal support, with sensory neglect of one side of the body, have cognitive problems and disturbed position sense, will likely need substantial help in the longer term. The degree of improvement that occurs in the first 2 weeks is useful for predicting the long-term outcome.

PARAPLEGIA

The origin of spinal injuries includes motor vehicle accidents in almost 50 per cent, falls in 20 per cent, sport in 15 per cent and acts of violence in a further 14 per cent, although these relative percentages change in communities with fewer motor vehicle accidents or with the introduction of legislated protective measures. Males suffer 82 percent of spinal injuries. The level of the injury is the cervical in 53 per cent, thoracic in 36 per cent, lumbar in 10 per cent.

Most spinal cord injuries are irreversible. At present there is no cure for such neurological damage. Unfortunately, such injury may mainly affect young adults. A normal life expectancy may be obtained for paraplegics when best care is provided. The spinal cord injury should not be a death sentence even in populous, rural and remote communities. The aim should be to rehabilitate these patients and to move them back to their families and the community. This is possible with education and training of the patients and close carers. Any movement of the patient in the early stages must be done according to the principles outlined in Chapter 5 so as not to increase the spinal cord injury. The management of the paraplegic patient encompasses the general rehabilitation already presented but its overall unique challenges justify a separate elaboration. The neglected spinal injury patient is a sorry sight and reflects poorly on the quality of medical and nursing care in a particular hospital. The care of the paraplegic patient is demanding on nursing time with 2-hourly turns essential from an early stage of care. If the patient is left to 4-hourly turns, pressure sores develop easily, which tend to enlarge rapidly. Poor bladder care with a chronically in-dwelling catheter leads to offensive infected urine and a small contracted bladder. Chronic deep pressure sores may cause underlying suppurating joints and osteomyelitis. Joint contractures result from lack of passive limb movement and poor treatment of spasticity. Eventually chronic pyelonephritis and chronic renal failure develop followed by death. Excellent nursing care is therefore a vital component of the care of spinal injury patients. The relatives should become involved in the day-to-day care of the patient to lessen the nursing burden. A paraplegic patient will need an inpatient stay of 4-5 months.

Practice point

The paralysed spinal patient can develop pressure sores in a few hours.

The aims of treatment for the patient with traumatic paraplegia are:
1. To prevent chest infections, urinary tract infection (UTI) (with the early establishment of a reflex bladder), chronic constipation, pressure sores, joint contractures, and deep venous thrombosis.
2. Rehabilitation to a craft.
3. Maintain morale of staff, patient and their family.
4. Give encouragement and hope. Explain to the patient the likely course and plan of treatment.
5. Keep the patient well-nourished and correct anaemia, keep haemoglobin >12 g/dl.
6. Keep the patient interested and occupied, e.g. reading material.

Skin care

The absence of pain, pressure and touch sensations place skin at great risk below the level of the spinal cord damage. In turn pressure causes skin ischaemia and underlying tissue infection, which may progress to septicemia and death. Pressure sores, however, are preventable. The staff should not massage cream, soap and water over areas of bony prominences, and the use of methylated spirits on the skin is not recommended. A correct posture is important to relieve pressure and the presence of kyphosis and scoliosis increases the risk of pressure sores. Regular turning and repositioning, particularly at night, is the correct management. Second hourly turning is required, and the patient should be encouraged to roll and reposition themselves at least at 6-8-hourly intervals. It is to be remembered that skin damage may result from:

- burns from heaters, cigarettes and hot taps,
- bed problems such as irregular turns, objects in the bed and poor positioning of body parts,
- incorrect use of equipment such as cushions and urinary condoms,
- incorrect use of chairs with poor posturing and unsuitable footplate height,
- poor technique with transfers,
- poor skin hygiene,
- skin moist with urine and faeces,
- poor subcutaneous fat padding due to a poor diet,
- spasms causing friction from bedclothes,
- poorly fitting clothing,
- bad habits such as an intake of drugs, alcohol and cigarette abuse.

While in bed, pillows are placed between and under the legs, the patient is laid on a sheep's wool blanket, the underside of the heels are padded (sheep's wool is ideal for this purpose), and creases are removed from the sheets, all of which help to prevent pressure sores. Early mobilisation in a wheelchair with or without callipers on the legs should be the goal. Special care should be taken over the thin skin over the sacral area, the malleoli, the sides of knees, and the iliac crests, which are danger zones for the development of pressure sores. An incipient sore is a reddened area - once identified, it is essential to avoid any pressure at that point until the area of redness resolves. The area needs to be kept dry, clean and free from pressure and gentle massage may help.

The treatment of an established sore is regular dressings with honey, pawpaw (papaya), eusol (hypochlorite) or saline. Large sores may require transposition flaps, rotation flaps or myocutaneous grafts to heal the defect once de-sloughed.

Bladder care

The commonest cause of early death is urinary tract infection (UTI). The correct management will protect the kidneys from damage. In most cases, the patient and relatives must have a disciplined approach to intermittent catheterisation. This is practical when the bladder has the capacity of greater than 400 ml of urine. Control over the bladder is lost following spinal cord injury and voluntary control over voiding is unlikely to return. Bladder management must be directed at protecting the kidneys from damage. A catheter on continuous drainage is needed during the period of spinal shock. Intermittent self-catheterisation is the goal for future care provided the bladder has an adequate capacity of 400 ml or more. A long-term suprapubic or urethral catheter will result in infected urine with a contracted bladder.

Other complications include urinary fistula, urethral stricture, bladder stone, and ascending infection. In order to avoid these problems, the natural cycle of voiding is imitated with regular catheterisation every 4-6 hours (up to every 6-8 hours in the chronic state) using a clean catheter (e.g. a boiled Jacques catheter), preferably with gloved hands. Infection is uncommon. This intermittent catheterisation is continued until the spinal cord recovers or an automatic bladder develops at 2-3 months.

At times an anticholinergic drug such as propantheline, or amitriptyline is used to minimise bladder irritability. Weekly urine cultures are carried out in the early stages to ensure that there is no infection. As part of the follow-up, an intravenous pyelogram is carried out to check on the kidney function at annual intervals. Ultrasound may also give useful information on any enlargement of the kidneys. Cystoscopy and micturating cystourethrogram (MCU) may also supply useful information.

If available, urodynamic pressure studies are helpful to check on the bladder responses to filling. If intermittent self-catheterisation is not feasible, e.g. elderly paraplegics or quadriplegics at C6 and above, an indwelling urinary catheter is left and changed at monthly intervals. The bladder complications in the spinal cord injury patient include UTIs, bladder overdistension and bladder calculi.

Automatic bladder

When the injury is above the conus, the bladder develops the micturition reflex. Condom drainage is applied and the reflex voiding is encouraged by getting the patient to stroke the inner thigh, or penis or applying suprapubic pressure when the bladder is full. A good fluid intake of 3 litres or more a day is helpful. The training is slow. Catheterisation is continued until the residual volume is less than 75 ml. A sphincterotomy may be required if the residual volume will not reduce below 75 ml.

Isolated bladder

The bladder is independent of spinal control and emptying depends on a local reflex which is much less effective than the spinal micturition reflex. Intermittent clean catheterisation is required and the bladder is emptied each time with suprapubic pressure. Infection is caused by persistent residual urine. These catheters do not need to be sterile, but can be washed in soap and water or light disinfectant after each use and are replaced regularly, depending on availability. The urine becomes colonised with bacteria but clinical infection is uncommon. The tip of the meatus and the hands are cleaned and the female will need a small mirror. The management of a UTI is to increase the frequency of catheterisation, and administer a course of antibiotics, e.g. sulphonamides. If this fails - sterile intermittent catheterisation with topical antibiotic bladder washouts are required.

Bowel care

The rehabilitation of the paraplegic (or the quadriplegic patient) requires a long-term attention to bowel management. Following the initial spinal shock, the patient may develop paralytic ileus. An enema should be given three times per week until bowel function returns, which usually takes 3-6 weeks. Oral medications may be required 12 hours before a bowel action and a suppository or enema might be given 30 minutes before evacuation. Sitting on the toilet 15 minutes after insertion of glycerine suppositories encourages the defaecation reflex.

The aim of long-term management is to ensure regular habit of a formed bowel motion at daily or second daily intervals. To achieve this, the patient requires a well-balanced high fibre diet with a good fluid intake. The bowel can be trained provided there is a disciplined routine. Constipation and diarrhoea are common problems and a manual disimpaction may become necessary.

Muscle and joint care

Each time the patient is turned the joints of the lower limbs should be put through their full range of passive movement. Turning patterns should be established:
- Thoracolumbar injury - left then right then prone. Avoid pillows under the hips in the prone position because flexion contractures will be promoted.

- Cervical spine injury - left supine, right supine.
- Home care.
- A suitable bed, toilet, and bath are organised.
- The patient is mobilised with crutches and with calipers on legs to support the knees and ankles.
- The patient is instructed to build up strength of the non-paralysed muscles.
- particularly the arms, with weight training and a bar suspended over the bed.
- Encourage the patient to get involved in paraplegic sport if available.
- Encourage the patient to develop craft skills.
- The wheelchair is initially used 2 hours per day, then 2 hours twice a day and gradually builds up.
- The patient should lift up the buttocks a few times every 15 minutes.
- Foam rubber cushions are placed beneath the buttocks in the wheel-chair.
- Development of pressure sores or UTI require admission to hospital.
- Occasionally amputation is required for grossly infected legs.

Injury level and functional capability

For rehabilitation purposes the level of the lesion refers to the last normal level of movement and sensation. This level indicates the future functional capabilities in the patient's rehabilitation.

- C5 - the patient can self-feed and brush his or her teeth with assistive devices. The patient can drive a powered wheelchair with a hand control unit.
- C6 - the patient pushes a manual wheelchair with vertical tips on the hand rim. There is potential independence in self-care activities by using a natural wrist tenodesis mechanism. If the patient does not have elbow flexion contractures, he is able to do pushups while sitting in a wheelchair. The patient is independent in sliding board transfers.
- C7 - the patient is competent with self-care activities and can use a manual wheelchair for locomotion.
- C8/T1 - the patient is fully independent with wheelchair excluding high level wheelchair activities. The patient can self-catheterise and insert rectal suppositories.
- T2/T10 - it is unlikely that this patient will achieve functional ambulation.

- T12/L1 - a borderline candidate for ambulation with orthosis, in the community.
- L2 downwards - common to walk with possible bilateral ankle and knee orthoses.

SPECIFIC COMPLICATIONS OF CHRONIC NEUROLOGIC DISABILITY

Chronic spasticity

The traumatic brain injured patient may be left with a range of physical disabilities including a spastic hemiplegia, an asymmetrical spastic quadriplegia and degrees of cerebellar incoordination. For these patients rehabilitation commences in the intensive or acute care unit. The nursing staff and the physiotherapists, if available, must ensure that the limbs are moved through the normal range each day.

In the first 2 weeks after the accident, the splinting may be necessary with antispasmodic drugs such as diazepam. Serial plaster of Paris circumferential casts changed every week can help maintain a reasonable limb posture in the spastic limb but need some experience to apply. In resistant cases epidural or relaxant anaesthetics may be diagnostic in assisting the separation of reversible spasticity from patients with contractures. Botulinum toxin injections are used in some units to modify spasticity and if this fails the orthopaedic surgeon may need to section tendons to allow a full range of joint movement.

Spasticity is common in the paralysed limbs of the spinal injury patient and is difficult to deal with in the developing world. Maintaining the passive range of movement helps to prevent contractures. Recurrent painful spasms, which can be triggered by cutaneous stimulation, can be very disabling. Oral diazepam or preferably baclofen if available can be helpful. Oral dantrolene sodium which is a muscle paralysing agent is also used in selected cases of severe spasticity, but has significant side effects. Selective motor neurectomy such as obturator nerve division for adductor spasm or tenotomies are helpful for intractable cases.

Injection of phenol into the selected motor nerves is an alternative. Botulinum toxin injected directly into spastic muscles is a major advance in the relief of this problem and helps to prevent contractures, but the injections wear off and need to be repeated. Selective dorsal rhizotomy (see cerebral palsy section in Chapter 9), and the insertion of a computer-driven infusion pump subcutaneously in the abdominal wall with delivery of continuous intraspinal baclofen or opiate are both effective in controlling severe spasticity. Much smaller intraspinal doses of baclofen compared with systemic doses are required and therefore side effects are minimised. Unfortunately, these treatments are expensive and generally unavailable in LMICs.

Heterotopic ossification

Brain injured or spinal cord injury patients who are immobile may develop heterotopic ossification in the soft tissues around the large joints (hips, shoulders, elbows and knees). This may severely restrict joint motion producing further disability. Diphosphonates and warfarin have been used to prevent the bone formation. Indomethacin may damp inflammation around the joints and an aggressive range of motion exercise is important to maintain as mobility of the joints and to try and prevent the problem. If joint deformity causes a significant functional impairment excision of the heterotopic ossification may be indicated.

Contractures

Joint contractures are a common result of chronic spasticity and immobility. Once established they are very difficult to treat. Examination under anaesthesia can help distinguish between fixed contracture and spasticity, which is eliminated by the relaxant anaesthesia. Orthopaedic procedures such as tenotomy, arthrodesis and osteotomies have a place in advanced cases.

Nutrition

The early nutritional requirements following TBI are described in Chapter 3. Adequate and good quality nutrition are important in the rehabilitation phase of any neurological disorder to help general well-being, promote wound healing, maintain skin health, and improve resistance to sepsis.

Psychological well-being

The sudden transition from a healthy, active person to a permanently disabled spinal injury patient, can cause unpredictable reactions in the patient and close relatives that require considerable understanding, counselling and education from the health care staff available. Complex grief reactions need careful management at this time. Poor motivation and depression supervene if the patient is sickly with pressure sores and other complications and is not receiving adequate care. This disturbs the rehabilitation process and the recovery is set back. Severe untreated depression may lead to suicide.

Secondary depression is easily missed unless you are considering it as a reason for poor progress. Maintenance of a positive and optimistic attitude among the staff and family is important in the boosting of the patient's self-confidence and morale.

Practice point

Pain and the suffering may also contribute to a depressive illness and the relief of pain is a key tenet of the rehabilitation program.

Sexual function

Once paraplegics return to home life, issues of sexuality surface. Some 30-75 percent of paraplegic males can obtain an erection but it is often short-lived and coitus incomplete. Unfortunately, very few paraplegics can ejaculate or experience orgasm. The ejaculation often occurs back into the bladder (retroejaculation). Testicular atrophy and loss of spermatogenesis is common following spinal cord injury. These factors render the individual infertile and may lead to marital discord. There may be better function than this with incomplete spinal lesions.

Prosthetic penile implants, which inflate to produce an erection can be implanted by urologists in advanced centres. There are also now implantable programmable electrical stimulators, which can be placed on the sacral nerve roots to produce sustained erection and ejaculation. Some paraplegics have been able to become fathers as a result of these techniques. Female paraplegics who are menstruating can become pregnant and give birth naturally. In complete paraplegia there is no vaginal sensation, so physical satisfaction during intercourse is absent.

Conclusion

Practice point

To achieve the best functional and psychological outcome for patients with neurological disability, surgeons in the tropics must be involved in the planning and implementation of a rehabilitation programme along with nurses, allied health professionals if they are available, and the relatives, while the patient is still in hospital, and they must ensure the continuance of this process after the patient is discharged.

MEDICOLEGAL ISSUES

Litigation is becoming an increasing problem facing the medical profession even in the developing world. Providing informed consent and frequent and detailed explanations to the patient and their family of procedures and other treatments and their possible complications and the likely effect of treatment is the best means of avoiding lawsuits. Clear, detailed written contemporaneous documentation of the patient's progress is a vital record for ongoing care but becomes a vital source of facts and opinions if litigation ensues.

Preparation of a medical report

Increasingly, medical practitioners are required to forward reports (Table 12.3, next page) on their patients to courts, medical tribunals, insurance companies and worker's compensation boards. These reports are important for the patient and their families. They can be done effectively provided the physician follows a protocol. The reports are usually requested some months after the patient's injury but the final report is best postponed until the patient has passed through 2 years of recovery. These reports should preferably be typed. The physician initially requires the hospital record, inpatient investigations, reports on inpatient treatment, and available reports from any other doctors. Ideally the patient and a relative should be interviewed. Many post-traumatic head injury patients are poor historians and some have a high level of denial. Relatives can be most helpful in alerting the physician to personality changes and their effects on the family.

Table 12.3 The contents of a medical report

The history of the accident

The examination on presentation

The inpatient treatment in intensive care and the wards

The positive investigations

The period of rehabilitation

The past family history

The past medical history

The educational and employment history

The physical examination

The opinion

The report should be objective, including the history of the accident, and the retrograde traumatic amnesia and the period of posttraumatic amnesia, together with the record of the Glasgow Coma Scale on presentation. The report includes the inpatient treatment, the list of investigations that were positive, the rehabilitation carried out and the length of stay in hospital. In addition, the report should note past medical history, the family history, educational and employment records. The final opinion should discuss the implications of each injury. The history of the accident should include the patient's description and, in the event of amnesia, a description from available records or relatives. The history should include the type of accident, the speed of impact, whether seatbelts or helmets were worn, and any record of alcohol or drugs complicating the event. The period of retrograde amnesia and posttraumatic amnesia (the time from the accident to that in which continuous memory returned) is a useful guide to the severity. The hospital notes are sometimes helpful in indicating the Glasgow Coma Scale on presentation. The report should include a list of all injuries evident on presentation.

The treatment that the patient received, including blood transfusions, resuscitation, mechanical ventilation, operations and rehabilitation, should be outlined with the hospital discharge date. The patient's past medical history may have a significant bearing on the final opinion. Evidence of previous medical conditions, previous operations and particularly previous accidents should be sought. The patient's family history should be reviewed as it may highlight the problems that could complicate the recovery. The patient's educational and employment history gives a guide to educational levels, educational potential and previous trade or professional qualifications that might form a basis for re-employment. A full physical examination is carried out including an assessment of the patient's behaviour and cognitive function. Personality changes are common in head injury patients and information from close relatives can provide a very useful history of these changes and their effects on the family.

The Folstein Mini-mental Status Examination (score of O to 30) is useful in identifying cognitive deficits. The report should include positive investigations with the date they were carried out, particularly CT scans, EEGs and plain X-rays of the skull. The opinion should be expressed concisely and objectively. It should be based on the information available. It should provide a final diagnosis and prognosis.

In the traumatic brain damaged patient, the report should consider:
1. The site of the organic brain damage
2. The period of posttraumatic amnesia and the Glasgow Coma Scale on admission
3. The treatment provided in hospital
4. The complications which affected the recovery and rehabilitation, e.g. pneumonia, deep vein thrombosis

5. The diagnosis should indicate areas of the brain that were damaged, e.g. diffuse axonal injury, frontal lobe damage, brain stem damage
6. The implications of such damage on the personality and behaviour of the patient should be defined. This might include the effect of the personality change on the patient's further education, domestic and social integration and the return to employment.

Epilepsy may have developed as a result of the organic brain injury and in some cases, there is an increased risk of epilepsy in the future. This should be discussed.

Any **deficit in the cranial nerves** should be addressed with long-term prognosis. Residual difficulties in speech, writing and balance should be included with the implications on the domestic life and future employment.

In cases where there is a degree of dependency it would be necessary to outline the number of hours per day of care required by a supervising adult. On many occasions the request for a medical report also includes a request on the rating of impairment, for the patient. This can be obtained from the American Medical Association's Guides to the Evaluation of Permanent Impairment, which the solicitor may be able to supply. If this is not available you should estimate the percentage disability in the affected areas.

Finally, at times it is necessary to indicate whether the patient is competent to look after his or her financial affairs in the event of an award. State what ongoing care is required.

Appendices

APPENDIX 1. HEAD CIRCUMFERENCE CHART FOR GIRLS[70]

**HEAD CIRCUMFERENCE
GIRLS
In utero 28-40 weeks, 0-12 months**

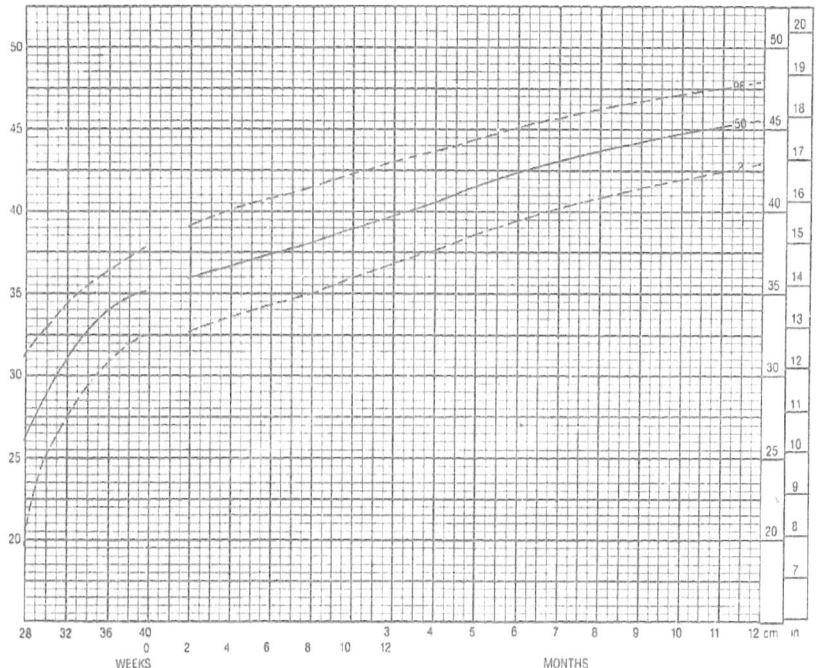

1-3 years

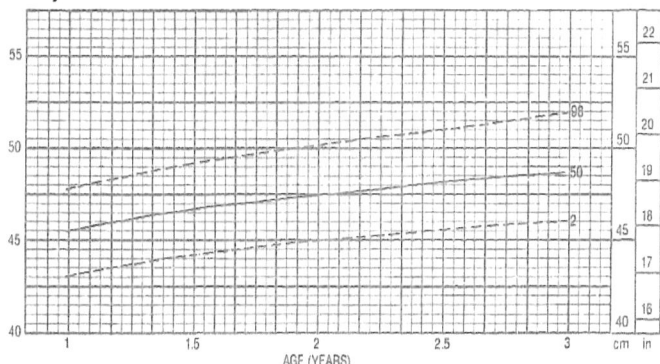

[70]Reproduced with permission from Pharmacia & Upjohn Pty Ltd, Rydalmere, NSW, Australia

APPENDIX 2. HEAD CIRCUMFERENCE CHART FOR BOYS[71]

HEAD CIRCUMFERENCE
BOYS
In utero 28-40 weeks, 0-12 months

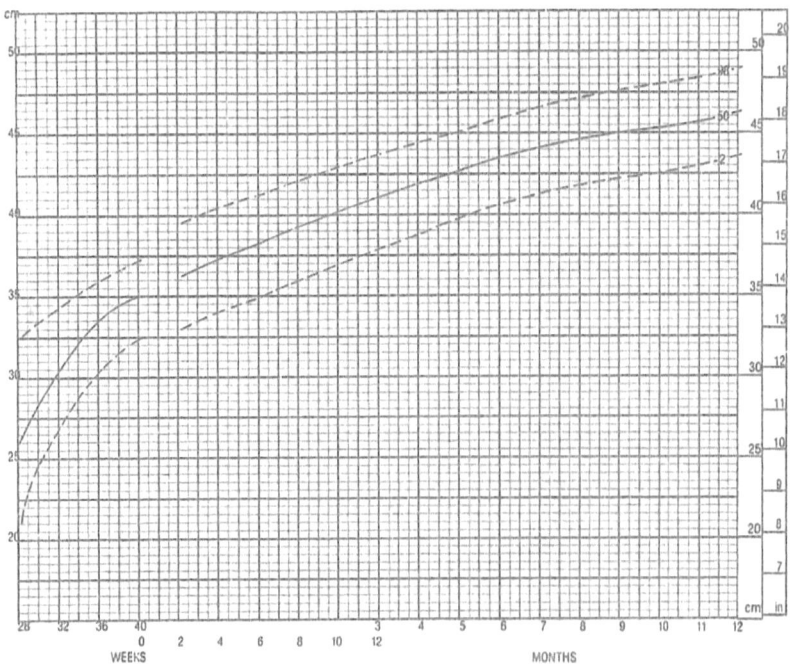

1-3 years

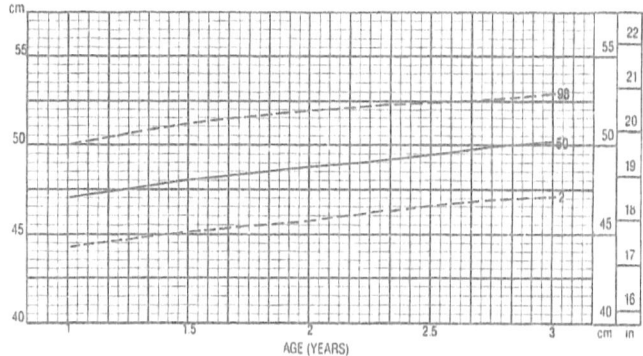

---

[71]*Reproduced with permission from Pharmacia & Upjohn Pty Ltd, Rydalmere, NSW, Australia*

APPENDIX 3. HEAD INJURY OBSERVATION CHART FOR CHILDREN

NORMAL COMA SCALE SCORES				
Age	Eyes Open	Verbal Response	Motor Response	TOTAL
0 - 6 months	4	2-3	4	10 - 11
6 - 12 months	4	3	5	12
1 - 2 years	4	4	5	13
2 - 4 years	4	4 - 5	6	14 - 15
> 4 years	4	5	6	15

DATE

TIME

COMA SCALE

Eyes Open	4	Spontaneous	
	3	To Speech	
	2	To Pain	
	1	None	
Best Verbal Response under 4 yrs.	5	Orientated	
	4	Words Confused	
	3	Vocal Sound Inappropriate	
	2	Cries Vocal Sounds	
	1	None None	
Best Motor Response	6	Obeys command	
	5	Localises Pain	
	4	Withdrawal	
	3	Abnormal Flexion	
	2	Extension	
	1	Nil	

TOTAL SCORE :

LIMB MOVEMENT

ARMS
- Normal power
- Mild Weakness
- Severe weakness
- Spastic flexion
- Extension
- No response

LEGS
- Normal power
- Mild weakness
- Severe weakness
- Extension
- No response

SEE ADDITIONAL OBSERVATIONS

PUPILS	RIGHT	SIZE
		REACTION
	LEFT	SIZE
		REACTION

PUPIL SCALE (mm)

1 •
2 •
3 •
4 ●
5 ●
6 ●
7 ●
8 ●

TEMPERATURE
- 41
- 40
- 39
- 38
- 37
- 36
- 35
- C

BLOOD PRESSURE
- 230
- 220
- 210
- 200
- 190
- 180
- 170
- 160
- 150
- 140
- 130
- 120
- 110
- 100
- 90
- 80
- 70
- 60
- 50
- 40

RESPIRATION
- 30
- 20
- 10

APPENDIX 3. *(Continued)*

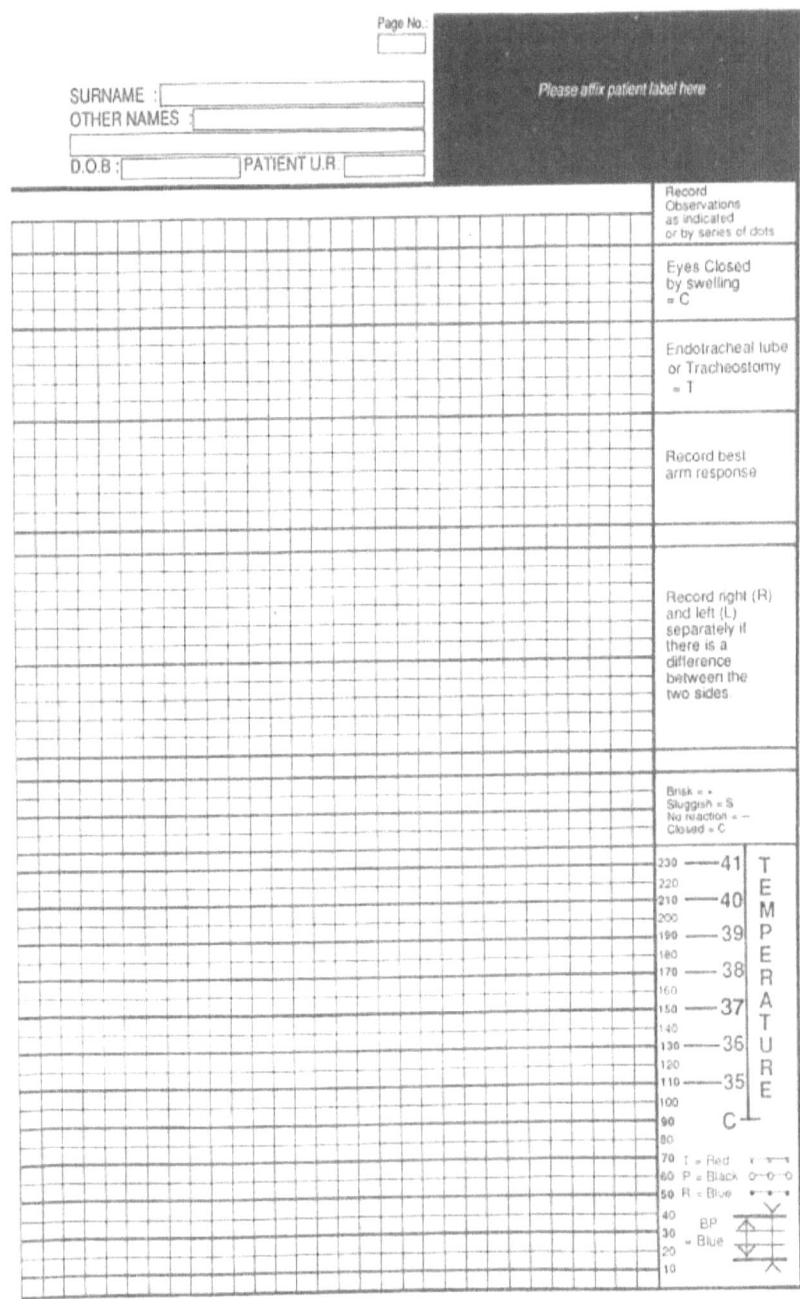

APPENDIX 3. *(Continued)*

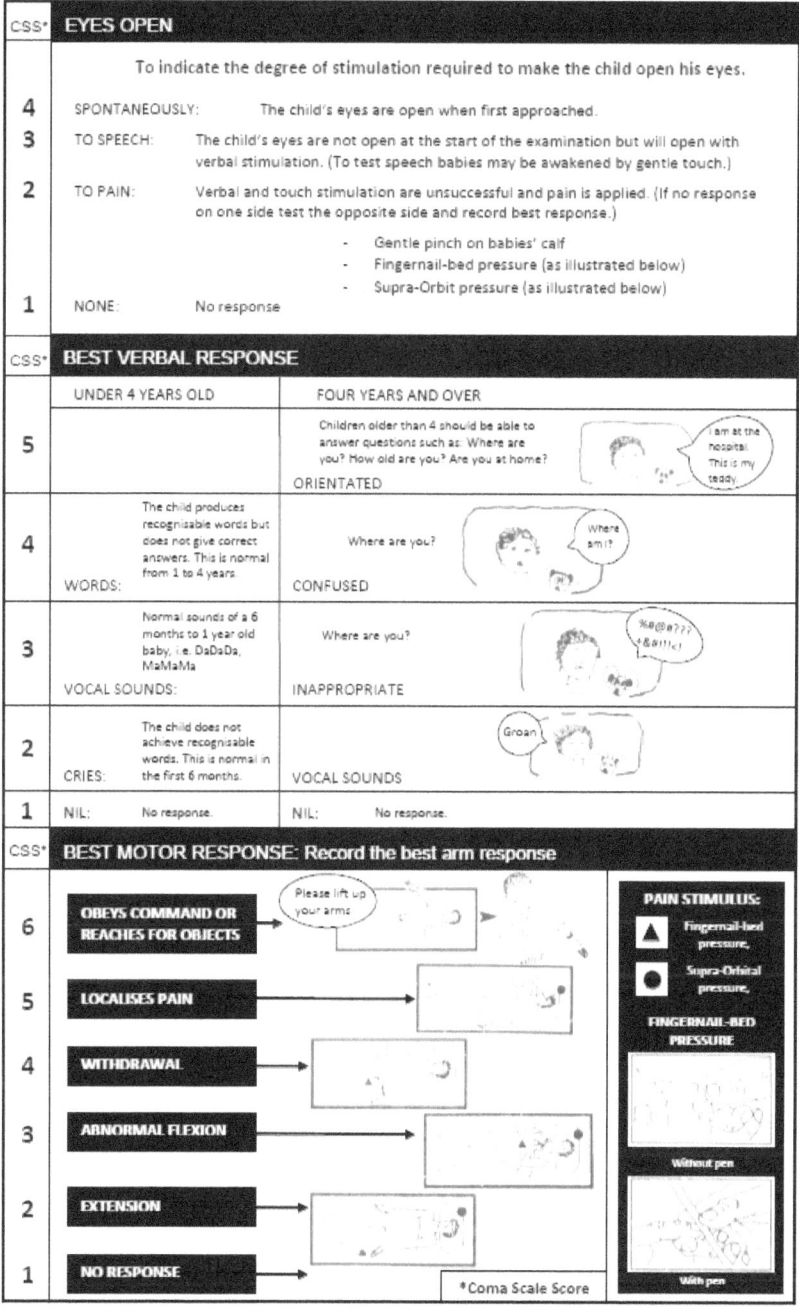

CSS*	EYES OPEN	
	To indicate the degree of stimulation required to make the child open his eyes.	
4	SPONTANEOUSLY:	The child's eyes are open when first approached.
3	TO SPEECH:	The child's eyes are not open at the start of the examination but will open with verbal stimulation. (To test speech babies may be awakened by gentle touch.)
2	TO PAIN:	Verbal and touch stimulation are unsuccessful and pain is applied. (If no response on one side test the opposite side and record best response.)
		- Gentle pinch on babies' calf
		- Fingernail-bed pressure (as illustrated below)
		- Supra-Orbit pressure (as illustrated below)
1	NONE:	No response

CSS*	BEST VERBAL RESPONSE	
	UNDER 4 YEARS OLD	FOUR YEARS AND OVER
5		Children older than 4 should be able to answer questions such as: Where are you? How old are you? Are you at home? ORIENTATED
4	The child produces recognisable words but does not give correct answers. This is normal from 1 to 4 years. WORDS:	Where are you? CONFUSED
3	Normal sounds of a 6 months to 1 year old baby, i.e. DaDaDa, MaMaMa VOCAL SOUNDS:	Where are you? INAPPROPRIATE
2	The child does not achieve recognisable words. This is normal in the first 6 months. CRIES:	VOCAL SOUNDS
1	NIL: No response.	NIL: No response.

CSS*	BEST MOTOR RESPONSE: Record the best arm response	
6	OBEYS COMMAND OR REACHES FOR OBJECTS	PAIN STIMULUS: ▲ Fingernail-bed pressure, ● Supra-Orbital pressure,
5	LOCALISES PAIN	FINGERNAIL-BED PRESSURE
4	WITHDRAWAL	
3	ABNORMAL FLEXION	Without pen
2	EXTENSION	
1	NO RESPONSE	*Coma Scale Score / With pen

APPENDIX 4. HEAD INJURY OBSERVATION CHART FOR ADULTS[72]

PATIENT IDENTIFICATION

U.R. No.

NAME

DATE OF OPERATION

RECORD OBS. AS SERIES OF DOTS OR AS INDICATED

DATE

TIME

LEVEL OF CONSCIOUSNESS

EYES OPEN
- SPONTANEOUSLY — 4
- TO SPEECH — 3
- TO PAIN — 2
- NONE — 1

EYES CLOSED BY SWELLING = C

BEST VERBAL RESPONSE
- ORIENTATED — 5
- CONFUSED — 4
- INAPPROPRIATE — 3
- INCOHERENT — 2
- NONE — 1

ENDOTRACHEAL TUBE OR TRACHEOSTOMY — T

BEST MOTOR RESPONSE
- OBEY COMMAND — 6
- LOCALISE PAIN — 5
- WITHDRAWS — 4
- ABNORMAL FLEXION — 3
- EXTENSION — 2
- NONE — 1

USUALLY RECORD BEST ARM RESPONSE

BLOOD PRESSURE (BLUE): 220, 210, 200, 190, 180, 170, 160, 150, 140, 130, 120, 110, 100, 90, 80, 70, 60, 50, 40, 30, 20, 10

TEMPERATURE (BLUE DOT): 40°C, 39, 38, 37, 36, 35, 34

PULSE RATE (RED DOT)

RESPIRATION (RED - OPEN CIRCLE)

PUPIL SCALE (mm): 1, 2, 3, 4, 5, 6, 7, 8

PUPILS
- RIGHT — SIZE, REACTION
- LEFT — SIZE, REACTION

- + REACTS
- S SLUGGISH
- — NO RESPONSE
- C EYE CLOSED

LIMB MOVEMENT

ARMS
- NORMAL POWER
- MILD WEAKNESS
- MOD WEAKNESS
- SEVERE WEAKNESS
- FLEXION TO PAIN
- EXTENSION TO PAIN
- NO RESPONSE

LEGS
- NORMAL POWER
- MILD WEAKNESS
- MOD WEAKNESS
- SEVERE WEAKNESS
- FLEXION TO PAIN
- EXTENSION TO PAIN
- NO RESPONSE

RECORD RIGHT (R) AND LEFT (L) SEPARATELY IF THERE IS A DIFFERENCE BETWEEN SIDES

USE A DOT IF EQUAL

* ADDITIONAL OBSERVATION RECORDED OVERLEAF

---

[72]Reproduced with permission from The Royal Melbourne Hospital, Melbourne, Australia

APPENDIX 5. ABBREVIATED WESTMEAD PTA SCALE (A-WPTAS)

ABBREVIATED WESTMEAD PTA SCALE (A-WPTAS)
GCS & PTA testing of patients with MTBI following mild head injury

Abbreviated Westmead PTA Scale (A-WPTAS)
incorporating Glasgow Coma Scale (GCS)

Date:		T1	T2	T3	T4	T5
Time						
Motor	Obeys commands	6	6	6	6	6
	Localises	5	5	5	5	5
	Withdraws	4	4	4	4	4
	Abnormal flexion	3	3	3	3	3
	Extension	2	2	2	2	2
	None	1	1	1	1	1
Eye Opening	Spontaneously	4	4	4	4	4
	To speech	3	3	3	3	3
	To pain	2	2	2	2	2
	None	1	1	1	1	1
Verbal	Oriented ** (tick if correct)	5	5	5	5	5
	Name	☐	☐	☐	☐	☐
	Place	☐	☐	☐	☐	☐
	Why are you here	☐	☐	☐	☐	☐
	Month	☐	☐	☐	☐	☐
	Year	☐	☐	☐	☐	☐
	Confused	4	4	4	4	4
	Inappropriate words	3	3	3	3	3
	Incomprehensible sounds	2	2	2	2	2
	None	1	1	1	1	1
GCS	**Score out of 15**	/15	/15	/15	/15	/15
	Picture 1	Show pictures (see over)				
	Picture 2					
	Picture 3					
A-WPTAS	**Score out of 18**		/18	/18	/18	/18

** must have all 5 orientation questions correct to score 5 on verbal score for GCS, otherwise the score is 4 (or less).

Use of A-WPTAS and GCS for patients with MTBI

The A-WPTAS combined with a standardised GCS assessment is an objective measure of post traumatic amnesia (PTA).

Only for patients with current GCS of 13-15 (<24hrs post injury) with impact to the head resulting in confusion, disorientation, anterograde or retrograde amnesia, or brief LOC. Administer both tests at hourly intervals to gauge patient's capacity for full orientation and ability to retain new information. Also, note the following: poor motivation, depression, pre-morbid intellectual handicap or possible medication, drug or alcohol effects. NB: This is a screening device, so exercise clinical judgement. In cases where doubt exists, more thorough assessment may be necessary.

Admission and Discharge Criteria:

A patient is considered to be out of PTA when they score 18/18.

Both the GCS and A-WPTAS should be used in conjunction with clinical judgement.

Patients scoring 18/18 can be considered for discharge.

For patients who do not obtain 18/18 re-assess after a further hour.

Patients with persistent score <18/18 at 4 hours post time of injury should be considered for admission.

Clinical judgement and consideration of pre-existing conditions should be used where the memory component of A-WPTAS is abnormal but the GCS is normal (15/15).

Referral to GP on discharge if abnormal PTA was present, provide patient advice sheet.

Target set of picture cards

PUPIL ASSESSMENT		T1		T2		T3		T4		T5		+	=	REACTS BRISKLY
		R	L	R	L	R	L	R	L	R	L	SL	=	SLUGGISH
Size												C	=	CLOSED
Reaction												-	=	NIL

Comments

Pupil Size (mm)

2   3   4   5   6   7   8

Shores & Lammel (2007) - further copies of this score sheet can be downloaded from http://www.psy.mq.edu.au/GCS

APPENDIX 6. INTERNATIONAL STANDARDS FOR NEUROLOGICAL CLASSIFICATION OF SPINAL CORD INJURY (ISNCSCI)[73]

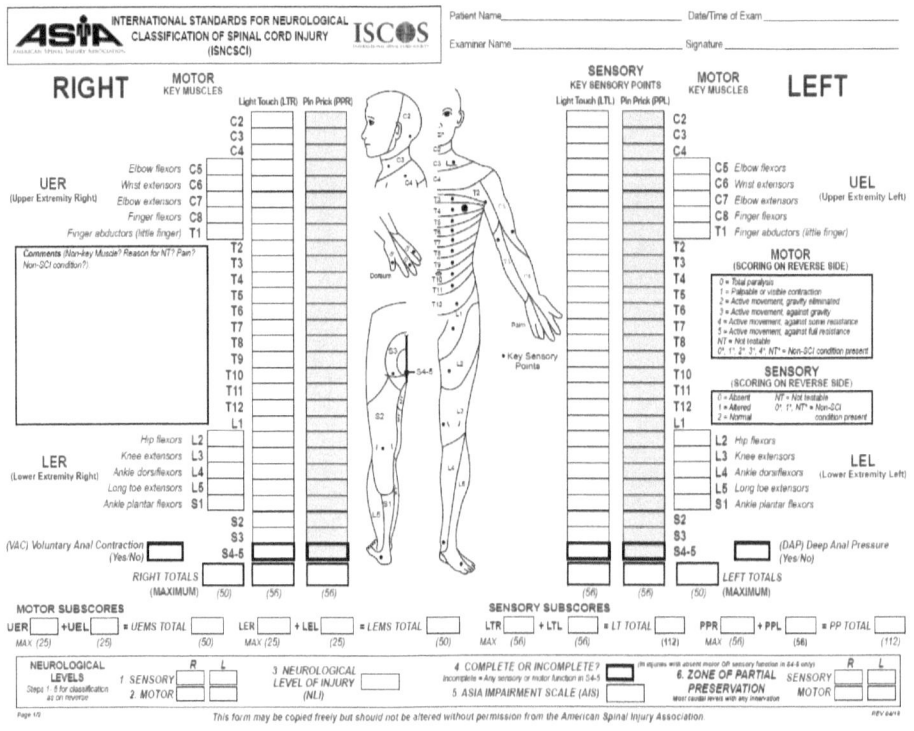

---

[73]Reproduced with permission from The Royal Melbourne Hospital, Melbourne, Australia

APPENDIX 6. *(Continued)*

Muscle Function Grading

0 = Total paralysis

1 = Palpable or visible contraction

2 = Active movement, full range of motion (ROM) with gravity eliminated

3 = Active movement, full ROM against gravity

4 = Active movement, full ROM against gravity and moderate resistance in a muscle specific position

5 = (Normal) active movement, full ROM against gravity and full resistance in a functional muscle position expected from an otherwise unimpaired person

NT = Not testable (i.e. due to immobilization, severe pain such that the patient cannot be graded, amputation of limb, or contracture of > 50% of the normal ROM)

0*, 1*, 2*, 3*, 4*, NT* = Non-SCI condition present *

Sensory Grading

0 = Absent   1 = Altered, either decreased/impaired sensation or hypersensitivity

2 = Normal   NT = Not testable

0*, 1*, NT* = Non-SCI condition present *

* Note: Abnormal motor and sensory scores should be tagged with a '*' to indicate an impairment due to a non-SCI condition. The non-SCI condition should be explained in the comments box together with information about how the score is rated for classification purposes (at least normal / not normal for classification).

When to Test Non-Key Muscles:

In a patient with an apparent AIS B classification, non-key muscle functions more than 3 levels below the motor level on each side should be tested to most accurately classify the injury (differentiate between AIS B and C).

Movement	Root level
Shoulder: Flexion, extension, abduction, adduction, internal and external rotation **Elbow:** Supination	C5
Elbow: Pronation **Wrist:** Flexion	C6
Finger: Flexion at proximal joint, extension **Thumb:** Flexion, extension and abduction in plane of thumb	C7
Finger: Flexion at MCP joint **Thumb:** Opposition, adduction and abduction perpendicular to palm	C8
Finger: Abduction of the index finger	T1
Hip: Adduction	L2
Hip: External rotation	L3
Hip: Extension, abduction, internal rotation **Knee:** Flexion **Ankle:** Inversion and eversion **Toe:** MP and IP extension	L4
Hallux and Toe: DIP and PIP flexion and abduction	L5
Hallux: Adduction	S1

ASIA Impairment Scale (AIS)

A = Complete. No sensory or motor function is preserved in the sacral segments S4-5.

B = Sensory Incomplete. Sensory but not motor function is preserved below the neurological level and includes the sacral segments S4-5 (light touch or pin prick at S4-5 or deep anal pressure) AND no motor function is preserved more than three levels below the motor level on either side of the body.

C = Motor Incomplete. Motor function is preserved at the most caudal sacral segments for voluntary anal contraction (VAC) OR the patient meets the criteria for sensory incomplete status (sensory function preserved at the most caudal sacral segments S4-5 by LT, PP or DAP), and has some sparing of motor function more than three levels below the ipsilateral motor level on either side of the body. (This includes key or non-key muscle functions to determine motor incomplete status.) For AIS C – less than half of key muscle functions below the single NLI have a muscle grade ≥ 3.

D = Motor Incomplete. Motor incomplete status as defined above, with at least half (half or more) of key muscle functions below the single NLI having a muscle grade ≥ 3.

E = Normal. If sensation and motor function as tested with the ISNCSCI are graded as normal in all segments, and the patient had prior deficits, then the AIS grade is E. Someone without an initial SCI does not receive an AIS grade.

Using ND: To document the sensory, motor and NLI levels, the ASIA Impairment Scale grade, and/or the zone of partial preservation (ZPP) when they are unable to be determined based on the examination results.

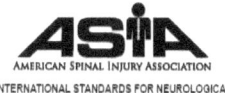

AMERICAN SPINAL INJURY ASSOCIATION

INTERNATIONAL STANDARDS FOR NEUROLOGICAL
CLASSIFICATION OF SPINAL CORD INJURY

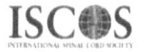

INTERNATIONAL SPINAL CORD SOCIETY

Page 2/2

Steps in Classification

The following order is recommended for determining the classification of individuals with SCI.

1. Determine sensory levels for right and left sides.
The sensory level is the most caudal, intact dermatome for both pin prick and light touch sensation.

2. Determine motor levels for right and left sides.
Defined by the lowest key muscle function that has a grade of at least 3 (on supine testing), providing the key muscle functions represented by segments above that level are judged to be intact (graded as a 5).
Note: in regions where there is no myotome to test, the motor level is presumed to be the same as the sensory level, if testable motor function above that level is also normal.

3. Determine the neurological level of injury (NLI).
This refers to the most caudal segment of the cord with intact sensation and antigravity (3 or more) muscle function strength, provided that there is normal (intact) sensory and motor function rostrally respectively.
The NLI is the most cephalad of the sensory and motor levels determined in steps 1 and 2.

4. Determine whether the injury is Complete or Incomplete.
(i.e. absence or presence of sacral sparing)
If voluntary anal contraction = No AND all S4-5 sensory scores = 0 AND deep anal pressure = No, then injury is Complete.
Otherwise, injury is Incomplete.

5. Determine ASIA Impairment Scale (AIS) Grade.
Is injury Complete? If YES, AIS=A
NO ↓
Is injury Motor Complete? If YES, AIS=B
NO ↓ (No voluntary anal contraction OR motor function more than three levels below the motor level on a given side, if the patient has sensory incomplete classification)
Are at least half (half or more) of the key muscles below the neurological level of injury graded 3 or better?
NO ↓   YES ↓
AIS=C   AIS=D

If sensation and motor function is normal in all segments, AIS=E
Note: AIS E is used in follow-up testing when an individual with a documented SCI has recovered normal function. If at initial testing no deficits are found, the individual is neurologically intact and the ASIA impairment Scale does not apply.

6. Determine the zone of partial preservation (ZPP).
The ZPP is used only in injuries with absent motor (no VAC) OR sensory function (no DAP, no LT and no PP sensation) in the lowest sacral segments S4-5 and refers to those dermatomes and myotomes caudal to the sensory and motor levels that remain partially innervated. With sacral sparing of sensory function, the sensory ZPP is not applicable and therefore 'NA' is recorded in the block of the worksheet. Accordingly, if VAC is present, the motor ZPP is not applicable and is noted as "NA".

Appendices

APPENDIX 7: FOLSTEIN MINI MENTAL STATE EXAMINATION (MMSE)

Patient score	Maximum score	Task
....	5	**Orientation** Ask the patient to name the (year) (season) (date) (day) (month)
....	5	Ask the patient where we are (country) (state) (city) (suburb) (hospital)
....	5	
....	3	**Registration** Name three objects (e.g. apple, book, coat), allotting one second to say each one. Then ask the patient to name all three objects after you have said them. Give one point for each correct answer. Continue until he or she repeats all three objects. Count the trials and record the number.
....	5	**Attention and calculation** Ask the patient to begin with 100 and count backwards by seven (stop after five answers: 93, 86, 79, 72, 65). Score one point for each correct answer. If the patient will not perform the task, ask him or her to spell 'world' backwards. Record the patient's spelling. Score one point for each correctly placed letter.
....	3	**Recall** Ask the patient to repeat the three objects above (see Registration). Give one point for each correct answer.
....	2	**Language** *Naming.* Show the patient a pencil and a watch and ask him or her to name them.
....	1	*Repetition.* Ask the patient to repeat the following: 'No ifs, ands, or buts'.
....	3	*Three-stage command.* Ask the patient to follow the three stage command" 'Take a paper in your right hand, fold it in half and put it on the table'.
....	1	*Reading.* Ask the patient to read and obey the following: 'Close your eyes'.
....	1	*Writing.* Ask the patient to write a sentence on a piece of paper.
....	1	*Copying.* Ask the patient to copy a design of intersecting pentagons which you have given him or her.
....	30	Total score

*A score below 22 is very suggestive of a significant cognitive problem.
Note that the patient needs to be literate to complete the test.
Adapted from: Folstein MF, Folstein S, McHugh PR. Mini-mental state: a practical method for grading the cognitive state of patients for the clinician. J Psychiatr Res 1975; 12: 189-198.

APPENDIX 8: DISABILITY RATING SCALE (RAPPAPORT)

Eye opening	0-3	
Verbal	0-4	
Motor response	0-5	
Toileting	0-3	
Feeding	0-3	Cognitive ability for self-care activities
Grooming	0-3	
Dependence	0-5	
Employability	0-3	

This gives ten degrees of disability

0	Nil
1	Mild disability
2-3	Partial disability
4-6	Moderate disability
7-11	Moderate/severe disability
12-16	Severe disability
17-21	Extremely severe disability
22-24	Vegetative state
25-29	Extreme vegetative state
30	Death

Appendices

Level I	No response to pain, touch, sound, or sight
Level II	Generalised reflex response to pain
Level III	Localised response. Blinks to strong light, turns toward/away from sound, responds to physical discomfort, inconsistent response to commands.
Level IV	Confused – agitated. Alert, very active, aggressive or bizarre behaviours, performs motor activities but behaviour is non-purposeful, extremely short attention span.
Level V	Confused – non-agitated. Gross attention to environment, highly distractible, requires continual redirection, difficulty learning new tasks, agitated by too much stimulation. May engage in social conversation but with inappropriate verbalisations.
Level VI	Confused – appropriate. Inconsistent orientation to time and place, retention span/recent memory impaired, begins to recall past, consistently follows simple directions, goal-directed behaviour with assistance.
Level VII	Automatic- appropriate. Performs daily routine in highly familiar environment in non-confused but automatic robot-like manner. Skills noticeably deteriorate in unfamiliar environment. Lacks realistic planning for own future.
Level VIII	Purposeful – appropriate.

Index

Index

Index

Index

Index

Index

Index

Index

Index

Index

www.ingramcontent.com/pod-product-compliance
Lightning Source LLC
Chambersburg PA
CBHW021347210526
45463CB00001B/1